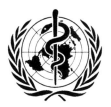

World Health Organization Classification of Tumours

WHO OMS

International Agency for Research on Cancer (IARC)

4th Edition

WHO Classification of Tumours of the Central Nervous System

Edited by

David N. Louis

Hiroko Ohgaki

Otmar D. Wiestler

Webster K. Cavenee

International Agency for Research on Cancer

Lyon, 2007

World Health Organization Classification of Tumours

Series Editors   Fred T. Bosman, M.D.
Elaine S. Jaffe, M.D.
Sunil R. Lakhani, M.D.
Hiroko Ohgaki, Ph.D.

WHO Classification of Tumours of the Central Nervous System

Editors   David N. Louis, M.D.
Hiroko Ohgaki, Ph.D.
Otmar D. Wiestler, M.D.
Webster K. Cavenee, Ph.D.

Layout   Sébastien Antoni
Marlen Grassinger

Printed by   Participe Présent
69250 Neuville s/Saône, France

Publisher   International Agency for
Research on Cancer (IARC)
69008 Lyon, France

This volume was produced in collaboration with and support from the

German Cancer Research Center

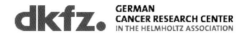

The WHO Classification of Tumours of the Central Nervous System
presented in this book reflects the views of a Working Group
that convened for an Editorial and Consensus Conference at the
German Cancer Research Center (DKFZ), Heidelberg
November 17-18, 2006.

Members of the Working Group are indicated
in the List of Contributors on pages 253-257.

Published by the International Agency for Research on Cancer (IARC),
150 cours Albert Thomas, 69372 Lyon Cedex 08, France

Distributed by
WHO Press, World Health Organization, 20 Avenue Appia, 1211 Geneva 27, Switzerland
(Tel: +41 22 791 3264; Fax: +41 22 791 4857; e-mail: bookorders@who.int).

Format for bibliographic citations:
Louis D.N., Ohgaki H., Wiestler O.D., Cavenee W.K. (Eds.): WHO Classification of
Tumours of the Central Nervous System.
IARC: Lyon 2007

IARC Library Cataloguing in Publication Data

WHO Classification of Tumours of the Central Nervous System
Edited by Louis D.N., Ohgaki H., Wiestler O.D., Cavenee W.K.

1. Central Nervous System Neoplasms – genetics
2. Central Nervous System Neoplasms – pathology
I. Louis, David N.

ISBN 978-92-832-2430-2

Contents

WHO Classification of Tumours of the Nervous System

TUMOURS OF NEUROEPITHELIAL TISSUE

Astrocytic tumours
Pilocytic astrocytoma	9421/1[1]
Pilomyxoid astrocytoma	*9425/3**
Subependymal giant cell astrocytoma	9384/1
Pleomorphic xanthoastrocytoma	9424/3
Diffuse astrocytoma	9400/3
Fibrillary astrocytoma	9420/3
Gemistocytic astrocytoma	9411/3
Protoplasmic astrocytoma	9410/3
Anaplastic astrocytoma	9401/3
Glioblastoma	9440/3
Giant cell glioblastoma	9441/3
Gliosarcoma	9442/3
Gliomatosis cerebri	9381/3

Oligodendroglial tumours
Oligodendroglioma	9450/3
Anaplastic oligodendroglioma	9451/3

Oligoastrocytic tumours
Oligoastrocytoma	9382/3
Anaplastic oligoastrocytoma	9382/3

Ependymal tumours
Subependymoma	9383/1
Myxopapillary ependymoma	9394/1
Ependymoma	9391/3
Cellular	9391/3
Papillary	9393/3
Clear cell	9391/3
Tanycytic	9391/3
Anaplastic ependymoma	9392/3

Choroid plexus tumours
Choroid plexus papilloma	9390/0
Atypical choroid plexus papilloma	*9390/1**
Choroid plexus carcinoma	9390/3

Other neuroepithelial tumours
Astroblastoma	9430/3
Chordoid glioma of the third ventricle	9444/1
Angiocentric glioma	*9431/1**

Neuronal and mixed neuronal-glial tumours
Dysplastic gangliocytoma of cerebellum (Lhermitte-Duclos)	9493/0
Desmoplastic infantile astrocytoma/ ganglioglioma	9412/1
Dysembryoplastic neuroepithelial tumour	9413/0
Gangliocytoma	9492/0
Ganglioglioma	9505/1
Anaplastic ganglioglioma	9505/3
Central neurocytoma	9506/1
Extraventricular neurocytoma	*9506/1**
Cerebellar liponeurocytoma	*9506/1**
Papillary glioneuronal tumour	*9509/1**
Rosette-forming glioneuronal tumour of the fourth ventricle	*9509/1**
Paraganglioma	8680/1

Tumours of the pineal region
Pineocytoma	9361/1
Pineal parenchymal tumour of intermediate differentiation	9362/3
Pineoblastoma	9362/3
Papillary tumour of the pineal region	*9395/3**

Embryonal tumours
Medulloblastoma	9470/3
Desmoplastic/nodular medulloblastoma	9471/3
Medulloblastoma with extensive nodularity	*9471/3**
Anaplastic medulloblastoma	*9474/3**
Large cell medulloblastoma	9474/3
CNS primitive neuroectodermal tumour	9473/3
CNS Neuroblastoma	9500/3
CNS Ganglioneuroblastoma	9490/3
Medulloepithelioma	9501/3
Ependymoblastoma	9392/3
Atypical teratoid / rhabdoid tumour	9508/3

TUMOURS OF CRANIAL AND PARASPINAL NERVES

Schwannoma (neurilemoma, neurinoma)	9560/0
Cellular	9560/0
Plexiform	9560/0
Melanotic	9560/0
Neurofibroma	9540/0
Plexiform	9550/0

[1] Morphology code of the International Classification of Diseases for Oncology (ICD-O) {614A} and the Systematized Nomenclature of Medicine (http://snomed.org). Behaviour is coded /0 for benign tumours, /3 for malignant tumours and /1 for borderline or uncertain behaviour.

* The italicised numbers are provisional codes proposed for the 4th edition of ICD-O. While they are expected to be incorporated into the next ICD-O edition, they currently remain subject to change.

Perineurioma
  Perineurioma, NOS   9571/0
  Malignant perineurioma   9571/3

Malignant peripheral
  nerve sheath tumour (MPNST)
  Epithelioid MPNST   9540/3
  MPNST with mesenchymal differentiation 9540/3
  Melanotic MPNST   9540/3
  MPNST with glandular differentiation 9540/3

TUMOURS OF THE MENINGES

Tumours of meningothelial cells
Meningioma   9530/0
  Meningothelial   9531/0
  Fibrous (fibroblastic)   9532/0
  Transitional (mixed)   9537/0
  Psammomatous   9533/0
  Angiomatous   9534/0
  Microcystic   9530/0
  Secretory   9530/0
  Lymphoplasmacyte-rich   9530/0
  Metaplastic   9530/0
  Chordoid   9538/1
  Clear cell   9538/1
  Atypical   9539/1
  Papillary   9538/3
  Rhabdoid   9538/3
  Anaplastic (malignant)   9530/3

Mesenchymal tumours
Lipoma   8850/0
Angiolipoma   8861/0
Hibernoma   8880/0
Liposarcoma   8850/3
Solitary fibrous tumour   8815/0
Fibrosarcoma   8810/3
Malignant fibrous histiocytoma   8830/3
Leiomyoma   8890/0
Leiomyosarcoma   8890/3
Rhabdomyoma   8900/0
Rhabdomyosarcoma   8900/3
Chondroma   9220/0
Chondrosarcoma   9220/3
Osteoma   9180/0
Osteosarcoma   9180/3
Osteochondroma   9210/0
Haemangioma   9120/0
Epithelioid haemangioendothelioma   9133/1

Haemangiopericytoma   9150/1
Anaplastic haemangiopericytoma   9150/3
Angiosarcoma   9120/3
Kaposi sarcoma   9140/3
Ewing sarcoma - PNET   9364/3

Primary melanocytic lesions
Diffuse melanocytosis   8728/0
Melanocytoma   8728/1
Malignant melanoma   8720/3
Meningeal melanomatosis   8728/3

Other neoplasms related to the meninges
Haemangioblastoma   9161/1

LYMPHOMAS AND HAEMATOPOIETIC NEOPLASMS

Malignant lymphomas   9590/3
Plasmacytoma   9731/3
Granulocytic sarcoma   9930/3

GERM CELL TUMOURS

Germinoma   9064/3
Embryonal carcinoma   9070/3
Yolk sac tumour   9071/3
Choriocarcinoma   9100/3
Teratoma   9080/1
  Mature   9080/0
  Immature   9080/3
  Teratoma with malignant transformation 9084/3
Mixed germ cell tumour   9085/3

TUMOURS OF THE SELLAR REGION

Craniopharyngioma   9350/1
  Adamantinomatous   9351/1
  Papillary   9352/1
Granular cell tumour   9582/0
Pituicytoma   *9432/1**
Spindle cell oncocytoma
  of the adenohypophysis   *8291/0**

METASTATIC TUMOURS

WHO grading of tumours of the central nervous system

P. Kleihues
D.N. Louis
O.D. Wiestler
P.C. Burger
B.W. Scheithauer

Histological grading is a means of predicting the biological behaviour of a neoplasm. In the clinical setting, tumour grade is a key factor influencing the choice of therapies, particularly determining the use of adjuvant radiation and specific chemotherapy protocols. Since its first publication in 1979, the WHO Classification of Tumours of the Nervous System has included a grading scheme that is a "malignancy scale" ranging across a wide variety of neoplasms rather than a strict histological grading system {1121, 1122, 2513}. WHO grading is widely used, having incorporated or largely replaced other previously published grading systems. Although it is not a requirement for application of the WHO classification for some tumours, including gliomas and meningiomas, numerical WHO grades are useful additions to the diagnosis. The WHO Working Group responsible for the 4th Edition has expanded its application to include additional entities; however, since the number of cases of some newly defined entities is limited, the assignment of grades is preliminary, pending publication of additional data and long-term follow-up.

Grading across tumour entities

Grade I lesions generally include tumours with low proliferative potential and the possibility of cure following surgical resection alone. Lesions designated grade II are generally infiltrative in nature and, despite low level proliferative activity, often recur. Some type II tumours tend to progress to higher grades of malignancy, for example, low-grade diffuse astrocytomas that transform to anaplastic astrocytoma and glioblastoma. Similar transformation occurs in oligodendroglioma and mixed gliomas. The designation grade III is generally reserved for lesions with histological evidence of malignancy, including nuclear atypia and brisk mitotic activity. In most settings, patients with grade III tumours receive adjuvant radiation and/or chemotherapy. The designation grade IV is

assigned to cytologically malignant, mitotically active, necrosis-prone neoplasms often associated with rapid pre- and postoperative disease evolution and a fatal outcome. Examples of grade IV neoplasms include glioblastoma, most embryonal neoplasms and many sarcomas as well. Although not an essential feature, widespread infiltration of surrounding tissue and a propensity for craniospinal dissemination characterize some grade IV neoplasms.

Grading of astrocytic tumours

Grading has been systematically evaluated and successfully applied to a spectrum of diffusely infiltrative astrocytic tumours. These neoplasms are graded in a three-tiered system similar to that of the Ringertz {1891}, St. Anne-Mayo {421} and the previously published WHO schemes {2513}. As currently defined by the WHO, tumours with cytological atypia alone are considered grade II (diffuse astrocytoma), those also showing anaplasia and mitotic activity are considered grade III (anaplastic astrocytoma), and tumours additionally showing microvascular proliferation and/or necrosis are WHO grade IV. This system is similar to the St. Anne/Mayo classification {421}, with the only major difference being grade I; in the WHO system, grade I is assigned to the more circumscribed pilocytic astrocytoma, whereas the St. Anne/Mayo classification assigns grade 1 to an exceedingly rare diffuse astrocytic tumour without atypia. St. Anne/Mayo grades 2 to 4 closely correspond to WHO II to IV. In the St. Anne/Mayo system {421}, the definition of histopathological features is important. Atypia is defined as variation in nuclear shape or size with accompanying hyperchromasia. Mitoses must be unequivocal, but no special recognition is given to their number or morphology. Since the finding of a solitary mitosis in an ample specimen does not confer grade III behaviour, separation of grade II from grade III tumours may be more reliably achieved by determination of MIB-1 labelling

indices {676, 876, 1574}. Endothelial proliferation is defined as apparent multi-layering of endothelium, rather than simple hypervascularity, or glomeruloid vasculature. Necrosis may be of any type; perinecrotic palisading need not be present. Simple apposition of cellular zones with intervening pallor suggestive of incipient necrosis is insufficient. The aforementioned criteria make their appearance in a predictable sequence, i.e., atypia followed in turn by mitotic activity and increased cellularity and finally microvascular proliferation and/or necrosis.

Tumour grade as a prognostic factor

WHO grade is one component of a combination of criteria used to predict a response to therapy and outcome. Other criteria include clinical findings, such as age of the patient, performance status and tumour location; radiological features such as contrast enhancement; extent of surgical resection; proliferation indices; and genetic alterations. For each tumour entity, combinations of these parameters contribute to an overall estimate of prognosis. Despite these variables, patients with WHO grade II tumours typically survive more than 5 years, and those with grade III tumours survive 2-3 years. The prognosis of patients with WHO grade IV tumours depends largely upon whether effective treatment regimens are available. The majority of glioblastoma patients, particularly the elderly, succumb to the disease within a year. For those with other grade IV neoplasms, the outlook may be considerably better. For example, cerebellar medulloblastomas and germ cell tumours such as germinomas, both WHO grade IV, are rapidly fatal if untreated, while state-of-the-art radiation and chemotherapy result in 5-year survival rates exceeding 60% and 80%, respectively.

WHO grades of CNS tumours

	I	II	III	IV
Astrocytic tumours				
Subependymal giant cell astrocytoma	•			
Pilocytic astrocytoma	•			
Pilomyxoid astrocytoma		•		
Diffuse astrocytoma		•		
Pleomorphic xanthoastrocytoma		•		
Anaplastic astrocytoma			•	
Glioblastoma				•
Giant cell glioblastoma				•
Gliosarcoma				•
Oligodendroglial tumours				
Oligodendroglioma		•		
Anaplastic oligodendroglioma			•	
Oligoastrocytic tumours				
Oligoastrocytoma		•		
Anaplastic oligoastrocytoma			•	
Ependymal tumours				
Subependymoma	•			
Myxopapillary ependymoma	•			
Ependymoma		•		
Anaplastic ependymoma			•	
Choroid plexus tumours				
Choroid plexus papilloma	•			
Atypical choroid plexus papilloma		•		
Choroid plexus carcinoma			•	
Other neuroepithelial tumours				
Angiocentric glioma	•			
Chordoid glioma of the third ventricle		•		
Neuronal and mixed neuronal-glial tumours				
Gangliocytoma	•			
Ganglioglioma	•			
Anaplastic ganglioglioma			•	
Desmoplastic infantile astrocytoma and ganglioglioma	•			
Dysembryoplastic neuroepithelial tumour		•		

	I	II	III	IV
Central neurocytoma		•		
Extraventricular neurocytoma		•		
Cerebellar liponeurocytoma		•		
Paraganglioma of the spinal cord	•			
Papillary glioneuronal tumour	•			
Rosette-forming glioneuronal tumour of the fourth ventricle	•			
Pineal tumours				
Pineocytoma	•			
Pineal parenchymal tumour of intermediate differentiation		•	•	
Pineoblastoma				•
Papillary tumour of the pineal region		•	•	
Embryonal tumours				
Medulloblastoma				•
CNS primitive neuroectodermal tumour (PNET)				•
Atypical teratoid / rhabdoid tumour				•
Tumours of the cranial and paraspinal nerves				
Schwannoma	•			
Neurofibroma	•			
Perineurioma	•	•	•	
Malignant peripheral nerve sheath tumour (MPNST)		•	•	•
Meningeal tumours				
Meningioma	•			
Atypical meningioma		•		
Anaplastic / malignant meningioma			•	
Haemangiopericytoma		•		
Anaplastic haemangiopericytoma			•	
Haemangioblastoma	•			
Tumours of the sellar region				
Craniopharyngioma	•			
Granular cell tumour of the neurohypophysis	•			
Pituicytoma	•			
Spindle cell oncocytoma of the adenohypophysis	•			

CHAPTER 1

Astrocytic Tumours

Pilocytic astrocytoma (WHO grade I)
A relatively circumscribed, slowly growing, often cystic astrocytoma occurring in children and young adults, histologically characterized by a biphasic pattern with varying proportions of compacted bipolar cells associated with Rosenthal fibers and loose-textured multipolar cells associated with microcysts and eosinophilic granular bodies/hyaline droplets.

Subependymal giant cell astrocytoma (WHO grade I)
A benign, slowly growing tumour typically arising in the wall of the lateral ventricles and composed of large ganglioid astrocytes (See Chapter 13, Tuberous sclerosis complex and subependymal giant cell astrocytoma).

Pleomorphic xanthoastrocytoma (WHO grade II)
An astrocytic neoplasm with a relatively favourable prognosis, typically encountered in children and young adults, with superficial location in the cerebral hemispheres and involvement of the meninges; characteristic histological features include pleomorphic and lipidized cells expressing GFAP and often surrounded by a reticulin network as well as eosinophilic granular bodies.

Diffuse astrocytoma (WHO grade II)
A diffusely infiltrating astrocytoma that typically affects young adults and is characterized by a high degree of cellular differentiation and slow growth; the tumour occurs throughout the CNS but is preferentially located supratentorially and has an intrinsic tendency for malignant progression to anaplastic astrocytoma and, ultimately, glioblastoma.

Anaplastic astrocytoma (WHO grade III)
A diffusely infiltrating malignant astrocytoma that primarily affects adults, is preferentially located in the cerebral hemispheres, and is histologically characterized by nuclear atypia, increased cellularity and significant proliferative activity. The tumour may arise from diffuse astrocytoma WHO grade II or *de novo*, i.e. without evidence of a less malignant precursor lesion, and has an inherent tendency to undergo progression to glioblastoma.

Glioblastoma (WHO grade IV)
The most frequent primary brain tumour and the most malignant neoplasm with predominant astrocytic differentiation; histopathological features include nuclear atypia, cellular pleomorphism, mitotic activity, vascular thrombosis, microvascular proliferation and necrosis. It typically affects adults and is preferentially located in the cerebral hemispheres. Most glioblastomas manifest rapidly *de novo*, without recognizable precursor lesions (primary glioblastoma). Secondary glioblastomas develop slowly from diffuse astrocytoma WHO grade II or anaplastic astrocytoma (WHO grade III). Due to their invasive nature, glioblastomas cannot be completely resected, and despite progress in radio/chemotherapy, less than half of patients survive more than a year, with older age as the most significant adverse prognostic factor.

Gliomatosis cerebri
A diffuse glioma (usually astrocytic) growth pattern consisting of exceptionally extensive infiltration of a large region of the central nervous system, with involvement of at least three cerebral lobes, usually with bilateral involvement of the cerebral hemispheres and/or deep gray matter, and frequent extension to the brain stem, cerebellum, and even the spinal cord. Gliomatosis cerebri most commonly displays an astrocytic phenotype, although oligodendrogliomas and mixed oligoastrocytomas can also present with the gliomatosis cerebri growth pattern.

Pilocytic astrocytoma

B.W. Scheithauer
C. Hawkins
T. Tihan
S.R. VandenBerg
P.C. Burger

Definition

A relatively circumscribed, slowly growing, often cystic astrocytoma occurring in children and young adults, histologically characterized by a biphasic pattern with varying proportions of compacted bipolar cells associated with Rosenthal fibers and loose-textured multipolar cells associated with microcysts and eosinophilic granular bodies/hyaline droplets.

ICD-O code   9421/1

Grading

Pilocytic astrocytomas correspond to WHO grade I.

Incidence

Pilocytic astrocytomas comprise approximately 5–6% of all gliomas {305} with an overall incidence of 0.37 per 100 000 persons per year. Pilocytic astrocytoma is the most common glioma in children, in whom the majority (67%) arise in the cerebellum {1625}.

Age and sex distribution

Pilocytic astrocytoma most commonly develops, without a clear gender predilection, during the first two decades of life with an age–adjusted incidence rate of 0.8 per 100 000 persons per year. From 0–14 years and 15–19 years, it comprises about 21% and 16% of CNS tumours, respectively {305}. In a study of 1195 paediatric tumours from a single institution, pilocytic astrocytoma was the single most common tumour (18%) in the cerebral compartment {1925}. In adults, these astrocytomas tend to appear one decade earlier (mean age 22 years) than low-grade diffusely infiltrating cerebral astrocytomas {648} but relatively few arise in patients older than 50 years.

Localization

Pilocytic astrocytomas arise throughout the neuraxis; however in the paediatric population more tumours arise in the infratentorial region. Preferred sites include the optic nerve (optic nerve glioma) {873}, optic chiasm/hypothalamus {1905},

thalamus and basal ganglia {1432}, cerebral hemispheres {592, 1061, 1766}, cerebellum (cerebellar astrocytoma) {405, 798}, and brain stem (dorsal exophytic brain stem glioma) {247, 249, 1769}. In the paediatric population, the most common supratentorial site is the hypothalamus/optic pathways followed by the thalamic/basal ganglia region {1925}. Pilocytic astrocytomas of the spinal cord are less frequent, but not uncommon {1482, 1835, 1939}, and in children represent about 11% of spinal tumours {1925}. Large hypothalamic, thalamic, and brain stem lesions may largely occupy the ventricle, their site of origin being difficult to define. In the spinal cord, these tumours tend to occur in older patients than at other sites and comprise a significant proportion (58%) of spinal astrocytic tumours {1482}.

Clinical features

Signs and symptoms

Pilocytic astrocytomas produce focal neurological deficits or non-localizing signs, e.g. macrocephaly, headache, endocrinopathy, or increased intracranial pressure due to mass effect or ventricular obstruction. Seizures are uncommon since the lesions infrequently involve the cerebral cortex {356, 592}. Given their slow rate of growth, the clinical presentation of pilocytic tumours is generally that of a slowly evolving lesion. Pilocytic astrocytomas of the optic pathways often produce visual loss. Proptosis may be seen with intraorbital examples. Early, radiologically detected lesions may be unassociated with visual symptoms or ophthalmologic deficits {873, 1333}. Hypothalamic/pituitary dysfunction, including obesity and diabetes insipidus, is often but not invariably apparent in large hypothalamic examples {1905}. Some hypothalamic-chiasmatic lesions of young children have been associated with leptomeningeal seeding and a poor outcome {1717}. It is unclear whether such tumours represent a distinct entity {388, 2245}.

Pilocytic astrocytomas of the thalamus generally present with signs of CSF obstruction or neurological deficits, such as hemiparesis, due to internal capsule compression.

Cerebellar pilocytic astrocytomas usually present in the first two decades with clumsiness, worsening headache, nausea and vomiting. Brain stem examples usually cause hydrocephalus or signs of brain stem dysfunction. In contrast to diffuse astrocytoma of the pons, which produces symmetric "pontine hypertrophy", pilocytic tumours of the brain stem are usually dorsal and exophytic or just into the cerebellopontine angle. Spinal cord examples produce non-specific signs of an expanding mass {1482, 1835, 1939}.

Neuroimaging

By either CT or MRI, pilocytic astrocytomas are well-circumscribed and contrast-enhancing {626, 1283}. Only a minority are calcified. Tumours of the optic nerve, being somewhat restrained in their outward expansion by the optic sheath, grow along the course of the nerve to produce a fusiform mass. Optic pathway lesions have only a limited capacity to spread posteriorly, for example from optic nerve to chiasm or from chiasm to optic tracts. Although sensitive neuroimaging may suggest extensive infiltration, the relative contributions of tumour tissue, edema and Wallerian degeneration to the observed T2 hyperintensity is unclear.

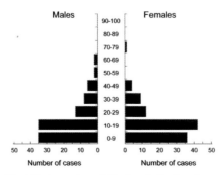

Fig. 1.01 Age and sex distribution of pilocytic astrocytoma, based on biopsies from 205 patients treated at the University Hospital, Zurich.

Pilocytic astrocytomas are found at all levels of the brain stem, are relatively discrete, often exophytic, and variably contrast enhancing {249, 1769}. Cyst formation is common. These characteristics distinguish them from diffuse astrocytomas (WHO grade II) of the basal pons which only show contrast enhancement after progression to anaplastic astrocytoma or glioblastoma. A diagnostically important feature suggesting pilocytic astrocytoma or some other WHO grade I lesion is cyst formation {1671A}, a common feature of cerebellar, spinal cord and cerebral hemispheric examples. Cysts may be either solitary and massive, the tumour being a mural nodule, or multiple, smaller and intratumoural.

Macroscopy

Most pilocytic astrocytomas are soft, grey and rather discrete. Intra- or paratumoural cyst formation is common. In spinal cord examples, syrinx formation may be conspicuous and can extend over many segments {1482, 1835}. Chronic lesions may contain calcium or haemosiderin deposits. Optic nerve tumours also often show collar-like involvement of the subarachnoid space {2153}. Primary diffuse leptomeningeal pilocytic astrocytoma is a rarity {194}.

Histopathology

This astrocytic tumour of low to moderate cellularity exhibits an often biphasic pattern with varying proportions of compacted bipolar cells with Rosenthal fibers and loose-textured multipolar cells with microcysts and granular bodies/hyaline droplets. Rare mitosis, hyperchromatic and pleomorphic nuclei, glomeruloid vascular proliferation, infarct-like necrosis and infiltration of leptomeninges are compatible with the diagnosis of pilocytic astrocytoma and are not signs of malignancy.

Due to heterogeneity of histologic features, smear preparations of pilocytic astrocytomas show considerable cytological variation. Basic cytologies are seen, often in combination. Compact portions of the tumour yield bipolar piloid cells, long, hair-like processes that often extend across a full microscopic field, and Rosenthal fibers. Their nuclei are typically elongate and cytologically bland. Due to their high content of refractile, eosinophilic fibrils, these cells are strongly glial fibrillary acidic protein (GFAP) immunopositive.

Cells derived from microcystic areas are often termed "protoplasmic astrocytes" and possess round to oval, cytologically bland nuclei, a small cell body and relatively short, cobweb-like processes which are fibril-poor and only weakly GFAP-positive. This growth pattern is typically associated with eosinophilic granular bodies and/or hyaline droplets. Less frequently seen are cells closely resembling oligodendrocytes. Cells indistinguishable from those of diffuse astrocytoma, WHO grade II, are often seen within peripheral, more infiltrative parts of the tumour. While many pilocytic astrocytomas are benign, some show considerable hyperchromasia and pleomorphism. Rare mitoses are seen in up to 30%. In occasional, often cerebellar tumours, a diffuse growth pattern overshadows more typical compact and microcystic features. In such cases, finding hyperchromatic nuclei or the occasional mitotic figure can cause confusion with high-grade diffuse astrocytoma. Less worrisome are obvious degenerative atypia with pleomorphism, smudgy chromatin, and nuclear-cytoplasmic pseudoinclusions, frequently seen in long-standing lesions. The designation 'pennies on a plate' describes the circumferential localization of multiple nuclei within large or giant cells {798}. Hyalinized and glomeruloid vessels are prominent features of pilocytic astrocytoma. Necrosis, when seen, is often infarct-like and non-palisading. Perivascular lymphocytes may also be seen. Since pilocytic astrocytomas to some extent overrun normal tissue, pre-existing neurons are sometimes trapped. Such lesions should be distinguished from ganglion cell tumours.

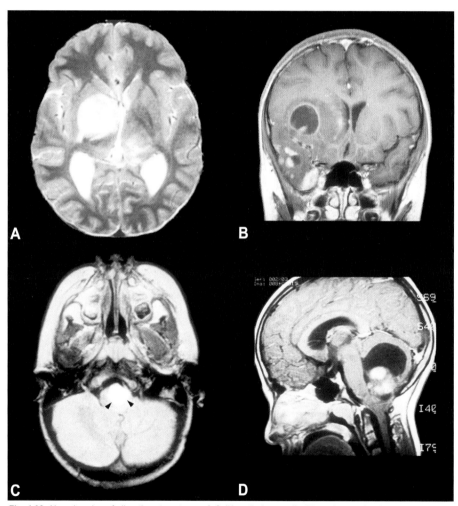

Fig. 1.02 Neuroimaging of pilocytic astrocytoma. **A** Solid, well-circumscribed hyperintense hemispheric lesion in a T2-weighted image. **B** Pilocytic astrocytoma of the frontal lobe presenting on T1 MRI as a hyperintense mural nodule with a large cyst. **C** Discrete pilocytic astrocytoma in the medulla (T1 MRI). **D** Cystic cerebellar lesion with a contrast-enhancing mural nodule.

Rosenthal fibers

These tapered corkscrew-shaped, brightly eosinophilic, hyaline masses are intracytoplasmic in location, a fact best seen on smear. Rosenthal fibers are most common in compact, piloid tissue. They appear bright blue on a Luxol fast blue (LFB) stain. Although helpful in diagnosis, their presence is not required. Lastly, Rosenthal fibers are neither specific to pilocytic astrocytoma nor indicative of neoplasia. They are often seen in ganglioglioma and are a common finding in chronic reactive gliosis. Densely fibrillar, paucicellular lesions containing Rosenthal fibers are as likely to be reactive gliosis as pilocytic astrocytoma. Ultrastructurally, Rosenthal fibers lie within astrocytic processes and consist of amorphous, electron-dense elements surrounded by intermediate (glial) filaments {475, 1246}. Being composed of α-B crystallin {704}, they lack GFAP immunoreactivity at all but their fibral rich periphery.

Eosinophilic granular bodies (EGB)

EGBs form globular aggregates within astrocytic processes. Brightly eosinophilic in H&E sections and PAS-positive, they show α-1-antichymotrypsin and α-1-antitrypsin immunoreactivity {1062}. EGBs are best seen in smear preparations. Their intracellular localization is usually not discernible in tissue sections. EGBs are an important diagnostic feature of several neoplasms, including ganglion cell tumours and pleomorphic xanthoas-

trocytoma, but again are not indicative of neoplasia. Occasional examples occur in diffusely infiltrating astrocytomas, usually after radiotherapy.

Vasculature

Pilocytic astrocytomas are highly vascular, as is evidenced by their contrast enhancement {626, 1283}. Although generally obvious in H&E sections, it is accentuated in Ulex europeus preparations or on immunostains for basement membrane (collagen IV, laminin) or endothelial cells (CD31, CD34). Also seen lining tumoural cyst walls and occasionally at a distance from the lesion, such glomeruloid vasculature should not prompt tumour misclassification or over-grading. Ultrastructural studies have shown fenestration of endothelium and a variety of abnormalities {2205}. Endothelial proliferation, a feature of high-grade diffuse astrocytic tumours, is generally not seen in conventional pilocytic tumours.

Regressive changes

Given the indolent nature and often slow clinical evolution of pilocytic astrocytomas, it is not surprising that regressive changes are seen. Markedly hyalinized, sometimes ectatic vessels are one such feature. When neoplastic cells are scant, it can even be difficult to distinguish the tumour from cavernous angioma with accompanying piloid gliosis. Evidence of previous haemorrhage (haemosiderin) further augments the likeness. Presentation

with acute haemorrhage is infrequent. Calcification, infarct-like necrosis, and lymphocytic infiltrates are additional examples of regressive changes {908}. On balance, calcification is an infrequent finding, only rarely seen in optic nerve or hypothalamic/thalamic tumours, or in superficially situated cerebral examples. Cysts are a common feature of pilocytic astrocytoma, especially in the locations specified above. Single or multiple, their fluid content is apparently rich in factors capable of stimulating vascular proliferation. Such neovascularity often lines cyst walls, thus explaining the narrow band of intense contrast enhancement seen at the circumference of some cysts. One frequently sees dense piloid tissue with accompanying Rosenthal fibers external to this vascular layer. When this layer is narrow and well defined from surrounding normal tissue, it may be considered reactive in nature. In other instances, the glial zone is more prominent, less well demarcated, and resembles tumour. Surgeons generally assume that the walls of large cysts are non-neoplastic and do not attempt resection of the cyst walls.

Tissue patterns

Although most pilocytic astrocytomas appear as a clearly defined clinical, radiologic, and pathologic entity, they exhibit a wide range of tissue patterns, sometimes several within the same lesion {257}. This is further complicated by a lack of tumour-specific immunohistochemical, cytogenetic and molecular markers. Some pathologists accept a wide range of patterns, whereas others are less accepting of what to them are unproven variants. The classic lesion consists of often alternating compact tissue composed of piloid cells and microcystic tissue rich in so-called protoplasmic astrocytes. This biphasic pattern is best seen in cerebellar tumours. Microcysts often contain peripherally vacuolated colloid. EGBs occur mainly in microcystic tissue, whereas Rosenthal fibers populate compact regions. A variant of the compact, piloid pattern occurs when the elongate cells are less compact but separated by mucin. In such cases, individual cell processes can be visualized and cell shape varies to include more full-bodied and pleomorphic, less obviously piloid cells. A distinctive lobular pattern results when leptomeningeal involvement engenders a

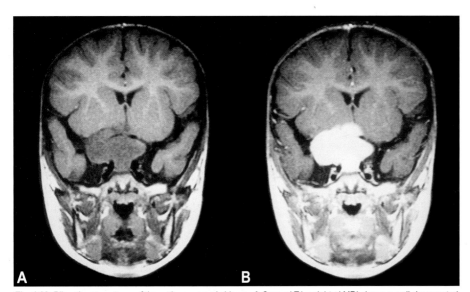

Fig. 1.03 Pilocytic astrocytoma of the optic nerve and chiasm. **A** Coronal T1-weighted MRI shows a well-demarcated lesion with (**B**) intense gadolinium (Gd)-enhancement. The tumour causes a compression and shift of the adjacent fronto-basal brain structures.

desmoplastic reaction. At this site, tissue texture varies but Rosenthal fibers are usually abundant.

Oligodendroglioma-like cells may be seen in pilocytic astrocytomas, especially in cerebellar examples. Arranged in sheets or dispersed within parenchyma, the overall appearance is that of an oligodendroglioma, particularly in a limited sample. It is the finding of foci of classic pilocytic astrocytoma that usually permits the correct classification of these lesions. A striking feature in some pilocytic astrocytomas is alignment of cells in prominent, regimented palisades. Such enfilades resemble those of what was termed the "primitive polar spongio-blastoma," which is thought to be more a tissue pattern than a defined tumour entity and is therefore no longer included in the WHO classification. Tumours with distinctive palisades, clusters, or organoid cell aggregates are examples of conten-tious lesions. The same is true of mucin-rich spindle cell neoplasms. Although astrocytomas in children are usually assigned to either the pilocytic or fibrillary type, in reality there are many which do not fit clearly into either category. In some instances, small biopsy size contributes to difficulties in classification.

Growth pattern

As a rule, pilocytic astrocytomas are macroscopically somewhat discrete. Thus, when anatomy permits, e.g. cerebellum or cerebral hemispheres, many can be removed *in toto* {592, 798, 1766}. Microscopically, however, many lesions are not well defined with respect to surrounding brain. Typical lesions permeate parenchyma for a distance of millimetres to several centimetres. As a result, neurons may be entrapped within the tumour. Nevertheless, as compared to diffuse gliomas, pilocytic tumours are relatively solid and do not aggressively overrun surrounding tissue. This property, evidenced by at least partial lack of axons on Bodian/Bielschowsky and NF protein immunostains, is of diagnostic value.

Pilocytic astrocytomas of the optic nerve and chiasm differ somewhat in their macroscopic and microscopic pattern of growth, often being less well-circumscribed and therefore difficult to stage, both macro- and microscopically. They share the same propensity for leptomeningeal involvement as seen in pilocytic tumours at other sites, but are somewhat more

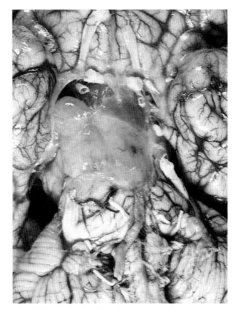

Fig. 1.04 Large pilocytic astrocytoma extending into the basal cisterns.

diffuse, especially within the optic nerve. This is evident when pathologists stage a lesion by analysis of sequential nerve margins. Microscopically, the lesion can be followed to a point beyond which it becomes less cellular but has no clearly defined termination.

There has been considerable discussion regarding a "diffuse" variant of pilocytic astrocytoma {692, 798, 1672}. Although some are simply classic pilocytic tumours in which the infiltrative edge is somewhat broader than expected or an artifact of plane of section, there are occasional, distinctly infiltrative lesions that mimic diffuse fibrillary astrocytoma. In two large studies, outcomes for children with "diffuse" pilocytic astrocytoma of the cere-bellum were favourable, thus confirming the notion that such tumours belong to the spectrum of pilocytic astrocytoma {798, 1672}. Regarding cerebellar astro-cytic tumours in neurofibromatosis type 1 (NF1), the relative incidence of diffuse vs. pilocytic examples and their natural history and prognosis, see Chapter 13. Bona fide infiltrating, diffuse astrocytomas represent up to 15% of astrocytic tumours of the cerebellum. Of these, most are high-grade tumours (WHO grade III and IV) {798}.

Infiltration of the meninges

Involvement of the subarachnoid space is a common finding in pilocytic astrocy-toma. It is not indicative of aggressive or

malignant behaviour, nor does it portend subarachnoid dissemination. In contrast, it is a characteristic, even diagnostically helpful feature. Leptomeningeal invasion occurs at any tumour site, but is particularly common in the cerebellum and optic nerve. In optic nerve, more so than in the cerebellum, the leptomeningeal compo-nent may be reticulin-rich. Another typical pattern of extraparenchymal spread is extension into perivascular spaces.

Distant spread and metastasis

Surprisingly, otherwise typical pilocytic astrocytomas very occasionally seed the neuraxis, rarely even before the primary tumour is detected {640, 1717, 1770}. The proliferation index in such cases varies but is usually low {1488}. Thus, this atypical behaviour of pilocytic astro-cytoma cannot be predicted {388}. The hypothalamus is the usual primary site. Even this finding is not necessarily an indicator of future aggressive growth, since both the primary lesion and the implants may grow only slowly {640, 1770}. Indeed, the implants may be asymptomatic and long-term survival is possible, even without adjuvant treatment {1770}. A related, less favourable lesion, the pilomyxoid astrocytoma {2245} typically occurring in the hypothalamic region, more often undergoes craniospinal spread. This lesion is discussed below.

Malignant transformation

As a group, pilocytic astrocytomas are remarkable in maintaining their WHO grade I {263A} status over years and even decades. As a rule, alterations over time are in the direction of regressive change rather than of anaplasia. One large study found the acquisition of atypia, particularly of increased cellularity, nuclear abnormalities and occasional mitoses, to be of no prognostic significance {2256}. There have, however, been rare examples of pilocytic astrocytoma under-going malignant transformation {476, 2256}. They often feature multiple mitoses per single high power field, endothelial proliferation and palisading necrosis. Such tumours should not be designated glioblastoma, since their prognosis is not uniformly grim. The designation anaplastic (malignant) pilocytic astrocytoma is preferred. Since most such tumours had previously been irradiated, radiation may be a factor promoting malignant change {476, 2256}.

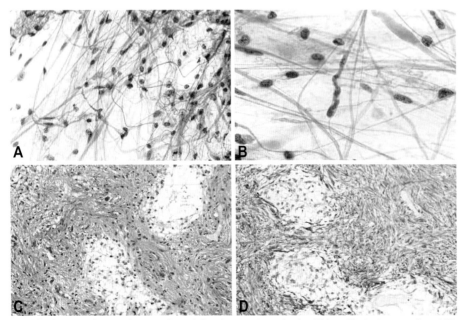

Fig. 1.05 Intraoperative squash preparations of pilocytic astrocytoma showing (**A**) long, bipolar tumour cells and (**B**) a Rosenthal fiber. **C,D** Typical biphasic pattern of compact, fiber-rich, GFAP-expressing areas and hypocellular areas with microcysts, lacking GFAP immunoreactivity.

Proliferation

Studies using the DNA S-phase marker bromodeoxyuridine have documented a generally low labelling index, typically less than 1% and only occasionally higher. Although in one study this index was of little prognostic value {930}, higher labelling was generally noted in young patients as was a tendency toward reduced labelling in subsequently obtained specimens. Indeed, tumour growth appeared to slow by about age 20. A more recent study of proliferative activity in both pilocytic and diffuse astrocytomas showed mitoses to vary from 0 to an exceptional 4 per 10 high-power fields and MIB-1 labelling indices to range from 0 to 3.9% (mean 1.1%) in pilocytic tumours {676}. The latter values overlapped with those of diffuse astrocytoma WHO grade II (mean 2.3%). Thus, MIB-1 labelling was of little use in differential diagnosis. These observations are in keeping with the facts that growth of the solid component of pilocytic astrocytomas is an infrequent cause of death and that such tumours show little tendency to progression and almost none to malignant transformation {2256}.

Genetic susceptibility

Pilocytic astrocytomas are the principal central nervous system neoplasm associ-ated with NF1. Optic nerve involvement, especially when bilateral, is the classic finding, but other anatomic sites, sometimes multiple, may also be affected. Approximately 15% of patients with NF1 develop pilocytic astrocytomas {1306}, particularly of the optic nerve. Conversely, up to one third of patients with a pilocytic astrocytoma at this location have NF1 {649}.

Genetics

Cytogenetic analyses of paediatric and adult pilocytic astrocytomas have been performed on approximately 132 tumours; the majority showed a normal karyotype {1007, 1985, 2092}. However, the possibility that these tumours harbour very small copy number changes, balanced translocations, and/or epigenetic alterations awaits future studies {1007}. To date, there has been no association between cytogenetic abnormalities and the location of the tumour. In some studies the majority of paediatric tumours with detectable abnormalities were from females {1985} and adults. A genome-wide study of 44 tumours with array-based comparative genomic hybridization (0.97Mb resolution) showed a non-random pattern of genetic alterations with whole chromosomal gains detected in 32% of tumours. Consistent with earlier studies demonstrating chromosomal gains, the most frequently affected chromosomes were 5 and 7 followed by chromosomes 6, 11, 12, 15, 17, 19, 20 and 22. In tumours of patients under 15 years with chromosomal gains, 50% had only one chromosome affected, whereas in tumours of patients over 15 years, all chromosomal gains were multiple. Smaller regions of chromosomal gain have involved a variety of loci on 1p, 2p, 4, 5q, 6q, 7q, 9q or 13q, and loss on 1p, 9q, 12q, 19, 20 or 22. There appears to be no role for either *TP53* mutations or aberrant PDGF signalling in the development of pilocytic astrocytomas when compared to the role of *TP53* mutations and increased expression of PDGF-A and PDGF-Rα as common, early events in the formation of diffuse-type astrocytomas {1311, 1621, 2194}. Gene expression analyses in sporadic pilocytic astrocytomas have demonstrated that these tumours are uniquely distinct from non-neoplastic white matter and other low-grade gliomas, and that they share similarities with fetal astrocytes {742} and oligodendroglial lineages {95, 369, 742, 1311}. Consistent with the presence of oligodendroglial progenitors, pilocytic astrocytomas, especially optic nerve tumours, contain significant numbers of O4 immunoreactive cells, and posterior fossa examples contain the highest number of A2B5+ glial progenitor cells {369}. Additional evidence for the relationship of pilocytic astrocytomas to gene expression associated with developmental processes is an expression analysis of 21 juvenile pilocytic astrocytomas by oligonucleotide microarray {2437}. Two potential subgroups differing in biologic behaviour were identified based on significant differences in the expression of genes involved in cell adhesion, cell growth regulation, motility, nerve ensheathment and angiogenesis. Neurogenesis seems to be one of the major biological processes affected, with detection of 18 deregulated genes including the up-regulation of four neurogenesis-related genes (SEMA5A, SCRG1, DPYSL3, and ASCL1), one central nervous system development-related gene (PTPRZ1), and achaetescute homologue-1 (ACSL1), a transcription factor involved in neurogenesis.

Pilocytic astrocytomas arising in NF1 patients are molecular genetically distinct from sporadic tumours {418, 740, 1136, 1619, 2070, 2194}. The archetypic change is loss of normal NF1 expression, allelic loss and genetic mutations resulting in constitutive RAS activation and down-stream hyperactivation of the mTOR pathway {417}. Pilocytic astrocytomas appear not to show aberrant promoter methylation of the *NF1* gene {505}. In addition, microsatellite analysis has shown a loss of heterozygosity on chromosome 10, including loss of *PTEN* and a homozygous deletion of $p16^{INK4a}$ in a small number of NF1 tumours {2194}. Sporadic pilocytic astrocytomas do not demonstrate loss of *NF1* gene expression and may even show its overexpression {1136, 1761, 2417}. Despite the apparently normal expression of NF1, sporadic tumours may activate RAS by other mechanisms {2071}. The paired overexpression of ErbB3 with SOX3 in sporadic pilocytic astrocytomas suggests that SOX10 may drive the over-expression of ErbB3 in the development of these tumours {15}. Pilocytic astrocytomas in NF1 also manifest dysregulation of methionine aminopeptidase-2 expression {418} as compared to over-expression of the matrilin-2 and EF-1α2 genes in the sporadic pilocytic astrocytomas {742, 2070}.

Pilocytic astrocytomas differ from the diffuse astrocytomas in their altered and increased expression of immune response genes {880} in addition to demonstrating their high content of proliferating microglia {1126}. Apolipoprotein D (apoD) is also expressed at 8.5 fold higher levels in pilocytic astrocytomas compared to diffuse gliomas {891,892}. Compared to low grade diffuse gliomas, pilocytic astrocytomas express increased levels of galectin-3 transcripts, a feature shared with glioblastomas {1575}. Pilocytic astrocytomas differ from glioblastoma by the expression of apoD, protease-serine-11 receptor, PLEKHB1, EF-1α1 and SPOCK1, whereas glioblastomas differ from pilocytic astrocytomas by expression of 5 genes involved in invasion and angio-genesis (fibronectin, osteopontin, YKL-40, keratoepithelin, fibromodulin) {368}.

Histogenesis

Having the capacity to form Rosenthal fibers, the hair-like, piloid cells of pilocytic astrocytomas are remarkably similar to reactive astrocytes surrounding various chronic lesions of the hypothal-amus, cerebellum and spinal cord. Similar cells are also found in the glial stroma of the normal pineal gland. Their histologic and cytologic resemblance makes such astrocytes prime candidates as precursors. Obviously, this simple notion does not take into consideration proto-plasmic astrocytes and microcystic forms of pilocytic astrocytoma rich in EGBs.

Prognostic and predictive factors

As a group, pilocytic astrocytomas are slowly growing masses which may stabi-lize at any point in their evolution. Rare examples even spontaneously regress {735}. Stability in tumour grade and differentiation is typically maintained for decades {118, 263A, 1666}. Long survival is the rule {565,1625}. Although the lesion may eventually prove fatal, there are few long-term studies documenting the ultimate outcome of patients with pilocytic astro-cytoma. As a rule, supratentorial examples and delay in radiotherapy, when needed, are associated with less-favourable progression-free survival {1102}. Recurrent hypothalamic and brain stem lesions can result in death, but usually only after a prolonged course with multiple local recurrences {592, 798, 1482, 1770, 1905}. Clinical "recurrence" in the short term is more often a reflection of cyst reformation than of enlargement of the solid tumour component. Generally, NF1-associated pilocytic astrocytomas remain stable or grow only slowly, especially those of the optic nerve {873, 1333, 1905}. One large series of paediatric pilocytic astrocytomas in NF1 found them to be less aggressive than non-syndromic lesions {1935}. One series suggesting that cerebellar examples in NF1 are more aggressive {908} should be viewed in light of the fact that a clear distinction between pilocytic and diffuse astrocytomas is not always achievable in this setting. Again, occasional NF1-associated pilocytic tumours spontaneously regress {1287}.

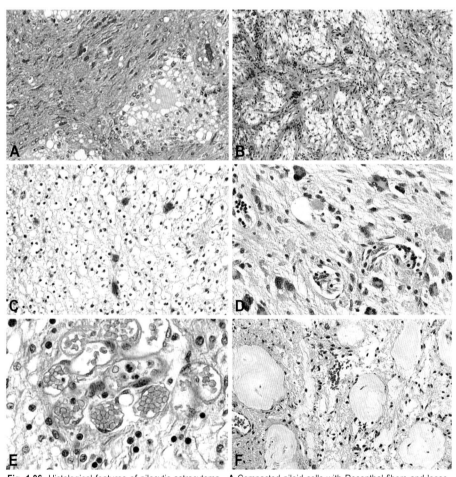

Fig. 1.06 Histological features of pilocytic astrocytoma. **A** Compacted piloid cells with Rosenthal fibers and loose-textured multipolar cells with microcysts. **B** A biphasic, compact and spongy pattern. **C** Tumour area with honeycomb cells resembling oligodendroglioma. **D** Marked nuclear atypia is not a sign of malignancy. Note the numerous eosinophilic granular bodies. **E** Vascular wickerwork pattern typically encountered in cerebellar lesions. **F** Tumour vessels with extensive hyalinization.

The definition and prognostic significance of lesions sometimes designated as "atypical" or "malignant" have been addressed {2256}. Such tumours often occur in the cerebellum and are more often solid than cystic {1909}. It is the varied presence of increased cellularity, mitotic activity, MIB-1 labelling, microvascular proliferation (glomeruloid and endothelial), and necrosis that generates concern. The rare mitosis (1-2/50 HPF) occurs in approximately 30% of pilocytic astrocytomas {676}. When seen in conjunction with significant nuclear atypia and increased cellularity, the designation atypical pilocytic astrocytoma has been applied but, in one large series {2256}, was not found to be of clinical significance. At present, there are no reliable, prognostically meaningful criteria of atypical pilocytic astrocytoma; this includes combined MIB-1 and p53 immunolabelling {2246}. Only when mitotic activity is expressed in terms of mitoses per single HPF and is associated with endothelial proliferation and/or palisading necrosis can the designation anaplastic (malignant) pilocytic astrocytoma be applied {2256}. Most such tumours are associated with aggressive behaviour, yet others are cured by resection with or without adjuvant radio- and/or chemotherapy. Classic pilocytic astrocytoma must be distinguished from pilomyxoid astrocytoma, a tumour which with rare exception {1158}, affects the hypothalamic/third ventricular region {354, 2245}. Prone to undergo craniospinal seeding, they are associated with a less favourable prognosis.

Pilomyxoid astrocytoma

Definition
A piloid neoplasm, closely related to pilocytic astrocytoma, that has a prominent mucoid matrix and angiocentric arrangement of monomorphous, bipolar tumour cells, typically without Rosenthal fibers or eosinophilic granular bodies/hyaline droplets.

ICD-O code
The provisional code proposed for the fourth edition is *9425/3*.

Grading
Pilomyxoid astrocytoma corresponds to a WHO grade II neoplasm.

Synonyms and historical annotation
Earlier reports refer to tumours with similar features as "infantile" pilocytic astrocytoma {968}. The term "pilomyxoid" was introduced in 1999 to describe its two distinct histological features {2247}.

The occasional phenotypical conversion of a pilomyxoid astrocytoma to a typical pilocytic astrocytoma supports a common origin for these two tumours {306}.

Incidence
The incidence of pilomyxoid astrocytoma is not known, but it comprises a small percentage of tumours historically classified as pilocytic astrocytoma.

Age and sex distribution
Pilomyxoid astrocytoma typically presents in the very young (median 10 months), but can occur in older children. They are rare in adults. Male:female distribution is roughly equal.

Localization
The hypothalamic/chiasmatic region is the most common location, although the tumour can occur in the thalamus {565, 2247}, cerebellum {565}, brain stem {565}, temporal lobe {2247} and spinal cord {1159}.

Clinical features
Pilomyxoid astrocytoma presents with non-specific signs and symptoms referable to its anatomic site. Radiological examination highlights a circumscribed mass with relatively distinct borders. On MRI scan, the tumour is typically hypointense on T1-, and hyperintense on T2-weighted images, and shows homogeneous contrast enhancement {68}. Evidence of CSF dissemination may be evident at presentation.

Macroscopy
Intraoperative reports often describe a solid, gelatinous mass {2247}. In at least some parts, the tumours may infiltrate parenchyma. Thus, a clear surgical plane may not be identified.

Histopathology
Pilomyxoid astrocytoma is dominated by a markedly mucoid matrix, monomorphous bipolar cells, and a predominantly angiocentric cell arrangement. The tumour typically has a compact, rather solid architecture, but some are infiltrative. The lesion is composed of relatively monomorphous, intermediate size, bipolar cells the processes of which may radiate from vessels in a pseudorosette fashion. Cells may be also aligned along the long axis of vessels. When strictly defined, the lesion does not contain Rosenthal fibers

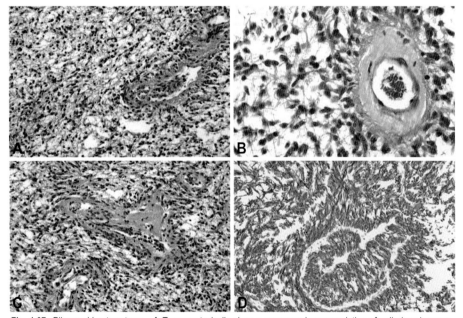

Fig. 1.07 Pilomyxoid astrocytoma. **A** Tumours typically show a monomorphous population of cells in a homogeneously myxoid background. **B** The prominent feature of pilomyxoid astrocytoma is the angiocentric arrangement of tumour cells. **C** The vascularity is often prominent with the above-mentioned angiocentric arrangement of tumour cells, but florid vascular proliferation is rare. **D** Tumours are typically diffusely and strongly positive for GFAP.

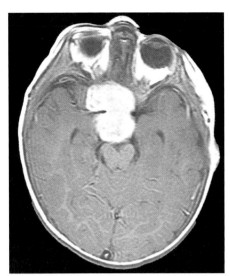

Fig. 1.08 Axial T1-weighted, gadolinium-enhanced image of pilomyxoid astrocytoma in a typical location.

or eosinophilic granular bodies/hyaline droplets. Mitotic figures can be present. Vascular proliferation, present in some cases, often takes the form of linear glomeruloid tufts associated with cystic degeneration. Rare examples may be focally necrotic. Limited pilomyxoid changes in an otherwise typical pilocytic astrocytoma do not warrant a diagnosis of pilomyxoid astrocytoma.

Immunohistochemical staining demonstrates strong, diffuse reactivity for GFAP, S-100 protein and vimentin. Some tumours are positive for synaptophysin, but staining for neurofilament protein or chromogranin is typically negative.

Proliferation

In limited studies of pilomyxoid astrocytomas, Ki-67 labelling indices were found to vary substantially, ranging from 2–20% {565, 1157, 2247}. There is considerable overlap of Ki-67 labelling indices in such tumours and pilocytic astrocytomas.

Genetic susceptibility

No genetic susceptibility has thus far been established, although two patients with NF1 and pilomyxoid astrocytoma have been reported {1097}.

Genetics

One report found no genetic abnormalities using conventional comparative genomic hybridization {1157}.

Histogenesis

The cell of origin for pilomyxoid astrocytoma is unclear. Some reports of pilomyxoid astrocytoma underscore the close relationship to pilocytic astrocytoma, thus implying a common astrocytic origin. An alternative suggestion that the tumour arises from radial glia in proximity to the optic tract remains to be substantiated {335}.

Prognostic and predictive factors

Pilomyxoid astrocytomas are more aggressive than pilocytic astrocytomas {565,1157,2247}. Local recurrence as well as cerebrospinal spread occur more often in pure pilomyxoid tumours than in pilocytic astrocytomas {2247}.

Pleomorphic xanthoastrocytoma

C. Giannini
W. Paulus
D.N. Louis
P. Liberski

Definition

An astrocytic neoplasm with a relatively favourable prognosis, typically encountered in children and young adults, with superficial location in the cerebral hemispheres and involvement of the meninges; characteristic histological features include pleomorphic and lipidized cells expressing GFAP and often surrounded by a reticulin network as well as eosinophilic granular bodies.

ICD-O code   9424/3

Grading

Pleomorphic xanthoastrocytoma corresponds histologically to WHO grade II. For lesions with significant mitotic activity (5 or more mitoses per 10 HPF) and/or with areas of necrosis, the designation "pleomorphic xanthoastrocytoma with anaplastic features" may be used {675}; when not completely excised, such tumours have an increased risk of early recurrence.

Synonyms and historical annotation

Before the introduction of immunostaining, pleomorphic xanthoastrocytomas were thought to represent mesenchymal neoplasms of the meninges and brain, partly because the lipidized neoplastic glial cells resemble "xanthoma" cells, and partly because many tumour cells produce a basement membrane. However, immunohistochemical and ultrastructural studies have clearly shown that the tumour cells

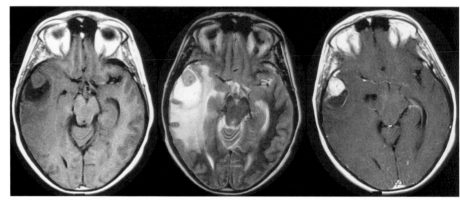

Fig. 1.10 T1, T2 and T1 with contrast of a typical PXA of the temporal lobe, presenting as a cystic tumour with a superficial enhancing mural nodule.

are neoplastic astrocytes, often with evidence of neuronal differentiation {678, 827, 1090}.

Incidence

Pleomorphic xanthoastrocytoma accounts for less than 1% of all astrocytic neoplasms. Since the initial description of 12 cases in 1979 {1090}, well over 200 additional cases have been reported {675}.

Age and sex distribution

This neoplasm typically develops in children and young adults. Two thirds of patients are less than 18 years old {674}, but manifestation in older patients, e.g. 62 and 82 years old {675, 1374} has also been reported. There is no documented gender bias, although one study reports these tumours appear more commonly in females {597}.

Etiology

No specific aetiologies have been implicated in the evolution of pleomorphic xanthoastrocytoma. The rare *TP53* mutations encountered do not suggest particular carcinogenic insults {673, 1067, 1702}. The occasional association with cortical dysplasia or with ganglionic lesions has suggested that their formation may be facilitated in malformative states {1243}. Given reports in patients with neurofibromatosis type 1 (NF1) {769, 1550}, a relation to defective NF1 function is possible.

Localization

A superficial location, involving the meninges and cerebrum ("meningocerebral") is typical of this neoplasm. Ninety-eight percent occur supratentorially, in particular the temporal lobe {675,1090}. Cases involving the cerebellum and spinal cord are also on record {683, 1557}, and two children with primary pleomorphic xanthoastrocytoma of the retina were reported {2484}.

Clinical features

Symptoms and signs

Because of the superficial cerebral location of the lesion, many patients present with a fairly long history of seizures. Cerebellar and spinal cord cases have symptoms that reflect the sites of involvement.

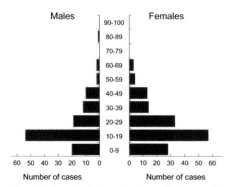

Fig. 1.09 Age distribution of patients with pleomorphic xanthoastrocytoma.

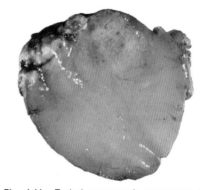

Fig. 1.11 Typical macroscopic appearance of a pleomorphic xanthoastrocytoma. The yellow areas correspond to xanthomatous parts of the tumour.

Neuroimaging

CT and MRI scans usually outline the tumour mass and/or its cyst. Perifocal edema is usually not pronounced, owing to the slow growth of the tumour.

Macroscopy

Pleomorphic xanthoastrocytomas are mainly superficial tumours attached to the meninges. They are frequently accompanied by a cyst, sometimes forming a mural nodule within the cyst wall. Invasion of the dura {436}, predominantly exophytic growth {1494}, multicentricity {1437} and leptomeningeal dissemination {1691} are exceptional.

Histopathology

The key histopathological features of the pleomorphic xanthoastrocytoma are well established {1205}. The adjective 'pleomorphic' refers to the variable histological appearance of the tumour, in which spindly elements are intermingled with mono- or multinucleated giant astrocytes, the nuclei of which show great variation in size and staining. Intranuclear inclusions are frequent {675}. In some cases, the neoplastic astrocytes are closely packed and assume an 'epithelioid' pattern {936}. The term 'xanthoastrocytoma' refers to the presence of large xanthomatous cells showing intracellular accumulation of lipids. This is usually in the form of droplets, which quite often occupy much of the cell body, pushing to the periphery cytoplasmic organelles and glial filaments that by conventional or GFAP stains generally make the astrocytic character easy to recognize. Granular bodies, intensely eosinophilic or pale, are almost a constant finding {675}. Focal collections of small lymphocytes, occasionally with plasma cells, are also frequent {675}. The third histological hallmark of pleomorphic xanthoastrocytoma is the presence of reticulin fibers best seen using silver impregnation. Not only reactive changes in the meninges result in the presence of reticulin fibers; the individual tumour cells may be surrounded by basement membranes that stain positively for reticulin, and these can be recognized ultrastructurally as pericellular basal laminae. Histological features of anaplasia, including significant mitotic activity (5 or more mitoses per 10 HPF) and necrosis are uncommon at initial presentation, respectively seen in 18% and 11% of cases in one series {675}. At recurrence,

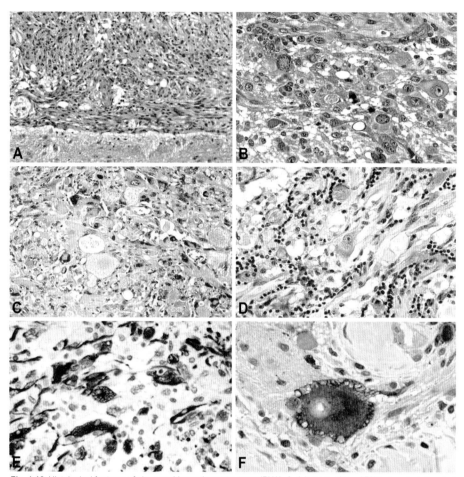

Fig. 1.12 Histological features of pleomorphic xanthoastrocytoma (PXA). **A** A leptomeningeal PXA, sharply delineated from the underlying cerebral cortex. **B** Granular bodies, intensely eosinophilic or pale, are almost a constant finding. **C** Tumour cells showing nuclear and cytoplasmic pleomorphism and xanthomatous change. **D** Mature ganglion cell and lymphocytic infiltrates in a PXA. From Kros *et al.* {1205}. **E** GFAP expression in large pleomorphic and xanthomatous cells. **F** Synaptophysin immunostaining in PXA cells. From Giannini *et al.* {678}.

tumours may show histological patterns similar to the original, or increasing anaplasia, in some cases being histologically indistinguishable from glioblastoma and featuring both necrosis and endothelial hyperplasia. Pleomorphism may cease to be a feature, and closely packed smaller cells may come to dominate the tumour. In addition, with increasing malignancy, the rich reticulin network may become fragmented or disappear completely {1088}.

Rarely, pleomorphic xanthoastrocytoma is part of a combination tumour in which it forms the glioma portion of a ganglioglioma {1725}. Exceptional is the occurrence of a combined pleomorphic xanthoastrocytoma/oligodendroglioma {1735}. Some highly vascularized forms have been denoted as 'angiomatous' {2170}.

Immunohistochemistry

Although the essential nature of pleomorphic xanthoastrocytoma is clearly and uniformly glial with nearly constant immunoreactivity for GFAP and S-100 protein {675, 678}, the tumour shows a significant tendency to exhibit neuronal differentiation. Expression of neuronal markers including synaptophysin, neurofilament, class III ß-tubulin and MAP2 has been reported with variable frequency {678, 1780}. This biphenotypic glioneuronal appearance in some cases has been confirmed ultrastructurally {827}. The haematopoietic progenitor cell and vascular endothelial cell associated antigen CD34 is frequently expressed in pleomorphic xanthoastrocytoma cells {1843}.

Proliferation

In most cases, mitotic figures are rare or

absent {675}. MIB-1/Ki-67 and PCNA labelling indices are generally lower than 1% {675, 1365, 2368}. S-phase fractions, as determined by flow cytometry, are also low {872, 2368}.

Genetic susceptibility

There are no distinct associations with hereditary tumour syndromes, with the exception of rare reports of pleomorphic xanthoastrocytoma in NF1 patients {1213, 1658}. Given the well-known association of NF1 with many different forms of astrocytomas, these occasional cases are not surprising. Familial clustering of pleomorphic xanthoastrocytoma has not been reported.

Genetics

Complex karyotypes have been documented, with gains of chromosomes 3 and 7, as well as alterations of the long arm of chromosome 1 {1314, 2002, 2003}. These cytogenetic changes, however, have also been reported in other types of astrocytoma. The tumours appear to be predominantly diploid {872, 2368}, occasionally with polyploid populations {872}, possibly due to subgroups of particularly bizarre, multinucleated tumour cells.

A CGH analysis of 50 cases revealed -9 as the chromosomal hallmark alteration (50% of cases), while less common recurrent chromosomal imbalances included +X (16%), -17 (10%), +7, +9q, +20 (8% each) and -8, -18, -22, +4, +5 and +19 (4% each) {2379}. Analysis of 10 tumours by array-based CGH indicated homozygous 9p21.3 deletions involving the *CDKN2A/p14^{ARF}/CDKN2B* loci in six cases (60%) {2379}. In four series with a total of 123 tumours, mutations in the *TP53* gene were found in only 7 cases (6%) {673, 1067, 1536, 1702}, being

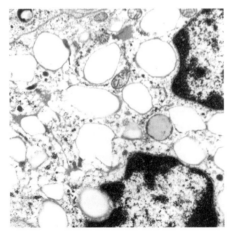

Fig. 1.13 Vacuolated cytoplasm in pleomorphic xanthoastrocytoma.

unrelated to absence or presence of histological features of anaplasia. Amplification of the *EGFR, CDK4* and *MDM2* genes were absent in a series of 62 tumours {1067}. These findings distinguish pleomorphic xanthoastrocytoma from diffusely infiltrating cerebral astrocytoma.

Histogenesis

The most popular hypothesis, originally proposed by Kepes *et al.* {1090}, postulates that pleomorphic xanthoastrocytoma originates from subpial astrocytes. This hypothesis would explain the superficial location of most pleomorphic xanthoastrocytomas, and is supported by ultrastructural features shared between subpial astrocytes and the neoplastic cells in pleomorphic xanthoastrocytomas, in particular the presence of a basal lamina surrounding individual cells. On the other hand, expression of neuronal markers {678} and the haematopoietic progenitor cell associated antigen CD34 {1843} in many

pleomorphic xanthoastrocytomas as well as the occasional association with cortical dysplasia suggests a more complex histogenesis and a possible origin from multipotential neuroectodermal precursor cells or from a pre-existing hamartomatous lesion {911, 1243}.

Prognostic and predictive factors

With some notable exceptions {1088, 2392, 2405}, pleomorphic xanthoastrocytoma behaves in a less malignant fashion than might be suggested by its highly pleomorphic histology {1090}. Cases with survival as long as 40 years after surgery have been published soon after the original description of this tumour {1671}. A series of 71 patients reported recurrence-free survival of 72% at 5 years and 61% at 10 years {675}. Recurrence-free survival curves, based on a review of previously published cases (n=121), are similar. The extent of the resection of the original tumour mass appears to be the most significant predictive factor, followed by a low mitotic index {675}. Both factors are independently predictive of recurrence-free survival.

Overall survival has been estimated as 81% at 5 years and 70% at 10 years {675}. Mitotic activity (more than 5 per 10 HPF) is the only independent predictor of survival. Necrosis, although significantly associated with survival, was not an independent predictor. A review of the previously published cases has also shown a significant association of necrosis with survival {675, 1667}.

No reliable correlation between *TP53* mutation and malignant progression or recurrence has been established in the few cases analysed to date {1536, 1702}.

Diffuse astrocytoma

A. von Deimling
P.C. Burger
Y. Nakazato
H. Ohgaki
P. Kleihues

Definition

A diffusely infiltrating astrocytoma that typically affects young adults and is characterized by a high degree of cellular differentiation and slow growth; the tumour occurs throughout the CNS but is preferentially located supratentorially and has an intrinsic tendency for malignant progression to anaplastic astrocytoma and, ultimately, glioblastoma.

ICD-O codes

Diffuse astrocytoma   9400/3
- Fibrillary astrocytoma   9420/3
- Gemistocytic astrocytoma   9411/3
- Protoplasmic astrocytoma   9410/3

Grading

Diffuse astrocytoma corresponds to WHO grade II. Although the gemistocytic variant appears to be particularly prone to progress to anaplastic astrocytoma and glioblastoma {1208, 1959, 2023}, the WHO Working Groups did not recommend assigning it a WHO grade III as for anaplastic astrocytoma {257, 2023}.

Synonyms and historical annotation

The term diffuse astrocytoma (WHO grade II) was proposed in the previous edition of the WHO Classification {1122}. The synonymous term 'low-grade diffuse astrocytoma (WHO grade II)' may be preferred. The designation 'well-differentiated astrocytoma' is not recommended since it could be confused with the pilocytic astrocytoma, which is usually more circumscribed and has a different age distribution, location and biology. 'Fibrillary astrocytoma' is commonly used for the most typical histological subtype of diffuse astrocytoma WHO grade II.

Incidence

Diffuse astrocytoma represents 10–15% of all astrocytic brain tumours, with an incidence rate of approximately 1.4 new cases / 1 million population a year {432}. Epidemiological data suggest that the incidence of astrocytoma in children has slightly increased during the past three decades in several Scandinavian countries and in North America {432, 807, 839, 2189}.

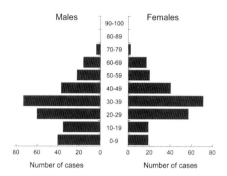

Fig. 1.14 Age distribution of diffuse astrocytoma WHO grade II, based on biopsies of 529 patients from the Tumour Registry of the University of California, San Francisco (courtesy of Ms Nancy Drungilas) and the Institute of Neuropathology, University Hospital Zurich.

Age and sex distribution

The age distribution of diffuse astrocytoma shows a peak incidence in young adults between ages 30 and 40. Approximately 10% occur below the age of 20, 60% between 20-45 years of age, and about 30% over 45 years of age with a mean of 34 years. There is a predominance of affected males (M:F ratio, 1.18:1).

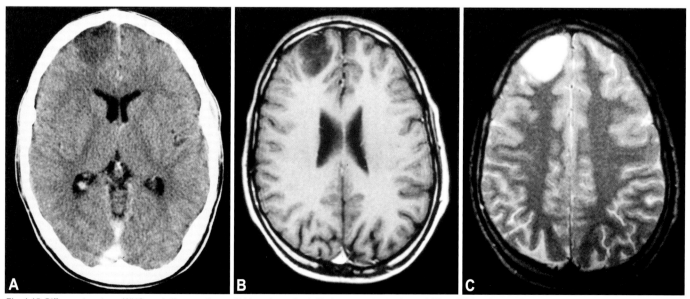

Fig. 1.15 Diffuse astrocytoma WHO grade II, presenting as (**A**) hypodense frontal lesion on contrast-enhanced CT, as (**B**) hypointense focus on gadolinium-enhanced MRI and (**C**) as well-delineated hyperintense lesion on T2-weighted MRI.

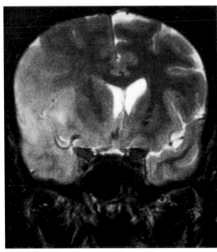

Fig. 1.16 T2-weighted MRI of a diffuse astrocytoma involving the fronto-temporal region with considerable mass effect. In the affected brain region, the cortex is enlarged but still recognizable.

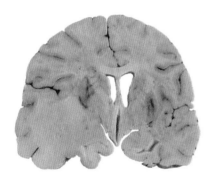

Fig. 1.17 Large fibrillary astrocytoma occupying the left temporal lobe, with extension to the Sylvian fissure. Note the homogeneous surface and the enlargement of local anatomical structures.

Localization

Diffuse astrocytoma may be located in any region of the CNS, but it most commonly develops supratentorially in the frontal and temporal cerebral lobes of both children and adults (one third of cases each). The brain stem and spinal cord are the next most frequently affected sites, while diffuse astrocytoma is distinctly uncommon in the cerebellum.

Clinical features

Symptoms and signs

Seizures are a common presenting symptom, although in retrospect subtle abnormalities such as speech difficulties, changes in sensation, vision, or some motor change may have been present earlier. With frontal lobe tumours, changes in behaviour or personality may be the presenting feature. Any such change may have been present for months before diagnosis, but symptoms may also be abrupt in onset.

Neuroimaging

On CT scans, diffuse astrocytoma most often presents as ill-defined, homogeneous masses of low density without contrast enhancement. However, calcification, cystic changes and even lower degrees of enhancement may be present early. MRI studies usually show hypodensity on T1-weighted and hyperintensity on T2-weighted images, with enlargement of the areas involved early in the evolution of the tumour. Gadolinium enhancement is uncommon in low-grade diffuse astrocytoma, but tends to appear during progression to anaplastic astrocytoma (WHO grade III).

Macroscopy

Because of their infiltrative nature, these tumours usually show blurring of the gross anatomical boundaries. There is enlargement and distortion, but not destruction, of the invaded anatomical structures, e.g. cortex and compact myelinated pathways. Local mass lesions may be present in either grey or yellow-white matter, but they have indistinct boundaries, and changes such as smaller or larger cysts, granular areas and zones of firmness or softening may be seen. Cystic change most commonly appears as a focal spongy area, with multiple cysts of varying size. Extensive microcyst formation may cause a gelatinous appearance. Occasionally, a single large cyst filled with clear fluid may be present. Tumours with prominent gemistocytes sometimes have single, large smooth-walled cysts. Focal calcification may also be present, and a more diffuse grittiness may be observed. Extension into contralateral structures, particularly in the frontal lobes, is also observed.

Histopathology

Diffuse astrocytoma is composed of well differentiated fibrillary or gemistocytic neoplastic astrocytes on the background of a loosely structured, often microcystic tumour matrix. In comparison to normal brain, cellularity is moderately increased and occasional nuclear atypia is a typical feature. Mitotic activity is generally absent, and a single mitosis does not yet allow the diagnosis of anaplastic astrocytoma.

The presence of necrosis or microvascular proliferation is incompatible with the diagnosis of diffuse astrocytoma. Phenotypically, neoplastic astrocytes may vary considerably with respect to their size, the prominence and disposition of cell processes, and the abundance of cytoplasmic glial filaments. The pattern may vary markedly in different regions of the neoplasm.

Histological recognition of neoplastic astrocytes using H&E staining on sectioned material depends mainly on nuclear characteristics. The normal astrocytic nucleus is oval-to-elongate, but on sectioning, occasional round cross-sections are seen. It is typically vesicular, with intermediate-sized masses of chromatin and often with a distinct nucleolus. Normal human astrocytes show no H&E stainable cytoplasm that is distinct from the background neuropil. Reactive astrocytes are defined by enlarged nuclei and the presence of stainable, defined cytoplasm, culminating in the gemistocyte, which has a mass of eosinophilic cytoplasm, often an eccentric nucleus, and a cytoplasm that extends into fine processes.

Differential diagnosis. The diffuse astrocytoma contains astrocytes that are increased in number and also usually in size, but are otherwise difficult to distinguish on an individual basis from the normal or reactive cells. In minor degrees of anaplasia, it is their number and, most commonly, the monotony of their morphology that is most helpful in recognising their neoplastic nature. Reactive astrocytes are rarely all in the same stage of reactivity at one time, so reactions reveal mixtures of astrocytes; some with enlarged nuclei, others with varying amounts of cytoplasm, most often on a somewhat rarefied background. With diffuse astrocytoma, almost all of the nuclei appear identical, and the background is at least of normal density, or shows increased numbers of cellular processes. Microcystic change may be present, but again most cells look like one another, without the admixture of gemistocytes more often seen as reactions to injury. Pre-existing cell types, e.g. neurons, are often entrapped.

Intraoperative diagnosis. The smear or 'squash' technique is often used during stereotaxic biopsies and yields similar findings, although estimating cellularity with this method is highly unreliable.

Many histological features are exaggerated and amplified, e.g. nuclear folds, abnormal chromatin pattern and astrocytic processes. On reducing the light by removing the top lens of the condenser, astrocytic processes are often emphasized. The presence of many round-to-oval nuclei with smooth chromatin can herald the presence of a mixed oligodendroglial component or, if the nuclei are less prominent, the background white matter. Histologically, there may be significant variation between tumours, and within the same lesion. According to the prevailing cell type, three major variants can be distinguished, but often a clear subclassification is not feasible.

Fibrillary astrocytoma

This most frequent histological variant of astrocytoma is predominantly composed of fibrillary neoplastic astrocytes. Nuclear atypia is a diagnostic criterion but mitotic activity, necrosis and microvascular proliferation are absent. A single mitosis does not allow the diagnosis of anaplastic astrocytoma. The occasional or regional occurrence of gemistocytic neoplastic cells is compatible with the diagnosis of fibrillary astrocytoma. Cell density is low to moderate. The cytoplasm is often scant and barely discernible, creating the appearance of naked nuclei. Nuclear atypia (i.e. enlarged, cigar-shaped, or irregular hyperchromatic nuclei) is a histological hallmark distinguishing tumour cells from normal and reactive astrocytes. Even prominent nuclear atypia is compatible with the diagnosis of diffuse astrocytoma WHO grade II so long as mitoses are very rare or absent. In more cellular lesions, neoplastic cell processes form a loose fibrillary matrix. Microcysts containing mucinous fluid are a characteristic feature and often dominate the histological picture. Cartilage formation is very rare {1089, 1412}.

Immunohistochemistry. Glial fibrillary acidic protein (GFAP) is consistently expressed, although to a variable degree and not by all tumour cells. In particular, small round cells with scanty cytoplasm and processes tend not to express GFAP. Often, GFAP immunoreactivity is restricted to a small perinuclear rim. The fibrillary matrix, which consists of a network of neoplastic cell processes (and entrapped reactive astrocytes), forms a diffuse GFAP-positive background {1123}. Vimentin, a 57 kDa intermediate filament protein,

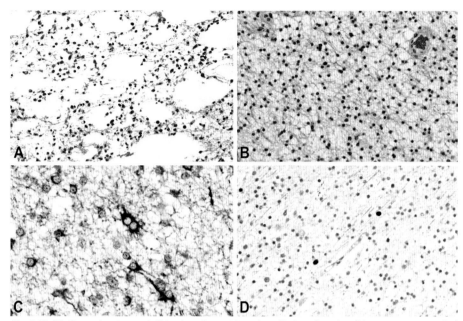

Fig. 1.18 Fibrillary astrocytoma. **A** Extensive microcyst formation. **B** A moderately cellular tumour composed of uniform fibrillary astrocytic cells with microcystic stroma. **C** Cytoplasm and processes showing GFAP immunoreactivity. **D** Low MIB-1 labelling index.

shows a pattern of immunoreactivity similar to that of GFAP, although vimentin immunoreactivity has a tendency to be seen mainly in the perinuclear region while GFAP is also expressed intensively in the cellular processes {815}. Vimentin-positive cells may lack GFAP expression. As vimentin is expressed early in astrogliogenesis, its presence in astrocytomas could indicate a lower degree of differentiation and there is a tendency for vimentin to be expressed more consistently in high-grade astrocytomas {1524}. Tumour cells usually show immunoreactivity to S-100 protein in the nucleus and in cell processes, but this feature has no diagnostic relevance {1114, 1123}. This is also true of the expression of B-crystallin {1055}.

Electron microscopy. Fibrillary neoplastic astrocytes are characterized by the presence of intermediate filaments ranging in diameter from 7 to 11 nm in the perikaryon and cell processes. However, these and other ultrastructural features are of limited diagnostic significance. In particular, they do not allow a distinction between tumour cells and reactive astrocytes.

Proliferation. Mitotic activity is typically absent in diffuse astrocytoma. Accordingly, the growth fraction, as determined by the Ki-67/MIB-1 labelling index, is usually less than 4%, with a mean of 2.5% {2369}.

Gemistocytic astrocytoma

This variant of astrocytoma is characterized by the presence of a conspicuous, though variable, fraction of gemistocytic neoplastic astrocytes. Gemistocytes should amount to more than approximately 20% of all tumour cells; the occasional occurrence of gemistocytes in a diffuse astrocytoma does not justify the diagnosis of gemistocytic astrocytoma. The mean size of the fraction of gemistocytes is approximately 35% {2370}. The cut-off value of 20% is somewhat arbitrary, but a useful criterion in borderline cases {1208, 2249}. The histopathological picture of gemistocytes is dominated by plump, glassy, eosinophilic cell bodies of angular shape. Stout, randomly oriented processes, forming a coarse fibrillary network, characterize the tumour cells, and are often useful to discriminate them from the minigemistocytes found in oligodendroglioma. The gemistocytic neoplastic astrocytes consistently express GFAP in their perikarya and cell processes. Expression of p53 protein and bcl-2 is frequently seen in gemistocytes {1586, 2373}. Nuclei are usually eccentric, with distinct nucleoli and densely clumped chromatin. Perivascular lymphocyte cuffing is frequent {261}. Electron microscopy confirms the presence of abundant, compact glial filaments in the cytoplasm and in cell processes.

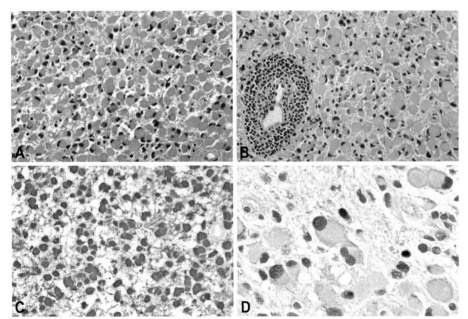

Fig. 1.19 Gemistocytic astrocytoma. **A** Tumour cells have a large eosinophilic cytoplasm with nuclei displaced to the periphery. **B** Characteristic feature of perivascular lymphocytic infiltrate. **C** Strong, consistent GFAP expression. **D** p53 accumulation is marked in nuclei of small and gemistocytic tumour cells.

Proliferation. The growth fraction, as determined by the Ki-67/MIB-1 labelling index, is usually less than 4%. The gemistocytic neoplastic astrocytes show a significantly lower rate of proliferation than the intermingled small-cell component {871, 1200, 1208, 1645, 2373, 2459}. However, microdissection discloses identical *TP53* mutations in both gemistocytes and non-gemistocytic tumour cells {1855}. Although the gemistocytic variant appears to be particularly prone to progress to anaplastic astrocytoma and glioblastoma {1208, 1959, 2023}, this does not justify a general classification as anaplastic astrocytoma {257, 2023}.

Protoplasmic astrocytoma

This rare variant is predominantly composed of neoplastic astrocytes showing a small cell body with a few flaccid processes with a low content of glial filaments and scant GFAP expression. Cellularity is low and mitotic activity absent. Mucoid degeneration and microcyst formation are common and characteristic features.
Nuclei are uniformly round to oval. GFAP immunostaining is variable and generally low. A clinico-pathological study indicates that protoplasmic astrocytoma is preferentially located in the fronto-temporal region {1796}. The mean size of the growth fraction as determined by the

MIB-1 labelling index was <1% {1797}. Immunohistochemical expression of p53, cyclooxygenase-2 and bcl-2 is limited to only a minority of tumours {1791,1797}. A FISH analysis indicated no allelic loss on chromosome 1p {1791}. This lesion is not well defined and is considered by some authors as an occasional histopathological feature rather than a reproducibly identifiable variant. When occurring in children, this neoplasm may be difficult to distinguish from pilocytic and pilomyxoid astrocytoma {1796,1959}.

Genetic susceptibility

Diffuse astrocytoma may occur in patients with inherited *TP53* germline mutations/ Li-Fraumeni syndrome (see Chapter 13) although affected family members more frequently develop anaplastic astrocytoma and glioblastoma. More recently, low-grade astrocytoma has been diagnosed in patients with inherited multiple enchondromatosis type 1 (Ollier disease; MIM No. 225795) which also predisposes to chondrosarcoma {605, 854}.

Genetics

TP53. A genetic hallmark of low-grade diffuse astrocytomas is frequent *TP53* mutation (>60%) {1634, 1851, 2371}. The frequency of *TP53* mutations does not significantly increase during malignant progression of low-grade astrocytomas

to secondary glioblastomas, indicating that this genetic change is an early event {2098, 2333, 2371, 2372}. In particular, in the gemistocytic variant, >80% of cases contain a *TP53* mutation {1634, 2370}.
PDGFR. Increased mRNA expression of the platelet-derived growth factor receptor α has been observed in astrocytic tumours of all stages, but gene amplification was only detected in a small subset of glioblastomas {814}.
Other genetic changes. Comparative genomic hybridization (CGH) analyses showed a gain of chromosome 7q and amplification of 8q as the most frequent genomic imbalance {1600, 2037}. The presence of LOH on 22q has been reported at a frequency of 17% {884} and chromosome 6 deletions in 14% of cases {1495}. LOH on 22q was found at one or more loci in 27–33% of grade II diffuse astrocytomas {776, 1558}. CGH after microdissecting small regions of tumours from paraffin sections and amplifying extracted DNA using degenerate oligo-nucleotide-primed polymerase chain reaction (DOP-PCR) in 30 grade II astrocytomas revealed that the most frequent copy number aberrations were gains on 7q, 5p, 9 and 19p, and losses on 19q, 1p and Xp {836}.
Promoter methylation. Approximately one third of low-grade astrocytomas show *p14^{ARF}* promoter methylation {1562}. *MGMT* promoter methylation was detected in approximately 50% of low-grade diffuse astrocytomas, and this was significantly associated with *TP53* mutations, in particular G:C->A:T transitions at CpG sites {1563}.
Gene expression profile. Gene expression patterns of low-grade diffuse astrocytoma are significantly different from those of normal brain tissues {879,880}, pilocytic astrocytoma {880}, oligodendroglioma {882} and glioblastoma {702}.

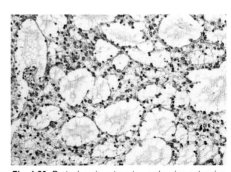

Fig. 1.20 Protoplasmic astrocytoma showing extensive mucoid degeneration.

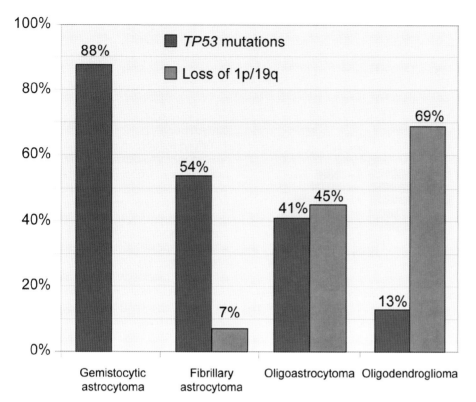

Fig. 1.21 *TP53* mutations are the genetic hallmark of low-grade astrocytomas in particular gemistocytic astrocytomas, whereas loss of 1p and 19q are frequent in oligodendrogliomas. Oligoastrocytomas commonly show either *TP53* mutations or loss of 1p/19q, with these changes being largely mutually exclusive. Modified from Okamoto *et al.* {1634}.

Prognostic and predictive factors

The mean survival time after surgical intervention is in the range of 6-8 years, with marked individual variation. The total length of disease is mainly influenced by the dynamics of malignant progression to glioblastoma, which tends to occur after a mean time interval of 4-5 years {1625, 2324, 2371}. Even in the presence of a *TP53* mutation in the first biopsy, long-term survival is possible in the absence of additional genetic alterations, e.g. LOH on 10 and 19q {1627}. Despite numerous correlative studies, there is currently no validated factor that unambiguously predicts in individual patients whether and how soon malignant progression to anaplastic astrocytoma and glioblastoma is likely to occur.

Clinical prognostic factors. Young age at diagnosis has been consistently predictive of a more favourable clinical course of patients with low-grade astrocytoma {1634, 2060}, while large tumour size appears to be a negative predictor {1046}. Gross total resection is significantly associated with longer survival {934, 1712, 2310}. Patients with low-grade astrocytoma who present with epilepsy as the single symptom appear to have a more favourable prognosis {2310}. Conversely, presentation with a neurological deficit is associated with worse prognosis than presentation with seizures or pressure symptoms alone {413}.

Proliferation. Analysis of a wide range of astrocytic tumours showed a gross correlation of proliferation with clinical outcome {870,1783}. A MIB-1/Ki-67 labelling index of >5% was found to constitute a threshold value for predicting shorter survival {974}.

Histopathological factors. Diffuse astrocytoma WHO grade II with a significant fraction of gemistocytes tend to undergo malignant progression more rapidly than the ordinary fibrillary astrocytoma {1208, 1634, 1712, 1713}, despite the fact that the majority of neoplastic gemistocytes are in a non-proliferative state (G0 phase of the cell cycle), suggestive of terminal differentiation {2373}. Some studies indicate that perivascular lymphocyte cuffing carries a somewhat more favourable prognosis {228,1670}, while others failed to note a correlation with patient survival {262, 928}. The presence of numerous microcysts appears to be associated with a somewhat better prognosis {2023}.

Genetic alterations. The presence of *TP53* mutations in low-grade astrocytoma has not been shown to be a predictor of clinical outcome {1634, 1713}, although some studies have found a shorter time interval before progression in patients with low-grade astrocytoma carrying a *TP53* mutation {2139, 2371}.

Anaplastic astrocytoma

P. Kleihues
P.C. Burger
M.K. Rosenblum
W. Paulus
B.W. Scheithauer

Definition

A diffusely infiltrating, malignant astrocytoma that primarily affects adults, preferentially located in the cerebral hemispheres, and that is histologically characterized by nuclear atypia, increased cellularity and significant proliferative activity. The tumour may arise from diffuse astrocytoma WHO grade II or *de novo*, i.e. without evidence of a less malignant precursor lesion, and has an inherent tendency to undergo progression to glioblastoma.

ICD-O code   9401/3

Grading

Anaplastic astrocytoma corresponds to WHO grade III {1120, 1121}.

Synonyms

These neoplasms are also referred to as 'malignant astrocytoma' and 'high-grade astrocytoma', but these terms are ambiguous as they are occasionally also applied to glioblastoma.

Age and sex distribution

Hospital-based data from the University of Zurich show a mean age of anaplastic astrocytoma at diagnosis of approximately 45 years, with a male/female ratio of 1.6:1. In a population-based study, the mean age at biopsy was 46 years, with male/female ratio of 1.1:1 {1625}, while population-based registry data from the USA {305} show a mean age at manifes-

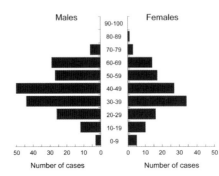

Fig. 1.22 Age distribution of anaplastic astrocytoma, based on biopsies of 319 patients treated at the University Hospital, Zurich.

tation of 51 years, with a male/female ratio of 1.31:1 {305}.

Localization

The localization of anaplastic astrocytoma corresponds to that of other diffuse infiltrating astrocytomas, with a preference for the cerebral hemispheres.

Clinical features

Symptoms and signs

Symptoms are similar to those of patients with diffuse astrocytoma WHO grade II. In some cases with a prior history of a diffuse grade II astrocytoma there are increasing neurological deficits, seizures and signs of intracranial pressure. Some patients have a shorter course, present without clinical evidence of a preceding astrocytoma WHO grade II.

Macroscopy

As diffuse astrocytoma WHO grade II, there is a tendency to infiltrate the surrounding brain without frank tissue destruction. This often leads to a marked enlargement of invaded structures, such as adjacent gyri and basal ganglia. Macroscopic cysts are uncommon, but frequently there are areas of granularity, opacity and soft consistency.

It is often difficult to grossly distinguish between anaplastic astrocytoma WHO grade III and a diffuse astrocytoma WHO grade II. On cut surface, the higher cellularity of the anaplastic astrocytoma produces a discernible tumour mass with a more clear distinction from surrounding structures than is the case in diffuse astrocytomas WHO grade II.

Histopathology

The principal histopathological features are those of a diffusely infiltrating astrocytoma with increased cellularity as compared to the grade II equivalent, distinct nuclear atypia and mitotic activity. Evaluation of the latter should be done in the context of sample size. In small specimens, such as are obtained at stereotactic biopsy, a single mitosis suggests significant proliferative activity. In such cases, Ki-67/MIB-1 immunohistochemistry may be helpful. In larger resection specimens, a single mitosis is not sufficient for WHO grade III designation {676}. Regional or diffuse hypercellularity is an important diagnostic criterion, but

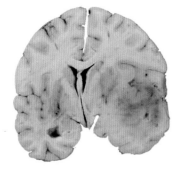

A

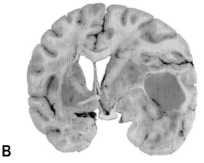

B

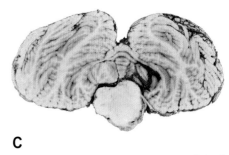

C

Fig. 1.23 Macroscopic appearance of anaplastic astrocytomas (**A**) in the right fronto-temporal region. Note the ill-defined borders with the adjacent brain structures. **B** Another lesion in a similar location contains a large cyst but no macroscopically discernible necrosis. **C** Anaplastic astrocytoma of the medulla with gross enlargement of local structures.

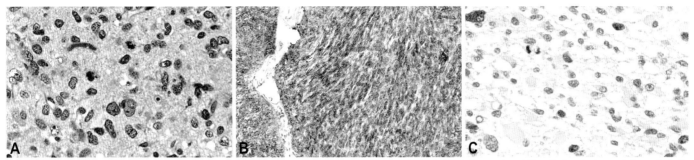

Fig. 1.24 Histological features of anaplastic astrocytoma. **A** Hypercellularity and hyperchromatic, irregular "naked nuclei" appearing within a fibrillary background. Several mitotic figures are evident. **B** GFAP immunoreactivity. **C** Several tumour cells show immunoreactivity for the proliferation marker MIB-1, including a cell in mitosis.

the diagnosis is still appropriate, even in the face of low cellularity if there is sufficient mitotic activity. With progressive anaplasia, nuclear morphology becomes more atypical, with increasing variations in nuclear size, shape, coarsening and dispersion of chromatin and increasing nucleolar prominence and number. Additional signs of anaplasia include multinucleated tumour cells and abnormal mitoses, but these are not required for grade III. By definition, microvascular proliferation (multilayered vessels) and necrosis are absent.

Proliferation

In contrast to diffuse astrocytoma WHO grade II, anaplastic astrocytoma displays mitotic activity. Growth fraction, as determined by the antibodies Ki-67/MIB-1, is usually in the range 5–10%, but may overlap with values for low-grade diffuse astrocytoma on one side and with glioblastoma on the other {376, 974, 1044, 1820}. Indices may vary considerably, even within a given tumour.

Genetics

From a clinical, morphologic and genetic point of view, anaplastic astrocytoma represents an intermediate stage on the route of progression to glioblastoma. It has a high frequency of *TP53* mutations and LOH 17p (50-60%), similar to that of diffuse astrocytoma (WHO grade II) {1620, 1634, 2332}. LOH 10q has been reported in 35-60% of anaplastic astro-cytomas {89,904}, and *PTEN* mutations in 18-23% of anaplastic astrocytomas {430, 2370}. LOH 22q occurs at a frequency similar to that of low-grade astrocytoma (20-30%) {776, 2332}, while LOH 19q is significantly more frequent (46%) than in low-grade diffuse astro-cytoma {2332}. LOH 6q occurs in approxi-mately one third of cases {1495}. *EGFR*

amplification is very uncommon in anaplastic astrocytoma (<10% of cases).

Histogenesis

Anaplastic astrocytomas are presumably derived from precursor cells committed to astrocytic differentiation. Their evolu-tion from diffuse astrocytoma WHO grade II and their progression to glioblastoma is morphologically well defined and is supported by molecular genetic findings. Less clear is whether all anaplastic astrocytomas develop from diffuse astrocytoma WHO grade II, since some cases present clinically *de novo*, without an identifiable precursor lesion. The pattern of genetic changes, in particular the high frequency (>70%) of *TP53* mutations {2371} would be compat-ible with the assumption that such tumours progressed rapidly from diffuse astrocytoma WHO grade II.

Prognostic and predictive factors

Anaplastic astrocytoma has a strong tendency to progress to glioblastoma. The pace of progression is variable, but population-based studies suggest a mean time interval of approximately 2 years {1620}. As in low-grade diffuse

astrocytoma and glioblastoma, increa-sing age is a negative prognostic factor. One study suggests that the survival of patients with *EGFR*-amplified anaplastic astrocytoma is significantly shorter {975}.

Glioneuronal tumour with neuropil-like islands

Rare infiltrating astrocytomas, usually WHO grade II or III, have focal, sharply delimited, round oval islands composed of a delicate, neuropil-like matrix with granular immunolabelling for synaptophysin. Save for one example situated in the cervico-thoracic spinal cord {770}, cases have arisen in the cerebrum (8 frontal, 1 bifrontal/callosal, 2 frontotemporal, 1 temporal, 3 parietal). The islands are rimmed in rosetted fashion, inhabited at highly variable density or traversed in streaming array by oligodendrocyte-like cells as well as larger, atypical forms showing at least focal nuclear reactivity for the neuron-associated NeuN or Hu antigens. Mature-appearing neurons of interme-diate or large size only exceptionally adjoin these loci, which are randomly distributed among the glial cells freely permeating the neuroparenchyma. The latter, often showing a high level of

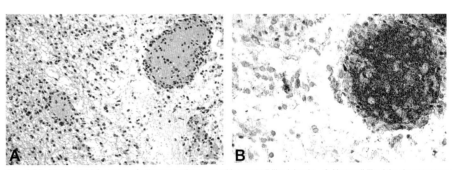

Fig. 1.25 Histological features of glioneuronal tumour with neuropil-like islands. **A** Neuropil-like islands appear as micronodules bordered or inhabited by oligodendrocyte-like cells and larger, more atypical cellular elements. These structures are surrounded by predominantly astroglial components of fibrillary or gemistocytic types. **B** Neuropil-like islands exhibit granular matrix immunoreactivity for synaptophysin.

atypia, consist mainly of GFAP-positive, fibrillary and gemistocytic elements identical to those populating conventional astrocytomas, but can include small numbers of GFAP/NeuN/ Hu-negative cells resembling oligodendrocytes. When present, mitotic activity is typically associated with the infiltrating glial components and may be conspicuous. The same can be said of complex microvascular proliferation and rarely necrosis. These anaplastic features may emerge on tumour recurrence. Aberrant nuclear immunoexpression of p53 is not uncommon and tends to be especially widespread among glial elements.

MIB-1/Ki-67 labelling activity, with occasional exceptions {1094}, is highest in regions of glial differentiation, generally modest (<4-5%) in examples of low histologic grade, and may be conspicuously elevated in tumours exhibiting features of anaplasia. Dramatically increased MIB-1/Ki-67 indices may also be encountered in recurrences {1792}.

CGH assessment of one example {1094} revealed 7q21.1-qter gain and 9p21-pter loss, non-specific abnormalities observed in some diffuse astrocytomas. PCR-based loss of heterozygosity assessment of 8 cases for chromosome 1p/19q deletions revealed intact 1p/19q status in 7, with 1 example exhibiting small interstitial deletions at 1p36 and 19q13 {99}, findings that distance these tumours from oligodendrogliomas (including variants with neurocytic rosettes). Losses of 1p and 22q have been observed in a rosette-forming glioneuronal tumour of the paediatric spinal cord {1874}; the relationship of this lesion to glioneuronal tumour with neuropil-like islands is unclear. Glioneuronal tumours with neuropil-like islands seem to behave in a manner comparable to neoplasms of diffuse astrocytic type when matched for WHO grade of their glial components.

Glioblastoma

P. Kleihues
P.C. Burger
K.D. Aldape
D.J. Brat
W. Biernat
D.D. Bigner

Y. Nakazato
K.H. Plate
F. Giangaspero
A. von Deimling
H. Ohgaki
W.K. Cavenee

Definition

The most frequent primary brain tumour and the most malignant neoplasm with predominant astrocytic differentiation; histopathological features include nuclear atypia, cellular pleomorphism, mitotic activity, vascular thrombosis, microvascular proliferation and necrosis. It typically affects adults and is preferentially located in the cerebral hemispheres. Most glioblastomas manifest rapidly *de novo*, without recognizable precursor lesions (primary glioblastoma). Secondary glioblastomas develop slowly from diffuse astrocytoma WHO grade II or anaplastic astrocytoma (WHO grade III). Due to their invasive nature, glioblastomas cannot be completely resected and despite progress in radio/chemotherapy, less than half of patients survive more than a year, with older age as the most significant adverse prognostic factor.

ICD-O code   9440/3

Grading

Glioblastoma and its variants correspond to WHO grade IV.

Synonyms and historical annotation

The term glioblastoma is used synonymously with "glioblastoma multiforme". Scherer {2013} and Kernohan {1093} were instrumental in developing the concept that glioblastoma is a malignant astrocytoma that sometimes develops by progression from a lower grade lesion.

Incidence

Glioblastoma is the most frequent brain tumour, accounting for approximately 12–15% of all intracranial neoplasms and 60-75% of astrocytic tumours {1260, 1625}. In most European and North American countries, the incidence is in the range of 3-4 new cases per 100 000 population per year {1260}. The incidence rate of glioblastoma in the USA, adjusted to the US Standard Population, is 2.96 new cases per 100 000 population per year {305}. The corresponding rate in a population-based study in Switzerland was 3.55 new cases, adjusted to the European Standard Population {1625}.

Age and sex distribution

Glioblastoma may manifest at any age, but preferentially affects adults, with a peak incidence at between 45 and 75 years of age. In a population-based study in the Canton of Zurich, Switzerland, the mean age of patients with glioblastoma was 61.3 years: more than 80% of patients were older than 50 years {1620}, whereas only 7 out of 715 cases (1%) were diagnosed in patients younger than 20 years old. The male:female ratio of glioblastoma patients is 1.26 in USA and 1.28 in Switzerland {1624}.

Localization

Glioblastoma occurs most often in the subcortical white matter of the cerebral hemispheres. In a series of 987 glioblastomas from the University Hospital

Zurich, the most frequently affected sites were the temporal (31%), parietal (24%), frontal (23%) and occipital lobes (16%). Combined fronto-temporal location is particularly typical. Tumour infiltration often extends into the adjacent cortex and through the corpus callosum into the contralateral hemisphere. Glioblastoma of the basal ganglia and thalamus is not uncommon, especially in children. Intraventricular glioblastoma is exceptional {1281}. Glioblastoma of the brain stem ('malignant brain stem glioma') is infrequent and often affects children {478}. Cerebellum and spinal cord are rare sites for this neoplasm.

Clinical features

The clinical history of the disease is usually short (less than 3 months in more than 50% of cases), unless the neoplasm has developed from a lower grade astrocytoma (secondary glioblastoma). Symptoms and signs of raised intracranial pressure (for example headache, nausea/vomiting with papilledema) are common. Up to one third of patients will experience an epileptic seizure. Non-specific neurological symptoms such as headache and personality changes can also occur.

Macroscopy

Despite the short duration of symptoms in many cases of glioblastoma, the tumours are often surprisingly large at the time of presentation, and may occupy much of a lobe. The lesion is usually unilateral, but those in the brain stem and corpus callosum can be bilaterally symmetrical. Supratentorial bilateral extension is due to rapid growth along myelinated structures, in particular across the corpus callosum and along the fornices toward the temporal lobes.

Glioblastomas are poorly delineated, the cut surface showing a variable colour with peripheral greyish tumour masses and central areas of yellowish necrosis from myelin breakdown. The peripheral hypercellular zone appears macroscopically as a soft, grey rim or a grey band of tumour tissue. However, necrotic tissue

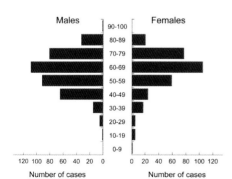

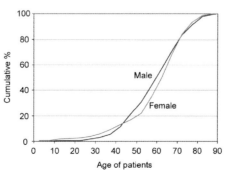

Fig. 1.26 Age and sex distribution of glioblastoma, based on 715 cases from a population-based study, Canton of Zurich, Switzerland.

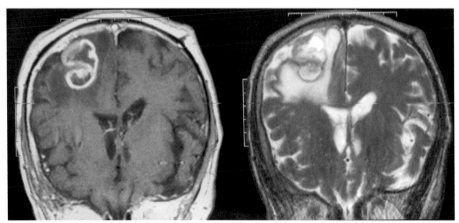

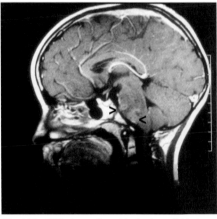

Fig. 1.27 Glioblastoma. **A** T1-weighted MRI with marked gadolinium-enhancement, indicating neovascularization and vascular permeability. **B** T2-weighted MRI reveals extensive perifocal edema.

Fig. 1.28 MRI of a malignant brain stem glioblastoma in a 6 year-old child. Arrows indicate foci of necrosis.

may also border adjacent brain structures without an intermediate zone of macroscopically detectable tumour tissue. The central necrosis may occupy as much as 80% of the total tumour mass. Glioblastomas are typically stippled with red and brown foci of recent and remote haemorrhages. Extensive haemorrhages may occur and evoke stroke-like symptoms, which are sometimes the first clinical sign of the tumour.

Macroscopic cysts, when present, contain a turbid fluid and represent liquefied necrotic tumour tissue, quite in contrast to the well-delineated retention cysts in diffuse astrocytomas WHO grade II.

Most glioblastomas of the cerebral hemispheres are clearly intraparenchymal with an epicentre in the white matter. Infrequently, they are largely superficial and in contact with the leptomeninges and dura and may be interpreted by the neuroradiologist or surgeon as metastatic carcinoma, or as an extra-axial lesion such as meningioma. Cortical infiltration may produce a preserved gyriform rim of thickened grey cortex overlying a necrotic zone in the white matter.

Spread and metastasis

Although infiltrative spread is a common feature of all diffuse astrocytic tumours, glioblastoma is particularly notorious for its rapid invasion of neighbouring brain structures {253}. A very common feature is extension of the tumour through the corpus callosum into the contralateral hemisphere, creating the image of a bilateral, symmetrical lesion ('butterfly glioma'). Similarly, rapid spread is observed in the internal capsule, fornix, anterior commissure and optic radiation.

These structures may become enlarged and distorted but continue to serve as a 'highway', allowing the formation of new tumour masses at their opposite projection site, thus leading to the neuroradiological image of a multifocal glioblastoma. Invading cells reside outside the contrast-enhancing rim of the tumour, thereby escaping surgical resection and evading high doses of radiation during radiotherapy. This likely represents the source for local recurrence usually seen after such therapy.

Despite its rapid, infiltrative growth, glioblastoma tends not to invade the subarachnoidal space, and consequently rarely metastasizes via the cerebrospinal fluid {688}. Extension within and along perivascular spaces is another typical mode of infiltration, but invasion of the vessel lumen seems to occur infrequently {142, 242}. Haematogeneous spread to extraneural tissues is very rare in patients without previous surgical intervention {1687, 1688}. Peritoneal metastasis via ventriculoperitoneal shunt has been observed {558}. Penetration of the dura, venous sinus and bone is exceptional {1708, 1776, 2095}.

Mechanisms of invasion

A number of molecular mediators of invasion in glioblastoma have been described, including activation of the TGF-ß and AKT pathways {1177, 2406}. Tumour hypoxia may also promote invasion through the activation of HIF-1α {1068}. An important aspect of glioblastoma invasion is the elaboration of a migration-enhancing extracellular matrix by tumour cells {1142}, as well as secretion of proteolytic enzymes which

permit invasion through this matrix. Consistent with this notion are recent gene expression profiling studies that identify a subset of tumours with elevated expression of extracellular matrix components as well as intracellular proteins associated with cell motility {608, 1742}. The interplay between the variety of matrix and growth factor receptors as well as activation of signalling pathways which facilitate tumour cell invasion is being recognized as a composite, dynamic consequence of altered cell-cell adhesion, proteolytic remodelling and synthesis of ECM, as well as selective expression and activation of integrins {136}. Activation of migration (seen at the leading edge of the neoplasm) appears to be associated with a decrease in proliferation rate {681}, which may have therapeutic consequences {2136}.

Multifocal glioblastomas

Although multifocality is not unusual when defined radiologically, the incidence of truly multiple, independent gliomas occurring outside the setting of inherited neoplastic syndromes is unclear. Even careful post-mortem studies on whole brain sections may not always reveal a connection between apparently multifocal gliomas, as the cells infiltrating along myelinated pathways are often small, polar and largely undifferentiated. In a careful histological analysis, Batzdorf & Malamud {114} concluded that 2.4% of glioblastomas are truly multiple independent tumours, a value similar to that reported by Russell & Rubinstein (2.3%) {1959}. In a post-mortem study, Barnard & Geddes {102} found that 7.5% of gliomas (including oligodendrogliomas) are multiple independent tumours and that in approximately 3% of these, tumour foci vary in their histological appearance. True multifocal glioblastomas are most likely polyclonal if they occur infra- and supratentorially, i.e. outside easily accessible routes like the cerebrospinal fluid pathways or the median commissures {1977}. Multiple independently arising gliomas would, by definition, be of polyclonal origin and their existence can only be proven by application of molecular markers which, in informative cases, allow a distinction between tumours of common or independent origin {141, 157, 1184}.

Primary and secondary glioblastoma

The terms primary and secondary glioblastoma were first used by Scherer in 1940 who noted: "From a biological and clinical point of view, the secondary glioblastomas developing in astrocy- tomas must be distinguished from 'primary' glioblastomas; they are probably responsible for most of the glioblastomas of long clinical duration" {2013}. The majority of glioblastomas (>90%) develop very rapidly with a short clinical history (usually <3 months), without clinical or histopathological evidence of a pre- existing, less malignant precursor lesion (primary or *de novo* glioblastoma). They typically develop in older patients (mean,

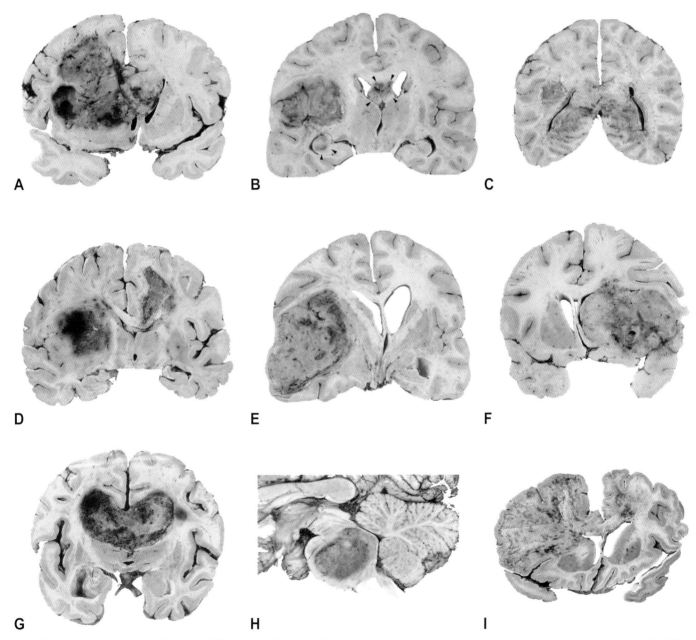

Fig. 1.29 Macroscopic features of glioblastoma (GBM). **A** Large GBM in the left frontal lobe extending into the corpus callosum and the contralateral white matter. **B,C** GBM of the left fronto-temporal region with invasion of the fornices, spread to the lower horn of the left ventricle and (**C**) extension to the corpus callosum and adjacent parieto-occipital structures. **D** GBM of the left basal ganglia and spread into the right hemisphere with formation of a cystic necrosis. **E** GBM of the left hemisphere with extensive necrosis occupying most of the tumour mass. **F** Right fronto-temporal GBM with mass shifting and subfalcial herniation. **G** GBM with unusual intraventricular location. **H** Malignant brain stem GBM in a child. **I** GBM of the left hemisphere with extensive necrosis and spread to the right frontal lobe via the corpus callosum.

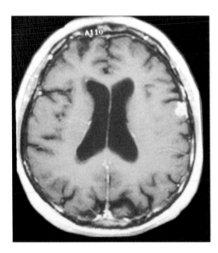
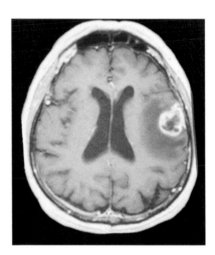

Small cortical lesion ➡ **Primary glioblastoma**

68 days

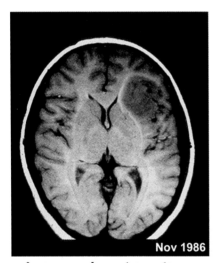

Nov 1986

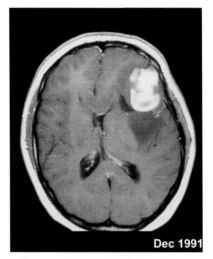

Dec 1991

**Low-grade astrocytoma
(WHO grade II)** ➡ **Secondary glioblastoma
(WHO grade IV)**

5 years

Fig. 1.30 Rapid evolution of a primary glioblastoma in a 79 year-old patient (upper). MRI shows a small cortical lesion that within 68 days developed into a full-blown glioblastoma with perifocal edema and central necrosis. This is in contrast to the development of secondary glioblastoma through progression from low-grade astrocytoma (lower).

62 years) {1620, 1625A}. Neuroimages of the dynamic growth of a primary glioblastoma and a secondary glioblastoma are shown in Fig. 1.30. Glioblastoma may also develop through progression from diffuse astrocytoma (WHO grade II) or anaplastic astrocytoma (WHO grade III); and these are termed "secondary glioblastomas". They are much less frequent than primary glioblastomas (<10% of all glioblastomas) {486, 1620, 1625A}, and typically develop in younger patients (mean, 45 years). The time to progression from diffuse astrocytoma WHO grade II to glio-

blastoma varies considerably, with time intervals ranging from less than 1 year to >10 years {1627}, the mean interval being 4–5 years {1625, 2371}. Survival of patients with secondary glioblastoma is significantly longer (median survival time, 7.8 months) than for those with primary glioblastoma (4.7 months), but this is likely to be the reflection of younger age of secondary glioblastoma patients {1620, 1625}. Primary and secondary glioblastoma constitute relatively distinct disease entities that evolve primarily through different genetic pathways, show different expression

profiles {1625}, and are likely to differ in response to therapy, but share a high frequency of LOH 10q, which is likely to be associated with the overall glioblastoma phenotype {620, 622, 1620, 1625A}.

Histopathology

Glioblastoma is an anaplastic, cellular glioma composed of poorly differentiated, often pleomorphic astrocytic tumour cells with marked nuclear atypia and brisk mitotic activity. Prominent microvascular proliferation and/or necrosis are essential diagnostic features.

As the term glioblastoma "multiforme" suggests, the histopathology of this tumour is extremely variable. While some lesions show a high degree of cellular and nuclear polymorphism with numerous multinucleated giant cells, others are highly cellular, but rather monotonous. The astrocytic nature of the neoplasms may be easily identifiable, at least focally, in some tumours, but difficult to recognize in others owing to the high degree of anaplasia. The regional heterogeneity of glioblastoma is remarkable and poses challenges to histopathological diagnosis on specimens obtained by stereotaxic needle biopsies {254}.

Tissue patterns

The diagnosis of glioblastoma is typically based on the tissue pattern rather than on the identification of certain cell types. The presence of highly anaplastic glial cells, mitotic activity and vascular proliferation and/or necrosis is required. The distribution of these key elements within the tumour is variable, but large necrotic areas usually occupy the tumour centre, while viable tumour cells tend to accumulate in the periphery. The circumferential region of high cellularity and abnormal vessels corresponds to the contrast-enhancing ring seen radiologically. Vascular proliferation is seen throughout the lesion, often around necrotic foci and in the peripheral zone of infiltration.

Secondary structures

The migratory capacity of glioblastoma cells within the CNS becomes readily apparent when they reach borders that constitute a barrier: tumour cells line up and accumulate in the subpial zone of the cortex, in the subependymal region, around neurons ("satellitosis"), and about vessels. Such patterns, known as "secondary structures" {2014}, result from the interaction of glioma cells with host brain structures, and are highly diagnostic. Secondary structures may be noted in other highly infiltrative gliomas such as gliomatosis cerebri and oligodendroglioma {2012, 2014}. This concept also extends to the adaptation of tumour cells to myelinated pathways, where the former often acquire a fusiform, polar shape. Identifying neoplastic astrocytes in the perifocal zone of edema and at more distant sites poses a challenge for the pathologist, in particular when dealing with stereotaxic biopsies {423}. A feature of many glioblastomas, especially the small cell variants, is the extensive involvement of the cerebral cortex. Secondary structures and most of the apparently multifocal glioblastomas reflect the pathways of migration of glioma cells in the CNS {1268}. The subependymal region may also be diffusely infiltrated, especially in the terminal stages of disease.

Epithelial structures

Occasionally, glioblastoma contains foci with glandular and ribbon-like epithelial structures {1932}. These elements have a large oval nucleus, prominent nucleolus and round, well-defined cytoplasms. They are also referred to as "adenoid" glioblastoma. Expression of GFAP in these areas may be reduced, but the astrocytic nature of these structures can usually be established unequivocally. Small cells with even more epithelial features and cohesiveness are less

common {1084}. A mucinous background and a 'mesenchymal' component (gliosarcoma) are not uncommon in such neoplasms.

Cellular composition

Few human neoplasms are as heterogeneous in composition as is glioblastoma. While poorly differentiated, fusiform, round or pleomorphic cells may prevail, more differentiated neoplastic astrocytes are usually discernible, at least focally {254}. This is particularly true of glioblastoma resulting from the progression of diffuse astrocytoma WHO grade II. The transition between areas that still have recognizable astrocytic differentiation and highly anaplastic cells may be either continuous or abrupt. A sudden change in morphology may reflect the emergence of a new tumour through the acquisition of one or more additional genetic alterations {620}.

Cellular pleomorphism includes the formation of small, undifferentiated, lipidized, granular and giant cells. In addition, there are often areas where bipolar, fusiform cells form intersecting bundles and fascicles prevail. The accumulation of highly polymorphic tumour cells with well-delineated plasma membranes and a lack of cell processes may mimic metastatic carcinoma or melanoma.

Small cell glioblastoma. Although small cells are common in glioblastoma, they are predominant or exclusive in a subset known as "small cell glioblastoma" {1720}. These tumours feature a highly mono-

morphic cell population characterized by small, round to slightly elongated, densely packed cells with mildly hyperchromatic nuclei, high nuclear: cytoplasmic ratio and modest atypia. GFAP immunoreactivity may be minimal. The tumours must be distinguished from poorly differentiated anaplastic oligodendrogliomas. Small cell glioblastoma has high proliferative activity.

Glioblastoma with oligodendroglioma component. Occasional glioblastomas contain foci that resemble oligodendroglioma. These areas are variable in size and frequency. Two large studies of malignant gliomas suggest that necrosis is associated with significantly worse prognosis in the setting of anaplastic gliomas with both oligodendroglial and astrocytic components {1474, 2301}: patients whose tumours had necrosis had a substantially shorter median overall survival compared to patients whose tumours did not (see Anaplastic oligoastrocytoma in Chapter 2). Such tumours should be classified as "glioblastoma with oligodendroglial component", although they may have a better prognosis than standard glioblastoma {799, 857, 1185}.

Multinucleated giant cells

Large, multinucleated tumour cells are often considered a hallmark of glioblastomas and occur with a spectrum of increasing size and pleomorphism. While typical, the presence of multinucleated giant cells is neither an obligatory feature nor associated with a more malignant

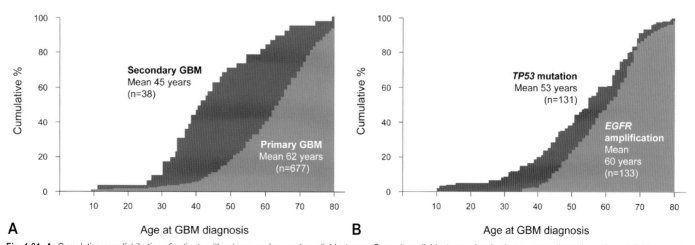

Fig. 1.31 A Cumulative age distribution of patients with primary and secondary glioblastomas. Secondary glioblastomas develop in younger patients than primary glioblastomas. **B** Cumulative age distribution of patients with glioblastoma with *TP53* mutations and those with *EGFR* amplification. *TP53* mutations are present in glioblastoma in all of the age groups of patients, whereas no glioblastoma in patients less than 35 years shows *EGFR* amplification. Modified from Ohgaki *et al.* {1620}.

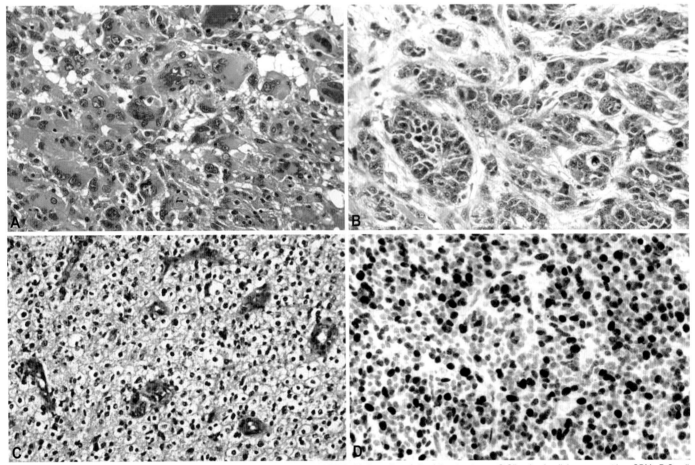

Fig. 1.32 Glioblastoma. **A** Glioblastoma with high degree of anaplasia. **B** Adenoid GBM with formation of glandular structures. **C** Oligodendroglial component in a GBM. **D** Small cell glioblastoma with very high MIB-1 labelling index.

clinical course {252}. Despite their malignant appearance, these cells are regarded as a type of regressive change. If multinucleated giant cells dominate the histopathological picture, the designation 'giant cell glioblastoma' is justified.

Gemistocytes

At the other extreme of glioblastoma differentiation are "gemistocytes" and the related "fibrillary astrocyte", recognizing that transition forms connect these two types. Gemistocytes have copious, glassy, non-fibrillary cytoplasm that appears to displace the dark, angulated nucleus to the periphery of the cell. Processes radiate from the cytoplasm, but are stubby and not long-reaching. GFAP staining is largely confined to the periphery of the cell, with the central hyaline organelle-rich zone remaining largely unstained. Perivascular lymphocytes frequently populate gemistocytic regions while often avoiding other

regions in the same neoplasm. When present in large numbers, particularly in a patient known to have a pre-existing glioma, these cells may represent a lower-grade precursor lesion within a secondary glioblastoma. Better-differentiated areas can sometimes be identified radiologically as a non-contrast-enhancing peripheral region and, in whole brain sections, as grade II to III astrocytomas clearly distinct from foci of glioblastoma {254, 2012}. Immunohistochemical studies have emphasized the low proliferation index of the neoplastic gemistocyte itself, despite the tendency of gemistocytic astrocytoma WHO grade II or III lesions to rapidly progress to glioblastoma {2373}. The proliferating component appears to be a population of cells with larger hyperchromatic nuclei and scant cytoplasm {2373}.

Granular cells

Large cells with a granular, periodic acid-Schiff (PAS) positive cytoplasm may

occur scattered within glioblastoma. In rare cases, they may dominate and create the impression of a granular cell tumour similar to that of the pituitary stalk or other tissues {457, 771}, where they are thought to be myogenic or Schwann-cell-derived (see Chapter 14). In the cerebral hemispheres transitional forms between granular cells and neoplastic astrocytes can be identified in some cases, but in others it is difficult to identify any conventional astrocytoma component. Although larger and more coarsely granular, the tumour cells also resemble macrophages. Given their lysosomal content the tumour cells may be immunoreactive for macrophage markers such as CD68. Occasional cells may have peripheral immunopositivity for GFAP, but most cells are negative {219, 655}. On the basis of both these findings it is most likely that the granular cells represent glioma cells with a distinct degenerative pathway.

Lipidized cells

Cells with a foamy cytoplasm are another feature occasionally observed in glioblastoma. In rare cases, they predominate, and the respective lesion has been designated 'malignant glioma with heavily lipidized (foamy) tumour cells' {1080, 1087, 1932, 2208}. The lipidized cells may be grossly enlarged {664}. If such lesions are superficially located in young people, the diagnosis of pleomorphic xanthoastrocytoma should be considered, particularly if the xanthomatous cells are surrounded by basement membranes positive on reticulin staining {1081}. Other lipid-rich lesions have epithelioid cytological features {1932}.

Perivascular lymphocytes

Perivascular lymphocyte cuffing occurs in a minority of glioblastomas, most typically in areas with a homogeneous gemistocytic component. The inflammatory cells have been phenotypically characterized on the basis of their immunoreactivity. CD8+ T-lymphocytes, which are MHC-class-I-restricted, prevail and occur in approximately 75% of tumours. CD4+ lymphocytes appear to be present in smaller numbers {185, 1937} while B-lymphocytes are detectable in less then 10% of cases {1937}. Expression of CD44 and ICAM-1 is observed in glioma cells, but not in tumour-infiltrating lymphocytes {1229}. Whether perivascular lymphocyte infiltration influences tumour growth is still a matter of dispute: while some studies indicate a beneficial effect {228, 1670}, others failed to note a correlation with patient survival. The presence or absence of lymphocytes is not used in prognostication {262, 928}. In addition to haemotogeneous lymphocytes, there are perivascular cells that are supposedly resident in the CNS; they express MHC class II antigens and immunoreactivity to PGM1 antibody, and may have a scavenger role {1101}.

Metaplasia

In general, this term refers to the reversible acquisition by a differentiated cell of morphological features typical of another differentiated cell type, and is most frequently observed as a preneoplastic lesion of epithelial tissues. However, the term is also used to designate aberrant differentiation in neoplasms. In glioblastoma, this reflects a high degree of genomic instability and is exemplified by foci displaying features of squamous epithelial cells, i.e. epithelial whorls with keratin pearls and cytokeratin expression {257, 1526}. Adenoid and squamous epithelial metaplasia are more common in gliosarcoma than in the ordinary glioblastoma {1084, 1526}. This is similarly true for the formation of bone and cartilage, which prevails in gliosarcoma and in a variety of childhood CNS neoplasms {1412}.

Microvascular proliferation

In addition to necrosis, the presence of microvascular proliferation (previously called endothelial cell proliferation) is a histopathological hallmark of glioblastoma. On light microscopy, classic microvascular proliferations typically appear as 'glomeruloid tufts', which are most commonly located in the vicinity of necrosis and appear directionally oriented to it. Histologically, microvascular proliferation in glioblastoma typically consists of multilayered, mitotically active endothelial cells together with smooth muscle cells/pericytes {751, 1547, 2396}.

Morphologically inconspicuous vessels have a MIB-1 labelling index of 2–4%, while proliferated tumour vessels have an index of >10% {2369}. A less common form of vascular malformation with a claim to the term endothelial proliferation is an intraluminal proliferation of cells in small and medium-sized vessels. Vascular thrombosis often occurs, and this may play a role in the pathogenesis of ischaemic tumour necrosis {1917}.

Proliferation

Proliferative activity is usually prominent, with detectable mitoses in nearly every case. Atypical mitoses are frequently present. Mitotic activity, however, can vary widely between tumours and also shows regional heterogeneity within a tumour. The growth fraction, as determined by the antibodies Ki-67/MIB-1, shows great regional variation. Mean values of 15–20% have been reported {260, 448, 974, 1044, 2038}. Tumours with small, undifferentiated, fusiform cells often show marked proliferative activity, in contrast to tumours composed of neoplastic gemistocytes, which typically have a lesser degree of proliferation {2373}. Despite the wide range of proliferation indices observed in glioblastoma, an association between proliferation index and clinical outcome has not been demonstrated {1527}.

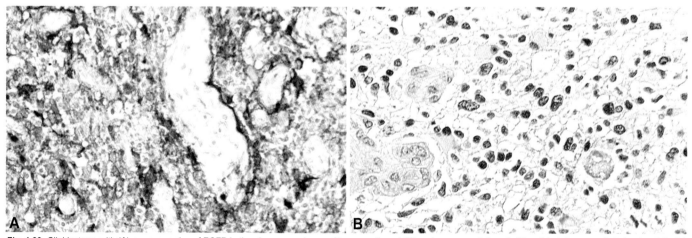

Fig. 1.33 Glioblastoma with (**A**) overexpression of EGFR in the plasma membrane of tumour cells and (**B**) nuclear accumulation of p53 protein in tumour cells but not endothelial cells.

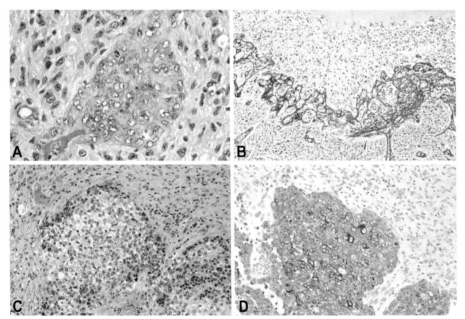

Fig. 1.34 **A** Microvascular proliferation in a glioblastoma with formation of a multilayered 'glomeruloid tuft'. **B** Reticulin stain showing a 'garland' of proliferated glioma vessels. **C** Focal squamous cell metaplasia in a glioblastoma characterized by (**D**) marked cytokeratin expression.

Angiogenesis

Glioblastomas are among the most vascularized tumours in humans. Glioblastoma vascularization occurs through several mechanisms including {583A} vessel co-option, e.g. adoption of pre-existing vessels by migrating tumour cells, {1371A} classical angiogenesis, e.g. sprouting of capillaries from pre-existing vessels by endothelial cell proliferation and migration and {10A} vasculogenesis, e.g. homing of bone marrow-derived cells that support vessel growth from the peripheral blood into the perivascular space {583A, 1371A}. Hypoxia is considered a major driving force of glioblastoma angiogenesis {10A} and leads to intracellular stabilization of the hypoxia master-regulator hypoxia-inducible factor 1-α (HIF-1α). HIF-1α accumulation leads to transcriptional activation of more than 100 hypoxia-regulated genes that control angiogenesis (VEGF, angiopoietin), cellular metabolism (carbonic anhydrase, lactate dehydrogenase), survival/apoptosis (BNIP) and migration (c-met, CXCR4). Vascular endothelial growth factor (VEGF) appears to be the most important mediator of glioma-associated vascular dysfunctions. VEGF is primarily produced by perinecrotic palisading cells as a consequence of cellular hypoxia. VEGF induces tumour angiogenesis, increases vascular permeability (edema) and regulates homing of bone marrow derived cells {10A}. In addition to endothelial cells, pericytes/smooth muscle cells and perivascular bone marrow derived cells participate in the vascular remodelling processes typically observed in glioblastoma.

These remodelling processes lead to microvascular proliferations that are a histopathological hallmark of glioblastoma.

Necrosis

Tumour necrosis is a fundamental feature of glioblastoma, and its presence is one of the strongest predictors of aggressive clinical behaviour in diffuse astrocytomas {252, 857, 1840}. Necrosis can be seen by neuroimaging as a non-enhancing core, which represents large areas of non-viable tumour tissue and may comprise more than 80% of the total tumour mass. These regions appear grossly as a yellow or white granular coagulum {250}. Microscopically, necrotic glioma cells can vaguely be identified, as well as the faded images of large, dilated necrotic tumour vessels. Areas of necrosis do not generally attract a large number of phagocytes. Occasionally, preserved tumour vessels with a corona of viable tumour cells are seen within extensive areas of necrosis. It is assumed that these large necroses are due to insufficient blood supply and are therefore ischaemic in nature.

A second form of necrosis that can be noted microscopically consists of multiple, small, irregularly-shaped band-like {2514} or serpiginous {257} foci, surrounded by radially oriented, densely packed, small, fusiform glioma cells in a 'pseudo-palisading' pattern, a histological hallmark of the glioblastoma {1261}. These pseudopalisading necroses are equally frequent in primary and secondary glioblastoma {2253}. The relationship of pseudopalisading necrosis to the larger regions of confluent necrosis has not been clearly defined, yet some have suggested that there is a temporal evolution. The central area of smaller pseudopalisading structures often consists of a fine fibrillary network without viable or necrotic glioma cells, whereas larger pseudopalisading structures always contain necrotic centres. Compared to adjacent tumour cells, pseudopalisading cells have higher rates of apoptosis and lower rates of proliferation {214}. They also are hypoxic and strongly express HIF-1α and its transcriptional target VEGF {2498}. Hypoxic upregulation of VEGF and other pro-angiogenic factors is considered to be responsible for the microvascular proliferation noted in glioblastoma {1760}. Many aspects of necrogenesis remain to be elucidated. It has been suggested that a sequence starting from small clusters of apoptotic cells leads to pseudopalisading necrosis and, eventually, large areas of ischaemic necrosis. Others have speculated that microscopic vaso-occlusion and thrombosis leads to hypoxia and hypoxia-induced cell migration to form pseudopalisading structures with central necrosis {1917}.

Apoptosis

Apoptosis, the programmed death of individual cells, is initiated through mechanisms that include death receptor (DR) ligation by members of the tumour necrosis factor (TNF) family, including TRAIL (TNF-related apoptosis-inducing ligand)/DR5 and FasL (CD95L)/Fas (CD95) {1660}. The higher levels of apoptosis seen in pseudopalisading cells may be due to increased expression or ligation of death receptors {214}. TRAIL induces apoptosis in glioblastoma by binding to DR5 and ultimately activating caspase-8 {767}. Both Fas and FasL levels are higher in astrocytomas than normal brain and correlate with tumour grade {2192, 2253}. Most Fas expression in glioblastoma is within pseudopalisading cells around necrosis and physical interactions between tumour cells expressing Fas and FasL may promote apoptosis. Compared to coagulative necrosis, the overall levels of cell death due to apoptosis are low in malignant gliomas, and apoptotic rates do not correlate with prognosis {1471, 2020}.

Histogenesis

The cellular origin of glioblastoma is a topic of considerable contemporary investigation and controversy. It has been thought for many years that the expression of markers of differentiated astrocytes by glioblastoma cells arose because of the de-differentiation of the cells after transformation. More recently, the cellular, biochemical and genetic heterogeneity that typify glioblastoma, together with the different clinical responses of histologically similar tumours has led to the notion that the tumours arise from the malignant transformation of either a bipotential precursor cell {2448} or an even more primordial cell, the neural stem cell {1422}. This idea has received considerable support because of the coincident anatomical position in the subventricular zone of the brain of dividing cells with stem-like properties and the development of glioblastoma. Moreover, cells with stem cell-like properties have been isolated from glioblastoma tumours and cell lines. These cells, termed brain tumour stem cells (BTSC), represent a small subpopulation but have the capacity of self-renewal as well as tumourigenic behaviour in animals. Thus, these BTSC may represent the descendants of a neural stem cell that was the target of a carcinogenic insult and that is seeding the tumour through its unlimited growth potential. While the accumulating data {1161, 1979, 2104, 2325} are consistent with this interpretation, direct proof remains to be found {1008A}.

Genetics

Malignant transformation of neuroepithelial cells is a multistep process driven by the sequential acquisition of genetic alterations. One would therefore expect that of all astrocytic neoplasms, glioblastoma should contain the greatest number of genetic changes, and this is indeed the case. On the basis of the different combinations of TP53 mutations, loss of heterozygosity (LOH) on chromo-

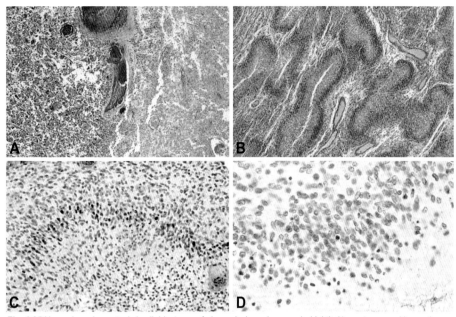

Fig. 1.35 Necrosis and apoptosis in glioblastoma. **A** Large ischaemic necrosis (right). Also note several large, thrombosed tumour vessels. **B** Multiple serpentine pseudopalisading necroses. **C** HIF-1α expression in perinecrotic palisading cells. **D** Apoptosis accumulating in pseudopalisading tumour cells (TUNEL).

somes 10 and 17p and EGFR amplification, the presence of subsets of glioblastomas with distinct genetic alterations {1257, 2341} has been correlated with clinical pathways to glioblastoma (see primary and secondary glioblastoma).

Epidermal growth factor receptor (EGFR)
The gene encoding EGFR, a cellular homologue of v-erbB {2284}, is located on chromosome 7. EGFR encodes a 170 kDa protein, which is a transmembrane receptor responsible for sensing its extracellular ligands, such as EGF and TGF-α, and for transducing this proliferation signal. EGFR is the most frequently amplified gene in glioblastoma {629}, and the amplified EGFR genes are typically present as double-minute extrachromosomal elements. EGFR amplification is associated with overexpression: all glioblastomas with EGFR amplification showed EGFR overexpression and 70–90% of those with EGFR overexpression showed EGFR amplification {158, 2252}. EGFR amplification occurs in approximately 40% of primary glioblastoma {513, 1620, 2435}, but rarely in secondary glioblastoma {1620, 2372}. In a population-based study, EGFR amplification was not detected in any glioblastoma from patients younger than 35 years {1620}. Amplification of the EGFR gene is often associated with structural alterations, and several major

truncated variants have been identified {1833}, the most common being variant III (EGFRvIII), also called de2-7EGFR or delta EGFR {2411}, which is present in 20-50% of glioblastomas with EGFR amplification {158, 2042, 2169}. EGFRvIII results from a non-random 801-bp in-frame deletion of exons 2-7 of the EGFR gene {607,2169}; it is structurally and functionally similar to v-erbB, and constitutively activated in a ligand-independent manner, leading to cell proliferation via the PI3-kinase, RAS and mitogen-activated protein kinase signalling pathways {351}. EGFRvIII is a promising target for therapy, since it is tumour-specific and occurs on the surface of glioblastoma cells with EGFR amplification {513, 1019, 2042}. EGFR point mutations are infrequent (3–5%) in glioblastomas of both European and Asian patients {624}.

PI3K/PTEN/AKT pathway
The EGFR, or other growth factor receptors, becomes activated upon binding of growth factors (EGF, TGF-α) and recruits PI3K (phosphatidylinositol 3-kinase) to the cell membrane. PI3K converts phosphatidynositol-4,5-bisphosphate (PIP2) to PIP3. PIP3 activates downstream effector molecules such as AKT and the mammalian target of rapamycin (mTOR), which results in cell proliferation and cell survival. The PTEN

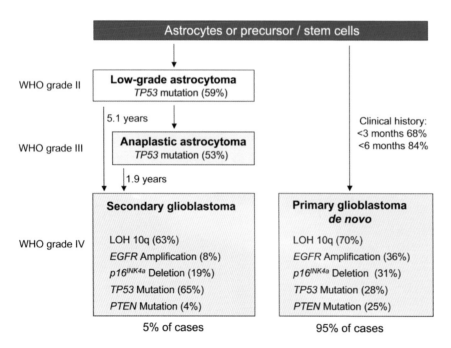

Astrocytes or precursor / stem cells

WHO grade II
Low-grade astrocytoma
TP53 mutation (59%)

5.1 years

WHO grade III
Anaplastic astrocytoma
TP53 mutation (53%)

1.9 years

Clinical history:
<3 months 68%
<6 months 84%

WHO grade IV

Secondary glioblastoma

LOH 10q (63%)

EGFR Amplification (8%)

p16^INK4a Deletion (19%)

TP53 Mutation (65%)

PTEN Mutation (4%)

5% of cases

**Primary glioblastoma
de novo**

LOH 10q (70%)

EGFR Amplification (36%)

p16^INK4a Deletion (31%)

TP53 Mutation (28%)

PTEN Mutation (25%)

95% of cases

Fig. 1.36 Timing and frequency of genetic alterations in the evolution of glioblastoma. Note that LOH 10q is frequent in both primary and secondary glioblastomas, and *TP53* mutations are early and frequent genetic alterations in the pathway leading to secondary glioblastoma. Modified from Ohgaki *et al.* {1620}.

(phosphatase and tensin homology) gene, located at 10q23.3 {1312, 2145}, encodes a protein with a central domain homologous to the catalytic region of protein tyrosine phosphatases, which is important in the function of protein phosphatase {1544, 2207} and 3'-phosphoinositol phosphatase activities {1377}. PTEN inhibits the PIP3 signal {1446}, thereby inhibiting cell proliferation. The amino terminal domain of PTEN is homologous to tensin and auxilin, which is important in regulating cell migration and invasion by directly dephosphorylating focal adhesion kinase (FAK) {2207}.
PTEN is mutated in 15-40% of cases {491,1139,2252}, and almost exclusively in primary glioblastoma {1620, 2252}. *PTEN* homozygous deletion may occur, but is rare in glioblastoma (<2%) {1140}. Of 78 *PTEN* mutations detected in glioblastoma, nonsense mutations (13%) and deletions or insertions leading to stop codons (32%) were equally distributed throughout the exons, whereas 33% were missense mutations leading to amino acid changes, preferentially located in exons 1-6, i.e. in the region homologous to tensin, auxilin and dual-specificity phosphatases {1620}. This suggests that cells with *PTEN* truncation at any site or *PTEN* missense mutations

in the region homologous to tensin/auxilin and dual-specificity phosphatases acquire a transformed phenotype.
The PIK3CA p110α catalytic subunit of PI3K is a 34kb gene located at 3q26.3 that consists of 20 exons coding for a protein of 124 kDa. *PIK3CA* mutations appear to be infrequent (<10%) in glioblastoma {225, 775, 1117A, 1141} except for one study which reported a 27% frequency {1978}. *PIK3CA* amplification also occurs in glioblastoma but studies vary significantly, with reported frequencies ranging from 0% to 64% {887, 1140, 1500}.

TP53/MDM2/p14^ARF pathway
The *TP53* gene (at 17p13.1) encodes a protein which plays a role in several cellular processes including the cell cycle, response of cells to DNA damage, cell death, cell differentiation, and neovascularization {188}. Following DNA damage, p53 is activated and induces transcription of genes such as p21Waf1/Cip1 {2079, 2159}. The *MDM2* gene (at 12q14.3-q15) encodes a 54 kDa protein, that binds to mutant and wild-type p53 proteins, thereby inhibiting the ability of wild-type p53 to activate transcription from minimal promoter sequences {1510, 1635}. Conversely, the transcription of the *MDM2* gene is induced by wild-type

p53 {97,2486}. In normal cells, this autoregulatory feedback loop regulates both the activity of the p53 protein and the expression of MDM2 {1743}. In addition, MDM2 promotes the degradation of p53 {792, 1212}. The *p14*^ARF (a part of the complex *CDKN2A* locus on chromosome 9p21) gene {1394, 2157, 2159, 2495} encodes a protein that directly binds to MDM2 and inhibits MDM2-mediated p53 degradation and transactivational silencing {1033, 1772, 2159, 2495}. Conversely, expression of p14^ARF is negatively regulated by p53 {2159}. Thus, loss of normal p53 function may result from altered expression of any of the *TP53*, *MDM2* or *p14*^ARF genes.
TP53 mutations are a genetic hallmark of secondary glioblastoma (>65%), and in almost all cases they are already present in precursor low-grade lesions or anaplastic astrocytoma {2371, 2372}. *TP53* mutations are significantly less frequent (approx. 25%) in primary glioblastoma {1620, 2372}. The distribution and type of *TP53* mutations also differs between primary and secondary glioblastoma: in the latter, 57% of mutations were located in the two hotspot codons 248 and 273; in the former, mutations were more equally distributed among the exons, with only 17% occurring in codons 248 and 273. G:C->A:T transitions at CpG sites were significantly more frequent in secondary than in primary glioblastoma {1620}, suggesting different molecular mechanisms underlying the acquisition of *TP53* mutations in these subtypes.
Amplification or overexpression of *MDM2* is an alternative mechanism for escaping p53-regulated control of cell growth. Amplification is observed in about 10% of those glioblastomas without *TP53* mutations {1844}, i.e. the primary glioblastoma {159}. Overexpression of MDM2 was observed immunohistochemically in more than 50% of primary glioblastomas {159}.
Loss of p14^ARF expression is frequent in glioblastoma (76%), and this correlated with homozygous deletion or promoter methylation of the *p14*^ARF gene {1562}. There was no significant difference in the overall frequency of p14^ARF alterations between primary and secondary glioblastomas (50% vs. 75%) {1562}. The analysis of multiple biopsies from the same patients revealed that *p14*^ARF methylation was already present in one third of low-grade astrocytoma {1562}.

p16^{INK4a}/CDK4/RB1 pathway

This signalling pathway is important for the control of progression through G1 into the S phase of the cell cycle {2054}. The *RB1* gene (at 13q14) encodes the 107 kDa retinoblastoma (RB1) protein. The CDK4/cyclin D1 complex phosphorylates the RB1 protein, thereby inducing release of the E2F transcription factor that activates genes involved in the G1->S transition {2079}. The *p16^{INK4a}* gene (at the *CDKN2A* locus, 9p21) encodes a protein that binds to CDK4 and inhibits the CDK4/cyclin D1 complex, thereby negatively regulating G1->S transition {2079}. Loss of cell cycle control may therefore result from altered expression of any of these genes, i.e. loss of p16^{INK4a} expression, overexpression/ amplification of CDKs or loss of RB function. In glioblastoma, *p16^{INK4a}* deletion and *RB1* alterations appear to be mutually exclusive {160, 265, 2282}. Inactivation of genes in this pathway is common in both primary and secondary glioblastoma {160} at an overall frequency of 40-50% {160, 1562}.

The *CDK4* gene (at 12q13-14) is amplified in about 15% of high-grade gliomas {1596,1846}, particularly in those without *p16^{INK4a}* deletion. A few tumours without *p16^{INK4a}* deletion or *CDK4* amplification had *CDK6* amplification, suggesting that the two proteins can functionally compensate for each other {386}.

LOH on 13q including the *RB1* locus was detected in 12% of primary and 38% of secondary glioblastoma {1564}. Promoter methylation of the *RB1* gene was significantly correlated with loss of RB1 expression and was found significantly more frequently in secondary (43%) than in primary glioblastoma (14%) {1565}. *RB1* promoter methylation was not detected in low-grade and anaplastic astrocytoma, indicating that it is a late event during astrocytoma progression {1565}.

Loss of chromosome 10

LOH 10 is the most frequent genetic alteration in glioblastoma, occurring in 60–80% of cases {904, 1048, 1620, 1626, 1832}. Many glioblastomas show loss of one entire copy of chromosome 10, but LOH studies identified at least 3 commonly deleted regions, i.e. 10p14-p15, 10q23-24, and 10q25-pter, suggesting the potential of several tumour-suppressor genes {632, 634, 904, 1048,

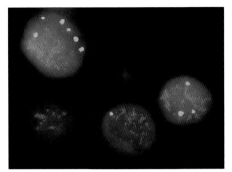

Fig. 1.37 *EGFR* amplification (many more red *EGFR* versus green centromere 7 signals) by FISH analysis in a small cell glioblastoma.

1832}. LOH 10q occurs at similar frequencies in primary and secondary glioblastoma {622, 1620}, with common deletions at 10q25-qter. LOH 10q25-qter is also directly associated with histologically recognized transition from low-grade or anaplastic astrocytoma to glioblastoma phenotypes {622}. In contrast, LOH 10p occurs almost exclusively in primary glioblastoma, leading to loss of entire chromosome 10, but very rarely in secondary glioblastoma {622}. LOH 10 is rare in lower grades of astrocytic tumours {167, 966}. There is a discrepancy between LOH for the chromosomal region containing the *PTEN* gene (75–95% of glioblastoma) and the frequency of *PTEN* mutations (30-44%) {2234}, suggesting the involvement of another not yet identified tumour suppressor gene(s) on 10q. The Deleted in Malignant Brain Tumours 1 (*DMBT1*) gene (at 10q25.3-26.1) is considered one of the candidate tumour suppressor genes on 10q {1508}. It is homozygously deleted in 13-38% of glioblastomas {1508,2123}. The genomic structure of *DMBT1* has recently been elucidated and points to a possible role in the evolution of chromosomal instability {1507}. Screening for genome wide chromosomal imbalances using array CGH revealed that loss of chromosome 10 was associated not only with changes in the expression of genes located on chromosome 10, but also with genome-wide differences in gene expression {1593}.

Loss of other chromosomal loci

LOH 1p was detected at a similar frequency in primary and secondary glioblastoma (12-15%). LOH 19q occurs in 20–25% of unselected glioblastomas

{2332, 2339, 2340}, and is significantly more frequent in secondary glioblastoma (54%) than in primary glioblastoma (6%) {1564}. Deletion mapping has narrowed the candidate region to the 19q13.3 region between the D19S412 and STD loci {1929}. LOH 22q occurs in 20–30% of gliomas of all grades {633, 966}, suggesting the presence of a tumour suppressor gene that plays a role in the early stages of astrocytoma progression. LOH 22q was significantly more frequent in secondary glioblastoma (82%) than in primary glioblastoma (41%) {1558}. Characterization of 22q deletions in primary glioblastoma identified two minimally deleted regions at 22q12.3-13.2 and 22q13.31, while 22 of 23 secondary glioblastomas affected shared a deletion in the same small (957 kb) region of 22q12.3, a region in which the human tissue inhibitor of metalloproteinases-3 (*TIMP-3*) is located. *TIMP-3* promoter methylation was observed at a significantly higher frequency in secondary than in primary glioblastoma and correlated with loss of TIMP-3 expression {1558}. Array CGH has revealed two small common and overlapping regions at 6q26 in glioblastoma and anaplastic astrocytoma {903}.

Co-presence of genetic alterations in glioblastomas

LOH 10q is not only the most frequent genetic alteration, but also typically co-presents with any of the other genetic alterations, consistent with it occurring late in disease progression {1620}. *EGFR* amplification is typically associated with *p16^{INK4a}* deletions {797, 802, 1620}, while *TP53* mutations, *EGFR* amplification and *PTEN* mutations show inverse associations {1620, 2114}. Analyses using array CGH in 50 primary glioblastomas revealed 3 major genetic subgroups, i.e. tumours with chromosome 10 loss and chromosome 7 gain, tumours with only chromosome 10 loss in the absence of chromosome 7 gain, and tumours without copy number change in chromosomes 7 or 10 {1489}.

Correlation between genetic alterations and histologic features

The small cell glioblastoma phenotype frequently shows *EGFR* amplification {255, 857, 1720}, *p16^{INK4a}* homozygous deletion {857}, *PTEN* mutations {857} and LOH 10q {1720}. Glioblastomas containing

>5% multinucleated giant cells were found to be associated with frequent TP53 mutations but infrequent EGFR amplification {857}.

Promoter methylation
O⁶-Methylguanine-DNA methyltransferase (MGMT) is a repair protein that specifically removes promutagenic alkyl groups from the O^6 position of guanine in DNA, thereby protecting cells against alkylating agents {713, 1399}. Loss of MGMT expression may be caused by methylation of promoter CpG islands {537, 1811}. *MGMT* promoter methylation is frequently present in glioblastoma (45-75%) {129, 801, 1034, 1563}, and was associated with longer survival of glioblastoma patients treated with temozolomide {801}. Secondary glioblastoma showed a higher frequency of *MGMT* promoter methylation than primary glioblastoma {129, 1563}. The presence of *MGMT* promoter methylation in low-grade astrocytomas is significantly associated with frequent G:C->A:T transitions. Promoter methylation of the *TP53*, *p14^ARF*, *RB1* and *TIMP-3* genes are also common in glioblastoma and were reported to be more frequent in secondary than primary glioblastoma {1562, 1563, 1565, 1886}.

Expression profiles
Based on gene expression patterns, glioblastoma can be distinguished from pilocytic astrocytoma {1886}, low-grade astrocytoma {999}, anaplastic astrocytoma {630} and oligodendroglioma {630}. However, expression patterns also vary significantly among glioblastoma cases {702, 1317}. This is particularly true for primary glioblastoma {702}, possibly due to a higher degree of genomic instability. Several studies using expression arrays revealed that glioblastoma typically shows overexpression of growth factor-related genes, and genes involved in cell migration {1870} and angiogenesis {702, 1317}. EGFR-overexpressing glioblastoma has a distinct global gene transcriptional profile, and the expression of 90 genes could distinguish EGFR-overexpressing from EGFR-nonexpressing glioblastoma {1487}. Primary and secondary glioblastoma also show different expression profiles {2122, 2271}.

Adult vs. paediatric glioblastomas
Glioblastoma in children has a genetic

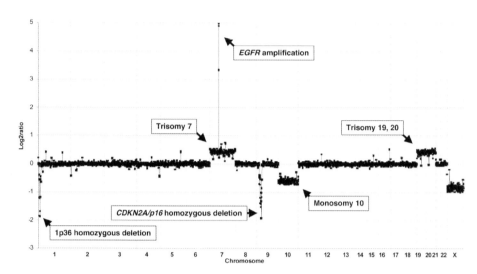

Fig. 1.38 1 Mb array-CGH profile of a male glioblastoma against female reference. Unpublished data from K. Ichimura and V.P. Collins.

profile distinct from that of glioblastoma of adult patients. Although paediatric glioblastoma usually develops *de novo*, the genetic pathway leading to primary glioblastoma in adults appears to be rarely involved in children, as reflected by high frequency of *TP53* mutations (approx 40%), and the low frequency of *EGFR* amplification (6%), *p16^INK4a* deletion (19%), and the absence of *MDM2* amplification {1585, 2180}. *TP53* mutations appear to be less frequent in high-grade gliomas (glioblastoma and anaplastic astrocytoma) in children <3 years old (12%) than older children (40%) {1767}. Microsatellite instability (MSI) due to DNA mismatch repair deficiency is rare in adult glioblastoma, but occurs in 27% of anaplastic astrocytoma and glioblastoma manifesting in children, and this phenomenon is associated with shorter survival. The frequency of *TP53* mutations was significantly lower in cases with MSI {49}. Comparative genomic hybridization revealed that chromosomal alterations significantly differ between paediatric and adult high-grade astrocytoma, and those characteristic for paediatric glioblastoma are +1q, +3q, +16p, -8q and -17p {1884}.

Genetic susceptibility
The occurrence of glioblastoma in more than one member of a family is sometimes seen. This is most often the case within the inherited tumour syndromes (see Chapter 13) that include the Turcot and Li-Fraumeni

syndromes, neurofibromatosis type 1 and multiple enchondromatosis {605, 1447, 2306}.

Prognostic and predictive factors
Despite progress in surgery, radiotherapy and chemotherapy of brain tumours, the overall survival of patients with glioblastoma remains extremely poor. In retrospective population-based studies from Switzerland and Canada, less than 20% of patients survived more than one year and less than 3% lived longer than 3 years {1620, 1625}. Clinical trials show a better outcome, with median survival rates of approximately 12 months, as they have a strong bias toward the recruitment of younger patients and those with higher preoperative Karnofsky performance scores, which are strong predictors of a more favourable clinical outcome.

Age
Virtually all therapy trials have shown that younger glioblastoma patients (<50 years at diagnosis) have a significantly better prognosis {252, 712}. In a large population-based study, age was the most significant prognostic factor; this persisted through all of the age groups in a linear manner {1620}. Patients with secondary glioblastoma survived significantly longer than those with primary glioblastoma {1620}, but this is likely due to their age rather than a reflection of different biological behaviour.

Histopathology

The presence and extent of necrosis are associated with shorter survival {252, 764, 857, 1744}.

Genetic alterations

Data on the prognostic value of *TP53* mutations in glioblastomas are contradictory, showing either no association or that the presence of *TP53* mutations was a favourable prognostic factor. In a large population-based study, the presence of *TP53* mutations was predictive of longer survival but this was not significant when adjusted for their usually younger age {1620}. There is no consistent correlation of *EGFR* amplification with survival, largely irrespective of the age at clinical manifestation {1620}. LOH 10 is the most frequent genetic alteration in glioblastoma and is associated with reduced survival {1620}. The presence of *PTEN* mutations is not associated with prognosis of glioblastoma patients {78, 1620, 2032, 2114}.

Biomarkers

YKL-40 (chitinase-3-like-1), a secreted protein of unknown function, is over-expressed in glioblastoma {2271}, and its expression is associated with LOH 10q, poorer radiation response, shorter time to progression and reduced overall survival {1708A}. It is typically co-expressed with matrix metalloproteinase-9 (MMP-9), and its detection in serum has been used to monitor patients for recurrent tumour growth {864}. One report showed that increased expression of GD3 synthase mRNA in combination with decreased GalNAcT message correlated with increased survival in glioblastoma patients {1613}. Insulin-like growth factor-binding protein-2 (IGFBP-2) and IGFBP-5 accumulate in glioma cells and the extent of expression correlated with histological grade {518, 2362}. IGFBP-2 enhances invasion {2361}, but there is currently no evidence that it is predictive of poorer outcome.

Mechanisms of treatment response

Glioblastoma is highly resistant to therapy, with only marginal survival increases in a small fraction of patients, even after aggressive surgical resection, external beam radiation therapy (both conformal and whole brain), and maximum tolerated doses for chemotherapy with agents such as temozolomide or nitrosourea. Over the

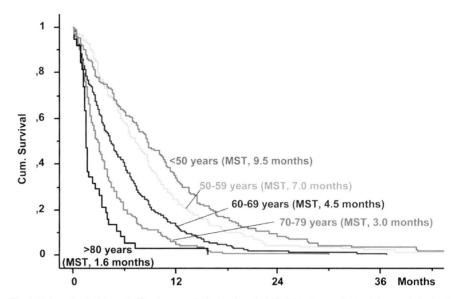

Fig. 1.39 Age of patient is a significant prognostic factor of survival of glioblastoma patients at the population level. Modified from Ohgaki *et al.* {1620}.

last 30–40 years, hundreds of clinical trials have had only marginal therapeutic success, although most brain tumour centres are observing a few long-term survivors among patients treated aggressively with multimodality therapy. Therapeutic resistance is due to: 1) poor drug delivery because of partial blood-brain-barrier preservation and high tumour interstitial pressure; 2) genome instability produced by point mutations, loss of heterozygosity, chromosome deletions and rearrangements, gene amplification, and epigenetic gene silencing which leads to broad genotypic and phenotypic heterogeneity resulting in clonal populations of cells resistant to any single therapeutic modality; 3) invasive properties of glioblastoma cells enabling malignant cells to cross the corpus callosum, spread even to the brain stem and spinal cord, and reside behind a completely intact blood-brain barrier; 4) the presence of a population of neural stem cell-like cells that may harbour resistance mechanisms that are distinct from those of the majority of non-stem-like tumour cells and that may contribute to cellular heterogeneity; and 5) retention of abundant DNA repair machinery that abrogates effectiveness of chemotherapy and radiotherapy.

Molecular abnormalities in glioblastoma provide specific mechanisms of resistance and susceptibility to therapy. The TP53 pathway inactivated by multiple mechanisms leads to a lack of apoptosis and cell cycle arrest. Mutations of the retinoblastoma pathway in both primary and secondary glioblastoma result in failure to provide appropriate cell cycle arrest. Although point mutations of the *Ras* gene in glioblastoma are rare, the Ras pathway is secondarily activated through IGFR, EGFR, and PDGFR signalling.

Downstream events such as silencing of the *NF1* tumour suppressor gene may also activate the Ras pathway to cause uncontrolled cellular proliferation. Similarly, the PI3K pathway may be activated by abnormal IGF1, EGF, or PDF signalling or downstream by abnormalities in the *PTEN* gene {1853}. These redundant signalling pathway abnormalities suggest that a single, specific, small-molecule signalling-pathway inhibitor might be expected to be ineffective in treating glioblastoma. This expectation has proven true in the testing of a large number of small-molecule inhibitors of signalling pathways in multiple glioblastoma xenografts. In a clinical trial of gefitinib, an EGF tyrosine kinase inhibitor, minimal responses were observed {1871}. On the other hand, testing individual glioblastoma biopsies for EGFRvIII and *PTEN* {1446} was able to identify patients responsive to the erlotinib or gefitinib EGFR kinase inhibitors. This may suggest that combinations of mutations common to glioblastoma may need to be targeted in these therapeutic approaches.

Recently, a population of neural stem-like glioma cells (SCLGCs) has been identified in glioblastoma {96, 643, 905, 2105}. These SCLGCs are highly tumourigenic in immunosuppressed mice, inducing intracranial tumours with a much smaller cellular inoculum than non-SCLGC cells from glioblastomas. Intracranial tumours induced by these SCLGCs had morphologic hallmarks of glioblastoma, such as markedly increased vascularity and endothelial cell proliferation, necrosis, and haemorrhage. These intracranial tumours responded to treatment with a neutralizing antibody to VEGF, bevacizumab, and the same humanized VEGF neutralizing antibody has showed a 60–65% response rate in a phase II trial in recurrent glioblastomas {2351}. Bao *et al.* {96} have shown that one of the mechanisms of radiation resistance may reside in the SCLGC population preferentially, and that the mechanism of radiation resistance is activation of the DNA checkpoint response. Bone morphogenic protein BMP4 causes a significant reduction of stem-like precursor cells of human glioblastoma and abolishes their tumour-initiating capacities *in vivo*.

Cellular immunotherapy or tumour vaccine approaches began decades ago, but have had little effect on the survival of glioblastoma patients. One of the mechanisms discovered for the failure of cellular immunotherapy was the production of TGF-β by glioblastoma cells, which caused a relatively profound immunosuppression that was evident at the time of diagnosis and prior to any therapy. Only recently has the cellular mechanism of the immunosuppression in glioblastoma patients been discovered. Fecci *et al.* {556, 557} showed that glioblastoma patients have a diminished population of CD4 cells, which although capable of normal immune function, are hindered in immune function by an increased number of regulatory T (Treg) cells in the CD4 compartment. Moreover, depletion of Treg cells in a syngenic murine animal model bearing intracranial tumours derived from a spontaneous astrocytoma resulted in immune rejection of the intracranial astrocytomas, with statistically significant survival increases. Removing Treg cells and targeting tumour-specific antigens such as EGFRvIII by pulsing autologous dendritic antigen-presenting cells and re-administering them to individual glioblastoma

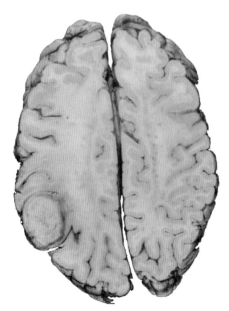

Fig. 1.40 Well-circumscribed, superficially located giant cell glioblastoma in the left parietal lobe.

patients are avenues that may have promise.

As molecular methods advance for obtaining comprehensive data from glioblastoma biopsies in real time on genetic abnormalities, gene expression, signalling and programmed cell death pathway status, hypoxia, SCLGC composition, and DNA repair protein levels and cellular distribution, subsets of patients that will respond to specific monotherapies should be identified. Examples are clinical tools such as recursive petition analysis (RPA) {1486} which identified patients surviving longest in RPA class III in the Stupp *et al.* {2166} EORTC/NCIC randomized trial of radiation therapy alone versus radiation therapy with temozolomide. Further analysis also showed the benefit of gross total surgical resection versus biopsy or partial resection {2302}. Another subset of patients within the Stupp et al. {2166} trial that had significantly better survival were those with methylation silencing of the methyl guanine-methyltransferase gene, whose gene product is known to repair the mono-DNA adduct at the O^6 position of guanine, a DNA adduct essential for the cytotoxic effect of temozolomide {801}.

Because of our knowledge of the molecular abnormalities in subsets of glioblastoma and the identification of patients likely to respond or be resistant to specific therapies, there is good reason to hope that much more progress in treating glioblastoma should be made in the next decade than has been made in the past 50 years. A multitude of new molecularly targeted therapies, such as monoclonal antibodies reactive with growth factors or their receptors, small-molecule signal transduction inhibitors, improvements in cellular immunotherapies, the use of neural stem cells as therapy or therapeutic carriers, and the targeting of tumour stem cells all bode well for improving glioblastoma therapy. Drug delivery will also be improved with methodologies such as convection-enhanced delivery and nanotechnology.

Giant cell glioblastoma

Definition
A histological variant of glioblastoma with a predominance of bizarre, multinucleated giant cells, an occasionally abundant stromal reticulin network and a high frequency of *TP53* mutations.

ICD-O code   9441/3

Grading
Giant cell glioblastoma corresponds histologically to WHO grade IV.

Synonyms and historical annotation
Because of the often prominent stromal reticulin network, giant cell glioblastoma was originally termed monstrocellular sarcoma {2513, 2514} but the consistent expression of GFAP has firmly established its astrocytic nature {972, 1120, 1959}.

Incidence
Giant cell glioblastoma is a rare variant that accounts for less than 1% of all brain tumours {1669} and up to 5% of glioblastoma {857,1669}.

Age and sex distribution
In a series of 55 cases, the mean age at clinical manifestation was 41 years, but the age distribution of this tumour covers a wider range than other diffuse astrocytomas and includes children {857, 1464, 1714}. Males and females are equally affected (M/F ratio, 1.1).

Clinical features
Symptoms and signs
Giant cell glioblastomas develop *de novo*

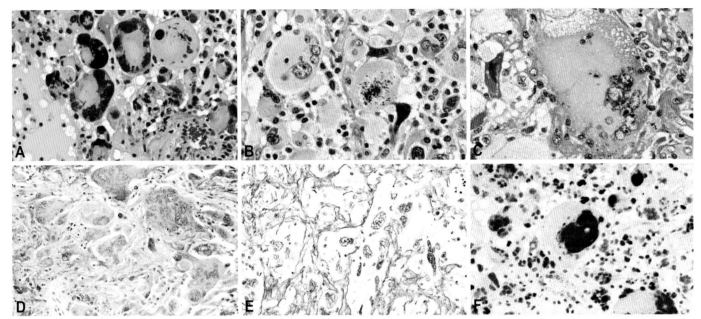

Fig. 1.41 **A** Giant cell glioblastoma consists of cells with variable size and shape. **B** An atypical mitotic figure in a giant cell. **C** A very large multinucleated giant cell. **D** Most but not all tumour cells express GFAP. **E** Marked stromal reaction (Bodian silver stain). **F** Tumour shows a high labelling index with MIB-1 antibody.

after a short preoperative history and without clinical or radiological evidence of a less malignant precursor lesion. Symptoms are similar to those of the ordinary glioblastoma.

Neuroimaging
Giant cell glioblastomas are distinctive because of their circumscription and firmness caused by the marked production of tumour stroma. They are often located subcortically in the temporal and parietal lobes. On CT and MRI, they may mimic a metastasis.

Histopathology
This type of glioblastoma has numerous multinucleated giant cells, smaller fusiform cells and, to a varying extent, a reticulin network {1398, 1959}. The giant cells often have extremely bizarre and grotesque appearances, and may measure more than 500 μm in diameter. They may be heavily lipidized {1812, 1959}. The number of nuclei ranges from a few to more than 20. They are often angulated, may contain prominent nucleoli and, on occasion, have cytoplasmic inclusions. Atypical mitoses are frequent, but the overall proliferation rate is similar to that of ordinary glioblastoma. Necrosis, often of a large geographic type or, more rarely a pseudopalisading one, is observed. Giant cells are immunopositive for S-100 protein, vimentin, class III ß-tubulin, p53

and EGFR, but their GFAP expression is highly variable {1057, 1714, 1966}. Neuronal markers are virtually negative, in contrast to pleomorphic xanthoastrocytoma {1408}. Occasionally, perivascular lymphocyte cuffing is noted. Microvascular proliferation is exceptional.

Genetics
Giant cell glioblastoma is characterized by frequent *TP53* mutations (75–90% of cases) and *PTEN* mutations (33%), but typically lacks *EGFR* amplification/overexpression and homozygous p16 deletion {1464, 1714, 1715}. These results indicate that giant cell glioblastoma occupies a hybrid position, sharing with

primary (*de novo*) glioblastoma a short clinical history, the absence of a less malignant precursor lesion and frequent *PTEN* mutations. In common with secondary glioblastoma that develops through progression from low-grade astrocytomas, they have a younger patient age at manifestation and a high frequency of *TP53* mutations {1715}.

Prognostic and predictive factors
Most giant cell glioblastomas carry a poor prognosis {884} but some reports indicate that the clinical outcome is somewhat better than that of ordinary glioblastoma {262,1398,2088}, possibly because of a less infiltrative behaviour.

Table 1.01 Clinical and genetic profile of the giant cell glioblastoma, in comparison with primary and secondary glioblastoma. Modified from Peraud *et al.* {1714, 1715}.

	Primary GBM	Giant cell GBM	Secondary GBM
Clinical onset	*de novo*	*de novo*	Secondary
Preoperative history	1.7 months	1.6 months	>25 months
Age at GBM diagnosis	55 years	42 years	39 years
Sex ratio M/F	1.4	1.1	0.8
PTEN mutation	32%	33%	4%
EGFR amplification	39%	5%	0%
TP53 mutation	11%	84%	67%
p16^{INK4a} deletion	36%	0%	4%

Gliosarcoma

Definition
A glioblastoma variant characterized by a biphasic tissue pattern with alternating areas displaying glial and mesenchymal differentiation.

ICD-O code   9442/3

Grading
Gliosarcoma corresponds histologically to WHO grade IV.

Synonyms and historical annotation
Gliosarcoma was originally defined as a glioblastoma in which the sarcomatous component was the consequence of malignant transformation of proliferating tumour vessels {560}. There is cytogenetic and molecular evidence for a monoclonal origin of both the glial and mesenchymal components.

Incidence
Gliosarcoma constitutes approximately 2% of all glioblastoma {559, 1444}, although a higher frequency (up to 8%) has also been reported {1521, 1991}.

Age and sex distribution
The age distribution is similar to that of glioblastoma, with preferential manifestation between ages 40 and 60 (mean, 52.1 years). Rare cases may occur in children, even in the very young {748, 1991}. Males are more frequently affected.

Localization
Gliosarcoma is usually located in the cerebral hemispheres, involving the temporal, frontal, parietal and occipital lobes in decreasing order of frequency. Rarely, gliosarcoma may occur in the posterior fossa and the spinal cord {291, 1587, 1601}. An unusual location of a gliosarcoma developing from an ependymoma has been identified {822}. Multifocal occurrence of gliosarcoma has also been reported {1668}.

Clinical features
Symptoms and signs
The clinical profile of the gliosarcoma is that of the primary glioblastoma, with symptoms of short duration which reflect the location of the tumour and increased intracranial pressure. Most tumours arise in the absence of recognized predisposing factors, but gliosarcoma has been associated with prior irradiation {1320, 1738}. Radiotherapy may also favour sarcomatous growth in a recurrent standard glioblastoma {32}

Neuroimaging
In cases with a predominant sarcomatous component, the tumour appears as a well-demarcated hyperdense mass with homogeneous contrast-enhancement that may mimic a meningioma. {794, 1387, 1975}. In cases with a prevalence of the gliomatous component, the radiological features are similar to those of glioblastoma.

Macroscopy
The high content of connective tissue gives the gross appearance of a firm, well-circumscribed mass that can be mistaken for a metastasis or, when attached to the dura, for a meningioma. Lesions less rich in connective tissue may have typical features of glioblastoma.

Histopathology
A mixture of gliomatous and sarcomatous tissues confer to gliosarcoma a striking biphasic tissue pattern. The glial portion is astrocytic in nature and anaplastic, mostly showing the typical features of a glioblastoma. Epithelial differentiation, manifest as carcinomatous features {1659} with gland-like or adenoid formations and squamous metaplasia {1084, 1526} may occur in the glial portions of selected cases. The sarcomatous component by definition shows signs of malignant transformation, e.g. nuclear atypia, mitotic activity and necrosis, and often demonstrates the typical pattern of fibrosarcoma, with densely packed long bundles of spindle cells. Occasionally, the histology resembles features of a malignant fibrous histiocytoma {1444, 1587}. A subset of cases may show additional lines of mesenchymal differentiation, e.g. the formation of cartilage {93}, bone {1412}, osteoid-chondral tissue {794, 2195}, smooth and striated muscle {101, 750} and even lipomatous features {2329}. The distinction between the two components is facilitated using combined histochemical and immunohistochemical staining. Collagen deposition in the mesenchymal part is well demonstrated by a trichrome stain. Similarly the reticulin staining shows abundant connective tissue fibers. This component does not express GFAP, which, on the contrary, is observed in the glial part. The demonstration of a clearly malignant mesenchymal GFAP-negative component is important to distinguish true gliosarcoma from glioblastoma with a florid fibroblastic proliferation (desmoplasia) elicited by meningeal invasion {1443}.

Genetics
Gliosarcoma contains PTEN mutations (38–45%), p16^{INK4a} deletions (38%), and TP53 mutations (23–24%), but shows infrequent EGFR amplifications (0–8%) {11,1856}, suggesting that they have a distinct profile, similar to that of primary glioblastoma, except for the infrequent EGFR amplification. Comparative genomic hybridization (CGH) in 20 gliosarcomas revealed that chromosomal imbalances commonly detected were gains on chromosomes 7 (75%), X (20%), 9q and 20q (15% each); and losses on chromosomes 10 and 9p (35% each) and 13q (15%) {11}. Similar genetic alterations have been found in the gliomatous and sarcomatous components, indicating a monoclonal origin.

Table 1.02 Genetic and clinical profile of the gliosarcoma in comparison with primary GBM. Modified from Reis et al. {1856}.

	Primary GBM	Gliosarcoma
Preoperative clinical history	1.7 months	2 months
Sex ratio M/F	1.4	1.65
Age at diagnosis	55 years	56 years
TP53 mutation	11%	23%
PTEN mutation	32%	38%
p16^{INK4a} deletion	36%	37%
MDM2 amplification	8%	5%
EGFR amplification	39%	0%

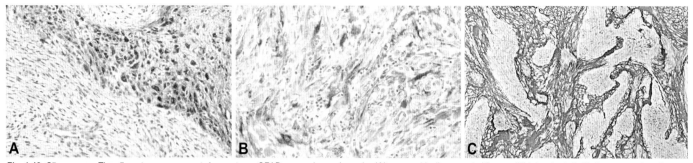

Fig. 1.42 Gliosarcoma. The gliomatous component shows strong GFAP expression and may be (**A**) geographically separated from or (**B**) intermingled with the sarcomatous tumour cells. **C** A biphasic tissue pattern denoting reticulin-rich sarcomatous and reticulin-free gliomatous elements.

Histogenesis

Originally, gliosarcoma was perceived as a collision tumour with a separate astrocytic component and an independent development of the sarcomatous portion from the proliferating vessels. Several immunohistochemical studies seemed to support that concept by demonstrating immunoreactivity to factor-VIII-related antigen {2028}, Ulex europaeus I agglutinin (UEA-I) {2111}, and monohistiocytic markers {718, 719, 1147}. Another hypothesis suggested that the sarcomatous portion results from advanced glioma dedifferentiation with subsequent loss of GFAP expression and acquisition of a sarcomatous phenotype {1008, 1443}. In a study using fluorescent *in situ* hybridization, two of three gliosarcomas showed identical numerical aberrations of chromosomes 10 and 17 in the glial and mesenchymal components, whereas in a third case, trisomy X was restricted to the chondrosarcomatous element {1695}. Similar cytogenetic patterns were also observed in both glial and mesenchymal components in a study using fluorescent *in situ* hybridisation and microsatellite allelic imbalance and cytogenetic analysis {526}. These results suggest that both components were derived from neoplastic glial cells. This view has further been supported by the observation of TP53 immunoreactivity in both tumour components {34}. Biernat *et*

al. {157} provided proof of a monoclonal origin by demonstrating that in two cases of gliosarcoma the gliomatous and sarcomatous components each contained an identical *TP53* mutation. Identical *PTEN* and *TP53* mutations were also detected in the gliomatous and sarcomatous tumour components of gliosarcoma {1856, 2359}. Monoclonality of both components of the gliosarcoma was also confirmed by identification of *p16* deletion and co-amplification of *MDM2* and *CDK4* in both tumour areas {1856}. These studies strongly support the view that the sarcomatous areas represent an aberrant differentiation of the glioblastoma cells, rather than coincidental development of two separate neoplasms.

Prognostic and predictive factors

It has been suggested that gliosarcoma has a somewhat more favourable prognosis {1387} than ordinary glioblastoma, but large clinical trials have failed to reveal significant differences in outcome {641, 1444, 1738}.

Gliofibroma

This is a very rare tumour that usually affects children. The age range of patients is from 11 days to 54 years (mean 14 years). It is more common in females (M:F=2:3). Gliofibroma frequently occurs in the cerebrum (36%) and the spinal cord (28%). In contrast to desmoplastic infantile astrocytoma, gliofibroma is not

dura-based and does not form large cystic tumours. It is a biphasic tumour composed of a glial component that ranges from a low-grade to high-grade level of differentiation, and a non-sarcomatous fibroblastic component. In contrast to gliosarcoma, the 'marbled' appearance of two tissue components is lacking. In some gliofibromas, collagen seems to be produced by the glioma cells themselves (desmoplastic astrocytoma) {612}, whereas in others it appears to be deposited by mesenchymal cells (mixed glioma/-fibroma) {1786}. Necrosis or vascular microproliferation is not a typical feature of gliofibroma {1786}. Cellularity, nuclear pleomorphism and increased mitotic activity are rarely present and may indicate more aggressive clinical behaviour; these tumours have been designated "malignant" or "anaplastic gliofibroma" {307, 1786}. Recently, the morphological variant with psammoma bodies has been described {1603}.

The prognosis of gliofibromas is usually favourable. The majority of the tumours has an indolent clinical course without evidence of recurrence or metastasis, even several years after resection. Occasionally, dissemination {278, 612, 2321} and/or death {612, 2067, 2119, 2321} has been reported, but most of these cases showed signs of cellular anaplasia or increased mitotic activity.

Gliomatosis cerebri

G.N. Fuller
J.M. Kros

Definition

A diffuse glioma (usually astrocytic) growth pattern consisting of exceptionally extensive infiltration of a large region of the central nervous system, with involvement of at least three cerebral lobes, usually with bilateral involvement of the cerebral hemispheres and/or deep gray matter, and frequent extension to the brain stem, cerebellum, and even the spinal cord. Gliomatosis cerebri most commonly displays an astrocytic phenotype, although oligodendroglioma and mixed oligoastrocytoma can also present with the gliomatosis cerebri growth pattern.

ICD-O code   9381/3

Grading

Gliomatosis cerebri (GC) is usually an aggressive neoplasm. The overall biologic behaviour corresponds to WHO grade III in a majority of cases. Several studies have demonstrated that, similar to all diffuse gliomas, substratification of gliomatosis patients by histologic subtype and grade using WHO criteria correlates with time to progression and overall survival {1718, 2320}. Given the extensive, multilobar nature of GC, diagnosis is typically confirmed through limited tissue biopsy; similar to diffuse gliomas in general, histologic subtyping and grading in this setting are subject to non-representative tissue sampling and undergrading.

Historical annotation

The term gliomatosis cerebri was coined by Nevin in 1938 to describe the extensive involvement of large areas of the brain by glial cells in the absence of a mass lesion {1584}. A number of names, such as glioblastomatosis and central diffuse schwannosis, were used in the early literature. The term gliomatosis cerebri is currently widely accepted. Uncertainty concerning histogenesis and whether GC warrants designation as a separate clinicopathologic entity apart from the other diffuse gliomas is reflected by the varying inclusion of GC under different rubrics in previous editions of the WHO

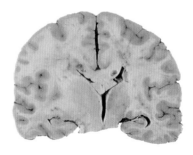

Fig. 1.44 Gliomatosis cerebri infiltrating the left hemisphere with enlargement of anatomic structures, in particular the thalamus.

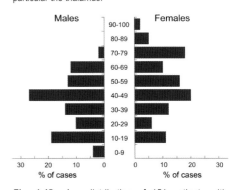

Fig. 1.45 Age distribution of 151 patients with gliomatosis cerebri. Modified from Jennings et al. {992}.

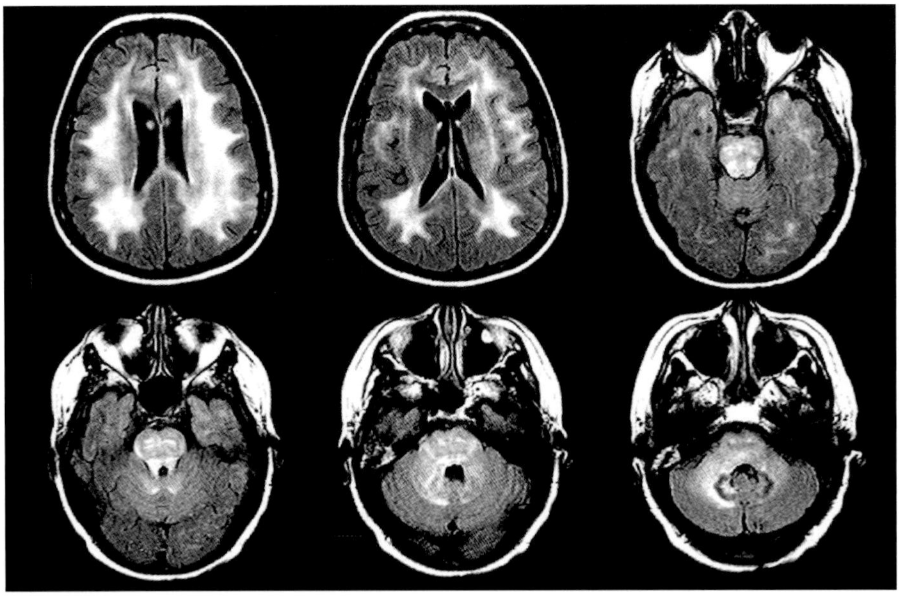

Classification {1121, 2513}. GC is currently viewed as a pattern of particularly extensive glioma infiltration. Early study of GC predated the advent of modern neuroimaging technologies by decades and consisted exclusively of autopsy examination. Contemporary MR imaging techniques (especially T2-weighted and FLAIR sequences), combined with biopsy, permit diagnosis during life.

Gliomatosis cerebri has been divided by some investigators into primary and secondary subtypes, with primary GC exhibiting extensive CNS involvement at the time of initial clinical presentation, and secondary GC consisting of progressive infiltration of the brain by a typical locally infiltrative diffuse glioma observed on clinical follow-up over time. Primary GC has been further divided by some investigators into type 1 (classical form), in which no tumour mass is present at initial clinical presentation, and

Fig. 1.43 MR imaging of gliomatosis cerebri, as seen on FLAIR sequences, reveals the characteristically extensive involvement of the central nervous system, which, in this case, includes the cerebral hemispheres bilaterally, the brain stem, and the cerebellum.

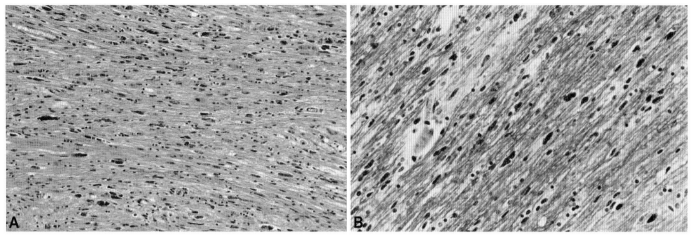

Fig. 1.46 Histological features of gliomatosis cerebri. **A** Diffuse infiltration of the corpus callosum with elongated tumour cells. **B** Tumour cell infiltration along the myelinated axons (Kluver-Barrera staining).

type 2, in which, in addition to extensive CNS involvement, a tumour mass is also present. In these schemes, primary, type 1 GC corresponds to classical GC. GC considered in the strict and classical sense would exclude secondary GC and type 2 GC, as defined above, as well as diffuse gliomas that by virtue of their anatomic location (e.g. in the region of junction of the frontal, temporal and parietal lobes) involve three cerebral lobes but are relatively localized in overall extent of CNS involvement.

Gliomatosis cerebri should be distinguished from two other types of gliomatosis, i.e. leptomeningeal gliomatosis and gliomatosis peritonei. Leptomeningeal gliomatosis is the widespread infiltration of the subarachnoid space by a diffuse glioma, most commonly an intra-axial glioma that has invaded the leptomeninges (secondary leptomeningeal gliomatosis), or, rarely, leptomeningeal spread of a glioma originating in an ectopic leptomeningeal glial or glio-neuronal rest (primary leptomeningeal gliomatosis). Gliomatosis peritonei is the presence of disseminated miliary foci of mature glial tissue throughout the peritoneal cavity, most commonly arising in association with an ovarian teratoma.

Incidence, age and sex distribution
In a review of 151 patients in which age at diagnosis was available, the age ranged from neonatal to 83 years, with the peak incidence between 40 and 50 years and males presenting somewhat earlier than females {992}. Both sexes were equally affected.

Localization
Virtually no anatomic site of the brain has been excluded from descriptions of GC. The most commonly involved areas, based on post-mortem studies {992}, are the cerebral hemispheres (76%), the mesencephalon (52%), the pons (52%), the thalamus (43%), the basal ganglia (34%), the cerebellum (29%), the medulla oblongata (13%), the hypothalamus, the optic nerves and chiasm, and the spinal cord (each at 9%). When GC involves the cerebral hemispheres, the centrum semiovale is always affected, whereas the cerebral cortex is infiltrated only in 19% of such cases, with spread to the leptomeninges in 17%. In 77% of cases of GC, the lesion is located bilaterally, and there is a predilection for the right side of the brain {2320}.

Clinical features
Symptoms and signs
The signs and symptoms vary considerably depending on the cerebral areas infiltrated and include changes in mental status such as dementia and lethargy, seizures (generalized and partial complex), headache, pyramidal symptoms (gait disturbances), cranial nerve dysfunction, signs and symptoms of increased intracranial pressure, spinocerebellar deficits, sensory deficits and paraesthesia, and visual disturbances {992, 2320}.

Neuroimaging
Diffuse enlargement of the involved cerebral structures, without tissue destruction or focal tumour mass formation, is seen both by CT scan and MR imaging, {458, 1809, 2086}. MRI gives superior results: on CT scans, GC may appear as only poorly defined, very subtle low density or isodensity, and the extent of involvement is typically smaller compared to T2-weighted or FLAIR MR sequences, on which signal hyperintensity reveals the full extent of the tumour and correlates best with post-mortem investigations {458, 2086}. FLAIR sequences are currently preferred over T2-weighted sequences by virtue of increased sensitivity and suppression of background "noise" from ventricular and subarachnoid space cerebrospinal fluid. Nevertheless, the ante-mortem diagnosis of gliomatosis cerebri can be difficult, especially in the case of limited tissue sampling of low-grade lesions by stereotactic biopsy. Proton MR spectroscopy may be of value in identifying target areas of denser tumour cellularity or higher grade tumour for subsequent sampling by stereotactic biopsy {2320}.

Histopathology
On macroscopic examination of autopsy or lobectomy specimens, involved regions of the brain are usually swollen and firm, with blurred distinction between grey and white matter but intact, recognizable gross anatomy. Classical histologic features include a proliferation of small glial cells with elongated, fusiform nuclei. A wide range of glial, predominantly astrocytic cellular morphologies can be seen, including larger tumour cells with irregular pleomorphic nuclei. Histological variation exists not only between different lesions, but also within the same

neoplasm. In some areas, the tumour cells are more obviously astrocytic, and gemistocytic forms may also be seen {1599}. Cases of GC exhibiting classical morphologic features of oligodendroglioma have also been described {90}. When infiltrating white matter, signs of demyelination may be present, but neurons and axons are intact {69}. Mitotic activity is variable and dependent on the extent of tissue sampling, but is typically low. Microvascular proliferation and necrosis are generally absent in classical (primary, type 1) GC at clinical presentation and during much of the disease course, but may appear in longer-surviving patients later in the clinical course through tumour progression. Perivascular cuffs of inflammatory cells are absent. GC should be distinguished from diseases in which prominent microglial cell proliferation is seen. Morphometric analysis has shown that most cellular parameters of cerebral gliomatosis are comparable to those of low grade astrocytoma {642}.

Immunohistochemistry

GFAP and S-100 protein immunostaining results are variable; in many cases, tumour cells exhibit strong positivity for both markers, whereas in others a majority of tumour cells are non-reactive {642, 2416}.

Proliferation

Proliferation in GC generally correlates with grade, as for other diffuse gliomas. Reported Ki-67 labelling indices range from <1 to 30% {403, 1104, 2187}.

Genetics

Molecular genetic characterization has lagged behind that of other types of diffuse gliomas. Secondary to the essential diagnostic criterion of widespread infiltration of extensive regions of the central nervous system, large surgical resections are generally not performed, and the amount of tissue available for scientific investigation is thus usually very small, often limited to stereotactic biopsy cores. Nevertheless, the data collected from surgical specimens and from the study of autopsy specimens suggest that the qualitative genetic abnormalities found in GC, such as TP53 mutation, are similar to those of diffuse astrocytoma, although occurring with a lower frequency {1419, 1420}. There is no definitive evidence for unique genetic alterations that distinguish gliomatosis from diffuse astrocytoma. As expected, for the limited number of cases studied of oligodendroglioma presenting with a GC pattern, an increased incidence of chromosome 1p deletion has been noted {1986}.

Histogenesis

Historically, the two competing hypotheses of gliomatosis origin were that: 1) it represents a subtype or subset of otherwise ordinary diffuse glioma characterized by exceptional infiltrative capacity, or 2) it results from the simultaneous neoplastic transformation of an extensive tissue field within the central nervous system ("field cancerization"). Central to this debate is the issue of clonality. Data from a majority of the limited number of studies available support a monoclonal origin for GC, with subsequent widespread diffuse glioma infiltration {1206,1419}.

Also integral to the issue of histogenesis is that of differentiation. Classical gliomatosis most commonly exhibits an astrocytic phenotype, as reflected by cellular morphology (elongated and/or pleomorphic nuclei) and immunopositivity for GFAP. Oligodendroglioma and mixed oligoastrocytoma can also present with the GC pattern of extensive brain infiltration, with exceptional cases involving the cerebral hemispheres bilaterally, the brain stem and the cerebellum {2211}. Such cases that exhibit classical morphologic features have been referred to as "oligodendrocytic GC" or "oligodendroglial GC" and, not surprisingly, tend to respond more favourably to treatment compared with astrocytic GC and to exhibit the favourable oligodendroglial genetic signature of chromosome 1p deletion {1299, 1986}. Thus, most investigators favour the interpretation of classical GC as exceptionally extensive involvement of a large contiguous region of the central nervous system by a diffuse, usually astrocytic glioma.

Prognostic and predictive factors

Median survival in gliomatosis patients is associated with younger patient age and higher Karnofsky performance status at clinical presentation, lower WHO grade and histologic subtype {1718, 2196}. The associations, however, are not unique to GC, and apply to diffuse gliomas in general.

CHAPTER 2

Oligodendroglial Tumours

Oligodendroglioma (WHO grade II)
A diffusely infiltrating, well-differentiated glioma of adults, typically located in the cerebral hemispheres, composed of neoplastic cells morphologically resembling oligodendroglia and often harbouring deletions of chromosomal arms 1p and 19q.

Anaplastic oligodendroglioma (WHO grade III)
An oligodendroglioma with focal or diffuse histological features of malignancy and a less favourable prognosis.

Oligoastrocytoma (WHO grade II)
A diffusely infiltrating glioma composed of a conspicuous mixture of two distinct neoplastic cell types morphologically resembling the tumour cells in oligodendroglioma and diffuse astrocytoma of WHO grade II.

Anaplastic oligoastrocytoma (WHO grade III)
An oligoastrocytoma with histological features of malignancy, such as increased cellularity, nuclear atypia, pleomorphism and increased mitotic activity.

Oligodendroglioma

G. Reifenberger
J.M. Kros
D.N. Louis
V.P. Collins

Definition
A diffusely infiltrating, well-differentiated glioma of adults, typically located in the cerebral hemispheres, composed of neoplastic cells morphologically resembling oligodendroglia and often harbouring deletions of chromosomal arms 1p and 19q.

ICD-O code   9450/3

Grading
Oligodendroglioma corresponds histologically to WHO grade II.
Histologically, oligodendroglial tumours comprise a continuous spectrum ranging from well-differentiated neoplasms to frankly malignant tumours. The WHO grading system recognizes two malignancy grades for oligodendroglial tumours: WHO grade II for well-differentiated tumours, and WHO grade III for anaplastic oligodendroglioma. Several recent studies have confirmed the WHO grading of oligodendroglial tumours as a significant predictor of survival {563, 680, 1269, 1625}. Several other systems have been used for grading of oligodendroglial tumours, including the four-tiered Kernohan {1093} and St Anne/Mayo systems {2074}, the Smith grading system {2115}, as well as three-tiered systems such as the Ringertz system {1891} and a three-tiered modification of the Smith scheme {1199,1202}.

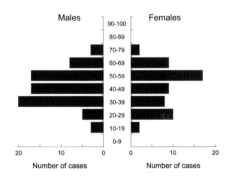

Fig. 2.01 Age and sex distribution of 130 patients with oligodendroglioma and anaplastic oligodendroglioma, based on combined biopsy series from the Universities of Düsseldorf (Germany) and Zürich (Switzerland).

In addition, a two-tiered system based on morphological and imaging criteria has been proposed {424}. Each of these grading systems is capable of distinguishing subsets of oligodendroglial tumours, but most studies suggest that there are basically two groups that differ prognostically, which is in line with the two-tiered WHO system.

Historical annotation
The first description of an oligodendroglioma was published by Bailey & Cushing {86} followed by the classic paper of Bailey & Bucy {83} on oligodendrogliomas of the brain.

Incidence
Adjusted annual incidence rates have been estimated to range from 0.27 to 0.35 per 100 000 persons {305, 1625}. Oligodendroglioma accounts for approximately 2.5% of all primary brain tumours and 5–6% of all gliomas {305, 1625}. The incidence of oligodendroglioma has significantly increased over the past years {305}, but this may primarily be due to the use of less stringent diagnostic criteria in recent years, possibly triggered by a desire not to impede any patient from gaining a benefit of chemotherapy {248}.

Etiology
Individual cases of oligodendroglioma in patients previously irradiated for other reasons have been documented {18, 383, 878}, but these account for an insignificant fraction of all oligodendroglial tumours. Although oligodendroglioma and oligoastrocytoma are among the most frequent types of CNS tumours to be induced experimentally in rats by chemical carcinogens such as ethylnitrosourea and methylnitrosourea, there is no convincing evidence of an etiological role for these substances in human gliomas. Some studies have reported the presence of viral genome sequences and proteins (SV40, BK and JC virus) in oligodendroglioma {460}; however, other authors failed to detect virus sequences {1913} and thus a viral etiology is uncertain at present.

Age and sex distribution
The majority of oligodendrogliomas arise in adults, with a peak incidence between 40 and 45 years of age {305, 1269, 1625}. Oligodendroglioma is rare in children, accounting for only 2% of all brain tumours in patients younger than 14 years {305}. Males appear to be affected slightly more frequently than females, with a ratio of 1.1:1 reported in a population-based series of 1559 patients {305}.

Localization
Oligodendroglioma arises preferentially in the cortex and white matter of the cerebral hemispheres. The frontal lobe is involved in 50–65% of the patients, followed with decreasing frequencies by the temporal, parietal and occipital lobes {1199, 2074}. Involvement of more than one cerebral lobe or bilateral tumour spread is common. Patients have been reported with oligodendroglioma in the posterior fossa {1663}, basal ganglia {1739}, brain stem {50} or spinal cord {599}, as well as primary leptomeningeal oligodendroglioma {1588}, and oligodendroglial gliomatosis cerebri {2196}.

Clinical features
Symptoms and signs
Approximately two thirds of the patients present with seizures. Further common presentations include headache and other signs of increased intracranial pressure, focal neurological deficits, and cognitive or mental changes {1269, 1642}. In older studies, intervals of more than 5 years between onset of symptoms and diagnosis were common, but modern neuroimaging has shortened the time to diagnosis {1642}.

Neuroimaging
On CT, oligodendroglioma usually appears as hypo- or isodense, well-demarcated mass lesions, usually located in the cortex and subcortical white matter. Calcification is common but not diagnostic. MRI studies typically demonstrate a hypointense lesion in T1-weighted images and a hyperintense lesion in T2-weighted

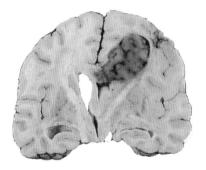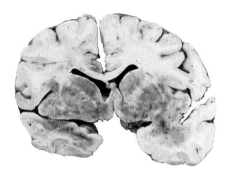

Fig. 2.02 **A** Well-circumscribed, partly haemorrhagic oligodendroglioma of the left frontal lobe. **B** Recurrent oligodendroglioma with bilateral, diffuse infiltration of the frontal and temporal lobes.

images which appears well-demarcated and shows little perifocal edema {1282}. Some tumours demonstrate heterogeneous features due to intratumoural haemorrhages and/or areas of cystic degeneration. Gadolinium enhancement has been associated with less favourable prognosis {2074}. Correlation with 1p/19q status revealed that oligodendrogliomas without 1p/19q deletions more often demonstrate mixed signal intensity on T1- and T2-weighted images {991, 1442}. One study suggested that 1p/19q deletions are associated with indistinct tumour borders on T1-weighted images, paramagnetic susceptibility and calcification {1442}, but these associations have not held true in other studies {991}.

Macroscopy

Oligodendroglioma usually appears as well-defined soft masses of greyish-pink colour. Cases with extensive mucoid degeneration may appear gelatinous. The tumour is typically located in the cortex and white matter, and infiltration of the overlying leptomeninges may be seen. Perifocal edema is uncommon.

Calcification is frequent and may impart a gritty texture to the tumour. Zones of cystic degeneration, as well as intratumoural haemorrhages, may be seen.

Histopathology

Oligodendrogliomas are diffusely infiltrating gliomas of moderate cellularity that are composed of monomorphic cells with uniform round nuclei and perinuclear halos on paraffin sections ('honeycomb' appearance). Additional features include microcalcifications, mucoid/cystic degeneration and a dense network of branching capillaries. Marked nuclear atypia and an occasional mitosis are compatible with the diagnosis of WHO grade II oligodendroglioma but significant mitotic activity, prominent microvascular proliferation or conspicuous necrosis indicate progression to anaplastic oligodendroglioma (WHO grade III).

Cellular composition

Oligodendroglioma is moderately cellular, although areas of increased cellularity, often in the form of circumscribed nodules, may occur in some otherwise well-

differentiated tumours. On the other hand, small biopsies may sometimes show only scattered oligodendroglioma cells, identifiable by their characteristic nuclei, infiltrating the brain parenchyma. The tumour cells have uniformly round nuclei that are slightly larger than those of normal oligodendrocytes and show an increase in chromatin density. Mitotic activity is either absent or low. In routinely formalin-fixed and paraffin-embedded material, the tendency of the tumour cells to undergo degeneration by acute swelling results in an enlarged rounded cell with a well-defined cell membrane and clear cytoplasm around a central spherical nucleus. This creates the typical honeycomb appearance which, although artifactual, is a helpful diagnostic feature when present. This artifact is seen neither in smear preparations nor in frozen sections, and may also be absent in rapidly fixed tissue and in paraffin sections made from frozen material.

Some oligodendrogliomas contain tumour cells with the appearance of small gemistocytes, which have a somewhat larger, often eccentric cytoplasm that is positive for glial fibrillary acidic protein (GFAP). These cells have been referred to as minigemistocytes or microgemistocytes. In rare tumours, GFAP-negative mucocytes or even signet-ring cells may be seen. Rare cases of oligodendroglioma consisting largely of signet-ring cells (signet-ring cell oligodendroglioma) have been described {1203}. Eosinophilic granular cells may also occur in some oligodendrogliomas {2202}. Reactive astrocytes are typically scattered throughout oligodendrogliomas and may be particularly prominent in the infiltration rim. These should not be confused with the neoplastic astrocytes in diffuse astrocytoma or oligoastrocytoma.

Calcifications

An important histological feature is the presence of microcalcifications, sometimes associated with blood vessels, within the tumour tissue proper as well as in the invaded brain. However, this feature is not specific for oligodendroglial tumours and, due to the generally incomplete tumour sampling, may sometimes not be found in the available tissue sections even if clearly demonstrated neuroradiologically. Areas characterized by extracellular mucin deposition and/or microcyst formation are frequent.

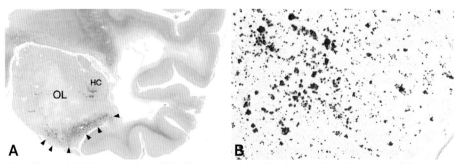

Fig. 2.03 **A** and **B** Oligodendroglioma (OL) of the temporal lobe with infiltration of the hippocampus (HC). Note the zone of calcification (arrows) at the periphery of the lesion and at higher magnification (**B**).

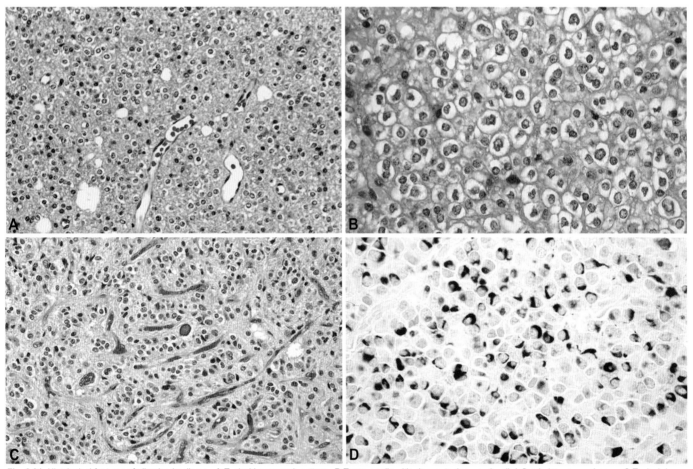

Fig. 2.04 Histological features of oligodendroglioma. **A** Typical honeycomb pattern. **B** Tumour cells with clear cytoplasm and well defined plasma membrane. **C** Typical dense network of branching capillaries. **D** Minigemistocytes with marked perinuclear immunoreactivity for GFAP.

Vasculature

Oligodendroglioma typically shows a dense network of branching capillaries resembling the pattern of chicken-wire. In some cases, the capillary stroma tends to subdivide the tumour into lobules. The tumours have a tendency for intratumoural haemorrhages.

Growth pattern

Oligodendrogliomas grow diffusely in the cortex and white matter. Within the cortex, tumour cells tend to form secondary structures such as perineuronal satellitosis, perivascular aggregates, and subpial accumulations. Circumscribed lepto-meningeal infiltration may induce a desmoplastic reaction. A rare growth pattern is the formation of parallel rows of tumour cells with somewhat elongated nuclei forming palisades reminiscent of the so-called polar spongioblastoma. Occasionally, perivascular pseudorosettes may be seen. These patterns are generally present only focally.

Immunohistochemistry

There is no immunohistochemical marker available that allows the specific and sensitive recognition of human oligodendroglial tumour cells. Oligodendroglioma shares with many other neuroectodermal tumours the expression of S-100 protein and the HNK1 (anti-Leu7, CD57) carbohydrate epitope {1529, 1553, 1847}. Immunoreactivity for γ-enolase is also frequent {1842}. GFAP may be present not only in intermingled reactive astrocytes but also in neoplastic oligodendroglial cells such as minigemistocytes and gliofibrillary oligodendrocytes {816, 1204, 1847}. The presence of GFAP in minigemistocytes and gliofibrillary oligodendrocytes has been corroborated by ultrastructural studies {816, 1201, 2434}. Some authors have suggested that these cells represent transitional forms between astrocytes and oligodendrocytes {816, 1201, 1204}. Alternatively, they may recapitulate a phenotype characteristic of a transient stage during oligodendroglial development {340, 957}. Vimentin is infrequently expressed in low-grade oligodendroglioma but more often found in anaplastic oligodendroglioma {455, 1165}. Cytokeratins are absent {1842}, although certain antibodies such as AE1/ AE3 may cross-react with other intermediate filament proteins, including GFAP, and thus give false-positive staining {1188}.

Oligodendroglioma is consistently positive for the microtubule-associated protein 2 (MAP2), a protein linked to the neuronal cytoskeleton in the mature central nervous system but also expressed in glial progenitor cells during development {179}. However, MAP2 immunoreactivity is also commonly seen in astrocytic gliomas as well as in neuronal and neurocytic tumours {179}. The oligodendrocyte lineage-specific transcription factors OLIG-1 and OLIG-2 are expressed not only in oligodendroglioma but also in the vast majority of other gliomas {1321,1887}. Similarly, SOX10, another transcription factor critically involved in oligodendroglial differentiation, is expressed in both oligodendroglioma and astrocytic tumours {95}.

A number of differentiation antigens that are specifically expressed by normal oligodendrocytes *in vivo* or *in vitro* have been identified. These include myelin basic protein (MBP), proteolipid protein (PLP), myelin-associated glycoprotein (MAG), galactolipids like galactocerebroside (GC) and galactosulphatide, and a number of gangliosides, as well as several enzymes such as carbonic anhydrase C, 2'-3'-cyclic nucleotide-3'-phosphatase (CNP), glycerol-3-phosphate dehydrogenase and lactate dehydrogenase (LDH). However, so far, none of these antigens has gained significance as a diagnostically useful marker for oligodendroglioma. They either are no longer expressed by neoplastic oligodendrocytes, e.g. MBP {1553,1842}, or they are expressed only in a minority of cases, e.g. MAG {1553}, GC {1075, 2178}, PLP and CNP {2178}, or their expression is not restricted to oligodendroglial tumour cells, e.g. carbonic anhydrase C {1554}.

Immunohistochemical expression of neuronal markers in oligodendroglioma is a complicated issue. Synaptophysin immunoreactivity due to residual neuropil is frequently seen, in particular at the infiltrating tumour borders. Such staining of tumour-infiltrated neuropil should not be mistaken as evidence for neuronal or neurocytic differentiation. However, some oligodendrogliomas, including cases with combined losses of 1p and 19q {1731}, may contain neoplastic cells that express synaptophysin and/or other neuronal markers, such as NeuN, neurofilaments and others {454, 1165, 1731, 2401}. 1p/19q

deletion analysis may be helpful to separate such cases from neurocytomas. Oligodendroglioma usually lacks nuclear p53 staining, a finding corresponding to the rarity of *TP53* gene mutations in these tumours. In fact, *TP53* mutation and p53 immunopositivity are mutually exclusive to 1p/19q deletion in oligodendroglial tumours {1226, 1625, 1634, 2432}.

Proliferation

Mitotic activity is low in WHO grade II oligodendroglioma, and labelling indices for proliferation markers are accordingly low, usually below 5%. Minigemistocytes are reported to be mostly MIB-1 negative and thus non-proliferative, whereas gliofibrillary oligodendrocytes are more commonly positive {1197}. Other proliferation markers, such as proliferating cell nuclear antigen (PCNA) {1854}, topoisomerase II α (Ki-S1) {1170} and minichromosome maintainance 2 (MCM2) protein {2400} also correlate with histological grade and survival in oligodendroglial tumours, but do not provide any clear advantages over MIB-1 staining.

Differential diagnosis

The differential diagnosis of oligodendroglioma includes both reactive and neo-plastic lesions. Among the former, oligodendroglioma needs to be distinguished from macrophage-rich processes such as demyelinating diseases or cerebral infarcts. In addition, increased numbers of oligodendrocytes sometimes seen in partial lobectomy specimens performed for intractable seizures should not be mistaken for oligodendroglioma.

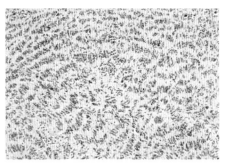

Fig. 2.06 Oligodendroglioma with a striking pattern of nuclear palisading.

Important neoplastic lesions that may mimic oligodendroglioma are clear cell ependymoma, neurocytoma and dysembryoplastic neuroepithelial tumour. These entities share with oligodendroglioma the presence of neoplastic cells with a uniform, round nucleus and clear cytoplasm, collectively referred to as oligodendroglial-like cells (OLC); these cells can readily be differentiated on the basis of their ultrastructural features {300}. In the routine diagnostic setting, immunostaining for neuronal markers, in particular synaptophysin, usually helps to distinguish neurocytoma from oligodendroglioma. However, rare cases of oligodendroglioma with deletion of 1p/19q and evidence of neurocytic differentiation have been reported {1731}. Clear cell ependymoma often shows at least focal perivascular pseudorosettes as well as dot- or ring-like EMA immunoreactivity, which helps to distinguish them from oligodendroglioma. Molecular analysis may be helpful since neurocytomas, clear cell ependymomas and DNTs lack 1p/19q losses. However, absence of 1p/19q deletion does not exclude an oligodendroglioma since a minor fraction of oligodendrogliomas in adults and the majority of paediatric oligodendrogliomas {1819} lack these deletions despite typical histology.

Pilocytic astrocytoma may occasionally mimic oligodendroglioma, however, at least foci of classic pilocytic features are usually present. A rare differential diagnosis is clear cell meningioma, which can readily be distinguished by abundant diastase-sensitive PAS positivity and immunoreactivity for EMA. Metastatic clear cell carcinoma differs from oligodendroglioma by its sharp tumour borders and immunoreactivity for cytokeratins and EMA.

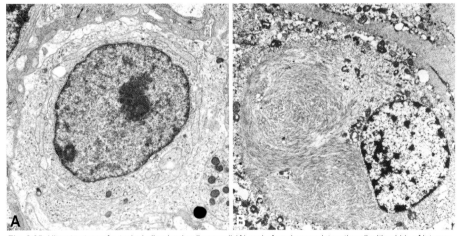

Fig. 2.05 Ultrastructure of a typical oligodendroglioma cell (**A**) and of a microgemistocytic cell with whirls of intermediate filaments (**B**).

Genetic susceptibility

Occasional familial clustering of oligodendroglioma has been reported: examples include two brothers {1681}, mother and daughter {1920}, twin sisters {1906} and a father and son {567}. Polymorphous oligodendroglioma has been reported in a brother and sister {1198}. Only occasional patients with an oligodendroglial tumour have been reported in families with hereditary cancer syndromes. In a survey of 47 families from Southern Sweden with BRCA1 mutations, one patient with an oligodendroglioma was reported {1001}. One patient with Turcot syndrome, who carried a germline mutation in exon 5 of the hPMS2 mismatch repair gene, developed two metachronous glioblastomas showing histological features of oligodendroglial differentiation {2228}. In addition, a child with retinoblastoma syndrome {18}, another child with oligodendroglioma and hereditary nonpolyposis colorectal cancer syndrome {1455}, and identical twins with oligodendroglioma and Ollier's disease have been documented {319}. Oligodendroglioma is rare in patients carrying a TP53 germline mutation (See Chapter 13). Studies of genetic polymorphisms, in as yet limited numbers of patients, have suggested that some polymorphisms are more frequently seen in patients with gliomas including oligodendroglioma; examples of positively correlated polymorphisms include the GSTT1 null genotype and polymorphisms in GLTSCR1 and ERCC2 {1074, 2460}.

Genetics

G-banded karyotypes of more than 60 oligodendrogliomas have been published {1379, 1829, 2237}. The vast majority showed normal or non-clonal karyotypes. A minor subset demonstrated simple clonal abnormalities, while occasional tumours had complex clonal karyotypes. Recently discovered is the frequent occurrence of an unbalanced translocation between chromosomes 1 and 19 [t(1;19) (q10;p10)] in oligodendroglioma {721, 989}, which appears responsible for the characteristic co-deletion of 1p and 19q in these tumours.

1p and 19q deletion. Concurrent deletion of chromosomal arms 1p and 19q constitutes the hallmark alteration in oligodendroglioma being found in up to 80% of cases {997, 1634, 1845}. Most tumours show losses of one entire copy of 1p and 19q due to an unbalanced t(1;19) (q10;p10) translocation {721, 989}, while partial deletions are rare in oligodendroglioma. 1p/19q deletions are more common in oligodendroglioma located in the frontal, parietal and occipital lobes as compared to locations in the temporal lobe, insula and diencephalon {1534, 2507}. The relevant tumour suppressor genes on these chromosomal arms are as yet unclear, although various candidates have been proposed. The CDKN2C gene at 1p32 showed point mutations or homozygous deletion in a minor fraction of anaplastic oligodendroglioma {1845}. Several other genes on 1p, including the calmodulin-binding transcription activator 1 gene the DNA fragmentation factor subunit ß gene, SHREW1, TP73 and RAD54, demonstrated reduced expression in 1p-deleted oligodendroglioma, sometimes associated with promoter hypermethylation but never with mutation {98, 480, 1429, 1430}. Reported candidate genes on 19q are p190RhoGAP {2429}, the myelin-related epithelial membrane protein gene 3 {31}, ZNF342 {860}, and the maternally imprinted PEG3 gene on 19q13.4 {2269}. However, none of these candidate genes has been definitively implicated.

Other genetic alterations. Several chromosomal aberrations other than 1p/19q deletion are found at more than random frequency in oligodendroglioma, most frequently gains on chromosome 7 and losses on chromosomes 4, 6, 11p, 14 and 22q {997, 1845}. Losses of chromosomes 9 and 10 are more common in anaplastic variants, although they can occasionally be detected in oligodendroglioma, including one case with a circumscribed 10q25-q26 deletion {1383}. In contrast to astrocytic tumours, loss of 17p and TP53 mutations are rare in oligodendroglial tumours and mutually exclusive to 1p/19q deletion {997, 1845}.

Epigenetic changes. Several genes have been demonstrated to be epigenetic silenced by aberrant promoter methylation in variable fractions of oligodendroglioma, including the tumour suppressors CDKN2A, p14ARF CDKN2B, and RB1, as well as DAPK1 (death-associated protein kinase 1), ESR1 (estrogen receptor 1), THBS (thrombospondin 1) and TIMP3 (tissue inhibitor of metalloproteinase 3) {1845}. MGMT promoter hypermethylation and reduced expression is also common, in particular among 1p/19q-deleted tumours {1506}.

Growth factors and receptors
About half of both WHO grade II and anaplastic oligodendrogliomas show strong expression of EGFR mRNA and protein in the absence of EGFR gene amplification {1849}. The simultaneous

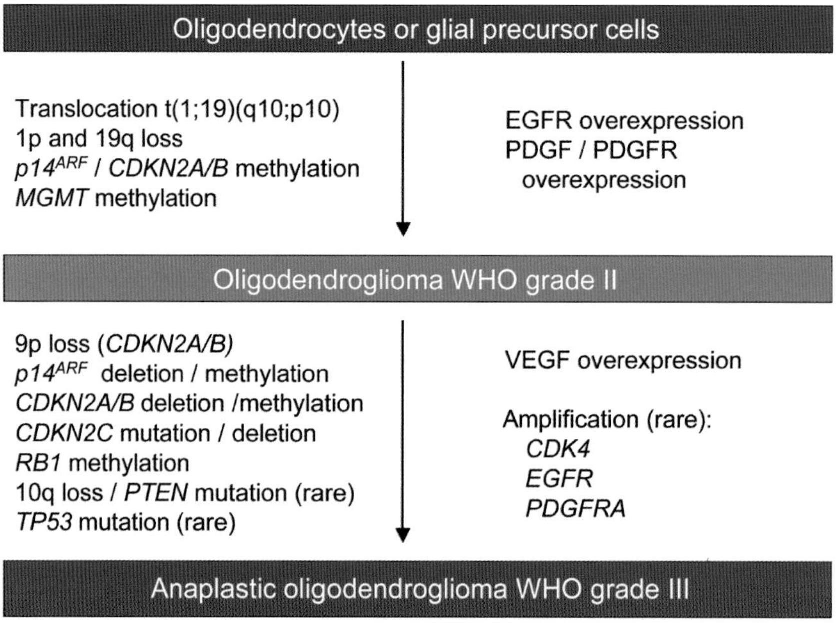

Fig. 2.07 Genetic alterations in oligodendroglial tumours.

expression of the mRNAs for the pre-pro-forms of EGF and/or TGFα indicates the possibility of auto-, juxta-, or paracrine growth stimulation via the EGFR system {512}. Several other growth factors, including basic FGF, PDGFs, TGFβ, IGF1 and NGF, have been reported to be involved in the regulation of proliferation and/or maturation of oligodendroglial cells {1845}. Platelet-derived growth factors A and B, as well as the corresponding receptors (PDGFR-α and PDGFR-β) are co-expressed in virtually all oligodendrogliomas {464}. Expression of vascular endothelial growth factor (VEGF) and its receptors play roles as angiogenic factors in oligodendroglial tumours, in particular in anaplastic oligodendroglioma {313, 347}.

Histogenesis

Although the designation of CNS neoplasms as oligodendroglial tumours implies a histogenesis from cells of the oligodendroglial lineage, evidence for this assumption is circumstantial and is based mainly on morphological similarities of the neoplastic cells in these tumours to normal oligodendrocytes. It is also not known whether human oligodendroglioma arises from neoplastic transformation of mature oligodendrocytes or immature glial precursors. Experimental data in transgenic mice suggests the likelihood that these tumours arise from progenitor cells {2082}, although it is interesting to note that an oligodendroglioma phenotype is commonly found in transgenic brain tumours, despite a variety of targeted cell types and oncogenic events {2391}. One suggested precursor cell has been the human equivalent of the rodent bipotential progenitor cell (designated O2-A progenitor), which may differentiate either into oligodendrocytes or type 2 astrocytes, but this hypothesis is unproven.

Prognostic and predictive factors

WHO grade II oligodendrogliomas are typically slowly growing tumours with relatively long survival times. A population-based study from Switzerland demonstrated a median survival time of 11.6 years and a 10-year survival rate of 51% {1625}. The Central Brain Tumour Registry of the United States has documented 5- and 10-year survival rates of 71% and 54%, respectively {305}. Estimates have varied markedly, however, with some studies documenting even longer median

overall survival times (e.g. over 15 years {1642}) and others shorter median survivals (e.g. 3.5 years {455}). Some of this variability may be accounted for by different diagnostic criteria (hence varying proportions of cases with 1p/19q loss) and differing treatment approaches. Malignant progression on recurrence is common, although it takes longer on average than in the setting of diffuse astrocytoma.

Clinical factors. Features associated with more favourable outcome include younger age at operation {2026, 2074}, frontal location {1199}, post-operative Karnofsky score {2026}, lack of contrast enhancement on neuroimaging {2074} and macroscopically complete surgical removal {455, 2074}.

Histopathology. Parameters that are associated with worse prognosis include necrosis, high mitotic activity, increased cellularity, nuclear atypia, cellular pleomorphism and microvascular proliferation (see anaplastic oligodendroglioma). The presence of minigemistocytes or gliofibrillary oligodendrocytes is not correlated to patient survival {1204}.

Proliferation. A number of studies have evaluated the prognostic significance of the Ki-67 (MIB-1) index {455, 800, 1197}. In general, higher proliferation rates (>3–5%), significantly correlate with worse prognosis. A study of 32 WHO grade II oligodendrogliomas {800} found that Ki-67 labelling indices of >3% were indicative of a worse prognosis, and a study of 89 oligodendroglioma patients documented a 5-year survival rate of 83% for patients whose oligodendroglioma had a MIB-1 labelling index of <5% but only 24% for patients with tumours displaying >5% MIB-1 positive cells {455}. Similar data {377} have discriminated two groups of patients with significantly different survival times when using a cut-off value of 5% MIB-1 positive cells. The value of measuring proliferation rates appears independent of patient age, tumour site, and histological grade {1197}.

Genetic alterations. Several retrospective studies have reported that 1p loss or combined 1p/19q loss is associated with longer patient survival in WHO grade II oligodendroglioma {563, 1039, 1226, 1994, 2113}. WHO grade II oligodendroglioma with 1p and 19q loss therefore appears to be a particularly slowly growing lesion, with survival times often

exceeding 10 years. In this regard, diagnostic testing for 1p and 19q status provides prognostic information in the setting of grade II oligodendroglioma. It is likely that 1p/19q status provides predictive as well as prognostic information in the setting of grade II oligodendroglioma; however, this has been more difficult to prove than in the setting of anaplastic oligodendroglioma because grade II oligodendroglioma shows less dramatic neuroradiological responses to therapy, requires long follow-up times for evaluation, and has high prevalence of 1p/19q loss. Nonetheless, small studies of low-grade oligodendroglioma patients treated with temozolomide have found that 1p loss is associated with objective radiological treatment response {846, 1300}. Such findings suggest that the longer survivals noted in such patients may reflect a combination of more indolent natural behaviour as well as greater therapeutic sensitivity.

Anaplastic oligodendroglioma

G. Reifenberger
J.M. Kros
D.N. Louis
V.P. Collins

Definition

An oligodendroglioma with focal or diffuse histological features of malignancy and a less favourable prognosis.

ICD-O code   9451/3

Grading

Anaplastic oligodendroglioma corresponds histologically to WHO grade III.

Anaplastic features that have been linked to malignancy in oligodendroglioma are similar to those in astrocytic gliomas, i.e. high cellularity, marked cytological atypia, high mitotic activity, microvascular proliferation and necrosis with or without pseudopalisading. Anaplastic oligodendroglioma usually shows several of these features. However, the individual impact of each parameter is not quite clear, although it has been argued that endothelial proliferation and mitotic activity are of particular importance {680}. Thus, the diagnosis of an anaplastic oligodendroglioma should require either the presence of conspicuous microvascular proliferation and/or high mitotic activity. In borderline cases, immunostaining for MIB-1 and attention to clinical and neuroradiological features such as rapid symptomatic growth and contrast enhancement may be helpful in assessing prognosis.

Incidence

Anaplastic oligodendroglioma accounts for approximately 1.2% of all primary brain tumours and adjusted annual incidence rates ranging from 0.07 to 0.18 per 100 000 population have been reported {305, 1625}. In population-based series, approximately 20–35% of oligodendroglial tumours are anaplastic oligodendrogliomas {305, 1625}.

Age and sex distribution

Anaplastic oligodendroglioma manifests preferentially in adults, with a peak incidence between 45 and 50 years of age {305, 1625, 2301}. Thus, patients with anaplastic oligodendroglioma manifest

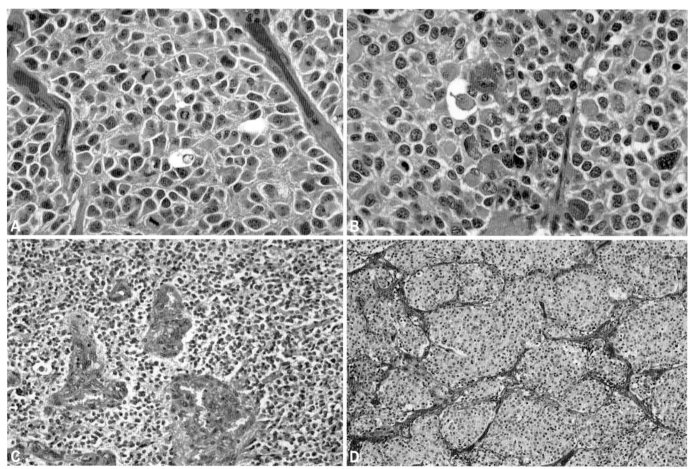

Fig. 2.08 A and **B** Anaplastic oligodendroglioma showing marked nuclear atypia and brisk mitotic activity. **C** Marked microvascular proliferation. **D** Highly cellular anaplastic oligodendroglioma with branching capillary network.

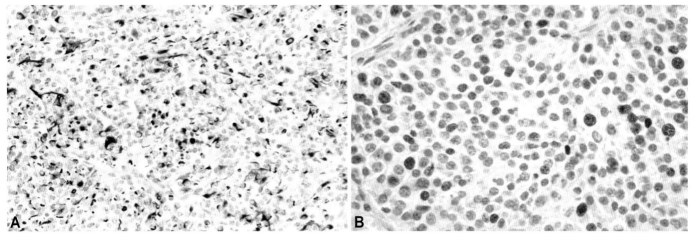

Fig. 2.09 Anaplastic oligodendroglioma. **A** Variable GFAP immunoreactivity. **B** High proliferative activity (MIB-1).

approximately 7–8 years later on average than patients with WHO grade II oligo-dendroglioma {305, 1625}. Anaplastic oligodendroglioma shows a slight male predominance, with a male:female ratio of 1.1:1 reported in a population-based series of 781 patients {305}.

Localization
Anaplastic oligodendroglioma shares with WHO grade II oligodendroglioma a preference for the frontal lobe, followed by the temporal lobe.

Clinical features
Symptoms and signs
Anaplastic oligodendroglioma may develop either *de novo* or by progression from a pre-existing WHO grade II oligodendro-glioma. The preoperative history of patients with *de novo* tumours is usually short with seizures being the most common presenting symptom {1269}. Some patients may present with long-standing signs, suggesting a pre-existing tumour of lower grade. The mean time to progression from WHO grade II oligodendroglioma to secondary anaplastic oligodendroglioma is approximately 6–7 years {1269, 1625}.

Neuroimaging
Anaplastic oligodendroglioma may show heterogeneous patterns, owing to the variable presence of necrosis, cystic degeneration, intratumoural haemorrhages and calcification. Contrast enhancement on CT and MRI is usual and may be patchy or homogeneous. Ring-enhancement is uncommon and, when present, heralds a poor prognosis {276}.

Macroscopy
The macroscopic features are similar to those of WHO grade II oligodendroglioma, except that anaplastic oligodendroglioma may demonstrate areas of tumour necrosis.

Histopathology
Anaplastic oligodendroglioma is a cellular, diffusely infiltrating glioma that may show considerable morphological variation. The majority of tumour cells demonstrate features that are reminiscent of oligo-dendroglial cells, i.e. rounded hyper-chromatic nuclei, perinuclear halos, and few cellular processes. Focal micro-calcifications are often present. Mitotic activity is usually prominent. Occasional tumours are characterized by marked cellular pleomorphism with multinucleated giant cells (polymorphic variant of Zülch {2514}), or have a conspicuous spindle-cell appearance. Rare cases with sarcoma-like tumour areas have also been observed {561, 1685}. Gliofibrillary oligo-dendrocytes and minigemistocytes are frequent in anaplastic oligodendroglioma; they do not argue against the diagnosis and are not of prognostic significance {1204}. The characteristic vascular pattern of branching capillaries is typically still recognizable, although pathological microvascular proliferation is often prominent. In addition, anaplastic oligo-dendrogliomas may feature areas of necrosis, including pseudopalisading necroses resembling those of glio-blastoma. However, if the tumour shows the typical cytological characteristics and other histological hallmarks of oligo-dendrogliomas, such as the branching capillary network and microcalcifica-

tions, classification as anaplastic oligo-dendroglioma WHO grade III is appropriate. A study on 1093 adults with newly-diagnosed high-grade gliomas showed that the presence of necrosis, in contrast to anaplastic oligoastrocytoma, is not indicative of shorter survival in patients with anaplastic oligodendro-glioma {1474}. Thus, if an anaplastic oligodendroglial tumour shows a significant astrocytic component, classification as anaplastic oligoastrocytoma is more appropriate and the presence of necrosis then is indicative of less favourable prog-nosis (see Anaplastic oligoastrocytoma). In such cases the presence of necrosis should be considered as a prognostically unfavourable.

Genetics
Chromosomal and array-based compar-ative genomic hybridization studies have revealed total losses of 1p and 19q in up to two thirds of anaplastic oligodendro-gliomas, which is slightly less common than in WHO grade II oligodendroglioma. Several studies identified additional chromosomal abnormalities in anaplastic oligodendroglioma; these include gains on 7 and 15q, as well as losses on 4q, 6, 9p, 10q, 11, 13q, 18 and 22q {997,1845}. Double minute chromosomes, a cyto-genetic hallmark of gene amplification, have been reported in occasional cases {2237}.
The average number of chromosomes involved in copy number abnormalities and loss of alleles is higher in anaplastic oligodendroglioma than in WHO grade II oligodendroglioma {166, 1850, 1907}, a finding in line with the hypothesis that

malignant progression is associated with the acquisition of multiple genetic abnormalities. Although the most frequent genetic alterations encountered in oligodendroglial tumours, i.e., 1p and 19q losses, differ significantly from those in astrocytoma, the current limited data on the genes involved in malignant progression indicate common molecular mechanisms. There is an increased incidence of deletions on the short arm of chromosome 9. The tumour suppressor locus CDKN2A at 9p21, which codes for $p16^{INK4A}$ and $p14^{ARF}$, is homozygously deleted in up to a third of anaplastic oligodendrogliomas, including tumours both with and without 1p/19q loss, albeit being somewhat more common in 1p/19q-deleted tumours {166, 276, 997, 1845}. Homozygous deletion or mutation of the CDKN2C gene at 1p32 has been observed in rare anaplastic oligodendrogliomas that do not carry CDKN2A deletions {896,1765}. Losses of 10q are infrequent occurring in only approximately 10% of cases {1993}. Mutations of the retained copy of the PTEN gene occur in about half of the cases with 10q loss, suggesting that there may be another progression-related gene target in the region {546, 997, 1845, 1993}. Anaplastic oligodendroglioma with loss of chromosome 10 and gain of chromosome 7 often lacks deletions on 1p and 19q. Rare tumours have activating mutations of the PI3KCA gene {225}. A small subset (<10%) of anaplastic oligodendrogliomas may demonstrate amplification of proto-oncogenes, including EGFR, PDGFRA, MYC, MYCN, CDK4, MDM2 and MDM4 {997,1845}. In addition, several genes have been shown to be epigenetically silenced in subsets of oligodendroglial tumours including anaplastic oligodendroglioma (see Oligodendroglioma).

Prognostic and predictive factors
Recent therapeutic advances have improved survival times of patients with anaplastic oligodendrogliomas. Reports antedating the advent of combined chemotherapy-radiotherapy—particularly those antedating the procarbazine, CCNU and vincristine (PCV) regimens—demonstrated relatively shorter survival times. For example, median survival has been reported to range from less than 1 year {455} to 3.9 years {2074}. A population-based analysis noted a median survival time of 3.5 years {1625}. Combination of chemotherapy-radiation therapy significantly prolongs progression-free survival (to approximately 2–2.5 years) and yields overall survival times of about 4–5 years {275, 2301}. In individual patients, notably longer survivals have been reported, typically in patients with 1p and 19q loss {276}. Indeed, prognosis is tightly linked to the allelic status of 1p and 19q {276}. In one large prospective trial, patients whose tumours lost 1p and 19q had markedly longer median survival times (>7 years compared to 2.8 years in patients whose tumours did not have 1p and 19q loss), and improvements in progression-free survival were most significant in this group {275}. Another large prospective trial showed that three-fourths of patients whose tumours had 1p and 19q loss were alive 5 years after diagnosis {2301}. Analysis of other genetic parameters, such as CDKN2A deletion, PTEN mutation or chromosome 10 loss, may also provide prognostic information {546,1845}, but the results of such analyses are less powerful than 1p/19q status and have not been as extensively validated.

In addition to 1p/19q status, better prognosis has been noted in younger patients, those with better performance status and those receiving more extensive resections {275, 2074, 2301}. On the other hand, ring enhancement on initial neuroimaging has also been reported to correlate with a lack of response to PCV chemotherapy and poor prognosis {276}. Most patients die from local tumour recurrence. Occasionally, patients may develop metastases via the CSF or even systemic metastases {1370,1461}. A rare complication of both oligodendroglioma and anaplastic oligodendroglioma is leptomeningeal 'oligodendrogliomatosis' {594,1755}. Occasional patients may present with primary leptomeningeal oligodendrogliomatosis in the absence of any solid tumour {1588}.

In addition to prognostic importance, molecular genetic analysis of 1p and 19q status appears to have predictive importance, providing information about the likelihood of response to therapy {276}. Although the use of 1p and 19q testing varies in terms of how results affect therapeutic decisions, 1p and 19q analysis is commonly performed {8}. Those anaplastic oligodendrogliomas that have allelic loss on the short arm of chromosome 1, or combined allelic losses on 1p and 19q, are typically sensitive to PCV chemotherapy, with many such tumours showing complete neuro-radiological responses to PCV {276}. Large prospective trials have shown improved responses to both radiation therapy alone and to combined radiation-PCV chemotherapy in patients whose tumours harbour 1p and 19q loss {275, 2301}. Responses to temozolomide as initial chemotherapy also appear related to 1p status {2206}. Overall, however, it remains unclear if improved responses are specific to particular therapies; more likely, tumours with 1p and 19q loss are biologically distinct entities that feature sensitivity to a variety of cytotoxic therapeutic approaches.

Oligoastrocytoma

A. von Deimling
G. Reifenberger
J.M. Kros
D.N. Louis
V.P. Collins

Definition

A diffusely infiltrating glioma composed of a conspicuous mixture of two distinct neoplastic cell types morphologically resembling the tumour cells in oligo-dendroglioma and diffuse astrocytoma of WHO grade II.

ICD-O code   9382/3

Grading

Oligoastrocytoma corresponds histo-logically to WHO grade II.

Historical annotation

Mixed oligoastrocytoma was first recog-nized as an entity by Cooper in 1935 {379}.

Incidence

Over the last 10 years the reported incidence of oligoastrocytoma has been increasing; this is probably a result of varying pathological criteria and to some degree increased recognition {248}, and must be interpreted with caution. Among 4859 patients with intracranial glioma registered by the Norwegian Cancer Registry between 1956 and 1984, mixed glioma accounted for 9.2% of the tumours {805}. Another study reported an incidence between 10 and 19% of supratentorial low-grade glioma {976}. In contrast, among 5216 gliomas registered from 1990–1992 by the Central Brain Tumour Registry of the United States of America, only 96 tumours were listed under the diagnosis mixed glioma (1.8%) {305}. The annual incidence was estimated as 0.1 per 100 000 individuals.

Age and sex distribution

Oligoastrocytoma usually develops in middle-aged indiviuals, with a median age at operation between 35 and 45 years {305,976,1625}. Males are affected slightly more frequently than females, with ratios of 1.3:1 in the Central Brain Tumour Registry of the United States {305} and 1.7:1 in a smaller series of 20 low-grade and 10 anaplastic oligo-astrocytomas {125}.

Etiology

DNA sequences similar to those of the JC virus, the etiologic agent of progressive multifocal leukoencephalopathy, have been detected in a human oligoastrocytoma and viral antigen was found to be expressed in the tumour cells {1859}. However, a possible role of the JC virus in the development of glial neoplasms requires further corroboration.

Localization

Oligoastrocytoma arises preferentially in the cerebral hemispheres. The order of site frequency parallels the relative sizes of the cerebral lobes: frontal, temporal, parietal, occipital {125, 1534, 2073}. Occasional oligoastrocytomas are encoun-tered in the brain stem, but cerebellar localization is very uncommon.

Clinical features

Symptoms and signs

Oligoastrocytoma presents with symptoms and signs similar to those described for astrocytomas and oligodendrogliomas, most commonly epileptic seizures, paresis, personality changes, and signs of increased intracranial pressure {125, 2073}.

Neuroimaging

Neuroradiologically, oligoastrocytoma demonstrates no specific features. In the series of Shaw et al. {2073}, calcifications were demonstrable in 14% of the tumours; however, the criteria used to define pure oligodendroglioma in this series were not clear.

Macroscopy

The macroscopical appearance of oligoastrocytoma does not usually allow their distinction from other WHO grade II gliomas. Only occasionally are there regional differences in colour and consis-tency reflecting areas of distinct cellular differentiation.

Histopathology

Oligoastrocytomas are moderately cellular neoplasms with no or low mitotic activity.

Microcalcifications and microcystic degeneration may be present but necrosis and microvascular proliferation are absent.

The diagnosis of oligoastrocytoma requires the recognition of neoplastic glial cells with convincing astrocytic or oligo-dendroglial phenotypes. Oligoastrocytoma may be divided into biphasic ("compact") and intermingled ("diffuse") variants {773}. In the biphasic variant, which is rare, distinct areas of oligodendroglial and astrocytic differentiation are juxta-posed. This histopathology should not be confused with that of classic oligoden-droglioma, in which the margins are often indistinguishable from fibrillary astro-cytoma. In the most common variant of mixed oligoastrocytoma, both oligo-dendroglial and astrocytic tumour cells are intimately mixed. A diffuse admixture in oligodendroglioma of GFAP-positive minigemistocytes and gliofibrillary oligo-dendrocytes should not prompt the diagnosis of oligoastrocytoma instead of oligodendroglioma. Only tumours in which fibrillary, protoplasmic or classic gemistocytic astrocytic cells are present, in addition to the oligodendroglial tumour cells, qualify for the diagnosis of oligo-astrocytoma. In the presence of numerous minigemistocytes, a careful search for an astrocytic component should be performed. A particular nosological problem are tumours composed of cells with phenotypical characteristics some-where in between those of oligodendroglial and astrocytic tumour cells.

The pronounced phenotypic heterogeneity of the astroglial and oligodendroglial cell lineages and a lack of reliable markers make it difficult to define diagnostic criteria. It has been recommended to assess the fractions of the two compo-nents, but opinions diverge, with the proposed minimum astroglial component ranging up to 50% {894, 1108}. In most instances the precise extent of each component is difficult to determine since tumour cells may not always be easily recognized as either oligodendroglial or astrocytic, i.e. they may have features of

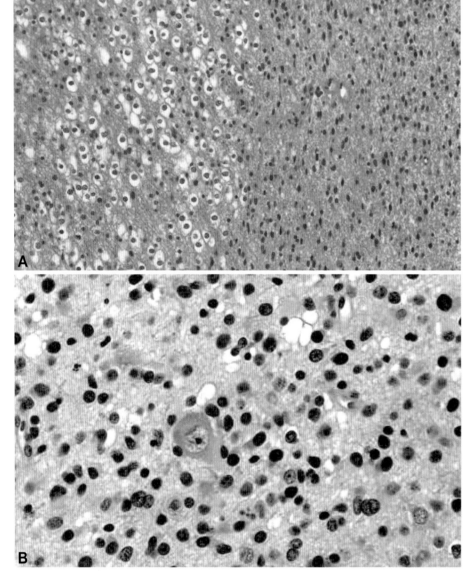

components. GFAP and vimentin expression are more consistently found in the astroglial component, compared with a more variable expression in the oligodendroglial tumour cells. In support of this immunohistochemical data, analysis of GFAP and its fragments by two-dimensional gel electrophoresis and Western blot analysis has allowed a discrimination of astrocytoma from oligodendroglioma {1357}. However, these techniques are not suitable as routine diagnostic methods and cannot be applied to oligoastrocytoma with a diffuse mixture of both cell types. Approximately one third of the oligoastrocytoma demonstrates nuclear p53 accumulation {125}.

Fig. 2.10 A Oligoastrocytoma with distinct components displaying oligodendroglial (left) and astrocytic (right) differentiation. **B** Oligoastrocytoma, intermingled ("diffuse") variant. Nuclear cytology ranges from rounded profiles with minimal atypia, crisp nuclear membranes, and small nucleoli to irregular, hyperchromatic forms.

Proliferation
Immunocytochemistry for the Ki-67 proliferation-associated nuclear antigen generally correlates well with the presence or absence of features of anaplasia in oligoastrocytoma, with an average value of less than 6% reported in a series of 20 tumours {448, 2083}. Expression of p21 correlated with outcome in oligoastrocytoma {796}.

Genetic susceptibility
Two family members with cerebral low-grade diffuse astrocytoma and cerebellar oligoastrocytoma have been reported {312}. Further, oligoastrocytoma was observed in identical twins {545}. Another study reported two siblings with glioblastoma and mixed oligoastrocytoma, respectively {2293}. No data are available on germline mutations in cases of familial clustering of oligoastrocytoma.

Genetics
The molecular genetic alterations underlying the oncogenesis and progression of oligoastrocytoma resemble those of oligodendroglioma and astrocytoma. About 30–50% of oligoastrocytomas are characterized by combined loss of genetic information on chromosomes 1p and 19q {1184, 1386, 1634, 1850}. The mechanisms leading to 1p and 19q deletions in oligoastrocytoma are likely to be similar to those in oligodendroglioma. About 30% of oligoastrocytomas carry mutations of the *TP53* gene {1386, 1534, 1634, 1850}. Oligoastrocytoma with *TP53* mutations tends not to have combined LOH on 1p and 19q, and vice versa {1386, 1534, 1850}. This suggests that

both lineages. Various studies have been undertaken to estimate interobserver concordance in gliomas with an oligodendroglial tumour component {378, 628, 1194}. Because of the poor delineation of the cell lineages causing considerable subjectivity in histological evaluation, interobserver variability for oligoastrocytoma is significantly larger compared to that for pure glioma {628, 1194}.

There is no specific grading scheme for oligoastrocytoma. The features that are commonly used for diffuse glioma, i.e., cellularity, mitotic activity, nuclear pleomorphism, microvascular proliferation

and necrosis, are also used for oligoastrocytomas. Necrosis and microvascular proliferation showed highest concordance in pathology panel review {1194}, and necrosis is considered a feature with independent prognostic value.

Immunohistochemistry
The oligodendroglial and astroglial components in oligoastrocytoma show the same immunoreactivity patterns as 'pure' oligodendroglioma and astrocytoma, respectively. There is no specific immunocytochemical marker that can be used for the reliable distinction of both

oligoastrocytomas are clonal neoplasms originating from a single precursor cell rather than representing composition tumours that had developed concurrently. Oligoastrocytoma of the temporal lobe is more frequently characterized by *TP53* mutations and less frequently by deletions of 1p and 19q than those from other localizations {528, 1534}. Taken together, these data indicate that tumours morphologically classified as oligoastrocytoma are genetically heterogeneous. One subset appears to be genetically related to oligodendroglial tumours, while another is genetically related to diffuse astrocytomas. The biological basis of the presence of two distinct glial phenotypes in each of these tumours remains to be elucidated.

Histogenesis

The histogenesis of oligoastrocytoma is unresolved, but derivation from a multipotent progenitor cell able to undergo astrocytic and oligodendroglial differentiation is a tenable hypothesis supported by transgenic mouse studies.

Prognosis and predictive factors

A median survival time of 6.3 years and 5- and 10-year survival rates of 58% and 32%, respectively, have been reported in a study of 60 patients with low-grade (Kernohan grade 1 and 2) oligoastrocytoma {2073}. A population-based study noted a median survival time of 6.6

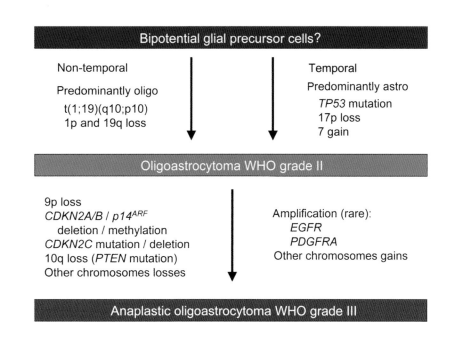

Fig. 2.11 Genetic alterations involved in the development of oligoastrocytoma and anaplastic oligoastrocytoma.

years and a 10-year survival rate of 49% {1634}. Factors associated with longer survival include younger age at operation (less than 37 years), gross total tumour resection, and postoperative radiation therapy {2073} as well as lower Ki-67 indices {2058}. Notably, as for oligodendroglioma, favourable prognosis appears associated with combined loss of 1p and 19q {528, 846}; a progression-

free survival time of 60 months was observed in patients whose tumours had 1p and 19q loss, compared with 30 months in patients whose tumours lacked these changes {528}. In a small series, response to temozolomide was also suggested to be associated with combined loss of 1p and 19q {846}.

Anaplastic oligoastrocytoma

A. von Deimling
G. Reifenberger
J.M. Kros
D.N. Louis
V.P. Collins

Definition

An oligoastrocytoma with histological features of malignancy, such as increased cellularity, nuclear atypia, pleomorphism and increased mitotic activity.

ICD-O code   9382/3

Grading

Anaplastic oligoastrocytoma corresponds histologically to WHO grade III.

Incidence

Precise epidemiological data on the incidence of anaplastic oligoastrocytoma are not available. The limited published data are confounded by the source of patients and the variability in the histological classification of these tumours. In a population-based series from Switzerland, only 11 tumours out of 987 (1%) oligodendroglial and astrocytic gliomas were diagnosed as anaplastic oligoastrocytoma {1625}. In a series of 285 supratentorial anaplastic gliomas in adults, anaplastic oligoastrocytoma accounted for 11 tumours (4%) {2419}. A single-institution review of 1093 patients with newly-diagnosed cerebral malignant gliomas in adults included 215 anaplastic oligoastrocytoma patients (20%); however, this high percentage may be an overestimate due to a consultation bias {1475}. In prospective trials on patients with anaplastic oligodendroglioma and anaplastic oligoastrocytoma, the latter accounted for 27% {2301} and 49% {275} of the cases.

Age and sex distribution

The incidence peaks in the fifth decade, with mean age at diagnosis of 44 years reported in 215 patients {1475}. The male to female ratio was 1.15:1 {1475}.

Localization

Anaplastic oligoastrocytomas are predominantly hemispheric tumours, with more

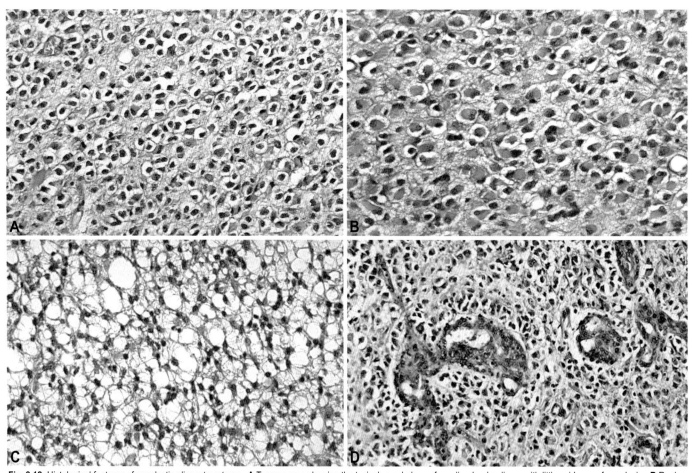

Fig. 2.12 Histological features of anaplastic oligoastrocytoma. **A** Tumour area showing the typical morphology of an oligodendroglioma with little evidence of anaplasia. **B** Region with marked nuclear atypia and numerous minigemistocytes. **C** Another area of the same tumour showing fibrillary astrocytic differentiation. **D** Marked microvascular proliferation in the same tumour.

than half of the tumours arising in the frontal lobe, followed by the temporal lobe.

Clinical features
Symptoms and signs
The clinical history of patients with anaplastic oligoastrocytoma is usually short. However, a preoperative history of several years may occasionally be encountered, suggesting a pre-existing low-grade glioma.

Neuroimaging
Anaplastic oligoastrocytoma usually shows contrast enhancement on CT and MRI.

Macroscopy
There are no consistent features that would allow the macroscopic distinction of anaplastic oligoastrocytoma from other anaplastic glioma types. Intra-tumoural haemorrhages may be seen, as well as areas of cystic degeneration and calcifications.

Histopathology
Anaplastic oligoastrocytomas are oligo-astrocytomas with histological features of anaplasia, including nuclear atypia, cellular pleomorphism, high cellularity, and high mitotic activity. In addition, microvascular proliferation may be present. The differential diagnosis of anaplastic oligoastrocytoma primarily includes anaplastic oligodendroglioma, anaplastic astrocytoma and glioblastoma. The identification of an astrocytoma component can be particularly challenging in a high-grade oligodendroglioma with considerable pleomorphism or in the presence of many gemistocytic cells, often in transition from minigemistocytes to classical gemistocytes.

Genetics
Anaplastic oligoastrocytoma typically exhibits the type and distribution of molecular lesions observed in oligo-astrocytoma, i.e. loss of 1p/19q or *TP53* mutations {1534}. With respect to progression-associated genetic abnor-malities, anaplastic oligoastrocytoma has been found to share many alterations that are also implicated in the progression of astrocytoma and oligodendroglioma, including allelic loss of 9p and homozygous deletion of *CDKN2A*, as well as allelic loss on chromosomes 10 and 11p {1850}. Individual cases of anaplastic oligoastrocytoma with amplification of the *EGFR* gene have been reported {1850}.

Prognostic and predictive factors
The prognosis of patients with anaplastic oligoastrocytoma is better than for patients with classical glioblastoma. A median survival time of 2.8 years and 5- and 10-year survival rates of 36% and 9%, respectively, have been reported for anaplastic oligoastrocytoma {2073} in a study of 11 patients treated by operation and postoperative radiation therapy. A study on 19 patients with anaplastic oligoastrocytoma treated by operation, irradiation, and PCV chemotherapy, however, noted a median survival time of 49.8 months {1108}. In this study, seven patients with anaplastic oligodendro-glioma treated in the same way showed a considerably longer median survival time of 76 months, most likely reflecting a subset of the cases with favourable genotype.

Important prognostic markers include necrosis and 1p status. One study of 180 patients with anaplastic oligoastrocytoma suggests that necrosis is associated with significantly worse prognosis {1474}. Anaplastic oligoastrocytoma with necrosis should be classified as "glioblastoma with oligodendroglial component" (see Glioblastoma chapter), although it may carry a better prognosis than standard glioblastoma {799,1185}. Some of these differences, however, may be related to 1p loss, since 1p loss was powerfully prognostic of improved progression-free and overall survival in a series of 48 anaplastic oligoastrocytomas {528}.

CHAPTER 3

Ependymal Tumours

Subependymoma (WHO grade I)
A slowly growing, benign neoplasm, typically attached to a ventricular wall, composed of glial tumour cell clusters embedded in an abundant fibrillary matrix with frequent microcystic change.

Myxopapillary ependymoma (WHO grade I)
A slowly growing ependymal glioma with preferential manifestation in young adults and almost exclusive location in the region of the conus medullaris, cauda equina and filum terminale of the spinal cord; typically characterized histologically by tumour cells arranged in a papillary manner around vascularized myxoid stromal cores.

Ependymoma (WHO grade II)
A generally slowly growing tumour of children and young adults, originating from the wall of the ventricles or from the spinal canal and composed of neoplastic ependymal cells.

Anaplastic ependymoma (WHO grade III)
A malignant glioma of ependymal differentiation with accelerated growth and unfavourable clinical outcome, particularly in children; histologically characterized by high mitotic activity, often accompanied by microvascular proliferation and pseudopalisading necrosis.

Subependymoma

R.E. McLendon
D. Schiffer
M.K. Rosenblum
O.D. Wiestler

Definition

A slowly growing, benign neoplasm, typically attached to a ventricular wall, composed of glial tumour cell clusters embedded in an abundant fibrillary matrix with frequent microcystic change.

ICD-O code   9383/1

Grading

Subependymoma corresponds histologically to WHO grade I.

Synonyms and historical annotation

Subependymoma was first described by Scheinker in 1945 {2005}. Alternative designations include subependymal astrocytoma and subependymal glomerate astrocytoma {617}, but the use of these terms is discouraged.

Incidence

The true incidence of subependymomas is difficult to determine, because these tumours frequently remain asymptomatic and are often found incidentally at autopsy. In two studies, they accounted for approximately 8% of ependymal tumours {1236, 2024}.

Age and sex distribution

Subependymomas develop in both sexes and in all age groups, but occur most frequently in middle-aged and elderly patients. The male:female ratio is approximately 2.3:1.

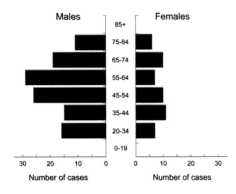

Fig. 3.01 Age and sex distribution of subependymoma, based on 167 cases. Data from CBTRUS 1995-2002.

Localization

The most frequent site is the fourth ventricle (50–60% of cases), followed by the lateral ventricles (30–40%). Less common sites include the third ventricle and septum pellucidum. In the spinal cord, subependymomas manifest as cervical and cervico-thoracic intramedullary or, rarely, extramedullary mass lesions {965}.

Clinical features

Symptoms and signs

Subependymomas may become clinically apparent through ventricular obstruction and raised intracranial pressure. Spontaneous intratumoural haemorrhage has been observed. Spinal tumours manifest with motor and sensory deficits according to the affected anatomical segment. Incidental detection of asymptomatic subependymomas at autopsy is not uncommon.

Neuroimaging

Subependymomas are sharply demarcated, nodular masses that are usually non-enhancing. Calcification and foci of haemorrhage may be apparent. Intramedullary examples are typically eccentric in location, rather than centrally positioned as is typical of intraspinal ependymomas. These lesions are hypo- to hyperintense on T1- and T2-weighted MRI, with minimal to moderate enhancement {1818}.

Macroscopy

These tumours present as firm nodules of variable size, bulging into the ventricular lumen. In most instances, the diameter does not exceed 1–2 cm. Intraventricular as well as spinal subependymomas are generally well demarcated. Large subependymomas of the fourth ventricle may cause brain stem compression.

Histopathology

Subependymomas are characterized by clusters of isomorphic nuclei embedded in a dense fibrillary matrix of glial cell processes with frequent occurrence of small cysts, particularly in lesions

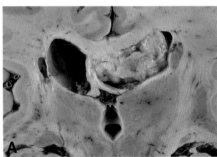

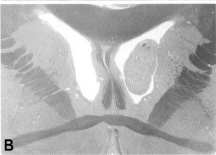

Fig. 3.02 **A** Subependymoma of the lateral ventricle originating from the roof of the lateral ventricle. **B** Subependymoma of the lateral ventricle.

originating in the lateral ventricles. Mitoses are rare or absent.

Tumour cell nuclei appear isomorphic and resemble those of subependymal glia. In solid tumours, occasional pleomorphic nuclei may be encountered, however, nuclear variation, sometimes of a disturbing quality, is the rule in multicystic tumours. Some subependymomas exhibit low-level mitotic activity, but this is exceptional. Calcifications and haemorrhage can occur. Prominent tumour vasculature may be accompanied by microvascular proliferation. Occasionally, cell processes are oriented around vessels, thus forming ependymal pseudorosettes. In some cases, subependymomas represent the most superficial aspects of a cellular ependymoma; such combined tumours are classified as mixed ependymoma/subependymoma and are graded based on the ependymoma component. On record are examples of subependymoma with melanin formation {1931}, rhabdomyosarcomatous differentiation {2257}, and sarcomatous transformation of

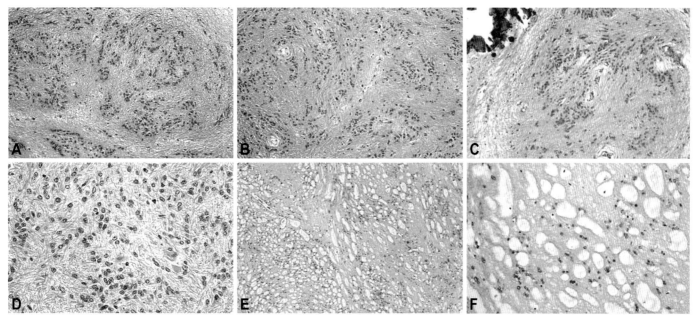

Fig. 3.03 Histological features of fourth ventricle subependymoma. **A** Lobular architecture and clustered nuclei. **B** Clustered nuclei and fibrillary stroma. **C** Clustered nuclei, lobular pattern and calcification. **D** Bland nuclei and abundant fibrillary stroma. **E** Microcystic degeneration. **F** High power of microcystic change.

vascular stromal elements {1351}. Immunoreactivity for GFAP is usually present, although to a variable extent, and positivity can be found for neuronal markers of low specificity (NCAM and neuron specific enolase) {2474}.

Electron microscopy
At the ultrastructural level, subependymomas show cells with typical ependymal characteristics, including cilia formation and microvilli, and sometimes with abundant intermediate filaments {76, 1528, 2018}

Proliferation
Mitotic activity is usually low or absent. Scattered mitoses and cellular pleomorphism are of no clinical significance {1342}. MIB-1 studies revealed labelling indices below 1%, compatible with the slow growth of this entity.

Genetic susceptibility
Rare familial cases have been described {1965}. The simultaneous clinical manifestation of infratentorial subependymomas in identical twins has been reported {355}.

Genetics
Consistent cytogenetic aberrations have not yet been uncovered {411A}. A molecular genetic analysis of 2 subependymomas for allelic deletions on chromosomes 10q and 22q and for point mutations of the *NF2* and *PTEN* tumour suppressor genes did not reveal any changes at these loci {504}.

Histogenesis
Proposed cells of origin include subependymal glia {76,1528}, astrocytes of the subependymal plate, ependymal cells {1959} and a mixture of astrocytes and ependymal cells {617, 2006}.

Development from subependymal glial precursors appears most likely.

Prognostic and predictive factors
Subependymomas carry a good prognosis. Surgical removal is usually curative in cerebral as well as spinal subependymomas. Recurrences have been reported following incomplete resection {2358}. Neoplasms with a mixed ependymoma and subependymoma morphology appear to follow a clinical course corresponding to the ependymoma component (WHO grades II-III).

Myxopapillary ependymoma

R.E. McLendon
M.K. Rosenblum
D. Schiffer
O.D. Wiestler

Definition

A slowly growing ependymal glioma with preferential manifestation in young adults and almost exclusive location in the region of the conus medullaris, cauda equina and filum terminale of the spinal cord; typically characterized histologically by tumour cells arranged in a papillary manner around vascularized myxoid stromal cores.

ICD-O code   9394/1

Grading

These slowly growing tumours have a favourable prognosis and correspond to WHO grade I. Anaplastic variants are virtually unknown.

Historical annotation

In his original description of 1932, Kernohan {1092} defined the distinct morphological properties and preferential location of this entity.

Incidence

Among all ependymomas, the frequency of myxopapillary variants is 9–13% {1236, 2024}. In the conus medullaris/cauda equina region, myxopapillary ependymomas constitute the most common intramedullary neoplasm having an approximate incidence of 0.08 in males and 0.05 per 100 000 persons per year in females {305}.

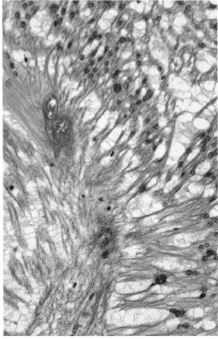

Fig. 3.05 Myxopapillary ependymoma showing radial perivascular arrangement of tumour cell processes.

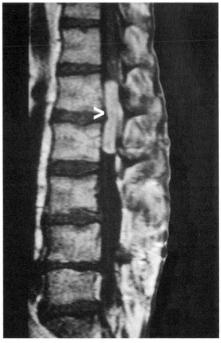

Fig. 3.06 MRI of a myxopapillary ependymoma of the filum terminale (arrow) presenting as a hyperintense spinal mass.

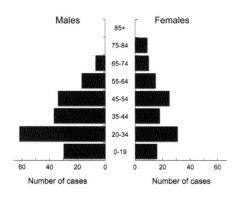

Fig. 3.04 Age and sex distribution of myxopapillary ependymoma, based on 311 patients. Data from CBTRUS 1995–2002.

Age and sex distribution

An average age at manifestation of 36 years has been reported, with a broad range between 6 and 82 years. In a study of 320 ependymomas of the filum terminale, 83% were of the myxopapillary type, with a male:female ratio of 2.2:1 {311}.

Localization

Myxopapillary ependymomas occur almost exclusively in the conus medullaris-cauda equina-filum terminale region. They may originate from ependymal glia of the filum terminale, involve the cauda equina, and only rarely invade nerve roots or erode sacral bone. Multifocal tumours have been described {1555}. Myxopapillary ependymomas can occasionally be observed at other locations, such as the cervical-thoracic spinal cord {2125}, the fourth ventricle {1322}, the lateral ventricle {1995}, or the brain parenchyma {2366}. Subcutaneous sacrococcygeal or pre-sacral myxopapillary ependymomas

represent a distinct subgroup. They appear to originate from ectopic ependymal remnants {909}. Intrasacral variants may masquerade clinically as chordoma.

Clinical features

Myxopapillary ependymomas are typically associated with back pain, often of long duration. MRI usually reveals a sharply circumscribed lesion with enhancement that is often bright. Extensive cystic change and haemorrhage may be apparent.

Macroscopy

Myxopapillary ependymomas display a lobulated, soft and greyish appearance. They are often encapsulated and do not usually exhibit grossly infiltrative properties.

Histopathology

Myxopapillary ependymomas are characterized by GFAP-expressing, cuboidal to elongated tumour cells radially arranged in a papillary manner around vascularized stromal cores. Some tumours, however,

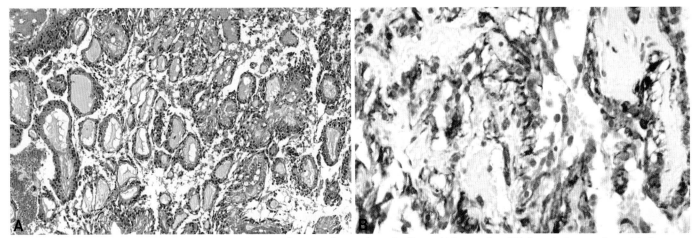

Fig. 3.07 Myxopapillary ependymoma of the cauda equina. **A** Layers of tumour cells around vessels with mucoid degeneration. **B** Perivascular tumour cells consistently express GFAP.

show minimal or no papillary areas and instead feature fascicles of more elongated cells. An Alcian-blue positive, myxoid matrix material accumulates between tumour cells and blood vessels, also collecting in microcysts. Alcian-blue positivity in small cystic spaces is particularly characteristic of those lesions lacking prominent papillary features. Mitotic activity is low, which correlates with a low MIB-1 labelling index {1787}.

Immunohistochemistry
Immunohistochemistry for GFAP, S-100 and vimentin are positive, whereas immunoreactivity for cytokeratins is typically absent. Co-occurrence of the tumour with lipoma {13} and paraganglioma {1071} has been described. Tumour entities to be distinguished from myxopapillary ependymomas include chordoma, myxoid chondrosarcoma, paraganglioma, mesothelioma and papillary adenocarcinoma. In these situations, immunoreactivity for GFAP and lack of cytokeratin expression confirm the diagnosis {366}.

Electron microscopy
The cells do not show polarity, but junctions of zonulae adherens type with cytoplasmic thickening and wide spaces containing amorphous material or loose filaments {1838, 2018, 2131}. Extracellular spaces, delineated by cells with basal membrane, contain projected villi {1838}. Few cilia, complex interdigitations and abundant basement membrane structures have been described, with a distinctive feature of some examples being aggregation of microtubules within endoplasmic reticulum complexes {844}.

Genetics
This entity has not yet been subjected to systematic molecular studies. A molecular genetic analysis of 6 myxopapillary ependymomas for allelic deletions on chromosomes 10q and 22q and for point mutations of the *NF2* and *PTEN* tumour suppressor genes did not reveal any changes at these loci {504}.

Prognostic and predictive factors
Prognosis is favourable, with more than 10-year survival after total or partial resection {2125}. Late recurrence and distant metastases may occur with incomplete resections in both adults {25} and children {553}. Subarachnoid dissemination has occasionally been observed {2423}. The subcutaneous sacrococcygeal myxopapillary ependymoma appears to be associated with a significant rate of regrowth and occasional distant metastases {909}.

Ependymoma

R.E. McLendon
O.D. Wiestler
J.M. Kros
A. Korshunov
H.-K. Ng

Definition

A generally slowly growing tumour of children and young adults, originating from the wall of the ventricles or from the spinal canal and composed of neoplastic ependymal cells.

ICD-O codes

Ependymoma	9391/3
- Cellular ependymoma	9391/3
- Papillary ependymoma	9393/3
- Clear cell ependymoma	9391/3
- Tanycytic ependymoma	9391/3

Grading

Ependymoma corresponds histologically to WHO grade II.

Incidence

In the United States, WHO grade II-III ependymomas have an approximate incidence of 0.29 in males and 0.22 per 100 000 persons per year in females {305}. There appears to be a racial disparity with an incidence of 0.35 in whites versus 0.14 in African Americans {305}. Ependymomas account for 2–9% of all neuroepithelial tumours, amounting to 6–12% of all intracranial tumours in children, and up to 30% of those in children younger than 3 years {495}. In the spinal cord, ependymomas are the most common neuroepithelial neoplasms, comprising 50–60% of spinal gliomas {2018} in adults, but are rare in children {73}.

Age and sex distribution

Ependymomas develop in all age groups, with a range from 1 month to 81 years {305} but incidence is greatly affected by histological type and location. Infratentorial ependymomas predominate in children, with a mean age at clinical manifestation of 6.4 years and a range of 2 months to 16 years {2358}. A second age peak at 30–40 years has been reported for spinal tumours. Supratentorial ependymomas affect paediatric as well as adult patients. Ependymomas appear equally distributed between males and females.

Etiology

The identification of SV40 virus large T antigen-related DNA sequences in a significant proportion of human choroid plexus papillomas and ependymomas received attention since it was thought possible to reflect latent infection following widespread use of SV40-contaminated polio vaccines during 1955–1962 {138, 883}. Natural SV40 strains have been also identified in human ependymomas {1270}. However, other investigators did not confirm these findings {2384}.

Localization

These tumours may occur at any site along the ventricular system and in the spinal canal. They most commonly develop in the 4th ventricle and in the spinal cord, followed by the lateral ventricles and the third ventricle {1788, 2024}. In adults, infratentorial and spinal ependymomas arise with almost equal frequency, whereas infratentorial ependymomas clearly predominate in young children {1222}. In the spinal cord, cervical and cervico-thoracic segments appear to represent primary sites. In contrast, the myxopapillary variant of ependymoma predominantly affects the conus-cauda equina region. Supratentorial parenchymal ependymomas may occur outside the ventricular system, particularly in children. Rare extraneural ependymomas have been observed in the ovaries {1160}, broad ligaments {127}, soft tissues, mediastinum and the sacrococcygeal area.

Clinical features

Symptoms and signs

Clinical manifestations are localization-dependent. Infratentorial ependymomas may present with signs and symptoms of hydrocephalus and increased intracranial pressure, such as headache, nausea, vomiting and dizziness. Involvement of posterior fossa structures may cause cerebellar ataxia, visual disturbance, dizziness and paresis. Patients with supratentorial ependymomas show focal neurological deficits, seizures and features of intracranial hypertension {495}. Head enlargement can be encountered in children below the age of two years. Spinal ependymomas present with motor and sensory deficits.

Neuroimaging

Gadolinium-enhanced MR scans demonstrate rather well circumscribed lesions with varying degrees of contrast enhancement. Ventricular obstruction or brain stem displacement and hydrocephalus are frequent accompanying features. Supratentorial tumours may exhibit cystic components. Intratumoural haemorrhage and extensive calcification are occasionally observed. Gross infiltration of adjacent brain structures and edema are rare. However, in supratentorial parenchymal ependymomas, the

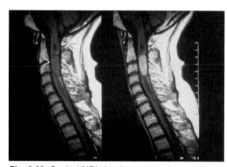

Fig. 3.09 Sagittal MRI showing an ependymoma in the upper cervical spinal cord (left, arrow) with marked gadolinium-enhancement (right), delineated on both sides by a typical cyst.

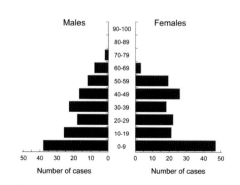

Fig. 3.08 Age and sex distribution of ependymoma, based on 298 cases. Data from Schiffer *et al.* {2024}.

neuroradiological distinction from other glioma entities constitutes a diagnostic challenge. MRI appears particularly useful for determining the relationship to surrounding structures and invasion along the CSF pathway and syrinx formation {636}.

Macroscopy

Ependymomas are typically soft tan masses with well-demarcated borders. Visible foci of haemorrhage or necrosis are uncommon. Macroscopically striking examples are the so-called "plastic ependymomas" which can fill the fourth ventricle, emerge out the foramina of Luschka or Magendie and surround the brain stem via subarachnoid growth {392}.

Histopathology

The most common, or classic, pattern of ependymoma is a well-delineated, moderately cellular glioma with a monomorphic nuclear morphology, characterized by round to oval nuclei with "salt and pepper" speckling of the chromatin. Mitoses are rare or absent. Apart from the nuclear aspects, key histological features are perivascular pseudorosettes and ependymal rosettes. Perivascular pseudorosettes originate from tumour cells arranged radially around blood vessels with perivascular anuclear zones of glial fibrillary protein (GFAP)-rich, fibrillary processes. True ependymal rosettes and ependymal canals are composed of columnar cells arranged around a central lumen. They develop in only a minority of cases. Areas of more extensive fibrillarity are frequently encountered. Regressive changes include regions of myxoid degeneration, intratumoural haemorrhage, calcifications and, occasionally, foci of cartilage and bone. Marked hyalinization of tumour vessels can be common and may precede calcification.

Occasional non-palisading, geographic foci of necrosis are compatible with the diagnosis of ependymoma WHO grade II. The tumour/parenchymal interface is typically sharp {2358} though evidence of infiltration may be encountered. In small samples, distinction from pilocytic astrocytoma can be difficult.

The following histopathological variants of ependymoma can be distinguished.

Cellular ependymoma

This variant is more common in extraventricular locations {2096} and shows conspicuous cellularity without a significant increase in mitotic rate. Pseudorosettes may be inconspicuous, and true ependymal rosettes may be absent. Lacking other properties of anaplasia, this variant is therefore classified as WHO grade II.

Papillary ependymoma

Ependymomas form linear, epithelial-like surfaces along their CSF exposures. Occasionally, exuberant growths arise in which fingerlike projections are lined by a single layer of cuboidal tumour cells with smooth contiguous surfaces and with GFAP-positive tumour cell processes; in contrast, choroid plexus papillomas and metastatic carcinomas form bumpy, hobnail cellular surfaces that do not feature extensive GFAP-positivity.

Clear cell ependymoma

Clear cell ependymomas display an oligodendroglia-like appearance with clear perinuclear halos. This variant appears to be preferentially located in the supratentorial compartment of young patients {596, 1479}. Clear cell ependymomas need to be distinguished from oligodendroglioma, central neurocytoma, clear cell carcinoma and haemangioblastoma. Ependymal and perivascular rosettes, immunoreactivity for GFAP and epithelial membrane antigen (EMA) and ultrastructural studies can be helpful in this differential diagnosis. Recent data suggest that clear cell ependymoma may follow a more aggressive course {596}. The clear cell tumour of the lateral ventricles previously classified as ependymoma of the foramen of Monro {2512} is now recognized as central neurocytoma in most instances (See Chapter 6).

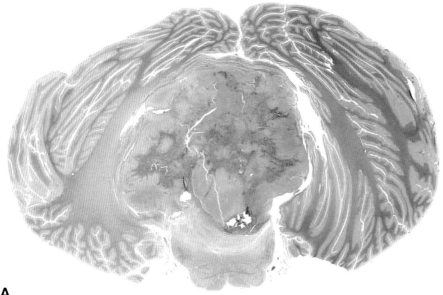

A

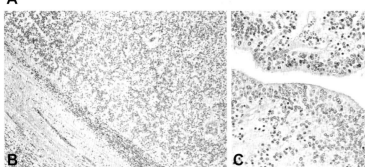

Fig. 3.10 **A** Ependymoma in a child, filling the entire lumen of the fourth ventricle. Note the displacement of the medulla, (**B**) the relatively clear demarcation from the cerebellar parenchyma and (**C**) the involvement of the ependymal lining in the neoplastic process.

Tanycytic ependymoma

Tanycytic tumours are most commonly found in the spinal cord. Their tumour cells are arranged in fascicles of variable width and cell density and only poorly intertwine. Nuclei exhibit the salt-and-pepper speckling of other ependymomas. The term tanycytic ependymoma has been chosen since its spindly, bipolar elements resemble tanycytes, the paraventricular cells with elongated cytoplasmic processes that extend to ependymal surfaces {585}. As ependymal rosettes are typically absent and pseudorosettes only vaguely delineated, the lesion may be misconstrued as an astrocytoma, particularly as pilocytic astrocytoma. Its ultrastructural characteristics, however, are ependymal.

Other patterns

Rare ependymoma variants include ependymoma with lipomatous differentiation {1952}, giant cell ependymoma {600}, ependymoma with extensive tumour cell vacuolation {826}, melanotic ependymoma {1931}, signet ring cell ependymoma {2515}, ovarian ependymoma {286, 732, 1127}, ependymoma with neuropil-like islands {661} and ganglioglioma with a tanycytic glial component {795}.

Immunohistochemistry

The great majority of ependymomas display GFAP immunoreactivity with a prominent reaction for GFAP usually observed in pseudorosettes. Immunoreactivity is more variable in the ependymal rosettes, ependymal canals and papillae where positive cells may alternate with unlabeled elements. Ependymomas typically express S-100 protein and vimentin {1114}. EMA immunoreactivity has been reported in a high percentage of ependymomas with a prominent signal along the luminal surface of ependymal rosettes or as dot-like cytoplasmic vacuoles representing microrosettes in scattered cells {1070}. However, dot-like EMA positivity is not specific to ependymomas and has been noted in glioblastomas. Focal immunoreactivity to cytokeratins can be seen in some cases {1393}, and thyroid transcription factor 1 (TTF-1) has been seen in ependymomas of the third ventricle {2481}. Expression of nestin, a neuro-developmental intermediate filament protein, may be strong in ependymomas

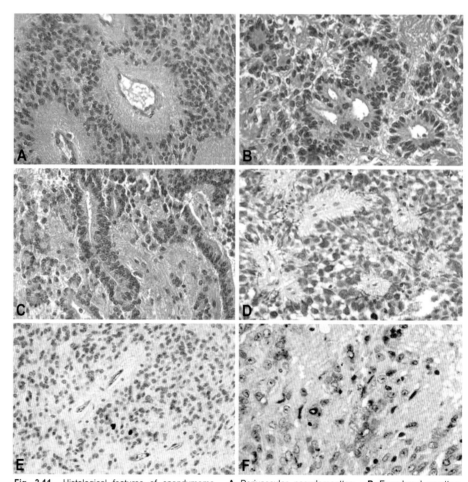

Fig. 3.11 Histological features of ependymoma. **A** Perivascular pseudorosettes. **B** Ependymal rosettes. **C** Ependymal canals. **D** GFAP immunoreactivity predominantly around tumour vessels. **E** Low MID-1 labelling index. **F** Ring-like and dot-like EMA positivities.

{48}. Ependymomas do not express most neuronal antigens, although reactivity to anti-NeuN has been described {1800}.

Electron microscopy

Ependymomas maintain characteristic ultrastructural properties of ependymal cells such as cilia in a 9+2 arrangement, blepharoblasts and microvilli located at the luminal surface, junctional complexes at the lateral surface and lack of a basement membrane at the internal surface. Cells may form microrosettes into which microvilli and cilia project. Junctional complexes (zonulae adherentes), irregularly linked by zonulae occludentes or gap junctions, and cell processes filled with intermediate filaments, may also be encountered {703}. A basal lamina may be present at the interface between tumour cells and vascularized stroma. Neuronal features are absent.

Growth pattern and invasion

Tumour expansion with formation of a clear-cut edge toward the adjacent nervous tissue is characteristic. From the fourth ventricle, ependymomas typically extend into the cerebellopontine angle and protrude into the cisterna magna. Sometimes, isolated tumour cells can be found in the adjacent tissue. Low cellular density may suggest parenchymal invasion. Infrequently, there is spread via the CSF, particularly from infratentorial lesions {1746, 2397} which may occur independent of grade. Several case reports describe extraneural metastases, mostly to the lungs.

Proliferation

Proliferation has been correlated with survival in most recent studies. Ki-67 labelling indices of less than 4% have been associated with significantly longer survival times than labelling indices (LIs) greater than 5% {1236, 1788, 2431}. However, the prognostic significance of the LI, particularly with regard to progression-free survival, has not yet been firmly established. Evaluation of tumour cell apoptosis has not yielded prognostically relevant information {2020}.

Histogenesis

Stem cells isolated from ependymomas indicate a radial glia phenotype. These findings suggest radial glia cells as a candidate cell of origin for ependymoma {2229}.

Genetic susceptibility

Spinal ependymomas are a major manifestation of neurofibromatosis type 2 (NF2), indicating a role for the *NF2* gene in these neoplasms. Other hereditary forms of ependymoma are uncommon. Two patients with Turcot syndrome and ependymomas have been reported {2261} and parental colon cancer is associated with a risk of ependymomas arising in offspring with a standardized incidence ratio of 3.70 {808}. A series of 10 brain tumour families exhibiting ependymomas has been reviewed {474}. Ependymomas have also been described, albeit uncommonly, in neurofibromatosis type 1 (NF1) {1890, 2303}. Very rarely, loss of a 22q11 locus has been found in patient constitutional DNA, raising the possibility of germline susceptibility {52}.

Genetics

Cytogenetic changes have been found in a significant fraction of ependymomas, with a 30% incidence of aberrations involving chromosome 22 as the most frequent change {761}. Monosomy 22 as well as deletions or translocations involving 22q appear to prevail and are more frequently identified in spinal cord tumours than in intracranial ones. Also commonly found are losses of 6q and 9q. Less frequently are losses of 3p14, 10q23 and 11q {877}. Gains of chromosome 7 are noted {1987} but *EGFR* is not amplified. Monosomy 13 was reported in eight cases, half of which occurred in paediatric patients {2162}.
Supratentorial tumours preferentially show loss of chromosome 9 {292, 723, 996, 2497}. Clear cell ependymomas, though mimicking oligodendroglial tumours focally, do not have 1p or 19q deletions but instead exhibit gains of chromosome 1q, and loss of chromosome

9, 3, and 22q {1875}. Childhood tumours tend to show balanced karyotypes, but gains of 1q correlate with anaplastic features in childhood posterior fossa ependymomas. Tumours exhibiting loss of chromosome 13 or 14q/14 show a strong association with spinal cord origin {292}.
At the molecular genetic level, ependymomas exhibit changes distinctive from most other gliomas. The *NF2* gene is clearly involved in ependymoma tumourigenesis, although initial studies yielded conflicting results, largely reflecting the increased incidence of *NF2* mutations in spinal ependymomas. For instance, a study of spinal cord tumours showed mutations of the *NF2* gene {170}, whereas others were unable to identify such mutations in a significant fraction of ependymomas from all locations {1951, 2342}. A subsequent analysis of 62 ependymal tumours revealed 6 cases with mutant *NF2*, all of which were localized in the spinal cord {504}. These data strongly indicate that ependymomas occur as genetically distinct subtypes, a finding that may also extend to clear cell ependymomas {1875}. The rhabdoid tumour suppressor gene *hSNF5/INI1* at 22q11 is not implicated in ependymoma tumourigenesis {1183}.
Disruptions of the *TP53* gene pathway are rare in paediatric ependymomas

{653,1621}, although inactivation of *CDKN2A* gene (deletions or promoter methylation) has been found in intra-cranial ependymomas {1453, 1942, 2229}. The promoters of the *RASSF1A* (3p21.3) and *HIC-1* (17p13.3) genes have been shown to be methylated in a large percentage of ependymomas, suggesting that down-regulation of these genes may play a role in ependymoma pathogenesis {760, 1468, 2355}. Amplification of *EGFR* was found in one of 68 ependymomas, although most showed EGFR overexpression on mRNA and protein levels {1453}. Adult ependymomas commonly exhibit *MDM2* amplification and/or overexpression {2186}.
A RNA expression profile of 39 ependymomas revealed *CLU, IGF2, RAF1, MMP12, PSAP* and *MSX1* to be highly expressed in these tumours. Gene expression levels could be correlated with chromosomal aberrations described including increased expression of *PRELP, EPHX1, FY* and *HSPA6*, located on chromosome 1q, and decreased expression of *COX7A2, COL10A1* and *TCP1* from chromosome 6q; *CNTFR, RAGA, TXN, AMBP* and *HSPA5* from chromosome 9; *TUBA2, PRDX2* and *LCP1* from chromosome 13; and *RANBP1, MCM5, EP300, G22P1, BZRP* and *MAPK12* from chromosomal arm 22q {1173}. Gene expression patterns also differ between

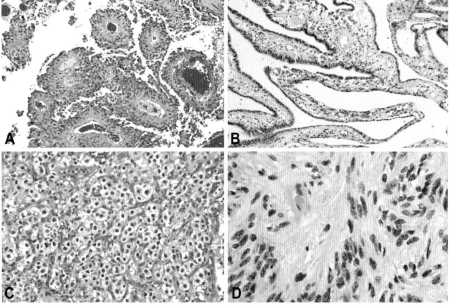

Fig. 3.12 A Papillary ependymoma with discohesive growth, pseudopapillae, and perivascular pseudorosettes. **B** Papillary ependymoma. Finger like projections are lined by single or multiple layers of cuboidal tumour cells with smooth contiguous surfaces. **C** Clear cell ependymoma. **D** Tanycytic differentiation.

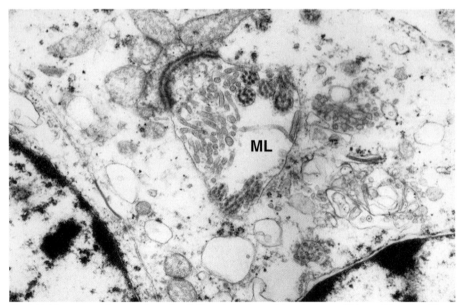

Fig. 3.13 Ultrastructural features of ependymal differentiation: intercellular microlumen (ML) containing microvilli and cillia, bordered by an elongate intercellular junction.

ependymomas from different sites of origin. Supratentorial tumours express high levels of various members of the EPHB, NOTCH, CYCLIN and CDK families, whereas spinal ependymomas show high-expression levels for multiple HOX family members {1173, 2229}.

Prognostic and predictive factors

The identification of parameters with prognostic value in ependymomas remains an important but controversial issue {2027}. The significance of histopathological properties has been confounded in many studies by the variable inclusion of spinal cord, brain stem and intraparenchymal tumours. The following factors have to be considered in order of importance:

Age and extent of resection. Children tend to fare worse than adults. To some extent, this difference may reflect the more common posterior fossa location in paediatric patients versus spinal location in adults. In addition, tumours with frank histopathological anaplasia may occur at a higher incidence in this age group. A multi-institutional retrospective analysis of 83 paediatric ependymoma patients revealed age below 3 years, anaplastic histopathological features and incomplete tumour resection as indicators of a poor outcome {865}. The Children's Cancer Group reported a 5-year progression-free survival of 50% in children with intracranial ependymomas {1899}. Children affected during the first two years of life carry a particularly dismal prognosis {1222, 1746}. In one adult series, survival at 5 and 10 years was 57% and 45%, respectively. Complete or near complete resection has emerged as an independent prognostic factor {981,1768}.

Location. Tumour site is usually identified as the most important prognostic factor. Supratentorial ependymomas are associated with better survival rates compared to posterior fossa neoplasms {534}. Spinal ependymomas show a significantly better outcome compared to cerebral lesions although late recurrences (>5 years) are common. Cerebrospinal dissemination indicates a poor prognosis.

Histopathological grading. A major and not completely resolved problem relates to the definition of reliable histopathological indicators of anaplasia. Of the features usually associated with anaplastic change in gliomas, only mitotic index, proliferation indices and foci of hypercellular, less differentiated tumour cells, appear to correlate with poor outcome in ependymomas {1171, 1236, 2027}. Many other histological parameters have been tested in various studies, with contradictory results {840, 1837}.

Anaplastic ependymoma

R.E. McLendon
O.D. Wiestler
J.M. Kros
A. Korshunov
H.-K. Ng

Definition
A malignant glioma of ependymal differentiation with accelerated growth and unfavourable clinical outcome, particularly in children; histologically characterized by high mitotic activity, often accompanied by microvascular proliferation and pseudopalisading necrosis.

ICD-O code   9392/3

Grading
Anaplastic ependymomas correspond histologically to WHO grade III.

Incidence
Incidence data vary considerably, due to the uncertainty regarding histological criteria of malignancy. Anaplastic changes are far more frequent in childhood intracranial ependymomas, particularly posterior fossa examples, than in those of the spinal cord {305}.

Clinical features
Signs and symptoms of anaplastic ependymomas are similar to those of ependymoma WHO grade II, but they usually develop more rapidly and may cause increased intracranial pressure at an early stage of the disease. MR images typically show contrast enhancement.

Histopathology
Anaplastic ependymomas show increased cellularity and brisk mitotic activity, often associated with microvascular proliferation and pseudopalisading necrosis. Perivascular pseudorosettes are a histological hallmark. Anaplastic ependymomas tend to remain well demarcated, but are occasionally frankly invasive. They often appear highly cellular and poorly differentiated, with pseudorosettes of narrow radial width. Geographic tumour necrosis (a particularly common phenomenon in posterior fossa ependymomas) is not a diagnostic feature of malignancy in the absence of vascular proliferation, frequent mitotic activity, or a high proliferation index {1172, 1236, 1837}. Poorly differentiated

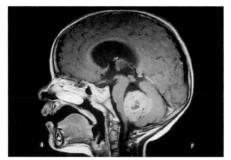

Fig. 3.14 Sagittal, gadolinium-enhanced, T1-weighted MRI of an anaplastic ependymoma of the fourth ventricle.

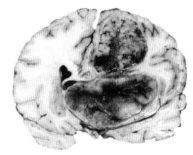

Fig. 3.15 Anaplastic ependymoma of the lateral ventricle in a four-year-old boy with extensive invasion of the right frontal lobe.

examples may be difficult to identify as ependymal in the absence of supporting ultrastructural evidence. By definition, embryonal components and ependymoblastic rosettes are not present (see Chapter 8).

Immunohistochemistry
The phenotypic profiles of anaplastic ependymomas resemble those of ependymoma, grade II, but GFAP expression may be reduced.

Genetics
Genetic alterations specifically encountered in anaplastic ependymomas are largely unknown. Although some lesions may develop through malignant progression from WHO grade II ependymomas, no underlying sequence of genetic

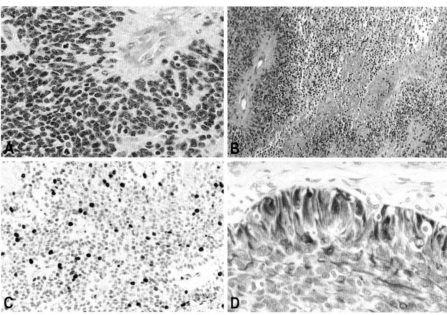

Fig. 3.16 Histological features of anaplastic ependymoma. **A** Poorly differentiated tumour cells with brisk mitotic activity. **B** Large foci of necrosis. **C** High MIB-1 labelling index. **D** Strong GFAP expression in an anaplastic ependymoma invading adjacent brain structures.

events has been identified. There is evidence for a putative tumour suppressor gene on chromosome 22 in familial anaplastic ependymomas {1595}. An analysis of 23 anaplastic ependymomas revealed loss of 10q in 4 cases {504}. A comparative genomic hybridization (CGH) study of 35 ependymomas showed that gain of 1q and loss of 9 and 13 were associated with WHO grade III tumours {835}. One array CGH study also identified two regions of gain on 1q (1q21.3-23.1 and 1q31.1-31.3); DUSP12 at 1q23 was proposed to be a "driver oncogene" for anaplastic ependymomas {1453}.

An RNA expression analysis of ependymomas was able to distinguish supratentorial WHO grade II and III tumours with 100% accuracy. However, infratentorial examples were more difficult to classify, with 5 of 18 tumour samples misclassified. The similar gene expression patterns of WHO grade II and III infratentorial malignancies may suggest that grade III tumours develop through progression {1173}.

Prognostic and predictive factors

An inconstant relationship between histology and outcome has emerged from the clinical studies {535, 577, 1458, 1930, 2431}. In two series with more than 200 cases, no correlation was observed between patient survival and classical histopathological signs of malignancy. However, a relationship with survival was evident when high cell density plus brisk mitotic activity {2022} or high cell density, vascular proliferation and/or cytologic atypia, were considered as independent variables {1171}. Age below 3 years, anaplastic histopathological features, incomplete tumour resection and evidence for CSF metastases have been proposed as indicators of an adverse outcome in children {865, 960}. Among spinal intramedullary tumours, extent of resection is most predictive of progression-free survival, with 12 of 21 treatment failures occurring after 5 years of follow-up in one study {705}. Paradoxically, a high frequency of imbalanced chromosomal regions, as revealed by CGH in ependymomas, does not indicate a high WHO grade {2004}. Several studies have suggested an association between p53 immunoreactivity and adverse outcome for ependymomas {1172, 2185, 2323}.

CHAPTER 4

Choroid Plexus Tumours

Choroid plexus papilloma (WHO grade I)
A benign, ventricular papillary neoplasm derived from choroid plexus epithelium.

Atypical choroid plexus papilloma (WHO grade II)
A choroid plexus papilloma with increased mitotic activity and greater likehood of recurrence.

Choroid plexus carcinoma (WHO grade III)
A frankly malignant choroid plexus neoplasm.

Choroid plexus tumours

W. Paulus
S. Brandner

Definition

Intraventricular, papillary neoplasms derived from choroid plexus epithelium.

ICD-O codes

Choroid plexus papilloma   9390/0
Atypical choroid plexus papilloma
                                  9390/1
Choroid plexus carcinoma   9390/3

Grading

Choroid plexus papilloma (CPP) corresponds to WHO grade I, atypical CPP to grade II, and choroid plexus carcinoma (CPC) to grade III.

Incidence

Although choroid plexus tumours account for 0.3–0.6% of all brain tumours, they represent 2–4% of those that occur in children under 15 years, and 10–20% of those manifesting in the first year of life. CPP outnumber CPC by a ratio of at least 5:1. Around 80% of CPC arise in children, in whom they constitute 20–40% of choroid plexus tumours. The average annual incidence is approximately 0.3 per 1 000 000 population per year {969, 1877, 2430}.

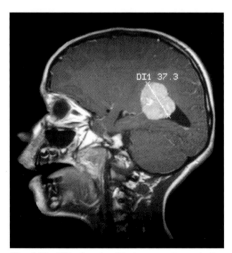

Fig. 4.01 MRI of a choroid plexus carcinoma in the lateral ventricle of a 5 year-old child with a *TP53* germline mutation.

Age and sex distribution

Around 80% of lateral ventricular tumours present in patients younger than 20 years, whereas fourth ventricle tumours are evenly distributed in all age groups. A meta-analysis found that median age was 1.5 years for the lateral and third ventricle, 22.5 years for the fourth ventricle, and 35.5 years for the cerebellopontine angle {2430}. Congenital tumours and fetal tumours have been observed in utero using ultrasound techniques. The overall male: female ratio is 1.2:1; this ratio is 1:1 for lateral ventricle tumours and 3:2 for fourth ventricle tumours.

Etiology

DNA sequences of the simian virus 40 (SV40) have been found in about 35% of brain tumours, including about 50% of choroid plexus tumours {138}. Since (i) surrounding brain tissue only rarely contains SV40 sequences, (ii) SV40 induces brain tumours in hamsters and in transgenic mice, (iii) SV40 large T antigen inactivates several tumour suppressor proteins including p53 and Rb, and (iv) SV40 large T antigen is capable of transforming human cells *in vitro*, it has been hypothesized that SV40 plays a role in the etiology of brain tumours, including choroid plexus tumours {138}. However, SV40 sequences in CPP were found only in populations that received SV40-contaminated polio vaccine between 1955 and 1963 (e.g. USA and Switzerland), but not in populations that did not use SV40-contaminated vaccine (e.g. Finland) {1623}. Because the incidence of brain tumours is not different among these nations, the data can be interpreted as reflecting a bystander infection caused by an intratumoural microenvironment that favours viral replication in humans with latent SV40 infection, rather than reflecting a causal role of SV40 {1623}.

Localization

CPP and CPC are confined to areas where choroid plexus is normally found, i.e. the lateral (50%), third (5%) and fourth (40%) cerebral ventricles, with two

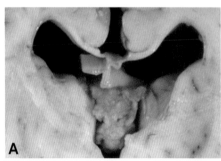
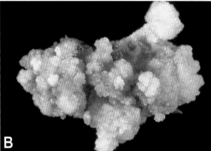

Fig. 4.02 A Choroid plexus papilloma arising in the posterior third ventricle producing partial obstruction with ventricle dilatation. B Villous architecture.

or three ventricles being involved in 5% of cases {969, 2163}. Primary manifestation in the cerebellopontine angle near the openings of the fourth ventricle is uncommon. Exceptional cases of ectopic locations, e.g. intraparenchymal, suprasellar or spinal epidural, are on record {1113, 1238, 1749}.

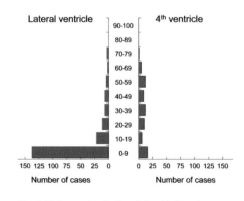

Fig. 4.03 Age *vs.* localization of choroid plexus tumours, based on a compilation of 264 published cases {2430}.

Clinical features

Symptoms and signs

Choroid plexus tumours tend to block CSF pathways. Accordingly, patients present with signs of hydrocephalus (in infants, increased circumference of the head) and raised intracranial pressure.

Neuroimaging

CT and MRI of CPP usually shows iso- or hyperdense, T1-isointense, T2-hyperintense, irregularly contrast-enhancing, well-delineated masses within the ventricles, but irregular tumour margins and disseminated disease may occur {731}. MRI features typical of CPC include large intraventricular lesions with irregular enhancing margins, heterogeneous signal on long TR/long TE images and short-TR images, edema in adjacent brain, hydrocephalus, and presence of disseminated tumour {1467}.

Macroscopy

CPP are circumscribed cauliflower-like masses that may adhere to the ventricular wall, but are usually well-delineated from brain tissue. Cysts and haemorrhages may occur. CPC are invasive tumours that may appear solid, haemorrhagic and necrotic.

Histopathology, immunohistochemistry and electron microscopy

Choroid plexus papilloma

Delicate fibrovascular connective tissue fronds are covered by a single layer of uniform cuboidal to columnar epithelial cells with round or oval, basally situated monomorphic nuclei. Mitotic activity is extremely low. Brain invasion, high cellularity, necrosis, nuclear pleomorphism and focal blurring of the papillary pattern are unusual, but may occur. CPP closely resembles non-neoplastic choroid plexus,

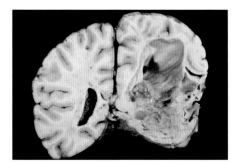

Fig. 4.04 Large choroid plexus carcinoma in the atrium of the right lateral ventricle with extensive invasion of the adjacent brain.

but cells tend to be more crowded, elongated or stratified instead of the normal cobblestone-like surface. Rarely, CPP may acquire unusual histological features, including oncocytic change, mucinous degeneration, melanization and tubular glandular architecture of tumour cells, as well as degeneration of connective tissue, such as xanthomatous change, angioma-like increase of blood vessels, and bone, cartilage or adipose tissue formation {64,236,1990}.

Cytokeratins, vimentin and podoplanin are expressed by virtually all CPP. The most common CK7/CK20 combination is CK7-positive and CK20-negative (74%), but the other three combinations are also possible {743}. Prominent staining for epithelial membrane antigen is typically not found. S-100 protein is present in 55–90% of cases. GFAP is absent from normal choroid plexus, but is present focally in 25–55% of CPP. Approximately 70% of CPP are positive for transthyretin (pre-albumin) {782}. Staining for synaptophysin has been reported to be strongly positive in normal and neoplastic choroid plexus epithelial cells {1083}, but this finding has not been confirmed by others {285,1696}.

Electron microscopy shows interdigitating cell membranes, tight junctions, microvilli, occasional apical cilia and a basement membrane at the abluminal pole.

Atypical choroid plexus papilloma

Atypical CPP is defined as CPP with increased mitotic activity. One study indicates that a mitotic index of two or more mitoses per 10 randomly selected HPF (one HPF corresponding to 0.23 mm^2) can be used to establish this diagnosis {983}. The same study showed that up to two of the following four features may also be present: increased cellularity, nuclear pleomorphism, blurring of the papillary pattern (solid growth) and areas of necrosis, but these features are not required for making a diagnosis of atypical CPP. Using these criteria, a series of 124 CPP had 19 cases of atypical CPP (15%).

Choroid plexus carcinoma

This tumour shows frank signs of malignancy. According to one study, frank signs of malignancy included at least four of the following five features: frequent mitoses (usually greater than 5 per 10 HPF), increased cellular density,

nuclear pleomorphism, blurring of the papillary pattern with poorly structured sheets of tumour cells, and necrotic areas. If brain tissue is available, diffuse brain invasion is common.

Immunohistochemically, CPC express cytokeratins, while positivity for S-100 protein and transthyretin is less frequent than in CPP. About 20% of CPC are GFAP-positive. Epithelial membrane antigen is usually not expressed {983}.

Differential diagnosis

Various immunostains have been recommended for the distinction between choroid plexus tumours and metastatic carcinomas. A microarray-based expression profiling study revealed inward rectifier potassium channel Kir7.1 and stanniocalcin-1 as markers of normal and neoplastic choroid plexus epithelial cells: immunostaining for Kir7.1 was seen in 17 of 23 (74%) choroid plexus tumours but in none of 100 other tumours, while an

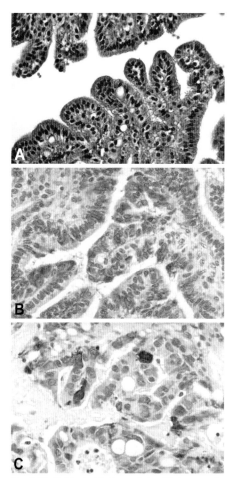

Fig. 4.05 Histological features of choroid plexus papilloma (**A**). Immunoreactivity for transthyretin (TTR) (**B**) and GFAP (**C**) in choroid plexus papillomas.

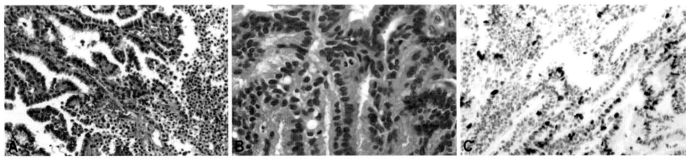

Fig. 4.06 Atypical choroid plexus papilloma. **A** A well-differentiated choroid plexus papilloma with an area of necrosis (lower right). **B** Prominent mitotic activity. **C** High Ki-67 (MIB-1) labelling.

antibody against stanniocalcin-1 stained 19 of 23 (83%) choroid plexus tumours but only 2% of other primary brain tumours and cerebral metastases {782}. Another study described membranous staining for the excitatory amino acid transporter-1 (EAAT1) in 23 of 35 (66%) choroid plexus tumours, but in none of 77 metastatic carcinomas {143}. Antibodies against transthyretin label most normal and neoplastic choroid plexus epithelia. However, up to 30% of CPP are negative, and other brain tumours as well as metastatic carcinomas may be positive {782}. The antibodies HEA125 and BerEP4 may be useful, because they label more than 95% of cerebral metastatic carcinomas, but only 10% of CPP or CPC {715}. Expression of carcinoembryonic antigen (CEA) suggests metastatic carcinoma {1698}, although occasional CPC are also positive {1056}. Due to overlapping clinical, histologic, ultrastructural or immunophenotypic features, differentiation between CPC and atypical teratoid/rhabdoid tumour (AT/RT) may be difficult. An immunohisto-chemical study suggested that staining

for INI1 protein is retained in the majority of CPC and lost in AT/RT {1016}.
Villous hypertrophy is a diffuse enlargement of the choroid plexus in both lateral ventricles with normal histological appearance, often associated with hypersecretory hydrocephalus. Ki-67/MIB-1 and neuroimaging may be useful in differentiating these lesions from monomorphous bilateral CPP {408, 533}.

Seeding and metastasis

Even benign CPP may seed cells into the CSF; drop metastases in the surroundings of the cauda equina may result. In contrast, CPC commonly produce frank metastases along CSF pathways, while exceptional cases of CPP with CSF-mediated metastases are also on record {1426, 2476}. Shunt-related metastases in the abdomen {482} and extracranial metastases in lung and tibia {793} are extremely rare.

Proliferation

Mean Ki-67/MIB-1 labelling indices for choroid plexus tumours have been reported as 1.9% (range, 0.2–6%) for

CPP, 13.8% (range, 7.3–60%) for CPC, and less than 0.1% for the normal choroid plexus {2296}. Another study described mean Ki-67/MIB-1 indices of 4.5% (range, 0.2–17.4) for CPP, 18.5% (range, 4.1–29.7%) for CPC, and 0% for the normal choroid plexus {285}.

Genetic susceptibility

CPC and, more rarely, CPP have been reported in about 20 families with germline *TP53* mutations or in families with unknown *TP53* status but with clustering of cancer suggestive of Li–Fraumeni syndrome {1210}. CPC has also been described in the rhabdoid predisposition syndrome, a familial cancer syndrome caused by germline mutations in the *INI1* (*SMARCB1/SNF5*) gene {2057}, but such cases may be difficult to distinguish from atypical teratoid/rhabdoid tumours. CPP represents a major diagnostic feature of Aicardi syndrome, a genetic but sporadic condition presumably linked to the X chromosome and defined by the triad of total or partial agenesis of the corpus callosum, chorioretinal lacunae

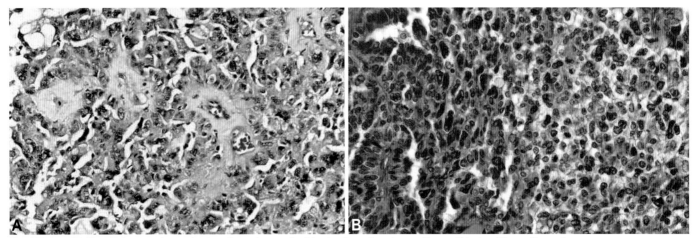

Fig. 4.07 **A** and **B** Choroid plexus carcinoma showing mitoses, increased cellular density, nuclear pleomorphism and blurring of the papillary pattern.

and infantile spasms {22}. In the setting of an X;17(q12;p13) translocation, hypomelanosis of Ito has been associated with the development of CPP in a few cases {2478}. Duplication of the short arm of chromosome 9, a rare constitutional abnormality, was associated with pathologically confirmed hyperplasia of the choroid plexus in one of two cases, and a CPP in another {1605}.

Genetics

Classical cytogenetics and FISH of CPP typically shows hyperdiploidy with gains particularly on chromosomes 7, 9, 12, 15, 17 and 18 {483}. CPC may exhibit loss of heterozygosity on chromosomes 1p, 1q, 3p, 5q, 9q, 10q, 13q, 18q and 22q {2480}. In a CGH study of 49 tumours, CPP frequently showed +7q (65%), +5q (62%), +7p (59%), +5p (56%), +9p (50%) and -10q (56%); while CPC mainly showed +12p, +12q, +20p (60%), +1, +4q, +20q (53%) and -22q (73%) {1885}. These data suggest that CPP and CPC may develop via different genetic pathways.

Some CPP and almost all CPC show immunohistochemical positivity for p53 {285,2451}, while *TP53* mutations are virtually absent in CPP and rare (< 10% of cases) in sporadic CPC {1621,2480}. Mutations in the *INI1* gene have been described in 6 of 18 apparently sporadic CPC {2056,2377, 2480}, but in none of 26 CPP {1533,2056}. However, given the histologic overlap between CPC and atypical teratoid/rhabdoid tumour, the frequency of *INI1* mutations in histologically unequivocal and immunohistochemically scrutinized CPC remains to be determined.

Notch3 signalling may play a role in the pathogenesis of choroid plexus tumours, because introduction of constitutively active Notch3 into periventricular cells of embryonic day 9.5 mice caused the formation of CPP; furthermore, in a small series of 7 human CPP there was nuclear translocation or overexpression of at least one Notch receptor (Notch1, Notch2, Notch3), suggesting Notch pathway activity {412}.

Prognostic and predictive factors

CPP can be cured by surgery, with a 5-year survival rate of up to 100%. In a series of 41 cases of CPP, five-year local control, distant brain control and overall survival were 84%, 92%, and 97%, respectively; local control at 5 years is better after gross total resection than after subtotal resection (100% *vs.* 68%) {1189}. A meta-analysis of 566 choroid plexus tumours revealed that one-, five-, and 10-year projected survival rates were 90%, 81% and 77% in CPP compared with only 71%, 41% and 35% in CPC {2430}. Malignant progression of CPP is rare, but has been described {344,1698}.

In a clinicopathological study of 52 patients, poor prognosis (recurrence and/or fatal outcome) correlated with the following pathological features: mitoses, necrosis, brain invasion, lack of immunoreactivity for transthyretin, and decreased expression of S-100 protein {1698}. Another study did not find evidence for prognostic relevance of brain invasion in otherwise benign CPP {1302}. In a series on 124 CPP, multivariate analysis revealed that increased mitotic activity (2 or more mitoses per 10 HPF), corresponding to atypical CPP, was the sole histological feature independently associated with recurrence, resulting in a 4.9-fold higher probability of recurrence after 5 years of follow-up {983}.

CHAPTER 5

Other Neuroepithelial Tumours

Astroblastoma
A rare glial neoplasm mainly affecting children, adolescents and young adults, composed of GFAP-positive cells with broad, non- or slightly-tapering processes radiating towards central blood vessels that often demonstrate sclerosis.

Chordoid glioma of the third ventricle (WHO grade II)
A rare, slowly growing, non-invasive, glial tumour located in the third ventricle of adults, histologically characterized by clusters and cords of epithelioid, GFAP-expressing tumour cells within a variably mucinous stroma typically containing a lympho-plasmacytic infiltrate.

Angiocentric glioma (WHO grade I)
An epilepsy-associated, stable or slowly growing cerebral tumour primarily affecting children and young adults; histopathologically characterized by an angiocentric pattern of growth, mono-morphous bipolar cells and features of ependymal differentiation.

Astroblastoma

K.D. Aldape
M.K. Rosenblum

Definition

A rare glial neoplasm mainly affecting children, adolescents and young adults, composed of GFAP-positive cells with broad, non- or slightly-tapering processes radiating towards central blood vessels that often demonstrate sclerosis.

ICD-O code

9430/3

Grading

The biological behaviour of astroblastoma is variable. In the absence of sufficient clinico-pathologic data, it is considered premature to establish a WHO grade at this time.

Historical annotation

Current conceptions of the astroblastoma as a circumscribed, vasocentric glial neoplasm with a predilection for relatively young subjects derive principally from the 1989 study of Bonnin and Rubinstein {195}, the term being originally applied by Bailey and Bucy {84} sixty years earlier to a disparate collection of, for the most part, infiltrating and aggressive gliomas mainly affecting the middle aged. The concept of the astroblastoma as a unified, distinct entity remains controversial.

Incidence

Since these are unusual tumours and uniform criteria have not been applied diagnostically, definitive epidemiological data are not available. However, astroblastomas appear to be most frequent in

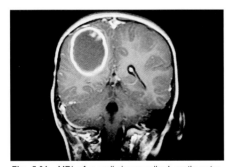

Fig. 5.01 MRI of a well-circumscribed cystic astroblastoma with edema and mass effects. The mural tumour component exhibits contrast enhancement.

children, adolescents and young adults {1959}.

Age and sex distribution

Combining three published series totalling 40 cases {195, 726, 2238} the median age was 11 years (range 1–58). Among these, there were 10 males and 30 females, suggesting a female predominance for this entity.

Localization

Astroblastomas typically involve, but are not restricted to, the cerebral hemispheres {895, 1959}.

Clinical features

They are visualized in CT and MR studies as well-demarcated, non-calcified, nodular or lobulated masses with frequent cystic change and conspicuous contrast enhancement {2048}.

Macroscopy

Tumour tissue is grey-pink or tan, its consistency depending on the extent of associated collagen deposition. Foci of necrosis or haemorrhage do not necessarily indicate anaplasia.

Histopathology

Tumours under consideration for a diagnosis of astroblastoma should be circumscribed at the histologic level and cannot contain elements of diffusely infiltrating astrocytoma, gemistocytic astrocytoma or conventional ependymoma. A well-defined or "pushing" margin is characteristic, although a narrow rim of neuroparenchymal permeation can be seen. Areas of perivascular structuring can be solid or loosely textured, the latter imparting regional pseudopapillary appearances. Unipolar cytoplasmic processes anchor neoplastic cells to stromal blood vessels in formations of radial ("cartwheel"), papillary or ribboned profiles. These columnar or subtly tapered processes are shorter and stouter than those of ependymal pseudorosettes and do not collect as a conspicuous fibrillary matrix. Polygonal

or spindled tumour cells surround gliovascular structures, either densely or as a rarefied population. Nuclei are rounded, oval or irregularly indented and can exhibit coarse chromatin clumping. A case manifesting signet-ring or adipocyte-like features has been reported {2171}. Progressive hyalinization of blood vessel walls is regularly seen and may result in large areas of fibrous overgrowth as well as regional tumour infarction.

Astroblastomas can be divided into well-differentiated and anaplastic (high-grade)

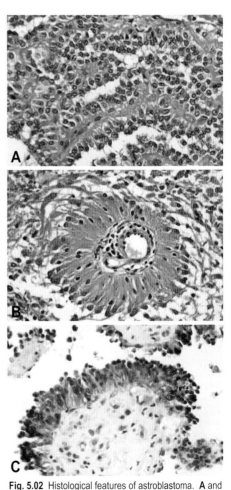

Fig. 5.02 Histological features of astroblastoma. **A** and **B** Anchoring of tumour cells to blood vessels by short, stout cytoplasmic processes. **C** Tumour cell processes radiating towards fibrovascular cores show strong immunoreactivity to GFAP.

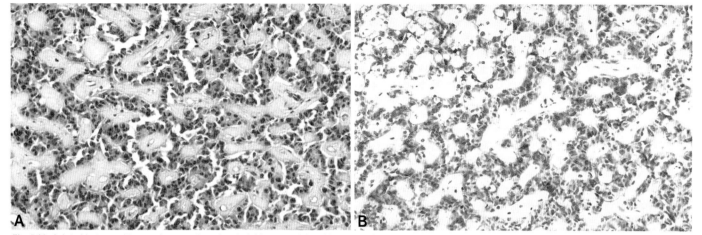

Fig. 5.03 A Astroblastoma with extensive vascular sclerosis (trichrome stain) and **B** variable GFAP immunoreactivity.

variants. The latter evidence conspicuous mitotic activity, cytologic atypia and architectural disorganization, i.e. a breakdown of the orderly perivascular structuring manifest throughout well-differentiated counterparts. Anaplastic (high-grade) examples may also exhibit complex microvascular hyperplasia and pseudopalisading necrosis. Necrosis without pseudopalisading may be encountered in either setting.

Immunohistochemistry
Cytoplasmic immunoreactivity for vimentin, S-100 and GFAP is characteristic, although the extent of labelling (particularly for GFAP) varies considerably {270, 1757, 1959}. Cell membranes may label for EMA {270, 977}, typically as a focal phenomenon. Limited immunoexpression of low molecular weight cytokeratins has been described {977}, other studies finding no CAM5.2 {270} or AE1/3 labelling {977}. Reactivity for NSE is inconstant {270, 895} and isolated cases have proven negative for synaptophysin {977}.

Electron microscopy
Regularly observed are intermediate filament-laden cell processes that form parallel or radial arrays terminating on perivascular basement membranes {895}. Compelling evidence of neuronal differentiation has not been forwarded, nor have ependymal features been encoun-

tered in most studied cases. Two reports examining ultrastructural features suggest an origin from tanycytes {1215, 1225}. These features included cell body polarization with investing basement membranes, apical cytoplasmic blebs capped by microvilli with "purse-string" pedicular constrictions, and lamellar cytoplasmic interdigitations ("pleatings"). Zonula adherens-type junctions framing occasional microrosettes and rare cilia were also identified in these cases.

Proliferation
Reported Ki-67 labelling indices vary between 1% and 18% {215,977}. A relationship between proliferation index and outcome has not been established in the literature, although elevated indices tend to be associated with high-grade histology.

Histogenesis
The histogenesis of astroblastomas is controversial, and the entity is not universally accepted. Bailey and Cushing considered these tumours to arise from embryonic cells programmed to become astrocytes. The presence of intermediate filaments on ultrastructural examination, lack of evidence of neuronal or, in most cases, ependymal differentiation, together with positive staining for GFAP and S-100 protein, suggest the possibility that the tumour is derived from a cell most similar to an astrocyte. The tanycyte, a cell with

features intermediate between astrocytes and ependymal cells, has been suggested as a cell of origin for astroblastoma on the basis of ultrastructural observations.

Genetics
DNA copy number aberrations identified by comparative genomic hybridization have been described for 7 cases {217} and the most common identified alterations in this small series (gains of chromosomes 19 and 20q) were not typical of either ependymoma or diffuse glial neoplasms. Conventional cytogenetic studies performed on two cases {215, 977} lead to the same overall conclusion. Although the number of cases studied to date is small, they are consistent with the concept that astroblastoma is distinct from conventional glial neoplasms.

Prognostic and predictive factors
Astroblastomas with low-grade histology have a better prognosis than those with high-grade features {195, 2238}. However, gross total resection of astroblastoma, even when high-grade, may result in a favourable outcome {195}. In general, however, anaplastic histology is associated with recurrence and progression {195, 2238}. In one study, only a single recurrence was noted (histologic features notwithstanding) in 14 informative cases treated by gross total resection at a mean follow-up of 24 months {215}.

Chordoid glioma of the third ventricle

D.J. Brat
B.W. Scheithauer

Definition

A rare, slowly growing, non-invasive, glial tumour located in the third ventricle of adults, histologically characterized by clusters and cords of epithelioid, GFAP-expressing tumour cells within a variably mucinous stroma typically containing a lymphoplasmacytic infiltrate.

ICD-O code 9444/1

Grading

This neoplasm corresponds histologically to WHO grade II.

Synonyms and historical annotation

In 1995, Wanschitz et al. {2365} described a solid, third ventricular tumour occurring in a 24-year-old woman and having histologic and immunohistochemical features of a chordoid glioma. The authors concluded the tumour was a meningioma with 'peculiar expression of GFAP'. Subsequent immunohistochemical and ultrastructural studies of similar cases have not supported a meningothelial derivation; rather, evidence indicates that they are glial in nature. Based on a series of eight third ventricular masses with identical histologic features, chordoid glioma was proposed as a distinct entity in 1998 {220}.

Incidence

These tumours are rare, but must enter into the limited differential diagnosis of a solid, contrast-enhancing third ventricular mass in an adult. Approximately 45 cases have been reported.

Age and sex distribution

Chordoid gliomas occur in adults, with the large majority presenting between 35 and 60 years (mean, 46 years) {220, 1690}. There is a 2:1 female predominance. Only one paediatric example, occurring in a 12-year-old male, has been reported {297}.

Localization

Chordoid gliomas occupy the anterior portion of the third ventricle, with larger tumours filling the middle and posterior aspects {1775}. They generally arise in the midline and displace normal structures in all planes as they enlarge. Neuroimaging descriptions, including reports of small, localized tumours, suggest that chordoid gliomas arise in the region of the lamina terminalis in the ventral wall of the third ventricle {1284, 1690}. In at least some instances, radiologic studies have demonstrated an intraparenchymal hypothalamic component.

Clinical features

Symptoms and signs

Most patients present with symptoms of obstructive hydrocephalus, including headache, nausea, and ataxia. Other tumours cause endocrine hypofunction, particularly hypothyroidism, and/or visual disturbances due to inferior displacement of the optic chiasm. Psychiatric and memory abnormalities have also been noted, presumably due to compression of the medial temporal lobes.

Neuroimaging

MRI typically demonstrates a bulky, well-circumscribed 2–4 cm, third ventricular mass. Aside from the uncommon finding of cystic change, the tumours are uniformly contrast-enhancing and appear contiguous with hypothalamic or suprasellar structures.

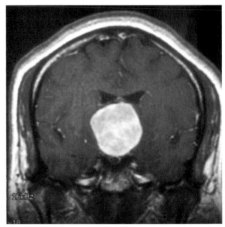

Fig. 5.05 MRI of a chordoid glioma of the third ventricle demonstrating a large contrast-enhancing, sharply delineated mass that fills the anterior third ventricle and compresses adjacent structures.

Histopathology

Chordoid gliomas are solid neoplasms composed of clusters and cords of epithelioid tumour cells within a variably mucinous stroma typically containing a lymphoplasmacytic infiltrate. Immunohistochemical and ultrastructural features indicate a glial derivation. The oval-to-polygonal epithelioid cells with abundant eosinophilic cytoplasm are embedded in a mucinous, often vacuolated stroma. In many instances, obvious but limited glial differentiation in the form of coarsely fibrillar processes can be seen {220}. Neoplastic nuclei are moderate in size, and relatively uniform. The majority of tumours lack mitoses; in the remainder, they are rare (<1 per 10 high-power fields). A stromal lymphoplasmacytic infiltrate, often with numerous Russell bodies, is a consistent finding. Chondroid differentiation has been described in one example {297}. Conforming to radiographic impressions, tumours are architecturally solid, and show little tendency to microscopic infiltration of surrounding brain structures. Reactive astrocytes, Rosenthal fibers and often chronic inflammatory cells including lymphocytes, plasma cells and Russell bodies are seen in adjacent non-neoplastic tissue.

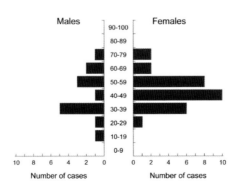

Fig. 5.04 Age and sex distribution of chordoid glioma of the third ventricle, based on 43 cases.

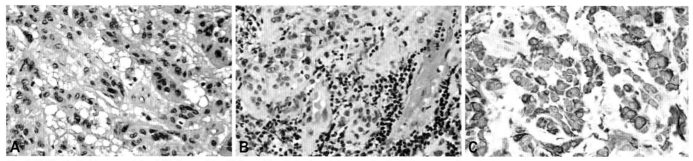

Fig. 5.06 Histological features of chordoid glioma of the third ventricle. **A** Cords and clusters of epithelioid tumour cells embedded in a mucinous matrix. **B** Solid arrangements of packed tumour cells and dense lymphoplasmacytic infiltrate. **C** Tumour cells with diffuse immunoreactivity for GFAP.

Immunohistochemistry

The most distinctive immunohistochemical feature of chordoid gliomas is their strong, diffuse reactivity for GFAP. Staining for vimentin is also strong, while S-100 protein immunoreactivity is variable. EMA staining can be seen focally, but it is usually more prominent in stromal plasma cells. Further, tumours show immunoreactivity for EGFR and the *NF2* gene product merlin, but no nuclear accumulation of the p53, p21 or MDM2 proteins {1848}.

Electron microscopy

On ultrastructural examination, parallels have been drawn with the morphology of ependymoma {1690} or the specialized ependyma of the subcommissural organ {303}. Features include intermediate filaments, intercellular lumina and apical microvilli, hemidesmosomes and basal lamina. In addition, some have been suggested to contain secretory granules {303}.

Proliferation

The proliferative potential of chordoid gliomas corresponds to that of a low-grade glioma. Mitoses are either very rare or absent, and the MIB-1 labelling index is low, with values of 0 to 1.5% in one study {220} and <5% in another {1848}.

Differential diagnosis

The strikingly 'chordoid' appearance of these neoplasms, with their eosinophilic clustered tumour cells in a blue mucinous matrix, is distinctive among other regional lesions, including chordoid meningioma, pilocytic astrocytoma, and ependymoma. While there are histological similarities between chordoid gliomas and chordoid meningiomas, the latter are GFAP-negative and EMA-positive {390}. In contrast to chordoid gliomas, chordoid meningiomas are typically dural-based. Histologic similarities include the clustering of epithelioid cells and the presence of a lymphoplasmacytic infiltrate, but the latter is often more prominent in meningiomas and may feature germinal centre formation.

Genetics

Analysis of 4 chordoid gliomas by comparative genomic hybridization revealed no chromosomal imbalances {1848}. None of the neoplasms contained genetic alterations of the *TP53* or *CDKN2A* genes. Similarly, no amplification of *EGFR, CDK4* or *MDM2* genes was found.

Histogenesis

The ultrastructural demonstration of microvilli and hemidesmosome-like structures in chordoid glioma has supported an ependymal histogenesis {303}.

Further evidence of ependymal or specialized-ependymal differentiation came from a report of abnormal cilia in a juxtanuclear location {1690}. The presence of a cytologic zonation pattern and secretory vesicles indicated a specialized ependymal differentiation as might be expected of cells derived from a circumventricular organ such as the lamina terminalis. Tanycytic derivation has been suggested based on ultrastructural studies and the occurrence of tanycytes in the lamina terminalis {1284, 1997}.

Prognostic and predictive factors

Chordoid gliomas are histologically low-grade. However, their location within the third ventricle and their attachment to hypothalamic and suprasellar structures often precludes a complete resection. Postoperative tumour enlargement has been noted in half of the patients undergoing subtotal resections. Among reported cases of chordoid gliomas, approximately 20% of patients died in the perioperative period or from tumour regrowth {1233}. The most frequent morbidity reported following neurosurgical resection is hypothalamic dysfunction.

Angiocentric glioma

P.C. Burger
A. Jouvet
M. Preusser
V.H. Hans
M.K. Rosenblum
A. Lellouch-Tubiana

Definition
An epilepsy-associated, stable or slowly growing cerebral tumour primarily affecting children and young adults; histopathologically characterized by an angiocentric pattern of growth, monomorphous bipolar cells, and features of ependymal differentiation.

ICD-O code
The provisional code proposed for the fourth edition of ICD-O is *9431/1*.

Grading
The lesion corresponds to WHO grade I.

Synonyms and historical annotation
Alternatively designated as "monomorphous angiocentric glioma" {2364} or "angiocentric neuroepithelial tumour" {1289}, this is a recently described lesion of uncertain relationship to other neoplasms exhibiting ependymal differentiation.

Incidence
Incidence figures are not yet available for this uncommon lesion.

Age and sex distribution
Three publications from France {1289}, the United States {2364} and Austria/Germany {1799A} have reported a total

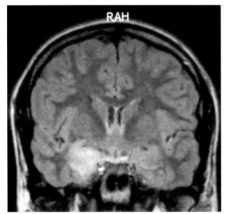

Fig. 5.07 Angiocentric glioma. The bright lesion with little mass effect is based largely in the amygdala of the gray matter.

of 26 patients. The age at surgery ranged from 2.3 to 70 years (mean, 17 years). Both sexes were equally affected (M/F ratio, 1.0).

Localization
A superficial, cerebrocortical location is typical. Reports to date indicate an excess of lesions involving the frontoparietal lobe (38% of cases) followed by temporal lobe including the hippocampus/parahippocampus (35%) and the parietal lobe (15%).

Clinical features
Symptoms and signs
Angiocentric gliomas are epileptogenic lesions, chronic and intractable partial epilepsy being especially characteristic. Most patients have a history of several years of pre-surgical epilepsy (mean, 7.5 years).

Neuroimaging
On fluid-attenuated inversion recovery (FLAIR) images, angiocentric gliomas are well delineated solid, hyperintense, non-enhancing cortical lesions that usually extend into the subcortical white matter {1799A}. Usually, there is a focal enlargement of the affected cortical gyrus. However, in one case, angiocentric glioma appeared radiologically as hippocampal and parahippocampal atrophy {1799A}. Calcifications are very rare. A stalk-like extension to an adjacent ventricle, hyperintense on T2-weighted MR and FLAIR images, is considered diagnostic {1289}. Sequential imaging indicates that these tumours are stable or very slowly growing {2364}.

Macroscopy
Gross features have not been detailed save for one temporal lobe example described at surgery as producing hippocampal enlargement with darkening and induration of the amygdala.

Histopathology
A unifying feature is the structuring of remarkably monomorphic, bipolar spindled cells oriented about cortical blood vessels (of all calibers) in mono- or multi-layered sleeves that extend lengthwise along vascular axes and as radial pseudorosettes of ependymomatous appearance. These cells often aggregate beneath the pia-arachnoid in horizontal streams or perpendicular, strikingly palisaded arrays, and can diffusely colonize the neuroparenchyma proper at variable density. Nuclei are slender, with granular chromatin stippling. Some examples exhibit regions of solid growth containing more conspicuously fibrillary elements in compact, miniature schwannoma-like nodules as well as rounded, epithelioid cells in nests and sheets interrupted by irregular clefts or cavities. The latter may contain paranuclear, round or oval eosinophilic densities with an internal granular stippling. These cytoplasmic structures correspond to EMA-immunoreactive microlumens (as seen in conventional ependymomas). Included neurons, interpreted as either entrapped {2364} or possibly intrinsic to the lesion {1289}, do not exhibit significant dysmorphism. Mitoses are unapparent or rare, and neither complex microvascular proliferation nor necrosis is seen, but one example exhibiting recurrence as a mitotically active, anaplastic astrocytoma-like lesion has been described {2364}.

In patients aged 35, 37 and 70 years at surgery, Alzheimer-type features were observed around and within tumours, including neurofibrillary tangles and plaque-like accumulations of hyperphosphorylated tau {1799A}.

Immunohistochemistry
Spindled and epithelioid tumour cells are reactive for GFAP, S-100, and vimentin, but do not label for neuronal antigens (synaptophysin, chromogranin or NeuN). Ependymomatous features are exhibited frequently in a dot-like, microlumen-type cytoplasmic labelling for EMA. Surface EMA expression may also be seen in epithelioid perivascular and subpial formations. Podoplanin immunoreactivity has been reported in some cases.

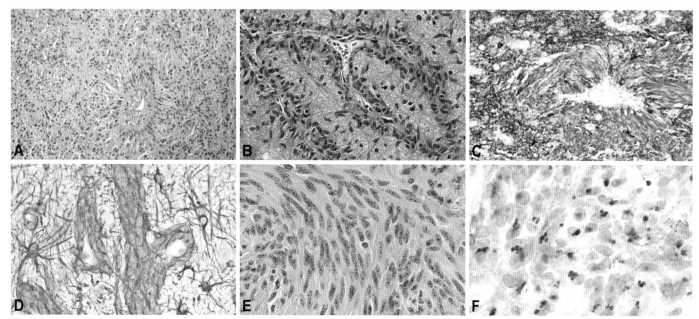

Fig. 5.08 Histological features of angiocentric glioma. **A** Elongated tumour cells forming occasionally perivascular pseudorosettes. **B** Perivascular rosettes. **C** Tumour cells in perivascular pseudorosettes express GFAP. **D** Longitudinally oriented GFAP-positive cells. **E** Compact areas that resemble schwannoma. **F** EMA-positive "dot-like" structures corresponding to microlumens.

Aberrant p53 expression and anomalous labelling patterns of included neurons for synaptophysin, chromogranin and NeuN have not been found.

Electron microscopy
Evidence of ependymal differentiation has been depicted in the form of tumoural microlumens filled with microvilli and cilia, and delimited by elongated intermediate junctions {2364}.

Proliferation
Reported MIB-1/Ki-67 labelling indices in primary neurosurgical material have ranged from 1% or less (most reported cases) to 5%. One anaplastic recurrence exhibited elevation of the labelling index to 10% (from 1% in the primary) {2364}.

Genetic susceptibility
Angiocentric gliomas have not been recorded in association with dysgenetic syndromes or in familial form.

Genetics
Using chromosomal comparative genomic hybridization (CGH), one in eight cases was found to have a loss at 6q24-q25. High-resolution array CGH revealed in one out of three cases a copy number gain at 11p11.2, containing the PTPRJ (protein-tyrosine phosphatase receptor type J) gene {1799A}.

Histogenesis
Angiocentric gliomas appear to differentiate along ependymal lines, but their cortical localization argues against an origin from native ependymocytes or tanycytes. It has been suggested that these tumours derive, via a maldevelopmental or neoplastic process, from the bipolar radial glia that span the neuroepithelium during embryogenesis and that may share ependymoglial traits or be capable of generating ependymocytes {1289}.

Prognostic and predictive factors
Angiocentric gliomas are stable tumours for which excision alone is generally curative. A possible antiepileptogenic effect of radiation therapy is described in one case without surgical resection {1799A}. The only angiocentric glioma reported as recurring (in anaplastic form) exhibited typical histologic features at presentation, affected an adult and had been subtotally resected {2364}.

CHAPTER 6

Neuronal and Mixed Neuronal-Glial Tumours

Dysplastic gangliocytoma of the cerebellum (Lhermitte-Duclos disease)

A benign cerebellar mass composed of dysplastic ganglion cells. (See Chapter 13, Cowden disease)

Desmoplastic infantile astrocytoma and ganglioglioma (WHO grade I)

Large cystic tumours of infants that involve superficial cerebral cortex and leptomeninges, often attached to dura, with a generally good prognosis following surgical resection; histologically composed of a prominent desmoplastic stroma with a neuroepithelial population, mainly restricted to neoplastic astrocytes (desmoplastic infantile astrocytoma, DIA) or to astrocytes together with a variable neuronal component (desmoplastic infantile ganglioglioma, DIG), in addition to aggregates of poorly differentiated cells, which are present in both.

Dysembryoplastic neuroepithelial tumour (WHO grade I)

Benign, usually supratentorial glial-neuronal neoplasms, occurring in children or young adults, characterized by a predominantly cortical location and by drug-resistant partial seizures; typically exhibiting a complex columnar and multinodular architecture and often associated with cortical dysplasia.

Gangliocytoma and ganglioglioma (WHO grade I)

Well-differentiated, slowly growing neuroepithelial tumours, composed of neoplastic, mature ganglion cells, alone (gangliocytoma) or in combination with neoplastic glial cells (ganglioglioma); the most frequent entity observed in patients with long-term epilepsy.

Papillary glioneuronal tumour (WHO grade I)

A relatively circumscribed, clinically indolent and histologically biphasic cerebral neoplasm composed of flat to cuboidal, GFAP-positive astrocytes lining hyalinized vascular pseudopapillae and synaptophysin-positive interpapillary collections of sheets of neurocytes, large neurons and intermediate size "ganglioid" cells.

Rosette-forming glioneuronal tumour of the fourth ventricle (WHO grade I)

A rare, slowly growing neoplasm of the fourth ventricular region, preferentially affecting young adults and composed of two distinct histological components, one with uniform neurocytes forming rosettes and/or perivascular pseudorosettes, the other being astrocytic in nature and resembling pilocytic astrocytoma.

Central neurocytoma and extraventricular neurocytoma (WHO grade II)

A neoplasm composed of uniform round cells with neuronal differentiation, typically located in the lateral ventricles in the region of the foramen of Monro (central neurocytoma) or brain parenchyma (extraventricular neurocytoma); affecting mostly young adults, and with a favourable prognosis.

Cerebellar liponeurocytoma (WHO grade II)

A rare cerebellar neoplasm of adults with consistent neuronal, variable astrocytic and focal lipomatous differentiation, and with a low proliferative potential; the tumour usually has a favourable clinical prognosis, although recurrences are frequent.

Spinal paraganglioma (WHO grade I)

A unique neuroendocrine neoplasm, usually encapsulated and benign, arising in specialized neural crest cells associated with segmental or collateral autonomic ganglia (paraganglia); consisting of uniform chief cells exhibiting neuronal differentiation forming compact nests (Zellballen), surrounded by sustentacular cells and a delicate capillary network; within the central nervous system, primarily affecting the cauda equina/filum terminale region.

Desmoplastic infantile astrocytoma and ganglioglioma

D.J. Brat
S.R. VandenBerg
D. Figarella-Branger
A.L. Taratuto

Definition

Large cystic tumours of infants that involve superficial cerebral cortex and leptomeninges, often attached to dura, with a generally good prognosis following surgical resection; histologically composed of a prominent desmoplastic stroma with a neuroepithelial population, mainly restricted to neoplastic astrocytes (desmoplastic infantile astrocytoma, DIA) or to astrocytes together with a variable neuronal component (desmoplastic infantile ganglioglioma, DIG), in addition to aggregates of poorly differentiated cells, which are present in both.

ICD-O code   9412/1

Grading

Histologically, desmoplastic infantile astrocytoma/ganglioglioma corresponds to WHO grade I.

Synonyms and historical annotation

The desmoplastic infantile astrocytoma (DIA) was originally defined in 1982 by Taratuto et al. {2216} as meningocerebral astrocytoma attached to dura with desmoplastic reaction. The lesion was further described as a superficial cerebral astrocytoma attached to dura {2217}, thus delineating a previously unrecognized entity. In 1993, it was included in the WHO Classification {1120} under the term 'desmoplastic

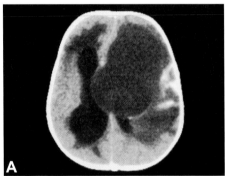
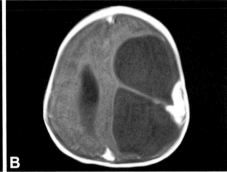

Fig. 6.02 A CT scan of a desmoplastic infantile ganglioglioma with a solid component involving the superficial parietal lobe and large cystic component that extends across the midline. **B** Post contrast axial MR image demonstrating a superficial enhancing component of a desmoplastic infantile ganglioglioma together with a large septated cystic component that enlarges the skull and displaces the midline.

cerebral astrocytoma of infancy'. In 1987, VandenBerg et al. {2314} described desmoplastic supratentorial neuroepithelial tumours of infancy with divergent differentiation ('desmoplastic infantile ganglioglioma', DIG), occurring in the same clinical setting. The histopathology of DIG differed from DIA by the presence of a neuronal component with variable differentiation, and this description also stressed the presence of immature neuroepithelial cell aggregates {2314}. Since both lesions have similar clinical and neuroimaging features, including a favourable prognosis, they have been categorized together as desmoplastic infantile astrocytoma/ganglioglioma in this and previous editions of the WHO classification.

Incidence

Desmoplastic infantile astrocytoma/gangliogliomas (DIA/DIG) are rare neoplasms of childhood. Their incidence can only be estimated from their frequency in institutional series. One series of 6500 CNS tumours from all ages reported 22 cases of desmoplastic infantile ganglioglioma (0.3%) {2312}. In a series of CNS intracranial tumours limited to the paediatric age group, 6 desmoplastic infantile astrocytomas were found, accounting for 1.25% of all childhood brain tumours {2217}. When studies have been limited to brain tumours of infancy,

DIA/DIG accounted for 16% of intracranial tumours {2511}.

Age and sex distribution

The age range for 84 reported cases of desmoplastic infantile astrocytoma/ganglioglioma is 1–24 months, with a male: female ratio of 1.5:1. The large majority of infantile cases present within the first year of life. Several non-infantile cases, with ages ranging from 5 to 25 years, have been reported. There is a strong male predominance in the non-infantile cases {645,1774}.

Localization

These tumours invariably arise in the supratentorial region and commonly involve more than one lobe, preferentially the frontal and parietal, followed by the temporal and, least frequently, the occipital.

Clinical features
Symptoms and signs

These are of short duration and include increasing head circumference, tense and bulging fontanelles, lethargy, and setting-sun sign. Occasionally, patients present with seizures, focal motor signs or skull bossing over the tumour.

Neuroimaging

On CT scans, DIA/DIG are seen as large, hypodense cystic masses with a solid isodense or slightly hyperdense superficial

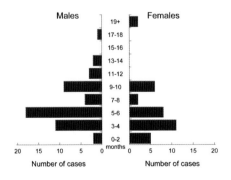

Fig. 6.01 Age (months) and sex distribution of desmoplastic infantile astrocytoma and ganglioglioma, based on 84 published cases.

portion that extends to the overlying meninges and shows contrast enhancement. The cystic portion is usually located deep, whereas the solid portion is peripheral. T1-weighted images on MRI are characterized by a hypointense cystic component with an isointense peripheral solid component that enhances with gadolinium. On T2-weighted images, the cystic component is hyperintense and the solid portion is heterogeneous. Edema is usually absent or moderate {2263}.

Macroscopy
These tumours are large, measuring up to 13 cm in diameter, and have deep uni- or multiloculated cysts filled with clear or xanthochromic fluid. The solid superficial portion is primarily extracerebral, involving leptomeninges and superficial cortex and is commonly attached to the dura, firm or rubbery in consistency, and grey or white in colour. There is no gross evidence of haemorrhage or necrosis.

Histopathology
Diagnostic features are those of a slowly growing superficial neuroepithelial tumour with three distinctive components: the main desmoplastic leptomeningeal component, the poorly differentiated neuroepithelial component and the cortical component. The desmoplastic leptomeningeal compo-

nent consists of a mixture of fibroblast-like spindle-shaped cells and more pleomorphic neoplastic neuroepithelial cells with eosinophilic cytoplasm both arranged in fascicles or in a storiform or whorled pattern. Reticulin impregnations show a prominent reticulin positive network surrounding almost every cell and mimicking a mesenchymal tumour. Astrocytes are the sole tumour cell population in DIA or the predominant neoplastic population, associated with neoplastic neurons, in DIG. Neoplastic neurons range from atypical ganglionic cells to small polygonal cell types {2311, 2314}. In addition to this desmoplastic leptomeningeal component, both DIA and DIG contain a population of poorly differentiated neuroepithelial cells with small, round, deeply basophilic nuclei and minimal surrounding perikarya. Such an immature component, lacking desmoplasia, may predominate in some areas. A cortical component devoid of desmoplasia may also be observed, and this neoplastic component is often multinodular, with some nodules being microcystic {1774}.

There is a sharp demarcation between the cortical surface and the desmoplastic tumour although Virchow-Robin spaces in the underlying cortex are often filled with tumour cells. Calcifications are common but mononuclear inflammatory

cells are not usually seen. Mitotic activity and necrosis are uncommon, but when present are mostly restricted to the population of poorly differentiated neuroepithelial cells {2311, 2312}. Some tumours may contain angiomatoid vessels, but microvascular proliferation is not evident {434, 1354}.

Immunohistochemistry
In the desmoplastic leptomeningeal component, fibroblast-like cells express vimentin. Most often, they also express GFAP, and a few express smooth muscle actin. In addition, most other neuroepithelial tumour cells react with GFAP. Therefore, astrocytes predominate in this component. Antibodies to type IV collagen react in a reticulin-like pattern around tumour cells {75, 405}. Expression of neuronal markers (synaptophysin, NF-H, class III ß-tubulin), is observed in the neoplastic neuronal cells but also in cells lacking apparent neuronal differentiation in routine stains {1703}.
In the poorly differentiated neuroepithelial component, cells react with GFAP {1589, 2219, 2312} and vimentin, but also with neuronal markers and MAP2 {1703, 1957, 2312}. Desmin expression may be encountered {1957} but epithelial markers (CAM 5.2, AE1/AE3, EMA) are lacking {1703}.

Electron microscopy
Astrocytic tumour cells are characterized by intermediate filaments typically arranged in bundles as well as scattered cisternae of rough endoplasmic reticulum and mitochondria. An extensive basal lamina surrounds individual tumour cells. Fibroblasts containing granular endoplasmic reticulum and well-developed Golgi complexes are also noted, particularly in collagen-rich areas {434, 1354, 2217}. The neuronal cells of DIG contain dense core secretory granules and may elaborate small processes containing neurofilaments. Immuno-electron microscopy has shown filamentous reactivity to NF-H in these neuronal cell bodies as well as processes lacking a basal lamina. The occurrence of Schwann cell differentiation remains unsettled {1156}.

Proliferation
Mitotic activity is rare and, when present, is mostly restricted to the undifferentiated, small cell population in DIG {2311, 2312}.

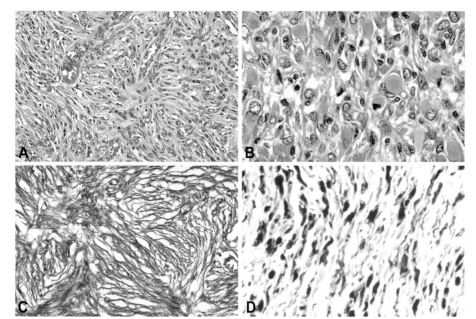

Fig. 6.03 Desmoplastic cerebral astrocytomas of infancy. **A** Neoplastic astrocytes arranged in streams, with a (**C**) marked desmoplastic component (reticulin stain). **B** Field of gemistocytic neoplastic astrocytes. **D** GFAP-expressing neoplastic astrocytes: the desmoplastic component remains unstained.

Ki-67 labelling indices reported in the literature range from less than 0.5% to 5%. The majority of Ki-67 labelling indices reported are less than 2% {1196}. In those unusual DIA/DIG that show histologic anaplasia, mitotic activity is readily identified, and Ki-67 indices up to 45% have been reported {437} Proliferation does not appear to be related to clinical behaviour in completely resected tumours but may predict more aggressive behaviour in subtotally resected cases. {437, 2220, 2235}. In three cases analyzed by flow cytometry, the S-phase fraction ranged from 3.7% to 12%, with a mean of 6.6% {2220}.

Genetics

Classic cytogenetic analysis has been carried out on only a limited number of cases. In each case, either a normal karyotype or non-clonal abnormalities were described, including alterations involving 1p, 3p, 3q, 5q, 7q, 9p, 11q, 14q, 17p, 21q and 22q {308}.
Molecular studies of DIA revealed no loss of heterozygosity on chromosomes 10 and 17 and no *TP53* mutations {1354, 2220}. A comparative genomic hybridization study of 3 cases of DIA and DIG did not reveal any consistent chromosomal gains or losses {1196}. One case of DIG showed a loss on 8p22-pter, while one DIA showed gain on 13q21 {308}. Hypermethylation of the *p14^ARF* gene was reported in one tumour {308}.

Histogenesis

The cellular origins of desmoplastic infantile astrocytomas and gangliogliomas have not been established. The presence of primitive small cell populations that express both glial and neuronal proteins might suggest that these are progenitor cells to the more differentiated neuro-epithelial components and supports the contention that DIA/DIG are embryonal neoplasms programmed to progressive maturation. The basal lamina-associated proteins that are seen in abundance in these neoplasms are known to inhibit cellular proliferation and to induce differ-

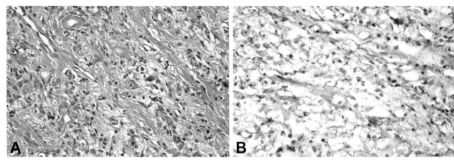

Fig. 6.04 Desmoplastic infantile ganglioglioma with (**A**) scattered ganglion cells and (**B**) marked synaptophysin immunoreactivity of ganglion cells and their processes.

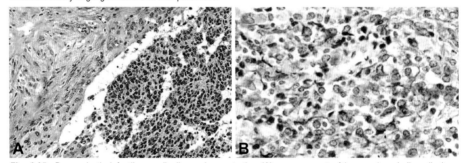

Fig. 6.05 Desmoplastic infantile ganglioglioma demonstrating (**A**) a component of low grade spindle cells in a collagen-rich matrix and a component of primitive small round blue cells and (**B**) the primitive, poorly differentiated component immunoreactive for neuronal marker MAP2.

entiation of human glioma cells *in vitro* {1354, 1961}. An origin from the specialized subpial astrocytes that form a continuous, limiting basal lamina investing their terminal processes could account for a comparable phenomenon occurring in desmoplastic infantile tumours and for their superficial localization {75, 1354}. The lack of genetic alterations typical of most diffuse astrocytomas suggests they are not related to these neoplasms.

Prognostic and predictive factors

Follow-up studies indicate that gross total resection results in long term survival in cases of DIA and DIG {2172}. In one study of eight patients with DIA (median follow-up, 15.1 years), six survived to the end of follow-up {2217, 2220}. In another study, no deaths or evidence of tumour recurrence were observed in 14 patients with DIG (median follow-up, 8.7 years) {2312}. Thus, surgery alone with total removal appears to offer local tumour control. In

cases of subtotal resection or biopsy, most tumours are stable or regrow slowly. Two tumours showed radiologic evidence of tumour regression following subtotal resection {2204}. Dissemination of these tumours through the CSF has been reported, but should be considered a rare event {437}
Long-term tumour control can be achieved by total surgical resection in DIA and DIG despite the presence of primitive-appearing cellular aggregates with mitotic activity or foci of necrosis. In two cases of DIG that showed frankly anaplastic features (high mitotic rate, microvascular proliferation and perinecrotic palisading tumour cells), there was no evidence of tumour recurrence following gross total resection {1219, 1220}. Tumour progression has been recorded in DIGs that could not be completely resected, including those with high prolif-erative indices and anaplastic features {437, 1156}.

Dysembryoplastic neuroepithelial tumour

C. Daumas-Duport
T. Pietsch
C. Hawkins
S.K. Shankar

Definition

Benign, usually supratentorial glial-neuronal neoplasms, occurring in children or young adults, characterized by a predominantly cortical location and by drug-resistant partial seizures; typically exhibiting a complex columnar and multinodular architecture and often associated with cortical dysplasia.

ICD-O code   9413/0

Grading

These lesions correspond histologically to WHO grade I.

Synonyms and historical annotation

This tumour entity was originally identified in patients who had undergone epilepsy surgery for the treatment of long-standing drug-resistant partial seizures. They showed unusual morphological features including cortical topography, multinodular architecture, a 'specific glioneuronal element' with a columnar structure, and foci of cortical dysplasia. Long-term follow-up demonstrated no clinical or radiological evidence of recurrence, even in patients with incomplete surgical removal. Moreover, several factors strongly suggested that these tumours might have a dysembryoplastic

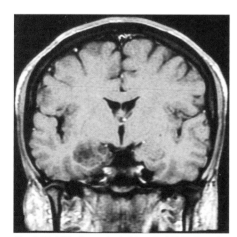

Fig. 6.06 MRI of supratentorial cortical DNT. Complex histological form with a pseudo-polycystic appearance (T1 post-contrast).

origin. Therefore the term "dysembryoplastic neuroepithelial tumour" (DNT) was proposed for these distinctive lesions {422}. In the WHO classification in 1993 {1120}, DNTs were included in the category of "neuronal and mixed neuronal-glial tumours". These histological criteria were based on the initial description of DNTs and allow only for the diagnosis of a morphological variant now referred to as the "complex form". A "simple form" of DNT with a unique glioneuronal element was later described {419}. It has been suggested that DNTs include a large spectrum of tumours that cannot be distinguished histologically from ordinary gliomas, and that the diagnosis of such "non-specific histological forms" requires that clinical presentation and imaging features be taken into consideration {419, 426, 858, 1689}. Furthermore, it has been demonstrated that DNTs are not exclusively located within the supratentorial cortex, but may also arise in various other supratentorial or infratentorial locations.

Incidence

Large variations are observed in the reported incidence of DNTs according to the surgical protocol and/or to the criteria used for their diagnosis. In epilepsy surgery, the incidence of "typical" DNTs was 12% in adults {1362} and 13.5% in children, while in series that included "non-specific" histological variants, DNTs were identified in 19–22% of the patients {426, 603, 1689}. Among all neuroepithelial tumours diagnosed in a single institution, DNTs were identified in 1.2% of the patients under 20 years of age and in 0.2% of those aged more than 20 years {1926}.

Age and sex distribution

Patient age at the onset of symptoms is an important diagnostic criterion. In about 90% of cases, the first seizure occurs before 20 years of age; however, ages of onset from 3 weeks {1649} to 38 years {1839} have been reported. At diagnosis, the patients are often in the

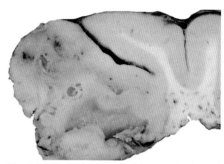

Fig. 6.07 Surgical specimen of the complex form of DNT showing the cortical topography of the lesion and several pseudo-cysts with the larger being an enlarged sulcus.

second or third decade of life, but detection of DNTs by imaging in children or young adults with recent onset seizures has become more common, and these tumours are increasingly operated on in the setting of paediatric neurosurgery {206, 298, 566, 691, 1602}. Males are more frequently affected.

Localization

DNTs may be located in any part of the supratentorial cortex, but they show a predilection for the temporal lobe, preferentially involving the mesial structures {315, 419, 420, 422, 426, 427, 451, 858, 1689, 1795}. In series based on general practice, the temporal lobe accounts for 50% or fewer of the cases {419, 2218, 2222}. DNTs have also been identified in the area of the caudate nucleus {310, 733} or lateral ventricle {1646}, the

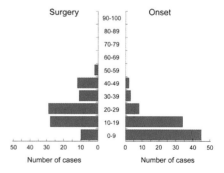

Fig. 6.08 Age distribution of dysembryoplastic neuroepithelial tumours, based on 92 cases from the Ste-Anne Hospital, Paris.

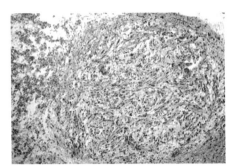

Fig. 6.09 Low-power micrograph of a cortical lesion showing a glial nodule within a specific glioneuronal element.

septum pelucidum {87, 774} the trigono-septal region {733}, the midbrain and tectum {1237}, and the cerebellum {422, 1216, 2464} or cerebellum and brain stem {619}. In total, 25 cases of extra-cortical examples were reported. In addition, four examples of multifocal DNTs have been reported, showing that these tumours may also be found in the region of the third ventricle, the basal ganglia and the pons {1290, 1296, 2404}.

Clinical features
Symptoms and signs
Patients who harbour supratentorial DNTs typically present with drug-resistant partial seizures, with or without secondary generalization and no neurological deficit. A congenital neurological deficit may, however, be observed in a minority of cases {315, 422, 426, 451, 566, 1602, 1689, 1795, 1839, 1928, 2218}. The duration of the seizures prior to surgical intervention can vary from weeks to decades, leading to variability in the age of the patients at pathologic diagnosis.

Neuroimaging
Cortical topography of the lesion, the absence of mass effect and no peri-tumoural edema are important criteria for differentiating between DNTs and gliomas. The tumours usually encompass the thickness of the normal cortex and, in a minority of the cases, the area of signal abnormality may also extend into the subcortical white matter {419, 426, 427, 566, 1234, 1653, 2140}. The cortical location of the lesion is better seen on MRI than on CT scan. DNTs appear hyperintense on T2-weighted and hypo-intense or, less often, iso-intense on T1-weighted images. These tumours may look like macrogyri but often have a pseudo-cystic or multi-cystic appearance {419, 426, 427, 1234, 2140}; however,

true cyst formations are uncommon and are usually small {2140}. In tumours that are located at the convexity, deformation of the overlying calvarium is often seen on imaging, and this finding further supports the diagnosis of DNT {419, 426, 427, 1234, 1839, 2140, 2218}. Calcifications are often seen on CT scan and may be voluminous. About one third of DNTs show contrast enhancement on CT scan or MRI, which often appears as multiple rings rather than homogeneous enhancement {1602, 2140}. Ring-shaped contrast enhancement may occur in a previously non-enhancing tumour {2140} and increased lesion size, with or without peritumoural edema, may also be observed on imaging follow-up. However, in DNTs, these changes are not signs of malignant transformation but are usually due to ischaemic and/or haemorrhagic changes {425, 993, 1653}.

Macroscopy
DNTs may vary in size from some milli-meters to several centimeters {1689}. In their typical location, they are often easily identified at the cortical surface and may show an exophytic development. However, the leptomeninges are not involved. The appearance of DNTs on cut sections may reflect the complex histoarchitecture of the lesion. The most typical feature is the viscous consistency of the glioneuronal component. This may be associated with multiple or single firmer nodules. The affected cortex is often expanded.

Histopathology
The histological hallmark of the classical DNT is the 'specific glioneuronal element', characterized by columns oriented perpendicularly to the cortical surface. They are formed by bundles of axons lined by small oligodendroglia-like cells. Between these columns, neurons with normal cytology appear to float in a pale, eosinophilic matrix. Associated with this element are scattered GFAP-positive stellate astrocytes. Depending on the amount of fluid extravasation, subtle variation from a columnar to an alveolar or a more compact structure may be observed {419}. Several histological forms of DNTs have been described but this subclassification has no clinical or therapeutic implication.

Simple form
In this morphological variant, the tumour consists of the unique glioneuronal element. It may show a patchy pattern {419}, owing to the juxtaposition of foci of tumour and of well-recognizable cortex.

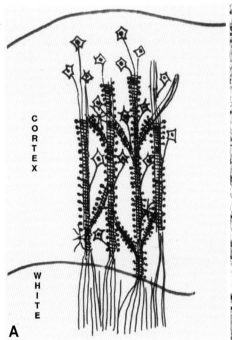
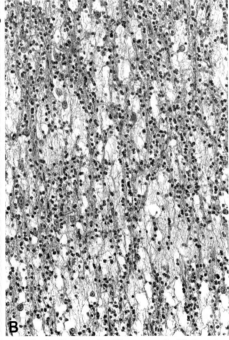

Fig. 6.10 A and **B** Bundles of axon (black) are attached to oligodendroglia-like cells while neurons float in the interstitial fluid. Histology shows the glioneuronal elements in a columnar orientation.

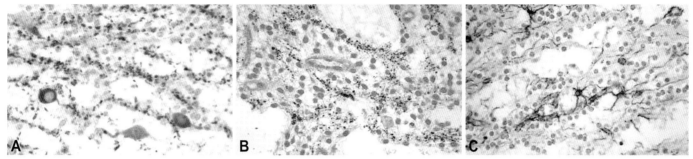

Fig. 6.11 Immunohistochemical features of dysembryoplastic neuroepithelial tumour. **A** Floating neurons showing immunoreactivity to MAP2. **B** Synaptophysin immunoreactivity of neuronal cell processes. **C** Scattered astrocytes evidenced by GFAP immunostaining.

Complex form

In this variant, glial nodules, which lend the tumour a characteristic multinodular architecture, are seen in association with the specific glioneuronal element. The heterogeneous appearance of these tumours is due to the presence of astrocytic, oligodendrocytic and neuronal components. These constituent cell populations may vary from case to case, and from area to area within the same tumour. The glial components seen in the complex forms of DNTs have a highly variable appearance: (i) they may form typical nodules, but may also show a rather diffuse pattern; (ii) they may closely resemble conventional categories of gliomas or may show unusual features; (iii) they often mimic low-grade gliomas, but may show nuclear atypia, rare mitosis, or microvascular-like proliferation and ischaemic necrosis; (iv) their microvascular network may also vary from poor to exuberant, including glomerulus-like formations. In these vessels, the endothelial cells may be hyperplastic and mitotically active. Within the glial components, frankly hamartomatous, usually calcified vessels are not uncommon {419, 426, 1839}. They may behave as vascular malformations

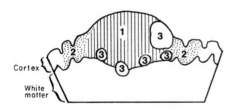

Fig. 6.12 Schematic representation of complex forms of DNTs. 1. Glioneuronal element; 2. cortical dysplasia; 3.glial nodules. Reproduced from Daumas-Duport et al. {422}.

and be responsible for haemorrhage {425, 566, 1653, 2140, 2240}.

On the basis of their similar clinical presentation, cortical topography, neuroradiological features and stability on long-term preoperative imaging follow-up, 'non-specific' histological variants of DNTs have been described {426}. As they lack the specific glioneuronal element and multinodular architecture these variants of DNTs are often histologically indistinguishable from low-grade gliomas, particularly when the cortical topography of the tumour is not apparent on non-representative samples. The diagnosis of these tumours thus requires that the clinical presentation and imaging appearance of the lesion be taken into consideration. Non-specific histological forms accounted for 20–50% of DNTs in three studies {426, 1689, 2299}. Although gliomas identified in patients with long-term epilepsy during epilepsy surgery are usually associated with a distinct benign prognosis {108, 181, 360, 1362}, the concept of 'non-specific' histological variants of DNTs remains controversial.

Cortical dysplasia

In association with the tumour, a dysplastic disorganization of the cortex may be observed in up to 80% of the cases with adequate sampling {1689, 1974, 2200, 2299}.

Neuronal populations of DNTs

Supratentorial cortical DNTs contain mature neurons. Both in the tumour itself and in the area of cortical dysplasia, the neurons may show various degrees of cytological anomalies. However, DNTs do not contain atypical neurons that resemble dysplastic ganglion cells, such as those found in gangliogliomas. Tumour cells with an oligodendrocytic appearance were found to occasionally

express neuronal markers and to exhibit axo-somatic synapses {831, 859, 2424}, suggesting that the so-called oligodendroglial-like cells of DNTs may show an early neuronal differentiation. However, recent results with in situ hybridization demonstrated that oligodendroglial-like cells transcribe myelin genes and express myelin oligodendrocyte glycoprotein protein, indicating oligodendroglial differentiation {2436}.

Cortical topography

The limits of the tumour most often coincide strikingly with that of the cortex. In other instances, the tumour seems also to involve the adjacent white matter, however, neurons may usually be identified even in the deeper part of the tumour and/or in the adjacent white matter, this likely reflecting disordered neuronal migration {426, 2427}.

Diagnostic criteria

The histological diagnosis of DNTs may be difficult, particularly with limited material. The typical columnar architecture of the specific glio-neuronal element may be obscured when the samples are not adequately oriented and, as a result of its semi-liquid consistency, this element may be lost because of inadvertent surgical aspiration and/or fragmentation during fixation. It is thus important that the diagnosis of DNT be taken into consideration whenever all of the following criteria are present: (i) partial seizures with or without secondary generalization, usually beginning before the age 20 years; (ii) no progressive neurological deficit; (iii) predominantly cortical topography of a supratentorial lesion, best demonstrated on MRI; and (iv) no mass effect on CT or MRI, except if related to a cyst, and no peritumoural edema {420,426,427}.

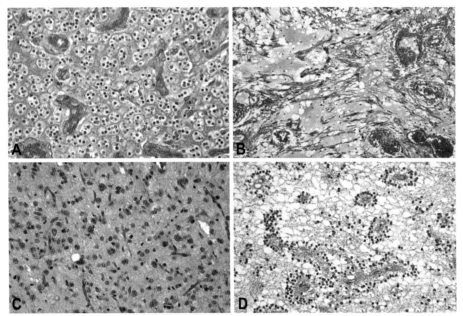

Fig. 6.13 Examples of glial components observed in cortical DNTs: **A** resembling oligodendroglioma, **B** resembling pilocytic astrocytoma, **C** showing marked nuclear atypia, **D** with small oligodendroglial-like cells forming perivascular pseudorosettes.

DNT versus low-grade diffuse gliomas.
The above clinical and radiological criteria help in distinguishing these benign tumours from diffuse gliomas. It is noteworthy that (i) in low-grade diffuse gliomas, infiltrative microcystic formation may mimic a "specific glioneuronal element, (ii) these tumours may occasionally exhibit so called "floating" neurons, (iii) oligodendroglioma may exhibit a nodular pattern and (iv) in the cortex, secondary architectural changes caused by the growth of gliomas may be difficult to distinguish from a dysplastic cortical disorganization.

DNT versus ganglioglioma
Gangliogliomas may also pose a difficult problem of differential diagnosis with DNTs because (i) the neoplastic ganglion cells of gangliogliomas may not be present in small or non-representative samples (ii), these tumours may show a multinodular structure, (iii) small gangliogliomas may show a predominant cortical topography and (iv) the clinical presentation of gangliogliomas is often similar to that of DNTs. A ganglioglioma should however be suspected when the tumour shows perivascular lymphocytic infiltration, a network of reticulin fibers and/or a large cystic component. Since gangliogliomas may undergo malignant transformation, their distinction from DNT

is important from a prognostic point of view. Nonetheless, examples of composite ganglioglioma and DNT have been reported and were considered to represent a transitional form between these two tumours {315, 828, 1789, 2084}.

Proliferation
MIB-1 labelling indices of DNTs have been reported to vary from 0% up to 8% focally {419, 426, 427, 1689, 1795, 2218}.

Genetic susceptibility
DNTs may occasionally occur in patients with neurofibromatosis type 1 (NF1) or with XYY syndrome {1041, 1207, 1290}.

Genetics
No deletion on 1p, 17p or 19q {621, 1004, 1793} and no *TP53* gene mutations {621} have been detected in DNTs.

Histogenesis
Several factors suggest that DNTs have a malformative origin, including the presence of focal cortical dysplasia and of ectopic neurons in the adjacent white matter, the young age at the onset of symptoms and bone deformity adjacent to the tumours {419, 422, 426, 427}. It was initially proposed that the sites in which these tumours are observed were in accordance with a hypothesis that DNTs may be derived from the secondary germinal

layers {422}. However, the notion of secondary germinal layers and, in particular, the hypothesis that the subpial granular layer may produce neurons and glial cells, is now obsolete. The histogenesis of DNT thus remains unsolved.

Prognostic and predictive factors
DNTs are benign. Their stability has been demonstrated in a study that included 53 patients for whom successive pre-operative CT or MRI was available with a mean duration of follow-up of 4.5 years {2140}. Long-term clinical follow-up usually demonstrates no evidence of recurrence, even in patients with partial surgical removal {419, 422, 426, 427, 566, 1116, 1274, 1362, 1839, 1981, 2140}. However, ischaemic or haemorrhagic changes may occur, with or without an increase in size of the lesion or peritumoural edema {425, 566, 993, 1653, 2140}. Risk factors for the development of recurrent seizures after operation at long-term follow-up were longer pre-operative history of seizures {66,810}, presence of residual tumour {1602} and presence of cortical dysplasia adjacent to DNT {1974}. Although more than 700 cases of DNT have to-date been reported (http://www.wnfs.org/re4-2/reviews4-2_3.htm), only two cases of malignant transformation, one of which occurred after radiation and chemotherapy, have yet been described {1958}; in addition, in both patients, the initial clinical presentation was atypical.

Ganglioglioma and gangliocytoma

A.J. Becker
O.D. Wiestler
D. Figarella-Branger
I. Blümcke

Definition

Well differentiated, slowly growing neuroepithelial tumours, composed of neoplastic, mature ganglion cells, alone (gangliocytoma) or in combination with neoplastic glial cells (ganglioglioma); the most frequent entity observed in patients with long-term epilepsy.

ICD-O codes

Gangliocytoma   9492/0
Ganglioglioma   9505/1
Anaplastic ganglioglioma   9505/3

Grading

Gangliocytomas and most gangliogliomas correspond to WHO grade I. Some gangliogliomas with anaplastic features in their glial component are considered WHO grade III (anaplastic ganglioglioma) {183, 1363}. Criteria for grade II have been suggested, but are not established {1363}.

Incidence

Available data indicate that gangliocytomas and gangliogliomas together represent 0.4% of all CNS tumours and 1.3% of all brain tumours {1030, 1363}. There are no population-based epidemiological data on gangliogliomas.

Age and sex distribution

The age of patients ranges from 2 months to 70 years. Data from five large series

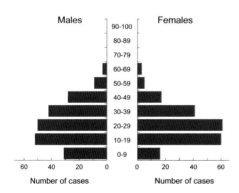

Fig. 6.14 Age and sex distribution of ganglioglioma patients, based on 418 cases from the German Neuropathology Reference Center for Epilepsy Surgery.

with a total of 626 patients indicate a mean/median age at diagnosis from 8.5 to 25 years. The male:female ratio varied from 1.1:1 to 1.9:1 {832, 1256, 1798, 2425}. In 99 cases involving only children, the mean age at diagnosis was 9.5 years, with 52% female patients {1002}. In a survey of the German Neuropathology Reference Centre for Epilepsy Surgery, the mean age of 124 children with gangliogliomas was 10.3 years, with 44% being female patients.

Localization

These tumours occur throughout the CNS, including cerebrum, brain stem, cerebellum, spinal cord, optic nerves, pituitary and pineal glands. The majority of gangliogliomas localize in the temporal lobe (>70%) {183, 832, 1256, 1798, 2425}. A distinct entity, dysplastic gangliocytoma of the cerebellum (Lhermitte-Duclos), is discussed in Chapter 13.

Clinical features

Symptoms and signs

Symptoms vary according to tumour size and site. Tumours in the cerebrum are frequently associated with a history of seizures ranging in duration from 1 month to 50 years before diagnosis, with a mean/median interval of 6–25 years {1256, 1798, 2425}. For tumours involving the brain stem or spinal cord, the mean duration of symptoms before diagnosis is 1.25 and 1.4 years, respectively {1256}. Gangliogliomas have been reported in 15–25% of patients undergoing surgery for control of seizures {2425, 2428}. They are the most common tumours associated with chronic temporal lobe epilepsy {1362}

Neuroimaging

CT shows a circumscribed solid mass or cyst with a mural nodule. The tumour may be calcified. Contrast enhancement is typical but may be faint or absent. Scalloping of the calvarium may be seen adjacent to superficially located cerebral tumours. MRI shows a T1-weighted hypointense, T2-weighted hyperintense circumscribed mass. Enhancement varies

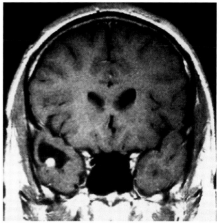

Fig. 6.15 MRI of a cystic ganglioglioma in the left temporal lobe with an intramural nodule.

in intensity from none to marked, and may be solid, rim or nodular {727, 1651}.

Macroscopy

Gangliogliomas are solid or cystic lesions, usually with little mass effect. Calcification may be observed. Haemorrhage and necrosis are rare.

Histopathology

Gangliocytomas are composed of irregular groups of large, multipolar neurons with often dysplastic features. The stroma consists of non-neoplastic glial elements and a network of reticulin fibers, often in perivascular location.

Table 6.01 Regional manifestation of gangliogliomas (GG) and other long-term epilepsy-associated tumours (LEAT). Other localizations include striatum and spinal cord. Data based on 413 GG and 802 LEAT.

Localization	GG	LEAT
Frontal	7%	12%
Parietal	3%	5%
Occipital	3%	3%
Temporal	86%	78%
Other	1%	2%
Multiple lobes	7%	7%

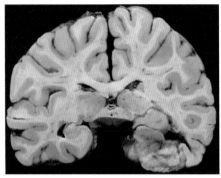

Fig. 6.16 Ganglioglioma of the right temporal lobe also involving the hippocampal formation.

The histopathological hallmark of gangliogliomas is a combination of neuronal and glial cell elements, which may exhibit marked heterogeneity. Dysplastic neurons should be characterized by (i) loss of cytoarchitectural organization, (ii) abnormal (subcortical) localization, (iii) clustered appearance, (iv) cytomegaly, (v) perimembranous aggregated Nissl substance or (vi) presence of bi- or multinucleated neurons (in up to 50% of cases). The glial component in gangliogliomas shows substantial variability, but constitutes the proliferative cell population of the tumour. It may include cell types resembling fibrillary astrocytoma, oligodendroglioma or pilocytic astrocytoma.

Table 6.02 Spectrum of long-term epilepsy-associated tumours. Data from the German Reference Center for Epilepsy Surgery, based on 1006 cases.

Entity		
Astrocytoma	Pilocytic	5%
	Diffuse	5%
	Anaplastic	3%
Cysts	Arachnoid	0.5%
	Epidermoid	1%
	Dermoid	0.1%
DNT		17%
Gangliocytoma		0.3%
Ganglioglioma	WHO I	44%
	WHO II	4%
	WHO III	0.6%
Meningioma		1%
NOS		4%
Oligodendroglioma	WHO II	3%
	WHO III	1%
Oligoastrocytoma	WHO II	3%
	WHO III	1%
Pleomorphic xanthoastrocytoma		3%
SEGA		1%
Other		1%

Rosenthal fibers and eosinophilic granular bodies are present in many cases. A fibrillary matrix is usually prominent and may contain microcystic cavities and/or mucous substance. Gangliogliomas may develop a reticulin fiber network apart from the vasculature. Occasional mitoses are compatible with the diagnosis of ganglioglioma. Necrosis is absent, unless the glial component is undergoing malignant progression. Additional histopathological features frequently identified in gangliogliomas are: (i) calcifications, either excessive or as neuronal/capillary incrustation; (ii) extensive lymphoid infiltrates along perivascular spaces or within the tumour/brain parenchyma; (iii) a prominent capillary network. In few cases, the latter manifests as malformative angiomatous component.

In anaplastic gangliogliomas, malignant change almost invariably involves the glial component {832, 1363, 1798, 2425}. Few cases have been observed in which a malignant glioma arises from the site of a previously resected ganglioglioma {183}.

The spectrum of gangliogliomas varies from a predominantly neuronal phenotype towards variants with a prominent glial population. Some tumours may also display a clear cell morphology, which raises the differential diagnosis of oligodendroglioma or dysembryoplastic neuroepithelial tumour. Ganglion cells may also be a component of extraventricular neurocytic tumours and papillary glioneuronal tumours.

Immunohistochemistry

Neuronal proteins, such as MAP2, NeuN, neurofilaments and synaptophysin are useful to demonstrate the neuronal component in gangliogliomas. The reactions usually demarcate the dysplastic nature of the neuronal cell types. There is still no specific marker available to differentiate dysplastic/neoplastic neurons from normal counterparts. Immunostains for the oncofetal CD34 antigen can be helpful. CD34 is not present in neural cells of the adult brain, but is consistently expressed in 70–80% of gangliogliomas, especially those variants emerging from the temporal lobe. CD34 immunoreactive neural cells are prominent not only in the solid tumour areas but also in peritumoural satellite lesions {178}. Staining for GFAP demonstrates the astrocytes that usually form the neoplastic glial

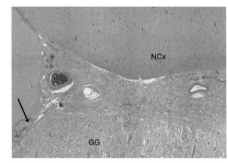

Fig. 6.17 Ganglioglioma (GG) with sharp demarcation towards the adjacent brain parenchyma (NCx) and infiltration into subarachnoid space (arrow).

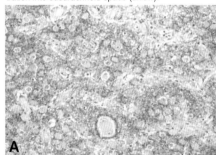

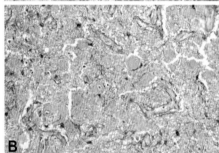

Fig. 6.18 Ganglioglioma. **A** Strong immunoreactivity to synaptophysin of ganglion cells and their processes. Note the binucleate neuron with synaptophysin staining of perisomatic synapses. **B** GFAP expression by neoplastic astrocytes.

element of gangliogliomas. In contrast to diffuse gliomas, MAP2 immunoreactivity is faint or absent in the astrocytic component of gangliogliomas {182}.

Electron microscopy

Neurons with dense core granules are characteristic and diagnostically useful ultrastructural features of these tumours. Synaptic junctions may be absent, or present in only small numbers {832, 1477}. Spherical protein bodies have been described in gangliogliomas {926}.

Proliferation

Mitotic figures are rare. Ki-67/MIB-1 labelling involves only the glial component, mean values ranging from 1.1 to 2.7% {832, 1363, 1798, 2425}.

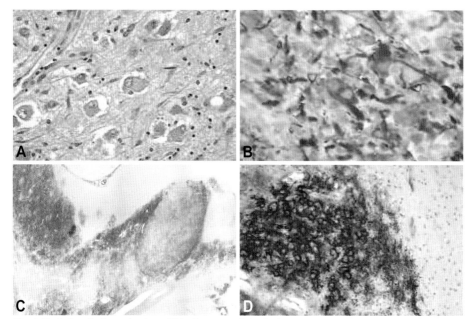

Fig. 6.19 A Ganglioglioma showing a biphasic pattern of dysplastic neurons and neoplastic glial cells. **B** MAP2 expression in dysplastic, occasionally binuclear neurons. **C** CD34 demarcates the tumour and demonstrates tumour satellites in adjacent brain parenchyma. **D** Focal expression of the stem cell epitope CD34 in a ganglioglioma.

Genetic susceptibility
A ganglioglioma of the optic nerve has been noted in a patient with neurofibromatosis type 1 {1465}. One case of spinal cord ganglioglioma was reported in a child with neurofibromatosis type 2 {2001}. A Peutz-Jeghers patient has also been described with a ganglioglioma {1862}.

Genetics
About thirty cases of gangliogliomas have been studied cytogenetically {148, 2135, 2353, 2467}. Chromosomal abnormalities were recorded in one third. Although structural and numerical abnormalities differ greatly between cases, gain of chromosome 7 was the most recurrent alteration. Correlation between cytogenetic data, grade and outcome was not fully addressed, but karyotype was abnormal in three cases with adverse outcome {978, 980, 2353}. Chromosomal imbalances were detected in 5/5 gangliogliomas by comparative genomic hybridization {2467}. Partial loss of chromosome 9p and gain of chromosome 7 were recurrent genetic events. In spite of gain of chromosome 7, abnormal EGFR expression was not recorded in 5/5 gangliogliomas {2467}. In a study of 14 cases (11 grade I and 3 grade III), TP53 mutation, PTEN mutation, CDK4 and EGFR amplification were not detected. CDKN2A deletion was observed in 2/3 anaplastic gangliogliomas {2334}. However, a TP53 mutation was reported in the recurrence of a grade I ganglioglioma {796}. Mutational analysis of the tuberous sclerosis 1 (TSC1) and TSC2 genes revealed sequence alterations in the TSC2 gene including polymorphisms in intron 4 and exon 41 to be significantly overrepresented in patients with gangliogliomas. A somatic mutation in intron 32 was identified in the glial portion but not in neurons of a ganglioglioma {121}.

Mutations in the coding region of the TSC1 and TSC2 genes have not been documented {121,1683}. A study of ezrin and radixin genes, coding for interaction partners of TSC1 and TSC2, was negative {1388}. Analysis of genes involved in the Reelin signalling cascade with a major role in neuronal development failed to uncover mutations of the cyclin dependent kinase CDK5, doublecortin DCX, TP53 and disabled-1, DAB-1 {120, 1031}. Although a Peutz-Jeghers patient with a germline mutation in the serine-threonine kinase LKB1 gene developed a ganglioglioma, LKB1 gene mutations were not recorded in the three sporadic gangliogliomas {1862}.

Histogenesis
The histogenesis of these intriguing neoplasms remains unresolved. An origin from a dysplastic, malformative glioneuronal precursor lesion with neoplastic transformation of the glial element has been hypothesized. A monoclonal origin was shown for 5 of 7 gangliogliomas by both methylation-based and transcription-based clonal analysis {2503}. Neoplastic transformation of subpial granule cells or of glial cells within hamartomas has also been discussed {1030, 2425}.

Prognostic and predictive factors
Gangliogliomas are benign tumours with a 7.5 year recurrence-free survival rate of 94% {1363}. Good prognosis is associated with temporal localization, complete surgical resection and long-standing epilepsy. Anaplastic change in the glial component, i.e. histological similarities to high-grade gliomas such as increased mitotic activity, prominent microvascular proliferation and necrosis, as well as high MIB-1 and TP53 labelling indices, may indicate aggressive behaviour and less favourable outcome {832, 1030, 1798}.

Central neurocytoma and extraventricular neurocytoma

D. Figarella-Branger
F. Söylemezoglu
P.C. Burger

Definition

A neoplasm composed of uniform round cells with neuronal differentiation, typically located in the lateral ventricles in the region of the foramen of Monro (central neurocytoma) or brain parenchyma (extraventricular neurocytoma); affecting mostly young adults, and with a favourable prognosis.

ICD-O codes

Central neurocytoma   9506/1
The provisional code for extraventricular neurocytoma proposed for the fourth edition of ICD-O is *9506/1*.

Grading

Central neurocytoma corresponds histologically to WHO grade II.

Synonyms and historical annotation

The term central neurocytoma was coined by Hassoun *et al.* {786} to describe a neuronal tumour with pathological features distinct from cerebral neuroblastomas, occurring in young adults, located in the third ventricle, and histologically mimicking oligodendroglioma. These tumours had been previously reported as ependymomas of the foramen of Monro or intraventricular oligodendrogliomas. Central neurocytomas were then reported in other intraventricular locations, mainly lateral and third ventricle but also the fourth. The term "central neurocytoma" should be restricted to

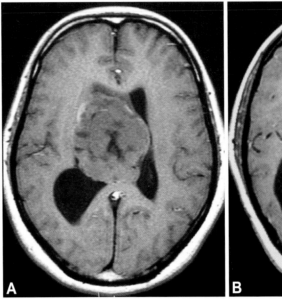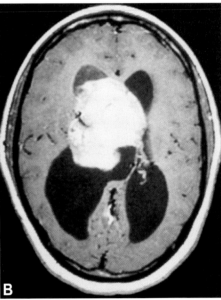

Fig. 6.21 MRI of central neurocytoma. **A** A large tumour of the lateral ventricle with heterogeneous hypointensity on T1-MRI. **B** A large contrast-enhancing central neurocytoma in the region of the foramen of Monro (gadolinium injection).

neoplasms located within the intracerebral ventricles. Subsequently, tumours mimicking central neurocytomas but occurring within the cerebral hemispheres ("cerebral neurocytomas"){1598} or the spinal cord {362, 2223} were documented. The term "extraventricular neurocytoma" is now given to neoplasms that arise within the central nervous system parenchyma and share histological features with the more common central neurocytomas but exhibit a wider morphological spectrum {666}. Notably, some tumours have neurocytic tumour cells but are not classified as central or extraventricular neurocytomas; for example, neurocytic differentiation has been reported in an increasing number of tumours with distinctive morphological features, some of them emerging as new entities such as cerebellar liponeurocytoma and papillary glioneuronal tumour {1153} or variants {301}.

Age and sex distribution

In analysis of 243 cases, age at clinical manifestation ranged from 8 days to 67 years (mean age, 29 years); 44% were diagnosed in the third decade of life, and

69% between the ages of 20 and 40 years. Both sexes are equally affected.

Incidence

Population-based incidence rates for central neurocytoma are not available. In large surgical series, incidence ranged from 0.25–0.5% {788} of all intracranial tumours.

Localization

Central neurocytomas are typically located supratentorially in the lateral ventricle(s) and/or the third ventricle. The most common site is the anterior portion of one of the lateral ventricles (50%), with a preference for the left, followed by combined extension into the lateral and third ventricles, and by a bilateral intraventricular location. Attachment to the septum pellucidum seems to be a feature of the tumour. Isolated third ventricular occurrence is rare.

Clinical features

Symptoms and signs
The majority of patients present with symptoms of increased intracranial

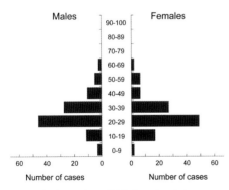

Fig. 6.20 Age and sex distribution of central neurocytoma excluding extraventricular neurocytoma, based on 243 patients.

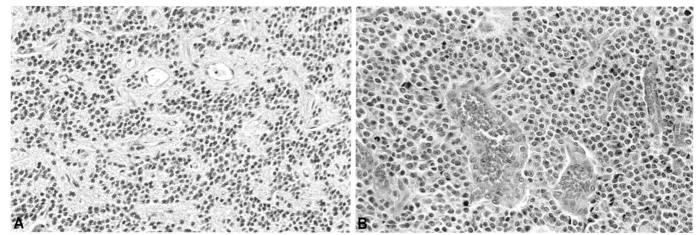

Fig. 6.22 Central neurocytoma. **A** Round cells and nucleus-free areas of neuropil. **B** Microvascular proliferation associated with mitotic activity.

pressure, rather than with a distinct neurological deficit. The clinical history is short (mean 3.2 months). Occasionally, visual and mental disturbances and hormonal dysfunction may be observed. Central neurocytomas may present as acute haemorrhage or as an incidental finding on imaging {788}.

Neuroimaging
On CT scans, mass are usually isodense or slightly hyperdense. Enhancement is observed after administration of contrast medium. Calcifications and cystic changes may be seen. MRI shows heterogeneous hypointensity on T1 and hyperintensity on T2-weighted images and FLAIR, with a well-defined margin and, in all cases, mild to strong enhancement after gadolinum injection {2491}.

Macroscopy
The intraventricular tumours are usually greyish and friable, with varying calcifications and occasional haemorrhage.

Histopathology
Neurocytoma is a neuroepithelial tumour composed of uniform round cells that show immunohistochemical and ultrastructural features of neuronal differentiation. Additional features include fibrillary areas mimicking neuropil, and a low proliferation rate. Central neurocytomas have a benign histological appearance. Various architectural patterns may be observed, even in the same specimen. They include an oligodendroglioma-like honeycomb appearance, large fibrillary areas mimicking the irregular "rosettes"

in pineocytomas, cells arranged in straight lines, or perivascular pseudo-rosettes as observed in ependymomas. Cells are isomorphous, having a round or oval nucleus with a finely speckled chromatin and an occasional nucleolus. Capillary-sized blood vessels, usually arranged in a linear arborizing pattern, give the tumours an endocrine appearance. Calcifications are seen in half the cases, usually distributed throughout the tumour. Rarer findings may include Homer Wright rosettes and ganglioid cells {1896, 2335}. The main differential diagnoses include oligodendroglioma, ependymoma, pineocytoma and dysembryoplastic neuroepithelial tumour. In rare instances, anaplastic histological features, including brisk mitotic activity {788, 2335, 2336} and microvascular proliferation, have been observed {1214, 2335, 2463}. In some cases, necrosis was associated with anaplastic features {1692, 2335, 2463}. Necrosis may also be observed in rare cases that are otherwise devoid of any malignant features, perhaps as a vascular effect {580, 821, 1214}.

Immunohistochemistry
Synaptophysin is the most suitable and reliable diagnostic marker, with immunoreactivity diffusely present in neuropil, especially in fibrillary zones and perivascular nuclei-free cuffs {580}. A significant number of nuclei are immuno-positive for NeuN in almost all cases {2128}. The mean labelling index was 74% in one series of 11 cases, with a significantly lower Ki-67 staining rate for cells expressing NeuN {525}. Chromogranin A

and neurofilament staining are usually absent except when ganglion cells are present {788}. In extraventricular neoplasms, intracytoplasmic and para-nuclear immunolabelling must be cautiously interpreted whenever other histological, immunohistochemical or ultrastructural evidence of neuronal differentiation is lacking. Of particular interest is the anti-Hu antibody because it labels the nuclei of neurocytes {734}. Although most reports find GFAP expressed only in trapped reactive astrocytes, the antigen has been detected by some authors in tumour cells {2127, 2272, 2335, 2336}.

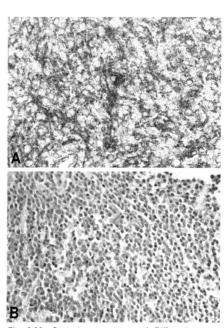

Fig. 6.23 Central neurocytoma. **A** Diffuse immunoreactivity to synaptophysin. **B** Nuclear NeuN expression.

Electron microscopy

Electron microscopy is required when expression of specific neuronal markers (synaptophysin, NeuN) is lacking or doubtful and in all extraventricular neoplasms mimicking central neurocytomas. Typically, central neurocytoma cells show regular round nuclei with a finely dispersed chromatin and a small distinct nucleolus in a few cells. The cytoplasm contains mitochondria, a prominent Golgi apparatus and some cisternae of rough endo-plasmic reticulum often arranged in concentric lamellae. Numerous thin and intermingled cell processes containing microtubules, dense core and clear vesicles, are always observed {300, 788}. Furthermore, well-formed or abnormal synapses may be present, but are not required for the diagnosis.

Proliferation

MIB-1 labelling indices are usually low, less than 2%. Tumours with indices greater than 2%, or in one series 3% {1815}, have been referred to as "atypical neurocytomas" and associated with a significantly shorter recurrence-free interval {1373, 2127}. Vascular proliferation may be present in these lesions. DNA flow cytometry performed in ten neurocytomas revealed diploidy in all {1103}.

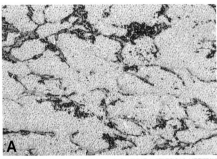

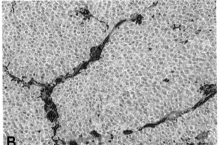

Fig. 6.24 Central neurocytoma, showing sheet-like growth composed of uniform round cells (**A**), and with endocrine appearance with linear arborizing capillaries (**B**).

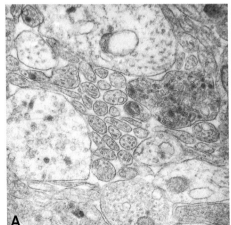
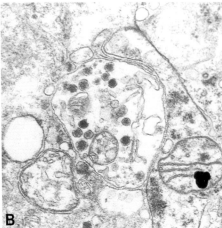

Fig. 6.25 **A** Ultrastructure of a central neurocytoma showing numerous cell processes filled with neurotubules and synaptic structures containing dense core granules and clear vesicles. **B** A neoplastic process containing dense-core vesicles in central neurocytoma.

Genetic susceptibility

One case of central neurocytoma, although originally reported as intraventricular cerebral neuroblastoma, was associated with von Hippel-Lindau disease {1707}.

Genetics

Though the molecular pathogenesis of central neurocytomas remains largely unknown, some genetic alterations, mainly chromosomal gains, have been reported. Gain on chromosome 7 was observed in 3 of 9 neurocytomas {2221}. However another study did not find *EGFR* amplification in central neurocytomas {2260} Gains on chromosomes 2p, 10q, 18q and 13q were found in over 20% of tumours studied {2468}. In two others, an isochromosome 17 and complex karyotype were reported {309, 979}. *TP53* mutations and *MYCN* amplification are rare or absent {621, 979, 1621, 2260, 2336}. There are two studies on loss of 1p and 19q: in one report, allelic loss on 1p and 19q was not detected {621}; in the other, 6 of 9 tumours showed loss at one or more loci on 1p, and 5 of the cases had 19q loss but the majority of informative markers are reported to be retained {2260}. These data suggest that central neurocytomas are genetically distinct from oligodendrogliomas. The expression profiles of cerebellar liponeurocytoma show a closer relationship to the central neurocytoma, however the lack of *TP53* mutations in central neurocytomas suggests the involvement of different genetic pathways {867}.

Histogenesis

Given the neuronal nature of the tumour and its location, central neurocytomas were previously thought to derive from the nuclei of the septum pellucidum {786}. However, the demonstration of both astrocytic and neuronal differentiation in some tumour cells by various approaches *in vivo* {2272, 2336} and *in vitro* {922, 2399} has suggested that they derive from neuroglial precursor cells having the potentiality of dual differentiation, although neuronal commitment largely predominate. This precursor cells might originate from the subependymal plate of the lateral ventricle {2336} or from circumventricular organs {1013}.

Prognostic and predictive factors

The clinical course of central neurocytoma is usually benign, with the extent of resection being the most important prognostic factor. Local recurrence is common in the face of incomplete removal, but the pace of residual tumour growth can be retarded by radiotherapy {1813, 1814}. Craniospinal dissemination is exceptional {524, 2258}. It is worth noting that histological findings alone cannot predict adverse outcomes {524, 1103}. Moreover, central neurocytomas showing aggressive histological features have been described in few patients {2335, 2336, 2463}. These features were not generally associated with poor prognosis. Central neurocytomas with a MIB-1 labelling index (LI) >2% {1373, 2127} or >3% {1815} have significantly shorter recurrence-free intervals. In one small study, cytological atypia had little relationship to MIB-1 index or length of survival {1373}. Involvement of periventricular parenchyma is associated with poor outcome in some cases {1103, 1896}.

Extraventricular neurocytoma

Extraventricular neurocytomas are well circumscribed, contrast-enhancing, and often have a cyst-mural nodule complex that is useful in distinguishing the tumour from histologically similar neoplasms such as oligodendroglioma. They present throughout the CNS. Histologically extraventricular neurocytomas may be identical to the densely cellular cytologically monomorphous central lesion, but are often more complex, less cellular,

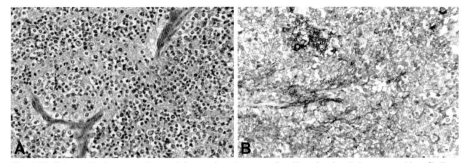

Fig. 6.26 Extraventricular neurocytoma. **A** Isomorphous tumour cells with perinuclear halos arranged in a fibrillary stroma. **B** Immunopositivity for synaptophysin in the cytoplasm and fibrillary stroma.

and more likely to contain ganglion cells or smaller ganglioid cells with nuclei that are larger and paler than those of neurocytes {218, 666}. Lower cellularity, in combination with perinuclear haloes, may create an appearance of oligodendroglioma. GFAP-positive glia are present, but it has been difficult to incriminate these as clearly neoplastic. Hyalinized vessels and dense calcification are common.

Cerebellar liponeurocytoma

P. Kleihues
L. Chimelli
F. Giangaspero
H. Ohgaki

Definition

A rare cerebellar neoplasm of adults with consistent neuronal, variable astrocytic and focal lipomatous differentiation, and with a low proliferative potential; the tumour usually has a favourable clinical prognosis, although recurrences are frequent.

ICD-O code

The provisional code proposed for the fourth edition of ICD-O is *9506/1*.

Grading

Histological features and data on postoperative survival available at the time the previous edition of the WHO Classification was published {1122} suggested that this tumour typically corresponded to WHO grade I. However, recurrences have been reported in almost 50% of cases, typically without histological features of malignant progression. Although the time to clinical progression is often long (mean, 6.5 years), relapse may also occur within a few months {990}. The current WHO classification therefore assigns the cerebellar liponeurocytoma to WHO grade II.

Synonyms and historical annotation

In 1978, Bechtel *et al.* {119} reported a case of lipomatous medulloblastoma in a 44-year-old man. Subsequently, 28 more cases were reported. The terms neurolipocytoma {517}, medullocytoma {667}, lipomatous glioneurocytoma {46}, and lipidized mature neuroectodermal tumour of the cerebellum {707} have also been proposed, so as to emphasize the similarity to central neurocytoma and the prognostic difference from the cerebellar medulloblastoma. In accordance with this, the WHO Classification in 2000 {1122} proposed the term 'cerebellar liponeurocytoma' since the label medulloblastoma could lead to unnecessary aggressive adjuvant therapy. This term is now largely accepted and is supported by genetic analyses that indicate that this lesion is not a variant of medulloblastoma

{867}. Clinical, morphological, immuno-histochemical, genetic and gene expression data strongly suggest that the cerebellar liponeurocytoma constitutes a rare but distinct clinico-pathological entity {241, 867, 2129}. Tumours with features of liponeurocytoma have also been observed in supratentorial locations; it remains to be shown whether these belong to the same clinico-pathological entity.

Age and sex distribution

In 29 patients with cerebellar liponeuro-cytoma published to date {23, 237, 867, 1441, 1657, 2300}, the mean age was 50 years (range 24-77 years), with a peak in the third to sixth decade of life. This is in sharp contrast with the age distribution of cerebellar medulloblastomas, more than 70% of which occur in children {885}. There is no significant gender predilection (13 males and 16 females) in patients with cerebellar liponeurocytoma {23, 237, 867, 1441, 1657, 2300}.

Clinical features

Symptoms and signs

Headache and other symptoms and signs of raised intracranial pressure, from either the lesion itself or obstructive hydrocephalus, are the most common presentations. Cerebellar signs referable to the location of the lesion are also frequent {1657}.

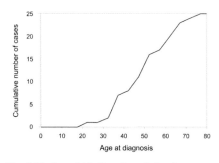

Fig. 6.27 Age distribution of cerebellar liponeurocytoma, based on 25 published cases.

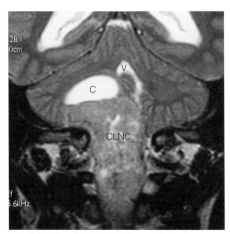

Fig. 6.28 T2-weighted MRI of a cerebellar liponeuro-cytoma (CLNC) with an adjacent cyst (C) and compression of the fourth ventricle (V).

Neuroimaging

MRI appearance is variable and may be related to the distribution and proportion of lipidized tissue. On T1-weighted MRI, the mass is generally hyperintense but heterogeneous. Hyperintense streaks on T2-weighted images have been associated with the macroscopic appearance of adipose tissue at surgery. Enhancement with gadolinium is usually heterogeneous, with areas of tumour demonstrating variable degrees of enhancement. Associated edema is minimal if present {24}.

Localization

Tumours are predominantly located in the cerebellar hemispheres, followed by a more central location in the vermis. Occasionally, they have been found in the cerebellopontine angle {23,867}.
Several cases resembling liponeuro-cytomas have been diagnosed in the supratentorial ventricular system, i.e. the typical location of central neurocytomas {1218}. However, these are rare lesions, amounting to approximately 3% of central neurocytomas {1449} while only two cases of cerebellar neurocytomas without adipose component have been reported {211, 520}. In one case, it was shown that the lipid vacuoles progressively accumulate and coalesce within

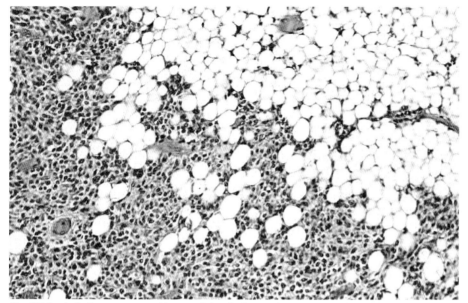

Fig. 6.29 Cerebellar liponeurocytoma with accumulation of adipocytes in a background of small round neoplastic cells.

cells retaining neurocytic features, indicating tumoural lipidization rather than true adipose metaplasia {658}. It remains to be seen whether these observations justify the delineation of central liponeurocytoma as a separate entity {658} and to what degree these lesions share histogenetic and biological characteristics with the cerebellar liponeurocytoma.

Histopathology

Biphasic in appearance, the tumour consists of isomorphic small neuronal cells with the cytology of neurocytes and focal lipomatous differentiation, characterized by lipidized cells resembling mature adipose tissue. Tumour cells have round or oval nuclei and often show a clear cytoplasm resembling neoplastic oligodendrocytes, but also have many morphological similarities to

medulloblastoma and clear cell ependymoma. Despite the cellularity of the lesion, tumour cells have a uniform cytological appearance, with absent or very few mitotic figures.

Immunohistochemistry

Neuronal differentiation is reflected by a consistent, diffuse expression of NSE, synaptophysin and MAP-2. Accordingly, several reported cases were diagnosed as neurocytoma or neuroblastoma rather than medulloblastoma. Focal GFAP expression by tumour cells, indicating astrocytic differentiation, is observed in the majority of cases {2129}. Immunoreactivity for neuronal markers and GFAP is also seen in the adipose cells, indicating an aberrant differentiation of tumour cells rather than an admixture of entrapped adipocytes. It is important to note that xanthomatous histiocytes, as

occasionally observed in ordinary medulloblastomas, are not considered evidence of lipomatous differentiation. Two reports mention additional immunoreactivity to desmin and morphologic features of incipient myogenic differentiation {119,707}.

Differential diagnosis

The most important differential diagnosis is that of medulloblastoma with lipidized cells {689, 1657, 2066}. In these lesions, the adipose tumour cells are usually more diffusely distributed, but may also show the typical clustering seen in the liponeurocytoma {237}. Most importantly, the growth fraction is in the range of 15–40%, which is incompatible with the diagnosis of liponeurocytoma. Cerebellar liponeurocytoma is a neoplasm of adults, while lipidized medulloblastomas also occur in children {689, 1657, 2066}. The distinction between these two lesions is crucial since medulloblastomas with lipidized cells require adjuvant radio/chemotherapy.

The small cell component of liponeurocytomas may also resemble neoplastic oligodendrocytes and clear cell ependymoma {947}.

Proliferation

The growth fraction of the small cell component, as determined by the Ki-67/MIB-1 labelling index, is usually in the range of 1–3% but may be as high as 6%, with a mean value of 2.5% {517, 1021, 2129}. In the adipose component, the MIB-1 labelling index is even lower.

Histogenesis

Immunoreactivity to neuronal antigens and GFAP includes cell bodies embracing fat globules. This suggests that the fat-containing cells result from lipomatous differentiation of tumour cells. The cell or

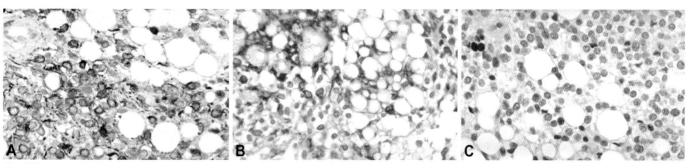

Fig. 6.30 Immunohistochemical features of cerebellar liponeurocytoma. **A** Small tumour cells and adipocytes focally express the neuronal marker MAP-2 (**A**) and GFAP (**B**). **C** Low MIB-1 labelling index reflecting the slow growth of liponeurocytomas.

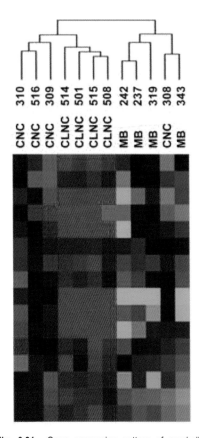

Fig. 6.31 Gene expression pattern of cerebellar liponeurocytomas (CLNCs), central neurocytomas (CNCs), and medulloblastomas (MBs). Cluster analysis suggests a relationship between cerebellar liponeurocytomas and central neurocytomas. Modified from Horstmann *et al.* {867}.

origin is most likely a precursor cell with preferential commitment to neuronal differentiation but a capacity for divergent, i.e. astrocytic and myogenic differentiation. An origin from the external granular layer of the cerebellum cannot be ruled out, although there is no evidence of a relationship to the cerebellar medulloblastoma and the histology as well as age at manifestation would be unusual for an embryonal neoplasm.

Genetics

Genetic analysis of 20 cerebellar liponeurocytomas collected by an international consortium revealed *TP53* missense mutations in 4 cases (20%), a frequency higher than in medulloblastomas (6%) {867}. There was no case with a *PTCH, APC*, or ß-catenin mutation, each of which can be present in subsets of medulloblastomas. FISH analysis of isochromosome 17q, a genetic hallmark present in 40% of cerebellar medulloblastomas, was not observed in any of the cases investigated. This supports the view that the cerebellar liponeurocytoma is a distinct tumour entity and not a variant of medulloblastoma. cDNA expression profiles showed a relationship to central neurocytoma, but the presence of *TP53* mutations, which are absent in central neurocytomas, suggests they develop through different genetic pathways {867}.

Prognostic and predictive factors

Because of the rarity of this tumour and the lack of systematic follow-up data, survival and recurrence rates must be interpreted with some caution. A review of published cases {23, 867} indicates that this lesion generally carries a favourable prognosis. Of 21 patients with follow-up data, 6 (29%) died within 6 months to 2 years, 5 (24%) died after 2–4 years and 10 (48%) survived 5–16 years after surgical intervention. The 5-year survival rate was 48% and the mean overall survival was 5.8 years.

However, 62% of patients developed a recurrence after periods ranging from 1 to 12 years (mean, 6.5 years) and in 3 patients there was a second relapse 1 to 5 years later (mean, 3 years). Despite being clinically progressive, recurrent liponeurocytomas did not show histological features of malignant progression. Early recurrence may even be associated with a relative increase in the lipomatous component {990}. There was no indication of age or gender affecting clinical outcome. Histopathological features predicting recurrence have not been identified.

Papillary glioneuronal tumour

Y. Nakazato
D. Figarella-Branger
A.J. Becker
B.W. Scheithauer
M.K. Rosenblum

Definition
A relatively circumscribed, clinically indolent and histologically biphasic cerebral neoplasm composed of flat to cuboidal, GFAP-positive astrocytes lining hyalinized vascular pseudopapillae and synaptophysin-positive interpapillary collections of sheets of neurocytes, large neurons and intermediate-sized "ganglioid" cells.

ICD-O code
The provisional code proposed for the fourth edition of ICD-O is *9509/1*.

Grading
Limited experience suggests that papillary glioneuronal tumours behave in a manner corresponding to WHO grade I lesions, but a rare example undergoing late biologic progression has been reported {924}.

Synonyms and historical annotation
The papillary glioneuronal tumour, listed in the 2000 WHO classification as a variant of ganglioglioma, was first established as a distinct clinicopathologic entity by Komori *et al.* in 1998 {1153}. Morphologically similar tumours were previously described under a variety of designations, including pseudopapillary ganglioglioneurocytoma {1154} and pseudopapillary neurocytoma with glial differentiation {1105}.

Incidence
To date, no population-based epidemiologic data regarding papillary glioneuronal tumour are available. However, they are rare neoplasms; only several dozen have been reported {226, 473}.

Age and sex distribution
These tumours occur over a wide range of ages. No gender predilection has been observed {208, 2273}. The mean age at presentation is 27 years, the oldest being 75 years, and the youngest being 4 years {103, 2273}.

Localization
Papillary glioneuronal tumours generally affect the cerebral hemispheres, with a predilection for the temporal lobe {226, 1153, 1790}. On MR and CT imaging, the tumours appear as demarcated, solid to cystic, contrast-enhancing masses with little mass effect. A cyst-mural nodule architecture may be seen.

Clinical features
Principal manifestations include headache and seizures. Disturbances of vision, gait, sensation, cognition and emotional affect may also be encountered. Haemorrhage as a presentation has been reported {238}.

Macroscopy
These tumours may be solid or often cystic lesions that exert variable, only occasionally considerable mass effect. Calcification may be observed. Haemorrhage and necrosis are rare.

Histopathology
Papillary glioneuronal tumour is characterized by prominent pseudopapillary architecture in which a single or pseudo-stratified layer of small, cuboidal glial cells with rounded nuclei and scant cytoplasm covers hyalinized blood vessels, as well as interpapillary sheets or focal collections of neurocytes and occasionally ganglion cells and/or medium-sized "ganglioid cells" {1153}. At the immunohistochemical level,

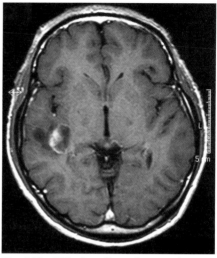

Fig. 6.33 MRI of papillary glioneuronal tumour presenting as a multicystic tumour with a gadolinium-enhanced solid component in the right temporal lobe.

vessels with mural hyalinization are ensheathed by a layer of small uniform, GFAP-positive cells with rounded nuclei and scant cytoplasm. In some cases, Olig2-positive, GFAP-negative glial cells surround this layer {2210}. These glial elements lack both nuclear atypia and mitotic activity. Interpapillary neuronal elements show a considerable variation in size and shape. Any combination of small neurocytes, intermediate-sized ganglioid cells and large ganglion cells can be found with accompanying neuropil; all are stained with antisera to synaptophysin, NSE and class III β-tubulin {1153, 2210}. The majority of neuronal cells are positive for NeuN, but NFP expression is mostly confined to larger ganglioid and ganglion cells {1153}. Membranous immunoreactivity for NCAM is also found {2297}, but chromogranin-A expression is lacking. In addition to neuronal elements, mini-gemistocytes with eccentrically placed nuclei and eosinophlic hyaline cytoplasm, showing intense GFAP-immunoreactivity, are occasionally noted in the interpapillary spaces {924, 2210}. Microvascular proliferation or necrosis is exceptional, even in cases with increased

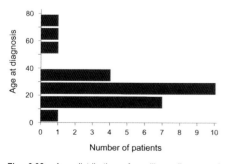

Fig. 6.32 Age distribution of papillary glioneuronal tumour, based on 25 published cases.

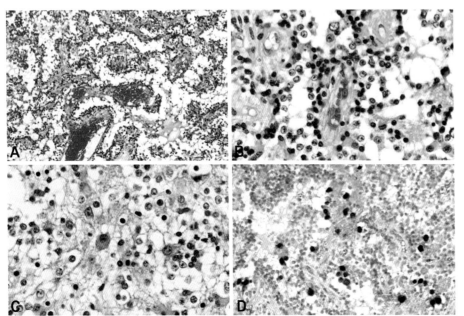

Fig. 6.34 Histological features of papillary glioneuronal tumour. **A** Layers of tumour cells around vessels, forming pseudopapillary structures. **B** A pseudopapilla covered by inner cells with hyperchromatic nuclei and outer cells with vesicular nuclei. **C** Neuronal cells of variable size and oligodendroglia-like cells. **D** Neuronal cells clearly shown by NeuN immunostaining.

proliferative activity. At the periphery of the lesion, scattered tumour cells are intermingled with gliotic brain tissue containing Rosenthal fibers, eosinophilic granular bodies, hemosiderin pigment, and microcalcifications, the result being a blurred tumour margin.

Electron microscopy

Few papillary glioneuronal tumours have been studied ultrastructurally. Three cell types have been reported, including astrocytic, neuronal and poorly differentiated, possibly glioneuronal progenitor cells {208, 1153}. Astrocytes, some elongate, contain bundles of intermediate filaments and are separated from vessels exhibiting thick collagen-rich adventitiae by a basal lamina. Minigemistocytes and OLIG-2-expressing oligodendrocyte-like cells may also be present {924}. Neurons vary in size; large forms with abundant organelles lie between the papillae, their neuronal processes filled with parallel microtubules, showed terminations containing clear vesicles and occasional synapses. The poorly differentiated cells contain mitochondria, ribosomes, occasional dense bodies, intermediate filaments and microtubules, but no well formed dense core granules. The relative proportion of neuronal and poorly differentiated cells vary from one case to another.

Proliferation

MIB-1 labelling indices are generally low, in the range of 1–2%. Only one tumour featuring minigemistocytes showed an increased (10%) labelling index in that unusual element {924}.

Genetic susceptibility

Papillary glioneuronal tumours reported to date have been sporadic in occurrence. No familial or syndrome-associated cases have been reported.

Genetics

In one series of 6 patients, 1p status was studied by FISH but showed no abnormality {2210}.

Histogenesis

The histogenesis of papillary glioneuronal tumours is unclear, but an origin from multipotent precursors capable of divergent glioneuronal differentiation is presumed. Paraventricular examples could derive from the subependymal matrix {1153}, while more superficially situated papillary glioneuronal tumours might arise from the secondary germinal layer.

Prognostic and predictive factors

The cyst formation, hyalinized vessels, and low proliferative activity are paralleled by a favourable clinical outcome. In most cases, gross total resection without adjuvant therapy results in recurrence-free, long-term survival. Only one example of tumour regrowth has been reported {924}.

Rosette-forming glioneuronal tumour of the fourth ventricle

J.A. Hainfellner
B.W. Scheithauer
F. Giangaspero
M.K. Rosenblum

Definition
A rare, slowly growing neoplasm of the fourth ventricular region, preferentially affecting young adults and composed of two distinct histological components, one with uniform neurocytes forming rosettes and/or perivascular pseudo-rosettes, the other being astrocytic in nature and resembling pilocytic astrocytoma.

ICD-O code
The provisional code proposed for the fourth edition of ICD-O is *9509/1*.

Grading
Both the benign histology and favourable postoperative course indicate that rosette-forming glioneuronal tumour (RGNT) corresponds to WHO grade I.

Synonyms and historical annotation
A lesion displaying features of RGNT was the subject of an early report of "dysembryoplastic neuroepithelial tumour (DNT) of the cerebellum" {1216}. Komori *et al.* described RGNT as a distinct entity, a variant of mixed glioneuronal tumour {1155}. Preusser *et al.* confirmed RGNT as a tumour entity {1799}. In 5 independent studies, a total of 17 cases have been reported {33, 952, 1003, 1155, 1799}.

Incidence
RGNT is a rare brain tumour, but population-based incidence rates are not yet available.

Age and sex distribution
The age range at disease manifestation is 12–59 years (mean, 33 years). Current data suggest a slight female predilection.

Localization
RGNTs arise in the midline, occupy the fourth ventricle and/or aqueduct, and may extend to involve adjacent brain stem, cerebellar vermis, pineal gland or thalamus. MR imaging reveals a relatively circumscribed, solid tumour of the fourth ventricular region showing high intensity on T2-weighted images, low intensity on T1, and focal/multifocal gadolinium

enhancement. Secondary hydrocephalus may be seen.

Clinical features
The presentation is most often with headache, a reflection of obstructive hydrocephalus, and/or ataxia. Cervical pain is occasionally experienced. Rare examples are asymptomatic and discovered as incidental imaging findings.

Macroscopy
RGNT involves primarily the cerebellum and wall or floor of the fourth ventricle. An intraventricular component is the rule, occasionally with aqueductal extension.

Histopathology
RGNTs are somewhat demarcated but some infiltration of brain stem and/or cerebellar parenchyma may be seen. They are characterized by a biphasic neurocytic and glial architecture {952, 1155, 1799}. The neurocytic component consists of a uniform population of neurocytes forming neurocytic rosettes and/or perivascular pseudorosettes. Neurocytic rosettes feature ring-like arrays of neurocytic nuclei around delicate eosinophilic neuropil cores. Perivascular

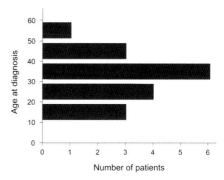

Fig. 6.35 Age distribution of RGNT, based on 17 published cases.

pseudorosettes feature delicate cell processes radiating toward vessels. Both, when viewed longitudinally, may assume columnar arrangement. Neurocytic tumour cells have spherical nuclei with finely granular chromatin and inconspicuous nucleoli, scant cytoplasm and delicate cytoplasmic processes. These neurocytic structures may lie in a partly microcystic, mucinous matrix. The glial component of RGNT typically dominates and in most areas resembles pilocytic astrocytoma. Astrocytic tumour cells are spindle to stellate in shape with elongate to oval nuclei and moderately dense

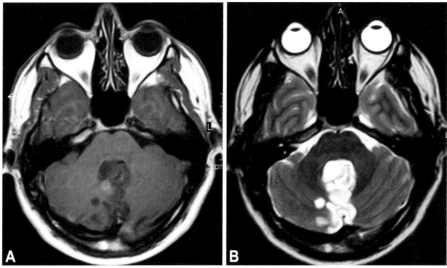

Fig. 6.36 A T1-weighted MR imaging shows low intensity of the tumour mass and focal gadolinium enhancement. **B** T2-weighted imaging demonstrates a relatively hyperintense, midline tumour, occupying the fourth ventricle and involving cerebellar vermis.

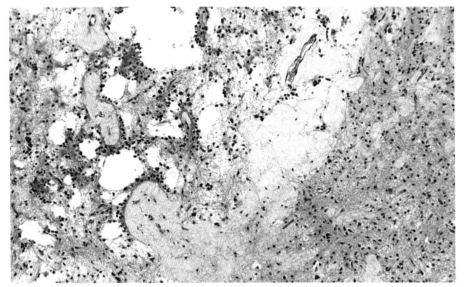

Fig. 6.37 RGNT consists of two components: neurocytic (left) and astrocytic (right).

chromatin. Cytoplasmic processes often form a compact to loosely textured fibrillary background. In areas the glial component may be microcystic, containing round to oval, oligodendroglia-like cells with occasional perinuclear halos. Rosenthal fibers, eosinophilic granular bodies, microcalcifications, and hemosiderin deposits may be encountered. Overall, cellularity is low. Mitoses and necroses are absent. Vessels may be thin-walled and dilated or hyalinized. Thrombosed vessels and glomeruloid vasculature may also be seen. Ganglion cells are occasionally present, but adjacent, perilesional cerebellar cortex does not show dysplastic changes.

Immunohistochemistry

Immunoreactivity for synaptophysin is present at the centers of neurocytic rosettes and in the neuropil of perivascular pseudorosettes {952, 1155, 1799}. In addition, both cytoplasm and processes of neurocytic tumour cells may express MAP-2 and neuron-specific enolase.

GFAP and S-100 immunoreactivity is present in the glial component, but absent in rosettes and pseudorosettes.

Electron microscopy

Astrocytic cells of the glial component contain dense bundles of glial filaments. Rosette-forming neurocytic cells are intimately apposed and feature spherical nuclei with delicate chromatin, cytoplasm containing free ribosomes, scattered profiles of rough endoplasmic reticulum, prominent Golgi and occasional mitochondria. Cytoplasmic processes, loosely arranged, form the centres of rosettes and contain aligned microtubules as well as occasional dense core granules. Presynaptic specializations may be seen and mature synaptic terminals may form surface contacts with perikarya and other cytoplasmic processes.

Proliferation

Mitoses are absent and Ki-67 labelling indices are low, being less than 3% in reported cases.

Genetic susceptibility

One reported patient with RGNT had a Chiari type I malformation {1155}. No other evidence of an underlying neurologic disorder or association with a familial tumour syndrome has been reported.

Histogenesis

Neuroimaging and histological investigations indicate that RGNTs arise from brain tissue surrounding the infratentorial ventricular system. An origin of RGNT from the subependymal plate, i.e. remnants of the periventricular germinal matrix in the mature mammalian brain, has been suggested {1155}.

Prognostic and predictive factors

The clinical outcome of these essentially benign lesions is favourable in terms of survival, but disabling postoperative deficits have been reported in approximately half of cases.

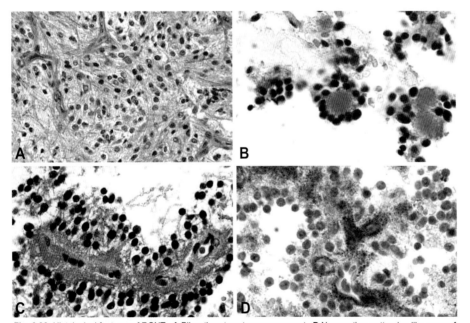

Fig. 6.38 Histological features of RGNT. A Pilocytic astrocytoma component. B Neurocytic rosette: ring-like array of neurocytic tumour cell nuclei around an eosinophilic neuropil core. C Perivascular pseudorosette with delicate cell processes radiating toward a capillary. D Synaptophysin immunoreactivity in the pericapillary area of a perivascular pseudorosette.

Spinal paraganglioma

B.W. Scheithauer
S. Brandner
D. Soffer

Definition

A unique neuroendocrine neoplasm, usually encapsulated and benign, arising in specialized neural crest cells associated with segmental or collateral autonomic ganglia (paraganglia); consisting of uniform chief cells exhibiting neuronal differentiation forming compact nests (Zellballen), surrounded by sustentacular cells and a delicate capillary network; within the central nervous system, primarily affecting the cauda equina/filum terminale region.

ICD-O code   8680/1

Grading

Paragangliomas of the filum terminale correspond histologically to WHO grade I.

Synonyms and historical annotation

The terminology surrounding paragangliomas is confusing. Early authors divided them into chromaffin and non-chromaffin on the basis of their reaction with chromic acid. However, since this reaction does not reliably reflect their functional activity, current terminology is based upon anatomic site, e.g. carotid body paraganglioma (chemodectoma), jugulotympanic paraganglioma (glomus jugulare tumour), etc. Usually, a descriptor of functional status is also appended, i.e. "functional" or "nonfunctional."

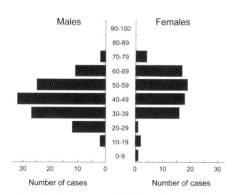

Fig. 6.39 Age and sex distribution of paraganglioma (spinal), based on 71 published cases.

Incidence and location

Paragangliomas of the CNS are uncommon. The vast majority present as spinal intradural tumours in the cauda equina region. Since the first description of cauda equina region paraganglioma in 1970 {1473}, more than 210 cases have been reported. For a complete list of 174 cases reported prior to 2003, see Gelabert-Gonzalez {656}. Altogether, paragangliomas of the cauda equine region comprise 3.4% to 3.8% of all tumours affecting this region {2420, 2461}. Other spinal levels are far less often involved; 14 paragangliomas were reported in the thoracic region, most being extradural with an intravertebral and paraspinal component {374, 2232} and 2 tumours involved the cervical region {174, 2177}. Intracranial paragangliomas are usually extensions of jugulotympanic paragangliomas {946}. However, rare examples of purely intracranial tumours have also been described. These include tumours of the sellar region {1549}, the cerebellopontine angle {443} and examples in cerebellar parenchyma {1794}, the fronto-temporal lobes {1857}, a functional paraganglioma of the temporo-parietal dura occurring 23 years after an adrenal phaeochromocytoma {1459} and one questionable pineal example {2117}.

Age and sex distribution

Cauda equina paragangliomas generally affect adults, their peak incidence being in the fourth through the sixth decades. Patient age ranges from 9 to 74 years (mean, 46 years), with a slight predominance in males (M:F 1.4:1). Jugulotympanic paragangliomas are more common in Caucasians, show a strong female predilection and occur mainly in the fifth and sixth decades {946}.

Clinical features

Symptoms and signs

As with other spinal tumours, cauda equina paragangliomas exhibit no distinctive clinical features. Most common presenting symptoms include a few-year history of low-back pain and sciatica. Sensory deficit, paraparesis and sphincter disturbances are infrequent, and full-blown cauda equina syndrome is uncommon. An unusual presentation is intracranial hypertension, a feature reported in 8 cases {94, 656, 1983}. Only 3 endocrinologically functional paragangliomas of the cauda equine region have been reported {656}. The few reported paragangliomas of the thoracic spine presented with signs of spinal cord compression, one example being functional {982}. About 36% of glomus jugulare paragangliomas extend into the cranial cavity {946}. These most often present with pulsatile tinnitus and lower cranial nerve dysfunction {946}: signs of catecholamine secretion may be seen.

Neuroimaging

Radiographically, cauda equina paragangliomas lack specific features {1303,2461}. Most appear as isodense, homogeneously enhancing masses on computed tomography (CT). However,

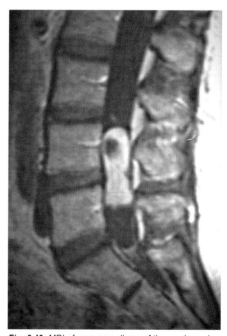

Fig. 6.40 MRI of a paraganglioma of the cauda equina with a cystic component.

since CT without contrast may miss the lesion, magnetic resonance (MR) imaging is the procedure of choice. MR images typically show a sharply circumscribed, occasionally partly cystic mass that is hypo- or isointense to spinal cord on T1-weighted images, markedly contrast-enhancing and hyperintense on T2-weighted images. The presence of serpentine, congested, ecstatic vessels and of a low signal intensity rim ("cap sign") on T2-weighted images are considered diagnostically helpful clues {1303, 2461}. Plain X-rays are usually non-informative, but rarely show erosion (scalloping) of vertebral laminae due to chronic bone compression.

Macroscopy

Cystic components may be found. An occasional tumour penetrates dura to invade bone. Most paragangliomas of the cauda equina are entirely intradural and are attached either to the filum terminale or less often to a caudal nerve root. As a rule, paragangliomas are oval to sausage-shaped, delicately encapsulated, soft, red-brown and measure 1.5 to 13 cm. Capsular calcification may be encoutered.

Histopathology

Tumours are well-differentiated, resembling normal paraganglia, composed of chief (type I) cells disposed in nests or lobules (Zellballen), surrounded by an inconspicuous, single layer of sustentacular (type II) cells. The Zellballen are surrounded by a delicate capillary network that may undergo sclerosis. The uniform round or polygonal chief cells possess central, round-to-oval nuclei with finely stippled chromatin and inconspicuous nucleoli. Degenerative nuclear pleomorphism ("endocrine anaplasia") is generally mild. Cytoplasm varies somewhat in quantity and is usually eosinophilic and finely granular. In some instances, it is amphophilic or clear. Sustentacular cells are spindle-shaped. Encompassing the lobules, their long processes are often so attenuated as to be undetectable by routine light microscopy and visible only on immunostains for S-100 protein. Nearly half of cauda equina paragangliomas contain mature ganglion cells, as well as cells transitional between chief and ganglion cells {256}. Such "gangliocytic paragangliomas" are also found in the duodenum and are

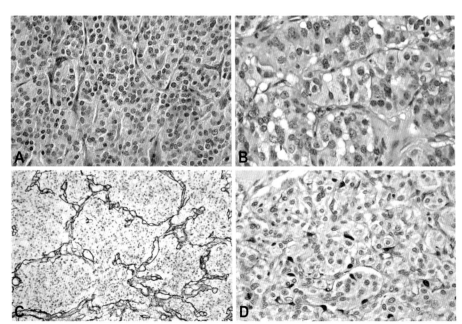

Fig. 6.41 Histological features of paraganglioma. **A,B** Typical Zellballen architecture. **C** Reticulin stain showing the septae delineating Zellballen. **D** Sustentacular cells identified by immunoreactivity to S-100.

analogous to phaeochromocytoma with neuronal differentiation. Some paragangliomas of the cauda equina region show architectural features reminiscent of carcinoid tumours, including angiomatous, adenomatous and pseudorosette patterns {2124}. Tumours composed predominantly of spindle {1520} and melanin-containing cells (melanotic paragangliomas) {638, 1520} have also been described at this site, as has oncocytic paraganglioma {1678}. Foci of haemorrhagic necrosis may occur and scattered mitotic figures can be seen. Neither these features nor nuclear pleomorphism are of prognostic significance {2124}.

Immunohistochemistry

Markers permit the identification of both chief and sustentacular cells. Neuron-specific enolase (NSE), although a sensitive marker of chief cells, lacks specificity, but synaptophysin and chromogranin {1132, 2124} are sensitive and reliable. Chromogranin A reactivity parallels the Grimelius (argyrophil) reaction {256}. Neurofilament proteins are also useful markers of chief cells. Expression of serotonin (5H-T) and of various neuropeptides (somatostatin, leu and metenkephalin) has been demonstrated in paraganglioma of the cauda equina region {1520, 2124}. Paranuclear cytokeratin immunoreactivity is particularly

prominent in cauda equina examples {330}. Sustentacular cells are uniformly reactive for S-100 protein and usually show staining for glial fibrillary acidic protein (GFAP) as well. Chief cells may also show variable S-100 immunoreactivity.

Electron microscopy

The distinctive ultrastructural feature of chief cells is the presence of dense core (neurosecretory) granules measuring 100 to 400 nm (mean, 140 nm) {531}. Depending on their cytoplasmic electron density, "light" and "dark" chief cells are recognized. Both feature interdigitation of cell processes and rudimentary junctions. A layer of basal lamina is present at the interface of Zellballen and surrounding stroma. In addition to well-developed Golgi, extensive smooth endoplasmic reticulum and lysosomes, chief cells may contain numerous atypical mitochondria as well as paranuclear whorls of intermediate filaments {531,2124}. Cytoplasmic crystalloids, hexagonal or quadrilateral in configuration and non-membrane-bound, are rarely seen {2469}. Sustentacular cells are characterized by an elongated nucleus with marginal chromatin, increased cytoplasmic electron density, relative abundance of intermediate filaments, and lack of dense core granules {531, 2124}.

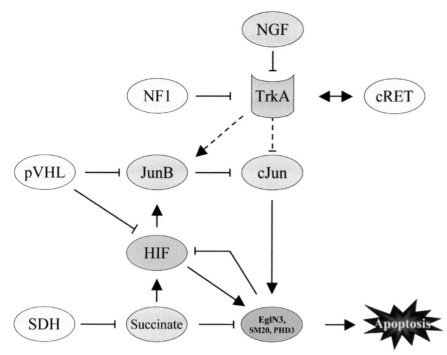

Fig. 6.42 Molecular pathways likely involved in paraganglioma pathogenesis. Mutant VHL fails to inhibit JunB, which would antagonize c-Jun. RET, which is the receptor for glial derived neurotrophic factor (GDNF), and NF1 act on the same pathway by modulating the NGF receptor TRK A, which all interact downstream with PHD, HIF-PH or EgIN3, enzymes that hydroxylate HIF1-α. Mutations of *cRET*, *NF1*, *VHL* and *SDH* decrease apoptosis during development, when NGF levels become limiting. Apoptosis is mediated by EgIN3, SM20 and PHD3. Adapted from Maxwell P. {1420A}.

Genetics

Systemic paragangliomas may be multifocal but to date there has been no reported association of cauda equina or other spinal paragangliomas. The concurrence of spinal paraganglioma with brain tumours {272, 373}, spinal epidural haemangioma {2398}, syringomyelia {2146} and intramedullary cysts {550} are notable, but these associations may be coincidental.

Several autosomal dominant inherited syndromes predispose to paraganglioma or phaeochromocytoma: von Hippel-Lindau disease (VHL), multiple endocrine neoplasia type 2 (*RET* mutations), neurofibromatosis type 1 (NF1) and mutations in subunits B, C, or D of the succinate dehydrogenase genes (*SDHB, SDHC, SDHD*) which form part of mitochondrial complex II. Multiple,

benign, head and neck paragangliomas are often caused by *SDHD* mutations while *SDHB* mutations are associated with phaeochromocytoma. To date, only four families with *SDHC* mutation have been identified.

Spinal paragangliomas are considered non-familial, but a study of 22 spinal paraganglioma showed an *SDHD* germline mutation in one patient with recurrent spinal paraganglioma and a cerebellar metastasis {1411}.

Histogenesis

The histogenesis of cauda equina paraganglioma is a matter of debate. Despite the fact that such cells have not been identified at this site, some authors favour an origin from paraganglion cells associated with regional autonomic nerves and blood vessels {1331}. Others

have suggested that peripheral neuroblasts normally present in the adult filum terminale undergo paraganglionic differentiation {272, 1959}. Jugulotympanic paragangliomas presumably arise from microscopic paraganglia within the temporal bone {1247}. Of interest, although perhaps not relevant to histogenesis, are reports of the coexistence of a paraganglioma and myxopapillary ependymoma in the cauda equina region {1071} and a biphasic tumour consisting primarily of paraganglioma and, to a lesser extent, ependymoma {272}.

Prognostic and predictive factors

Tumour location is often more relevant than histology in determining the prognosis of paragangliomas {1133}. For example, the metastasis rate of para-aortic paraganglioma is high (28 to 42%), whereas that of carotid body tumours is only 2 to 9% {1133}. Nearly half of the glomus jugulare tumours recur locally {1248} but only 5% metastasize {1247}. Several studies have demonstrated a correlation of MIB-1 labelling and malignant behaviour in phaeochromocytoma {231, 358}. In contrast, tumour vascularity is of no significance {1630}. The vast majority of cauda equina paragangliomas are slowly growing and curable by total excision. Based on long-term follow-up, it is estimated that 4% will recur following gross total removal {2164}. CSF seeding of spinal paragangliomas has occasionally been documented {373, 1901, 2164, 2239}. Metastasis outside the CNS (bone) has been reported only once {1520}. Although it is not possible to predict the biological behaviour of cauda equina paraganglioma on the basis of histologic criteria alone, truly anaplastic and metastasizing extraneural paragangliomas have been shown to be either devoid or markedly depleted of sustentacular cells {1132, 1133}. One case report of a recurring and metastasising spinal paraganglioma has confirmed this finding {2239}.

CHAPTER 7

Tumours of the Pineal Region

Pineocytoma (WHO grade I)
A rare, slowly growing, grossly demarcated pineal parenchymal neoplasm occurring mainly in adults and composed of relatively small, uniform, mature-appearing pineocytes often forming large pineocytomatous rosettes.

Pineal parenchymal tumour of intermediate differentiation (WHO grades II or III)
A pineal parenchymal neoplasm of intermediate-grade malignancy, affecting all ages and composed of diffuse sheets or large lobules of uniform cells with mild to moderate nuclear atypia and low to moderate level mitotic activity.

Pineoblastoma (WHO grade IV)
A highly malignant primitive embryonal tumour of the pineal gland, preferentially affecting children, frequently associated with CSF dissemination, and composed of dense, patternless sheets of small cells with round to somewhat irregular nuclei and scant cytoplasm.

Papillary tumour of the pineal region
A rare neuroepithelial tumour of the pineal region in adults, characterized by papillary architecture and epithelial cytology, immunopositivity for cytokeratin and ultrastructural features suggesting ependymal differentiation.

Pineocytoma

Y. Nakazato
A. Jouvet
B.W. Scheithauer

Definition
A rare, slowly growing, grossly demarcated pineal parenchymal neoplasm occurring mainly in adults and composed of relatively small, uniform, mature-appearing pineocytes often forming large pineocytomatous rosettes.

ICD-O code   9361/1

Grading
Pineocytomas correspond histologically to WHO grade I {1010, 1014}.

Incidence, age and sex distribution
Pineal region tumours account for less than 1% of all intracranial neoplasms, of which approximately 14–27% are of pineal parenchymal origin {1163, 1841}. Of these, based upon previous criteria, pineocytomas represent 14–60%. Pineocytomas occur throughout life, but most frequently affect adults (mean age: 38 years) {199, 337, 818, 1014, 1452, 1480, 1841, 2031, 2456}. There is no sex predilection.

Localization
Pineocytomas typically remain localized to the pineal area where they compress adjacent structures, including the cerebral aqueduct, brain stem and cerebellum. Protrusion into the posterior third ventricle is often seen.

Clinical features
Symptoms and signs
Clinically, it is not possible to differentiate pineocytoma from other pineal region lesions. Signs and symptoms vary, and relate to increased intracranial pressure, neuro-ophthalmologic dysfunction (Parinaud syndrome), changes in mental status, brain stem dysfunction, or cerebellum as well as hypothalamic-based endocrine abnormalities {199, 337, 851, 1014, 1163, 1841, 2031}. The majority of patients exhibit neuro-ophthalmologic signs, particularly Parinaud syndrome {337, 554, 851, 1163}. In rare cases, the presentation may be with intratumoural haemorrhage ("pineal apoplexy") {851}.

Neuroimaging
On CT scans, pineocytomas are usually globular, demarcated masses, measuring less than 3 cm in diameter. They appear hypodense and homogeneous, but some show peripheral calcification or occasional cystic changes {333, 2031}. Most tumours exhibit homogeneous contrast enhancement. Accompanying hydrocephalus is a common feature {1561}. On MRI, the tumours tend to be low or isointense on T1 and hyperintense on T2-weighted images with strong, homogeneous contrast enhancement {1169, 1561}.

Macroscopy
Pineocytomas are well-circumscribed lesions with a grey-tan, homogeneous or granular cut surface {199, 818}. Degenerative changes, including cyst formation and foci of haemorrhage may be present {1452}.

Histopathology
Pineocytoma is a well-differentiated, moderately cellular neoplasm composed of relatively small, uniform, mature cells resembling pineocytes. It grows primarily in sheets or ill-defined lobules, and often also features large pineocytomatous rosettes composed of abundant, delicate tumour cell processes.
The majority of nuclei are round-to-oval with inconspicuous nucleoli, and finely dispersed chromatin. Cytoplasm is moderate in quantity and homogeneously eosinophilic. Processes are conspicous

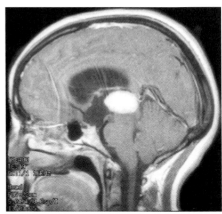

Fig. 7.02 Pineocytoma showing rounded contours and homogeneous enhancement on a T1-weighted MRI.

and short, often ending in club-shaped expansions that are optimally demonstrated on neurofilament, Bodian or Bielschowsky stains. Mitotic figures are lacking in all but occasional large specimens (fewer than 1/10 HPF) {1014}. Pineocytomatous rosettes vary in number and size, their anucleate centres being composed of delicate, enmeshed cytoplasmic processes resembling neuropil {199, 1014, 1608, 2031}. Nuclei surrounding the periphery of the rosette are not regimented. In some pineocytomas, large ganglion cells and/or multinucleated giant cells with bizarre nuclei are seen {199, 818, 1221, 1452, 2031}. Mitotic activity of this pattern is still low in spite of their ominous nuclear appearances. The stroma of pineocytoma consists of a delicate network of vascular channels lined by a single layer of endothelial cells and supported by scant reticulin fibers. Microcalcifications are occasionally seen.

Immunohistochemistry
Pineocytoma cells usually show strong immunoreactivity for synaptophysin, NSE and NFP. Also reported is variable staining for other neuronal markers, including class III ß-tubulin, tau protein, PGP 9.5, chromogranin and the neuropeptide serotonin {363, 1012, 1014, 1221, 1608, 2456}. Photosensory differentiation is associated with immunoreactivity for retinal S-antigen and rhodopsin {1452,

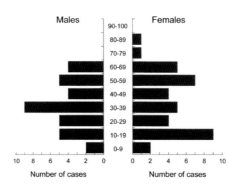

Fig. 7.01 Age and sex distribution of pineocytoma based on 72 cases.

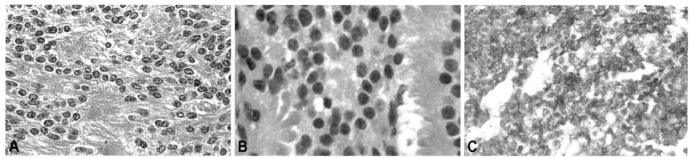

Fig. 7.03 Histological features of pineocytoma. **A** Pineocytomatous rosettes with nucleus-free spaces filled with a fine meshwork of cell processes. **B** High magnification shows tumour cells with irregular hyperchromatic nuclei and prominent processes with bulbous extensions. **C** Diffuse staining for synaptophysin.

1608, 1716}. In tissue culture, pineocytoma cells are also capable of synthesizing serotonin and melatonin {574}.

Electron microscopy

Pineocytomas are composed of clear and varying numbers of dark cells joined with zonulae adherents {787, 818, 1012, 1480}. Cells extend tapering processes which occasionally terminate in bulbous ends. Their cytoplasm is relatively abundant and contains well-developed organelles, including smooth and rough endoplasmic reticulum, Golgi complex, mitochondria, multivesicular bodies and lysosomes. Pineocytoma cells share numerous ultrastructural features with normal mammalian pineocytes, such as paired twisted filaments {785, 1012}, annulate lamellae {787}, 9+0 cilia {787, 1012, 1480}, microtubular sheaves {787, 1012}, fibrous bodies {787, 1012}, vesicle-crowned rodlets {787, 818, 1012, 1480}, heterogeneous cytoplasmic inclusion {787}, membrane whorls {787, 1012} and mitochondrial as well as centriolar clusters {1012}. Membrane-bound, dense-core granules and clear vesicles are present in both cytoplasm and cellular processes, the latter showing occasional synapse-like junctions {787, 818, 1012, 1480}.

Genetics

Cytogenetic studies have suggested that monosomy or loss of chromosome 22, deletions in the distal 12q region, and partial deletion or loss of chromosome 11 are related to tumour progression {130, 1821}. A relationship between the *RB1* gene and pineocytoma has not been established. A microarray analysis of pineocytoma has shown high-level expression of genes coding for enzymes related to melatonin synthesis (*TPH1, HIOMT*), and also genes involved in retinal phototransduction (*OPN4, RGS16, CRB3*), such reactivities indicating bi-directional neurosecretory and photosensory differentiation {572}.

Histogenesis

The histogenesis of pineal parenchymal tumours is linked to the pineocyte, a cell with photosensory and neuroendocrine functions. The ontogeny of the human pineal gland recapitulates the phylogeny of the retina and the pineal organ {1481}. During late stages of intrauterine life and

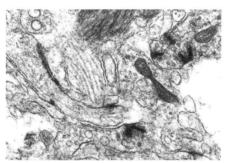

Fig. 7.04 Electron micrograph of pineocytoma. Terminal cell processes show synaptic vesicles and rods.

the early post-natal period, the human pineal gland consists primarily of cells arranged in rosettes similar to those of the developing retina. These feature abundant melanin pigment as well as cilia with a 9+0 microtubular pattern. By the age of three months, the number of pigmented cells gradually decreases so that pigment becomes undetectable by histochemical methods {1481}. As differentiation progresses, cells strongly immunoreactive for NSE accumulate. By postnatal age one year, pineocytes predominate. To a variable extent, pineal parenchymal tumours mimic the developmental stages of the human pineal gland.

Prognostic and predictive factors

The clinical course of pineocytomas is characterized by a lengthy interval (4 years in one series) between the onset of symptoms and surgery {199}. In series of strictly classified tumours, no pineocytomas have been shown to metastasize {554, 2030}. The 5-year survival rate of pineocytoma patients has ranged from 86% {2030} to 100% {554}, there being no relapses following gross total resection {554}. The prognosis of patients with pineocytomas with divergent differentiation, including glial, neuronal and retinoblastic elements, appears to be similar to that of conventional pineocytomas {1452}.

Pineal parenchymal tumour of intermediate differentiation

Y. Nakazato
A. Jouvet
B.W. Scheithauer

Definition

A pineal parenchymal neoplasm of intermediate-grade malignancy, affecting all ages and composed of diffuse sheets or large lobules of uniform cells with mild to moderate nuclear atypia and low- to moderate-level mitotic activity. Without justification, the few rare tumours showing coexistent patterns of both pineocytoma and pineoblastoma have occasionally been included in this category.

ICD-O code   9362/3

Grading

Pineal parenchymal tumour of intermediate differentiation (PPTID) may correspond to WHO grade II or III, but definite grading criteria have yet to be established.

Synonyms and historical annotation

The category of PPTID {1012, 1480, 2031} first introduced by Schild *et al.* in 1993 has since come to include mixed pineocytoma/pineoblastoma, and tumours such as "malignant pineocytomas" {818} and "pineoblastomas with lobules" {199}. This has obscured the value of the designation, and is not recommended terminology.

Incidence

PPTID comprises at least 20% of all pineal parenchymal tumours. The reported incidence of 0% to 60% reflects the frequent misdiagnosis of this pineal parenchymal tumour and/or the inclusion of mixed pineocytoma-pineoblastoma and other unusual pineal parenchymal tumours.

Age and sex distribution

PPTID occurs at all ages, including childhood to adult life, with a peak incidence in early adults (mean; 38 years; range, 1–69) {851, 1014, 1452, 2031}. There is a slight female preponderance.

Clinical features

The presentation of PPTID, the largest subgroup of pineal parenchymal tumours {1014}, is like that of pineocytoma, i.e. combinations of increased intracranial pressure, Parinaud's syndrome, ataxia and occasional diplopia. When defined according to histologic pattern {2031}, it is clear that cerebrospinal metastases occur in a minority.

Macroscopy

The gross appearance PPTID is similar to that of pineocytoma. The tumours are circumscribed, soft in texture and lacking gross evidence of necrosis.

Histopathology

PPTID are either diffuse (neurocytoma-like) or somewhat lobulated tumours characterized by moderately high cellularity, mild to moderate nuclear atypia, and low to moderate mitotic activity. Preliminary studies suggest that tumours corresponding to grades II and III can be distinguished on the basis of mitotic activity and neurofilament protein immunoreactivity {554, 1014}. PPTID include transitional cases in which typical pineocytomatous areas are associated with a diffuse pattern. Occasional giant cells, Homer Wright rosettes or ganglion cells may infrequently be seen.

Immunohistochemistry shows synaptophysin and neuron-specific enolase positivity {1012, 1014, 1608}. Variable labelling is also seen with antibodies to neurofilament protein, chromogranin A, retinal S-antigen and S-100 protein {1012, 1014, 1608, 2276, 2456}.

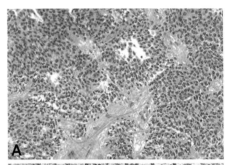

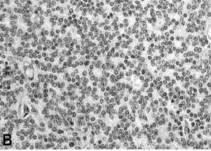

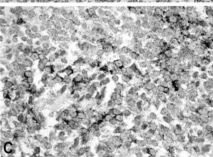

Fig. 7.06 **A** Highly cellular pineal parenchymal tumour of intermediate differentiation. Note the absence of rosettes and the tendency to form nucleus-free perivascular spaces. **B** Moderate cellularity, nuclear pleomorphism, and formation of small rosettes. **C** Focal chromogranin staining of a pineal parenchymal tumour of intermediate differentiation.

Proliferation

PPTID is a potentially aggressive neoplasm. Reflecting the difficulty encountered in making the diagnosis, often in a small biopsy, is the wide range of reported mitotic indices in a large published series, being 0/10 HPF in 58%, 1–2 in 28%, 3–6 in 14%, and rarely higher {1014}. Similarly, the mean MIB-1 labelling index reportedly ranges from 3 to 10% {1608, 1883, 2276}.

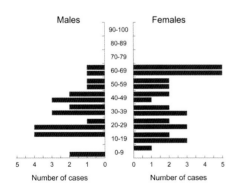

Fig. 7.05 Age and sex distribution of PPTID, based on 58 cases.

Genetics

By comparative genomic hybridization, frequent chromosomal changes have been identified in pineal parenchymal tumours. An average of 3.3 gains and 2 losses has been noted {1883}. The most common chromosomal imbalances in PPTID are +4q, +12q, and -22. In a real-time RT-PCR analysis, the expression of 4 genes (*PRAME*, *CD24*, *POU4F2* and *HOXD13*) in PPTID is distinctly high, almost the same level as in pineoblastoma, and in contrast to the low expression of these genes in pineocytoma {572}.

Histogenesis

Strong evidence indicates that pineal parenchymal tumours arise from pineocytes or their precursor cells. The close kinship among pineocytoma, PPTID and pineoblastoma is supported by a number of shared clinical, morphologic and genetic features {572, 1012, 1014, 1452, 1480, 1608, 2031}. The very occurrence of rare mixed tumours (pineocytoma-pineoblastoma) confirms the existence of a spectrum from pineocytoma through PPTID to pineoblastoma.

Prognostic and predictive factors

The five-year survival of patients with PPTID is 39% to 74% {554}. Only very occasional examples of PPTID are associated with central nervous system or extraneural metastases {2031}. One series found the first relapse to be local in 22% and spinal-leptomeningeal in 4% {554}. Factors affecting the survival of pineal parenchymal tumours are morphological subtype as well as histologic grading according to presence or absence of necrosis, mitotic index and NFP immunostaining {1014}.

Pineoblastoma

Y. Nakazato
A. Jouvet
B.W. Scheithauer

Definition

A highly malignant primitive embryonal tumour of the pineal gland, preferentially affecting children, frequently associated with CSF dissemination, and composed of dense, patternless sheets of small cells with round to somewhat irregular nuclei and scant cytoplasm.

ICD-O code   9362/3

Grading

Pineoblastomas correspond histologically to WHO grade IV.

Incidence

Pineoblastomas are rare, comprising approximately 40% of all pineal paren-chymal tumours.

Age and sex distribution

They may occur at any age, but most present in the first two decades of life (mean age, 18.5 years) with a distinct predilection for children {818, 851, 1010, 1014, 1452, 2456}. No gender preference is apparent.

Clinical features

Symptoms and signs

The clinical presentation of pineoblastoma is similar to that of other tumours of the pineal region. The interval between initial symptoms and surgery may be shorter than one month {199}. Median post-surgical survivals vary from 24 to 30 months {818, 1452}.

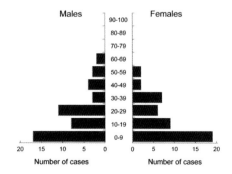

Fig. 7.07 Age and sex distribution of pineoblastoma based on 93 cases.

Neuroimaging

In contrast to pineocytoma, the CT appearance of pineoblastoma is that of a large, lobulated or poorly-demarcated, homogeneous mass, which is hyperdense after contrast enhancement. Calcification is infrequent. On T1-weighted MRI scan, pineoblastomas are hypo-to isointense, but they show heterogeneous contrast enhancement {333, 1561}. Extensive cystic change is rare.

Macroscopy

Pineoblastomas are soft, friable and poorly demarcated {199, 2456}. Haemor-rhage and/or necrosis may be present, but calcification is rarely seen. Infiltration of surrounding structures, including lepto-meninges, is common, as is craniospinal dissemination {199, 452, 554, 818, 851, 1278, 1452}.

Histopathology

Representing the most primitive of pineal parenchymal tumours, pineoblastomas are composed of highly cellular, pattern-less sheets of densely packed small cells with round to somewhat irregular nuclei and scant cytoplasm. Pineocytomatous rosettes are lacking, but Homer Wright and Flexner-Wintersteiner rosettes may be seen. Pineoblastomas resemble other small cell, or primitive neuroectodermal tumours of the CNS. The cells feature a high nuclear: cytoplasmic ratio, hyper-chromatic nuclei with an occasional, small nucleolus, scant cytoplasm, and indistinct cell borders. The diffuse growth pattern is only interrupted by occasional rosettes. Flexner-Wintersteiner rosettes indicate retinoblastic differentiation, as do highly distinctive but infrequently occuring fleurettes. Mitotic activity varies, but is generally high, and necrosis is common. Only rarely does one encounter mixed tumours showing a biphasic pattern with alternating areas resembling pineo-cytoma and pineoblastoma. The former must be distinguished from overrun normal parenchyma. Microcalcifications may be seen. Silver impregnations for pineal parenchymal cells demonstrate

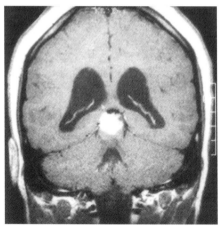

Fig. 7.08 On T1-weighted MRI, pineoblastoma shows homogeneous contrast enhancement.

scant cytoplasm and relatively few processes {453}. Melanin production as well as cartilaginous and rhabdomyoblastic differentiation are encountered in rare pineoblastomas referred to as "pineal anlage tumours" {818, 1608}.

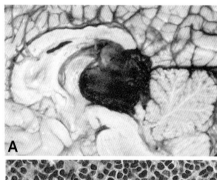

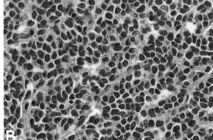

Fig. 7.09 A Large, haemorrhagic pineoblastoma. B Highly cellular pineoblastoma showing undifferentiated small cell histology.

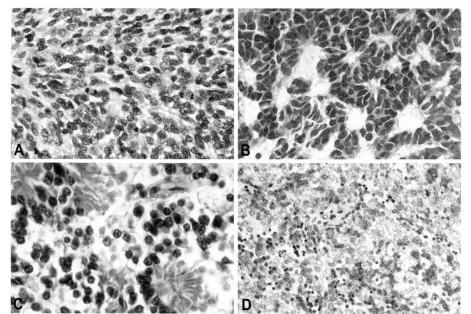

Fig. 7.10 Histopathological features of pineoblastoma. **A** High cellularity with numerous mitotic figures. **B** Homer Wright and Flexner-Wintersteiner rosettes. **C** Fleurettes. **D** Focal expression of retinal S-antigen.

Immunohistochemistry

The immunophenotype of pineoblastomas is similar to that of pineocytomas and includes reactivity for neuronal, glial and photoreceptor markers. Positivity for synaptophysin, NSE, NFP, class III ß-tubulin and chromogranin A may be seen, as can retinal S-antigen staining {1014, 1452, 1608, 1716, 2456}. Reactivity for GFAP and αB crystallin, should prompt the exclusion of entrapped reactive astrocytes. Average MIB-1 indices are high {1608, 1883}.

Electron microscopy

Characterized by a relative lack of significant differentiation, the fine structure of pineoblastoma is similar to that of any poorly differentiated neuroectodermal neoplasm. Cells have round to oval with slightly irregular nuclei and abundant euchromatin as well as heterochromatin. Cytoplasm is scant and contains polyribosomes, few profiles of rough endoplasmic reticulum, small mitochondria, as well as occasional microtubules, intermediate filaments, and lysosomes {1403, 1480, 1608}. Dense core granules are rarely seen in the cell body {1403, 1480}. Cell processes, poorly formed and short, may contain microtubules as well as scant dense core granules {1403}. Bulbous endings are not identified {1480}. Junctional complexes of zonula adherens and zonula occludens type may be present between cells and processes {1012, 1403, 1480, 1608}. Synapses are absent {1608}. Cilia with a 9+0 microtubular pattern are occasionally seen {1403}. Rarely, cells radially arranged around a small central lumen may be encountered {1608}.

Genetic susceptibility

Pineoblastomas may be seen in patients with familial (bilateral) retinoblastoma, an occurrence termed "trilateral retinoblastoma syndrome" {438, 1118} and have also been reported in patients with familial adenomatous polyposis {637, 907}. The rare association of pineoblastoma with embryonal rhabdomyosarcoma has been reported in an infant {380}.

Genetics

In 7 pineoblastomas studied, no consistent cytogenetic changes have been identified {1313}. In yet another analysis of pineoblastoma, both monosomy 22 and a missense *INI1* mutation were found {154}. No aberrations of the *TP53* and *Waf1/p21* genes have been detected {2274, 2275}. Pineoblastomas are known to occur in patients with *RB1* gene abnormalities; their prognosis is significantly worse than that of sporadic cases {1762}. A comparative genomic hybridization analysis of three pineoblastomas has shown an average of 5.6 chromosomal changes, including 2.3 gains and 3.3 losses {1883}. The most common chromosomal imbalance in pineoblastoma is -22; in addition, high-level gains are identified on 1q12-qter, 5p13.2-14, 5q21-qter, 6p12-pter, and 14q21-qter. In a microarray analysis of pineal parenchymal tumours, 7 genes were expressed in only pineoblastoma: HOXD13, PITX2, POU4F2, Hist1H3D, Hist1H4E, DSG1 and TERT, thus implicating cellular growth, junctional modification and immortalization {572}.

Histogenesis

Pineoblastomas share morphologic and immunohistochemical features with cells of the developing human pineal gland and retina. Evidences for this ontogenic concept include the finding of interphotoreceptor retinoid-binding protein and its mRNA in one mixed pineocytoma/pineoblastoma, and the occasional concurrence of bilateral retinoblastoma and pineoblastoma (trilateral retinoblastoma syndrome) {53, 438}.

Prognostic and predictive factors

With the exception of pineocytomas, all other pineal parenchymal tumours are potentially aggressive, as demonstrated by the occurrence of craniospinal seeding and, rarely, of extracranial metastases {372, 818, 2031}. Extent of disease at the time of diagnosis, as determined by CSF examination and MRI of the spine, directly affects the survival of patients with pineoblastoma. Extent of resection and radiotherapy also affect prognosis {1278}. Metastases of the pineal tumour within the CNS and vertebral column are the most common causes of death {1397}. The prognosis for patients with sporadic and familial trilateral retinoblastoma is dismal, survival being less than one year after diagnosis {438, 1397}. Occasionally, the pineal tumour remains asymptomatic and is discovered on routine imaging studies; in such instances, the outcome is better {438, 1397}. In one series, projected 1-, 3- and 5-year survival rates of pineoblastoma patients treated by various modalities are 88%, 78% and 58%, respectively {2031}.

Papillary tumour of the pineal region

A. Jouvet
Y. Nakazato
B.W. Scheithauer
W. Paulus

Definition
A rare neuroepithelial tumour of the pineal region in adults, characterized by papillary architecture and epithelial cytology, immunopositivity for cytokeratin and ultrastructural features suggesting ependymal differentiation.

ICD-O code
The provisional code proposed for the fourth edition of ICD-O is *9395/3*.

Grading
The biological behaviour of papillary tumour of the pineal region (PTPR) is variable and may correspond to grades II or III, but histological grading criteria remain to be defined.

Synonyms and historical annotation
Based on a series of 6 cases of tumours with identical histology features, PTPR was described as a distinct entity in 2003 {1011}. An origin from specialized ependymal cells of the subcommissural organ was suggested. It is highly likely that some PTPRs were previously reported as "papillary pineocytoma" {2267, 2317}, pineal parenchymal tumour {1014}, choroid plexus tumour {1192, 1567}, ependymoma {1679} and even papillary meningioma {28}.

Incidence
Since these tumours are rare, incidence data are not available.

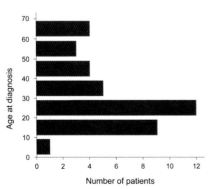

Fig. 7.11 Age distribution of papillary tumour of the pineal region, based on 38 published cases.

Age and sex distribution
Among 38 PTPR reported to date, examples have been identified in both children and adults {572, 573, 781, 1011, 1091, 1217, 2080}. Ages have ranged from 5 to 66 years (mean, 32 years). No sex predilection has been noted.

Localization
Papillary tumours of the pineal region arise exclusively in the pineal region.

Clinical features
Symptoms are non-specific, may be of short duration and include headache due to obstructive hydrocephalus. On neuroimaging, PTPRs appear large, well circumscribed, and occasionally feature a cystic element. CT shows them to be hypodense and variably contrast enhancing. MRI scans show a low T1 signal, increased signal on T2-weighted images, and contrast enhancement.

Macroscopy
PTPR present as relatively large (2.5–4 cm), well-circumscribed tumours indistinguishable grossly from pineocytoma.

Histopathology
PTPR is an epithelial-appearing tumour with papillary features and more densely cellular areas, often exhibiting ependymal-like differentiation (true rosettes and tubes). In papillary areas, the vessels are covered by layers of large, pale to eosinophilic columnar cells. In cellular areas, cells with a somewhat clear or vacuolated cytoplasm, and occasionally an eosinophilic, PAS-positive, cytoplasmic mass, may also be seen. Nuclei are round to oval, with stippled chromatin; pleomorphic nuclei may be present. Mitotic activity ranges from 0–10 per 10 HPF. Necrotic foci are often seen. Microvascular proliferation is usually absent. Instead, vessels are often hyalinized when seen, there is a clear demarcation between the tumour and the adjacent pineal gland.

Immunohistochemistry
The most distinctive immunohistochemical feature of PTPRs is their reactivity for keratins (KL1, AE1/AE3, CAM5.2, CK18), particularly in papillary structures. In contrast to ependymoma, only focal GFAP expression may be seen. PTPRs also stain for vimentin, S-100 protein, NSE, MAP2, N-CAM and transthyretin {781, 2080}. Focal membrane or dot-like EMA staining can sometimes be seen

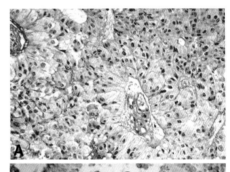

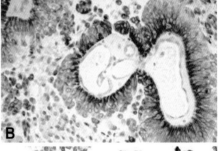

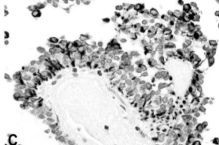

Fig. 7.12 Histological features of papillary tumour of the pineal region. **A** The tumour is characterized by papillary architecture and epithelial cytology. In papillary areas, the tumoral cells are large and columnar or cuboidal. **B** Expression of cytokeratin (KL1) in tumoral cells with strong immunoreactivity particularly in papillary structure. **C** A distinct immunoreactivity for cytokeratin CAM5.2.

{1011, 1217}. NFP immunolabelling is never seen, while the neuroendocrine markers synaptophysin and chromogranin A are sometimes weakly and focally expressed {1011}. The majority of PTPR are characterized by absence of staining for membranous Kir 7.1 or cytoplasmic stanniocalcin-1, both of which are frequently seen in choroid plexus tumours {781}.

Proliferation

Mitotic activity is moderate (range 0–10 per 10 HPF) {573, 781, 1011}. The Ki-67/MIB-1 labelling index is also moderate {573, 1217, 2080}, highest indices being seen in tumours of young patients {573}. The prognostic significance of proliferation indices has yet to be established.

Genetic susceptibility

At present, no syndromic association or evidence of genetic susceptibility has been documented.

Genetics

In one comparative genomic hybridization study of 5 tumours, chromosomal imbalances were found in 4 cases; the most common changes were loss of chromosomes 10 (4 cases) and 22q (3 cases) as well as gain of chromosomes 4 (4 cases), 8, 9, and 12 (each in 3 cases) {781}.

Histogenesis

Immunohistochemical findings (cytokeratin -positivity) and ultrastructural demonstration of ependymal, secretory, and neuro-endocrine organelles suggest that PTPR may originate from remnants of the specialized ependymal cells of the subcommissural organ (SCO) {1011}. Further support for a putative origin from specialized ependymocytes of the SCO comes from a DNA microarray study showing high expression of genes expressed in the SCO, namely ZFH4, RFX3, TTR, and CGRP {572}.

Prognostic and predictive factors

In a retrospective multicentre study of 31 patients, tumour progression occurred in 72% of cases, while the 5-year estimates for overall survival and progression-free survival were 73% and 27%, respectively. Incomplete resection and marked mitotic activity (5 or more mitoses per 10 HPF) tend to be associated with decreased survival and recurrence {573}.

CHAPTER 8

Embryonal Tumours

Medulloblastoma (WHO grade IV)
A malignant, invasive embryonal tumour of the cerebellum with preferential manifestation in children, predominantly neuronal differentiation, and an inherent tendency to metastasize via CSF pathways.

Central nervous system primitive neuroectodermal tumours (WHO grade IV)
A heterogeneous group of tumours occurring predominantly in children and adolescents. They may arise in the cerebral hemispheres, brain stem or spinal cord, and are composed of undifferentiated or poorly differentiated neuroepithelial cells which may display divergent differentiation along neuronal, astrocytic, and ependymal lines. CNS/supratentorial PNET is an embryonal tumour composed of undifferentiated or poorly differentiated neuroepithelial cells. Tumours with only neuronal differentiation are termed cerebral neuroblastomas or, if ganglion cells are also present, cerebral ganglioneuroblastomas. Tumours that recreate features of neural tube formation are termed medulloepitheliomas. Tumours with ependymoblastic rosettes are termed ependymoblastomas. Features common to all CNS PNET variants include early onset and aggressive clinical behaviour.

Atypical teratoid/rhabdoid tumour (WHO grade IV)
A highly malignant CNS tumour predominantly manifesting in young children, typically containing rhabdoid cells, often with primitive neuroectodermal cells and with divergent differentiation along epithelial, mesenchymal, neuronal or glial lines; associated with inactivation of the *INI1/hSNF5* gene in virtually all cases.

Medulloblastoma

F. Giangaspero
C.G. Eberhart
H. Haapasalo
T. Pietsch
O.D. Wiestler
D.W. Ellison

Definition

A malignant, invasive embryonal tumour of the cerebellum with preferential manifestation in children, predominantly neuronal differentiation, and an inherent tendency to metastasize via CSF pathways.

ICD-O codes

Medulloblastoma	9470/3
- Desmoplastic/nodular medulloblastoma	9471/3
- Medulloblastoma with extensive nodularity	*9471/3*
- Anaplastic medulloblastoma	*9474/3*
- Large cell medulloblastoma	9474/3

Grading

Medulloblastomas correspond histologically to WHO grade IV.

Incidence

The annual incidence has been estimated at 0.5 per 100 000 children less than 15 years {304, 2154}. In the United States, whites are more frequently affected than African-Americans {1438}.

Age and sex distribution

The peak age at presentation is 7 years. Seventy percent of medulloblastomas occur in individuals younger than 16 {67, 1898}. In adulthood, 80% of medulloblastomas arise in the 21–40 years age group {690, 885}. This tumour rarely occurs beyond the fifth decade of life. Approximately 65% of patients are male.

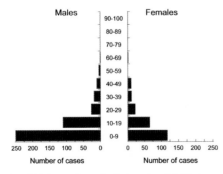

Fig. 8.01 Age and sex distribution of medulloblastoma, based on 651 cases.

Etiology

Different polyomaviruses have been discussed as possible causative agents. In experimental animals, cerebellar neoplasms with a phenotype similar to that of human medulloblastoma have been induced in hamsters by perinatal intra-cerebral injection with JC virus {1413, 2510}, and in rats by retrovirus-mediated transfection of fetal rat brain cells with the large T antigen of SV40 {510}. Other models of medulloblastoma-like PNETs have been produced using transgenic mice that express SV40 large T antigen under the influence of different promoters {635}. Some studies have demonstrated a high frequency of detection of JC virus DNA sequences and its viral oncoproteins, T-antigen and agnoprotein, by immunohistochemistry in human medulloblastoma {461, 1095, 1211}. SV40 sequences have also been identified in medulloblastomas {883}. However, these findings have not been confirmed by others in independent larger series {1913, 2384}. Therefore, the role of polyomavirus infections in the development of medulloblastomas remains unclear.

An increased risk for medulloblastoma was found in children born before term (standardized incidence ratio 3.1) {1445}. A protective function of folate substitution in maternal diet against the development of medulloblastoma in children was claimed in an earlier study {244}, but was not confirmed in a more recent study {245}.

Localization

At least 75% of childhood medulloblastomas arise in the vermis, and project into the fourth ventricle. Involvement of cerebellar hemispheres increases with the age of the patient. Most tumours located in the hemispheres are of the desmoplastic/nodular subtype {243}.

Clinical features

The presenting clinical manifestations include truncal ataxia, disturbed gait, intracranial hypertension secondary to obstruction of CSF-flow and lethargy, headache and morning vomiting. On computerized tomography (CT) or magnetic resonance imaging (MRI), medulloblastomas appear as solid, intensely contrast-enhancing masses.

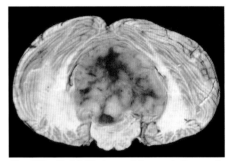

Fig. 8.02 Medulloblastoma of the cerebellar vermis compressing the brain stem.

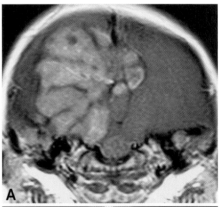

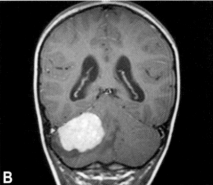

Fig. 8.03 A Grape-like appearance of medulloblastoma with extensive nodularity in a 18-month-old child.
B MRI appearance of desmoplastic/nodular medulloblastoma in an adult patient. Note the hemispheric location and the well-circumscribed appearance.

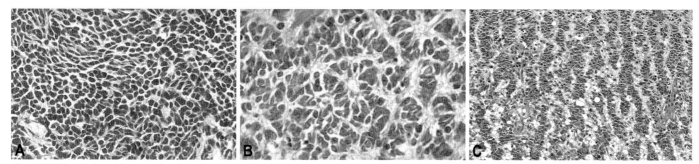

Fig. 8.04 Histopathological features of medulloblastoma. **A** Typical arrangement of sheets of undifferentiated tumour cells. **B** Area with Homer Wright (neuroblastic) rosettes. **C** Arrangement of tumour cells in parallel rows.

Medulloblastomas involving the peripheral cerebellar hemispheres in adults may occasionally appear as extra-axial lesions simulating meningiomas or vestibular nerve schwannomas {124}. A nodular, "grape-like" pattern on MRI characterizes the medulloblastoma with extensive nodularity, because of its distinctive and diffuse nodular architecture {669, 1551}. CSF-borne metastases are seen as foci of nodular or diffuse contrast enhancement in the leptomeninges or on the ventricular surface. They are present in one third of patients at presentation.

Macroscopy
The majority of medulloblastomas arise in the region of the vermis and appear as pink or grey masses that can fill the fourth ventricle. Medulloblastoma occurring in the cerebellar hemispheres tends to be firm and more circumscribed than the classic variant. Small foci of necrosis can be evident but extensive necrosis is rare.

Histopathology
Medulloblastoma is composed of densely packed cells with round-to-oval or carrot-shaped hyperchromatic nuclei surrounded by scanty cytoplasm. Neuroblastic (Homer Wright) rosettes, which are observed in less than 40% of cases, are often associated

with marked nuclear pleomorphism and high mitotic activity. Spongioblastic features, characterized by tumour cell nuclei arranged with their long axes in parallel, can be encountered. Nuclear size and pleomorphism in medulloblastomas may be variable {1435}, which has led to the concept of anaplasia. Although usually numerous, mitoses are infrequent in about 25% of the cases {251}. The most common type of differentiation in medulloblastoma is neuronal, most commonly manifesting as immunopositivity for neuronal markers such as synaptophysin. In addition, small groups of frankly neurocytic cells or ganglion cells are found in approximately 5% of medulloblastomas. Glial differentiation is unusual, and takes the form of scattered small groups of cells with an astrocytic phenotype. Vascular hyperplasia as exemplified by the glomeruloid neovascularization of high-grade gliomas is rare. Areas of necrosis are quite uncommon, but when present necrotic zones may show pseudopalisading similar to that observed in glioblastomas. Tumour in the subarachnoid space may elicit a considerable desmoplastic reaction with ribbons or small clusters of neoplastic cells entrapped among collagenous fibers.

Desmoplastic/nodular medulloblastoma
Synonym: Desmoplastic medulloblastoma
This variant is characterized by nodular, reticulin-free zones ('pale islands') surrounded by densely packed, highly proliferative cells with hyperchromatic and moderately pleomorphic nuclei which produce a dense intercellular reticulin fiber network {257, 668, 1059}. This characteristic pattern may be present only focally. The nodules, which represent regions of neuronal maturation, exhibit a reduced nuclear cytoplasmic ratio, a fibrillary matrix and uniform cells with a neurocytic appearance. Accompanying this maturation are negligible mitotic activity and increased apoptosis. Medulloblastomas showing only an increased amount of collagenous and reticulin fibers without the nodular pattern are not classified as the desmoplastic/nodular variant.

Medulloblastoma with extensive nodularity
The medulloblastoma with extensive nodularity, which was previously designated "cerebellar neuroblastoma", occurs in infants and differs from the related desmoplastic/nodular variant by having an expanded lobular architecture, due to the fact that the reticulin-free zones become unusually enlarged and rich in

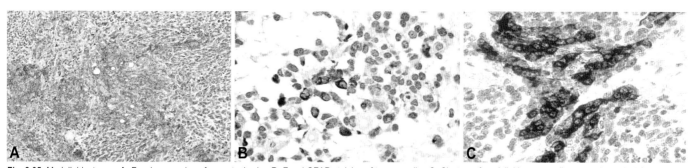

Fig. 8.05 Medulloblastoma. **A** Focal expression of synaptophysin. **B** Focal GFAP staining of tumour cells. **C** Clusters of medulloblastoma cells expressing retinal S-antigen.

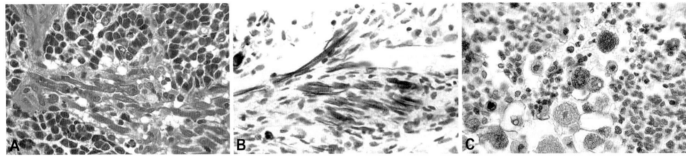

Fig. 8.06 Medulloblastoma with myogenic differentiation, showing (**A**) striated muscle fibers with brisk mitotic activity, (**B**) anti-fast-myosin immunostaining of highly differentiated, striated myogenic cells and (**C**) biphasic pattern of small undifferentiated medulloblastoma cells and large rhabdomyoblasts immunostaining for myoglobin.

neuropil-like tissue. Such zones contain a population of small cells with round nuclei, which resemble the cells of a central neurocytoma and exhibit a streaming pattern. The internodular component is markedly reduced in some areas {669, 2183}. Following radiotherapy and/or chemotherapy, medulloblastomas with extensive nodularity may occasionally undergo further maturation to tumours dominated by ganglion cells {433} .

Anaplastic medulloblastoma
Marked nuclear pleomorphism, nuclear moulding, cell-cell wrapping and high mitotic activity, often with atypical forms, are characteristics of this variant. Apoptosis is also prominent. Although all medulloblastomas show some degree of atypia, these changes are particularly pronounced and widespread in anaplastic medulloblastomas. The presence of such features only in focal areas is not sufficient to define the lesion as an anaplastic medulloblastoma.
Histological progression over time, from non-anaplastic to anaplastic medulloblastoma, has been described in several studies, and a transition can be even observed within a single specimen, as inferred from the presence of differing

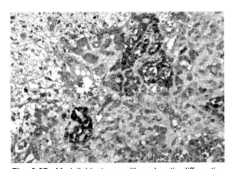

Fig. 8.07 Medulloblastoma with melanotic differentiation. Melanotic cells commonly appear as tubular epithelial structures.

degrees of cytological atypia or anaplasia in one tumour {230, 498, 670, 671, 1255}.

Large cell medulloblastoma
The large cell variant represents approximately 2–4% of medulloblastomas. The term derives from its monomorphic cells with large, round, vesicular nuclei, prominent nucleoli and variable amount of eosinophilic cytoplasm {230, 498, 670, 1255}. The cells lack cohesiveness, and mitotic and apoptotic figures are abundant. Large cell and anaplastic medulloblastomas have considerable cytological overlap. The large cell medulloblastoma frequently contains anaplastic regions, and in several studies, a combined large cell/anaplastic category has been proposed {230, 1292, 1435}.

Myogenic differentiation
Synonym: medullomyoblastoma
(ICD-O: 9472/3)
Medulloblastoma with myogenic differentiation was previously termed medullomyoblastoma. However, genetic changes in medulloblastoma with myogenic differentiation are similar to those in other medulloblastomas, suggesting that this is not a distinct entity {806, 1292}. The descriptive term "medullomyoblastoma" therefore describes any variant (classic, desmoplastic/nodular, etc.) of medulloblastoma containing focal rhabdomyoblastic elements {806, 1292}. This population of spindle-shaped cells is admixed with scattered or clumped large oval cells, which have hyaline eosinophilic cytoplasm {2116}. Occasionally, elongated 'strap cells' with the cross-striations of skeletal muscle are evident {1830}. The rhabdomyoblastic component is immunoreactive for desmin {855, 2029}, myoglobin {471, 855, 2116}, and fast myosin {1026}, but not smooth muscle α-actin {855, 2029}. Ultrastructural

studies demonstrate thick and thin filaments arranged in sarcomeres and Z-band material characterizes the rhabdoid element {855, 1026, 2029, 2116}.

Melanotic differentiation
Synonym: Melanocytic medulloblastoma (ICD-O: 9470/3)
Medulloblastoma with melanotic differentiation was previously termed melanocytic medulloblastoma. However, groups of melanotic tumour cells can occur in different variants of medulloblastoma and therefore this is not regarded as a separate variant. The phenotype of the melanotic tumour cells varies; they may appear undifferentiated, like the PNET component, or epithelial and form tubules, papillae {117, 479, 647} or cell clusters {187, 755, 1000}. They usually immunolabel with antibodies to S-100 protein {117, 647}, but they may also be immunonegative, as described for cells of the ocular pigment layer at very early stages of development {479}. Ultrastructural analysis of some tumours has verified that the pigment is oculocutaneous melanin with distinct melanosomes {187, 479, 647, 1000}. However, neuromelanin may occur in some of these lesions {1047}.

Immunohistochemistry
The frequent differentiation of the medulloblastoma along neuronal lineage manifests immunophenotypically as expression of neuronal antigens. Class III β-tubulin, microtubule-associated protein 2, neuron specific enolase (NSE) and synaptophysin, are demonstrated, at least focally, in many medulloblastomas {1063, 1396}. Homer Wright rosettes and the pale islands of the desmoplastic/nodular medulloblastomas are immunoreactive for these markers {251, 364, 1064}. Neurofilament protein expression occurs less commonly. {1396}. Particularly in the large cell variant,

synaptophysin immunoreactivity may have a characteristic dot-like appearance. In this variant, immunoreactivity for neurofilaments and chromogranin may also be demonstrated.

Cells positive for GFAP are often found among the undifferentiated cells of classic medulloblastomas; however, they mostly show the typical spider-like appearance of reactive astrocytes and tend to be more abundant near blood vessels. These cells are usually considered entrapped astrocytes, though the observation of similar cells in extra-cerebral metastatic deposits raises the possibility that at least some represent well-differentiated neoplastic astrocytes. Cells showing GFAP immunoreactivity and the cytological appearance of bona fide neoplastic elements can be observed in approximately 10% of cases of classic medulloblastoma {514}. The pale islands of the desmoplastic/nodular medulloblastoma may show fibrillary, GFAP-positive cells {1064}. However, GFAP-positive tumour cells can also be found in the inter-nodular areas of large cell and anaplastic medulloblastomas. Focal GFAP immonureactivity has been documented in large cell medulloblastoma, but is rare {514}.

The immunophenotype of the medulloblastoma also includes reactivities for vimentin, nestin {2254}, neuronal cell adhesion molecules {579, 615, 1505}, nerve growth factors {2199} and even photoreceptor-associated proteins, such as rodopsin and retinal S-antigen {407, 956, 1396}. Nuclear INI1 expression is retained in all medulloblastoma variants.

Electron microscopy

In areas of neuroblastic differentiation, such as rosettes and pale islands, the cells elaborate neurite-like cytoplasmic processes joined by specialized adhesion plaques, and are laden with microtubules in parallel array. Dense-core vesicles and synapses may also be observed {1058, 1531}. Abundant intermediate filaments may be noted in areas of glial differentiation. Tissue from histologically and immunohistochemically undifferentiated areas may reveal few, if any, specific ultrastructural features.

Apoptosis

Apoptosis is a major contributor to cell loss in medulloblastomas. Apoptotic indices generally parallel mitotic indices

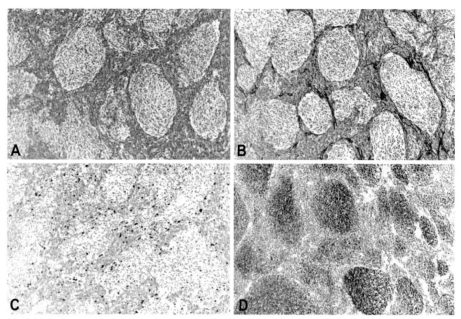

Fig. 8.08 Desmoplastic/nodular medulloblastomas. **A** Pale nodular areas surrounded by densely packed hyperchromatic cells. **B** Reticulin stain showing the reticulin-free pale islands. **C** MIB-1 staining shows that the proliferative activity predominates in the highly cellular, internodular areas, whereas (**D**) neuronal differentiation, shown by immunoreactivity to NSE, occurs in the pale islands.

in histological preparations {2020}, with the notable exception of the apoptosis that characterizes nodules in desmoplastic medulloblastomas, which have a low growth fraction {514}. The proportion of nuclei in apoptosis is in the range of 1–4% {239, 1989, 2019}, and does not appear to differ significantly between classic and desmoplastic variants {1784}, despite the regional variation seen in desmoplastic/nodular tumours. Various regulators of apoptosis have been studied in medulloblastoma. Bcl-2 inhibits apoptosis in many conditions, and is expressed in approximately 30% of all medulloblastomas, though Bcl-2 immunoreactivity appears to be more frequent (67%) in desmoplastic tumours {2021,2040}. Bcl-2 expression is found in the internodular regions of desmoplastic

tumours, and thus correlates inversely with markers of neurocytic differentiation {499,2040}. Caspase-8 is involved in death receptor-mediated apoptosis, and its CpG island is hypermethylated in a significant proportion (62–100%) of medulloblastomas {625}. Survivin is a member of the inhibition of apoptosis gene family, and also regulates the cell cycle. It is expressed in a wide range of neoplasms, including medulloblastoma {186}. REN is a putative tumour suppressor that antagonises the effects of Shh on the proliferation of cerebellar granule cells. In this paradigm, REN promotes growth arrest and apoptosis by enhancing the activity of caspase-3. Loss of REN has been implicated in the development of medulloblastoma {65}.

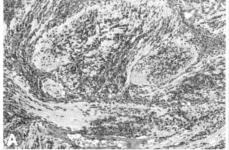 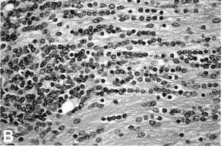

Fig. 8.09 **A** Medulloblastoma with extensive nodularity has a lobular architecture with large elongated reticulin-free zones. **B** These zones contain small round neurocytic cells in the fibrillary background.

Proliferation

Cell turnover in most medulloblastomas is high; indices of proliferation and apoptosis can be as high as in any other malignant neuroepithelial tumour {239}. However, for an embryonal tumour, these measures can be unexpectedly low in some classic tumours, and foci of differentiation in medulloblastomas, such as the nodules of the desmoplastic variant or groups of ganglion cells, may contain no mitotic activity and a negligible growth fraction by Ki-67 immunolabelling {514}. In contrast, particularly large numbers of mitotic figures and apoptotic bodies are hallmarks of the large cell and anaplastic medulloblastoma {498, 1435}. The mitotic index for childhood medulloblastomas is usually in the range of 0.5–2% {685, 1435}. The growth fraction, as assessed by Ki-67 immunolabelling, is generally >20% {1435, 2019}.

Genetic susceptibility

Several cases of medulloblastoma have been reported in monozygotic twins {331} as well as in dizygotic twins and siblings {150, 890, 2458} or other relatives {2344}. Associations with other brain tumours {552} and extraneural malignancies, including Wilms' tumour {1643,1822}, have also been observed. Moreover, medulloblastomas have been diagnosed in several familial cancer predisposition syndromes (see Chapter 13), including patients with *TP53* germline mutations (Li-Fraumeni syndrome), *PTCH1* mutations (the naevoid basal cell carcinoma syndrome or Gorlin syndrome; NBCCS {1249}, and *APC* mutations (Turcot syndrome), CBP (Rubinstein-Taybi syndrome) {2227} and *SUFU* {2226}. Occasionally, medulloblastomas develop in the setting of complex malformations, e.g. intestinal malrotation, omphalocele, and bladder extrophy {1615}, and Coffin-Siris syndrome (mental retardation, deficiency of postnatal growth, joint laxity, brachydactyly of the fifth digit with absence of the nail bed) {1910}. Some studies suggest that relatives of patients with medulloblastomas have an increased risk of developing other childhood tumours, particularly leukaemia and lymphoma {551, 1224}.

Genetics

Modern molecular cytogenetic strategies, such as comparative genomic hybridization (CGH), fluorescence *in situ* hybridization (FISH) and spectral karyotyping, have superseded conventional cytogenetic analysis over the last 10 years, though some findings made in the era of chromosomal analysis remain biologically relevant. The most common cytogenetic abnormality in medulloblastomas is isochromosome 17q, which is present in about 30–40% of tumours {164, 722}. In the majority of cases, the breakpoint is in the proximal portion of the short arm, so that the resultant structure is dicentric. Both loss of 17p and gain of 17q, which result from isochromosome 17q, can also occur independently {1590}. Whether generated as part of an isochromosome 17q, an interstitial deletion or monosomy 17, loss of 17p appears to be an indicator of poor prognosis {1255, 1590}. Other abnormalities detected by early cytogenetic studies were on chromosomes 6, 7, 8 and 11 {151}. It was noted that loss of chromosome 6 occurred independently of isochromosome 17q, a finding reinforced in recent studies that have shown an association between loss of chromosome 6 and Wnt pathway activation {2244}. In contrast, trisomy 7 is common and associated with isochromosome 17q {151}. Double minutes and homogeneously staining regions are demonstrated in medulloblastomas and are particularly linked to amplification of the *MYCC* gene {39, 163}. Amplification of *MYCC*, which is present in 5–10% of tumours, has been associated with the large cell and anaplastic variants and a poor outcome {501, 1255}.

Common genetic gains

Chromosomal gains of the *MYCC* locus (8q24) have been identified in primary medulloblastoma using Southern blot, FISH, and CGH. The frequency of amplification varies, ranging from 4% to 17% {39, 79, 502, 1454, 1573, 2015}. The frequency of *MYCN* amplification is also variable, but generally falls into a similar range {39, 502, 1454}. *MYC* amplicons are even more common in medulloblastoma cell lines and xenografts than in primary tumours, suggesting MYC might promote growth outside the normal tumour milieu {163}. Consistent with this concept, amplification of *MYCC* or *MYCN* is associated with the aggressive large cell tumour variant and with poor clinical outcomes {39, 79, 502, 2015}, *MYC* gene amplification has been reported in 3 of 6 medullomyoblastomas using FISH {806, 1292}. Additional chromosomal loci commonly gained in medulloblastoma that include potential oncogenes include 7q21 (*CDK6*) {1454}, 5p15 (*hTERT*) {502, 1454} and 14q22 (*OTX2*) {197,466}. All three of these oncogenes have also been shown to be overexpressed and associated with worse clinical outcomes. The *PIK3CA* gene, a member of the PI3

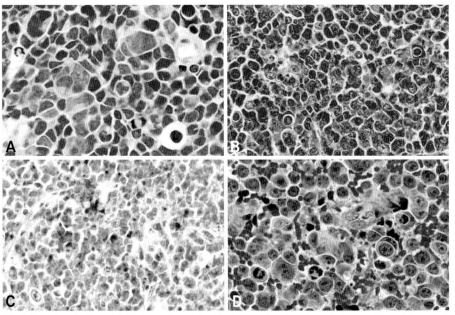

Fig. 8.10 **A** Anaplastic medulloblastoma characterized by increased nuclear size and pleomorphism. **B** Large cell medulloblastoma displaying pleomorphic, large nuclei with prominent nucleoli. **C** Large cell medulloblastoma displaying dot-like immunoreactivity for synaptophysin. **D** Large cell medulloblastoma showing enlarged vesicular nuclei, prominent nucleoli, and moderate cytoplasm. Tumour "cell wrapping" is also prominent.

kinase pathway, was found to be amplified in one study {2259} and activated by mutation in another {225}.

Common genetic losses

Two compilations of metaphase chromosome CGH data from over 200 medulloblastoma cases found that the chromosomal arms most commonly lost were 17p (23–28%), 16q (16–17%), 8p (15–22%), 10q (21%) and 11q (11–16%) {502,1881}. Array CGH studies have identified similar large regions of loss, and have begun to more precisely localize smaller deletions {888, 1454, 1938}. Studies of loss of heterozygosity (LOH) by both RFLP and microsatellite analysis, as well as FISH analyses, disclose that deletion or recombination of material on chromosome arm 17p is seen in 38–54% of cases {1145, 1255, 1428, 2016}. In the majority of cases, most of the short arm is missing with breakpoints in the 17p11 region {2016}. In occasional cases, partial 17p deletions have been identified, mapping the smallest overlapping region of deletion to 17p13.3 {1145, 1428}. As *TP53* is located on 17p13 and is mutated in a variety of human tumours, this gene was initially considered as a candidate gene. *TP53* mutations have been identified in only a small subset (5–10%) of medulloblastomas {16, 38, 1621}, but the p53 pathway can be altered in up to 21% of cases by other mechanisms such as *INK4A/ARF* deletion {602}. Nonetheless, because of the low incidence of mutations and the localization of the smallest region of deletion to 17p13.3 (distal to *TP53* at 17p13.1), *TP53* is not considered a major target of chromosome 17p loss. One potential tumour suppressor gene in the 17p13.3 region is *HIC1*, which is commonly hypermethylated in medulloblastoma {1919,2356}. While hypermethylation of *HIC1* is not significantly associated with LOH at the locus, it does appear to correlate with decreased transcription. *REN*, a negative regulator of the Hedgehog pathway located at 17p13.2, is also frequently deleted in medulloblastoma and appears to suppress the growth of tumour cells {463}.

Candidate genes on chromosome 10q

Two candidate genes have been studied in detail on 10q: *PTEN* and *DMBT1*. The tumour suppressor gene *PTEN*, located on 10q23, encodes a dual specificity

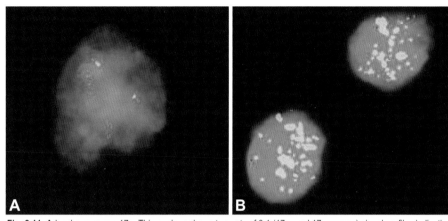

Fig. 8.11 A Isochromosome 17q. This nucleus shows two sets of 3:1 (17q - red:17p - green) signal profiles indicating loss of 17p and gain of 17q. **B** *MYC* amplification. These nuclei show multiple clumped *MYC* signals (green). The red signals from centromeric probes indicate chromosome 8 copy number.

phosphatase frequently deleted in cancers. Most studies have only identified rare medulloblastoma cases in which PTEN is lost {778, 1454}. In one report, however, differential PCR identified homozygous loss of *PTEN* in 30% (7 of 23) of medulloblastomas {915}. *PTEN* promoter methylation may represent a more common mechanism by which this tumour suppressor is down-regulated {778}. *DMBT1* was initially cloned in a medulloblastoma cell line following identification of a homozygous deletion at 10q25.3-26.1 using representational difference analysis {1508}. It contains multiple scavenger receptor cysteine-rich (SRCR) domains, but its role in tumour pathogenesis remains unclear. Intragenic homozygous deletions were detected in 2/20 medulloblastomas in the initial study, while two later reports found such deletions in 7/23 and 5/24 cases {915, 1674}. Mutations, however, were not detected in *DMBT1* {1674}.

The Hedgehog signalling pathway

Another tumour suppressor locus, *PTCH*, is located on the long arm of chromosome 9, where allelic losses have been described in 10–18% of medulloblastoma cases {2015, 2035}. *PTCH* is altered in NBCCS, which predisposes patients to develop basal cell carcinoma and medulloblastomas of the desmoplastic variant {2035}. *PTCH* is an inhibitor of the Hedgehog signalling pathway. It is the human homologue of the Drosophila segment polarity gene *PATCHED*, and it plays an important role in the development of the central nervous system and in tumourigenesis {588, 1401}. Hedgehog

signalling is particularly important in cerebellar development; as a pathway ligand, Sonic Hedgehog (SHH), is secreted by Purkinje cells, and is a major mitogen for cerebellar granule cell progenitors in the external granular cell layer {2382}. Activation of the pathway occurs by binding of Hedgehog ligand to PTCH, which stops PTCH from inhibiting SMO, and thereby activates Gli transcription factors {588}. The Hedgehog pathway can thus be aberrantly activated, at least in theory, by loss of PTCH function, or increased activity of SHH, SMO or Gli factors. Inactivating mutations of the *PTCH* gene, most of which result in truncated proteins, have been identified in approximately 8% of sporadic medulloblastomas {1747, 1816, 2345, 2433, 2516}. This seems to be the most common genetic mechanism of Hedgehog pathway activation in medulloblastoma, but other genes in the pathway can also be altered. A potentially activating point mutation in exon 2 of the *SHH* gene was identified in 1/14 medulloblastomas in one study {1648}, but not in others {2407, 2516}. An amplicon containing *SHH* has also been reported, suggesting increased gene dosage as another mechanism for increased activity {1454}. Mutation analysis of the *SMO* gene in medulloblastomas uncovered two cases with missense mutations {1252, 1852}, one being an activating mutation at position 1604 in exon 9. Others, however, have failed to identify *SMO* mutations in medulloblastoma {2516}. An inactivating mutation of *PTCH2*, a human homologue of *PTCH* located on chromosome 1p32-34, has been reported in a single case of medulloblastoma {2118}. *SUFU*, another hedgehog pathway inhibitor, has been found to be mutated in the germline of a small number of medulloblastoma patients {2226}. Array-based expression studies have in general supported the concept that Hedgehog signalling is active in a subset of medulloblastomas, and that this developmentally critical pathway is associated with the desmoplastic/nodular medulloblastoma subtype {1773, 2244}. Hedgehog pathway activity also appears to regulate expression of oncogenic ErbB-4 isoforms {570}.

APC and the Wnt signalling pathway

The adenomatous polyposis coli (APC) gene was originally identified as the target of germline mutations causing familial adenomatous polyposis (FAP), a syndrome of inherited predisposition to colon cancer {1751}. Some FAP patients also develop medulloblastoma, a condition known as Turcot syndrome {762}. The APC protein is a negative regulator of the Wnt pathway. It forms a complex with glycogen synthase kinase 3b (GSK-3ß) and Axin, and together they regulate the activity of ß-catenin {588,1751}. In the absence of Wnt ligands, GSK-3ß phosphorylates the N-terminal domain of ß-catenin and thereby targets it for degradation. When ligands are present, the APC/GSK-3ß/Axin complex is inactivated, allowing ß-catenin to enter the nucleus, where it binds TCF cofactors and positively regulates transcription of pathway targets {588, 1751}. While germline mutations in APC underlie medulloblastoma formation in Turcot syndrome patients, somatic APC mutations in sporadic medulloblastoma are relatively rare, with only 3–4% of tumours containing sequence changes {881, 1146}. Unlike the APC alterations in FAP patients, which result in a truncated, non-functional protein, the sequence changes identified to date in sporadic medullo-blastoma are missense mutations of undetermined functional significance.

Clear involvement of the Wnt pathway in the evolution of sporadic medulloblastomas was first indicated by the presence of ß-catenin mutations predicted to activate signalling by ablating inhibitory phosphorylation sites in 3/67 (4.5%) cases {2517}. Three other studies detected similar ß-catenin mutations in 5 to 10% of sporadic medulloblastoma {503, 881, 1146}. Finally, point mutations have been reported in the *Axin* gene in sporadic medulloblastoma {81, 411, 2472}. These studies suggest that the Wnt pathway is activated in a significant fraction of medulloblastoma. Indeed, if one uses nuclear immunopositivity for ß-catenin as a marker, between 18% and 25% of medulloblastoma show evidence of Wnt activity {503, 516, 2472}. This correlates fairly well with a recent expression array study, in which 6 of 46 medulloblastoma (13%) were classified into a Wnt subgroup {2244}.

The Notch signalling pathway

Like Hedgehog and Wnt, Notch is a pathway that plays a critical role in patterning of multiple organs, including the brain, and in the regulation of neural stem cells {1264}. In the cerebellum, Notch2 is known to promote the proliferation of external granular cell layer progenitor cells {2121}. Elevated levels of Notch signalling have been found in human medulloblastoma and medulloblastoma cell lines {548, 757}. *Notch2* gene amplification could account for this in 15% of cases {548}. γ-secretase inhibitors, which block Notch pathway activity, slow medulloblastoma growth, and appear to deplete stem-like medulloblastoma cells {547, 757}.

Neural transcription factors

Many transcription factors implicated in the development of the brain appear to be deregulated in medulloblastoma. In general, however, the altered expression of these proteins is not associated with copy number changes or mutations of the loci in question. PAX5 and PAX6 mRNA was detected in 70% and 78% of medulloblastomas by *in situ* hybridization {1182}. The lack of expression of the *PAX5* gene in normal neonatal cerebellum and its upregulation in medulloblastoma indicates that it may play a role in development of medulloblastoma. Other neural transcription factors found to be expressed in medulloblastomas include the granule cell marker ZIC, and transcription factors of the NEUROD family {269, 1773, 1940, 2470}. SOX transcription factors are also expressed in medulloblastoma, with increased levels of SOX4 most commonly reported {1272, 1573, 2471}. REST, a repressor of neural differentiation, is also overexpressed in medulloblastoma, and seems to cooperate with proproliferative oncogenes to promote tumour formation {631, 2167}.

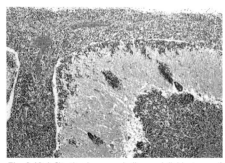

Fig. 8.12 Infiltration by a cerebellar medulloblastoma of the subarachnoidal space. Note clusters of tumour cells in the molecular layer, particularly in the subpial region.

Histogenesis

Bailey and Cushing recognized the medulloblastoma as a distinct clinicopathological entity in 1925 {85}. They assumed a derivation from medulloblasts, i.e. undifferentiated, proliferating embryonal cells with the capacity to differentiate into spongioblasts and neuroblasts. The existence of such precursor cells was postulated, but not unequivocally identified, in subsequent neuro-anatomical studies of the developing nervous system {2313}. The histogenesis of medulloblastoma has been controversial for over 75 years. There are two main hypotheses: One view suggests that medulloblastoma originate from the external granular layer (EGL) of the cerebellum, which forms during embryogenesis by migration of undifferentiated cells from the roof of the fourth ventricle to the surface of the fetal cerebellar cortex, where they give rise to cells which later form the internal granular layer neurons {2313}. This view is supported by the observation that the proliferation of precursor neurons in the external granular layer of the cerebellum is controlled by sonic Hedgehog {2382}, by analysis of murine medulloblastoma models based on Hedgehog activation {1107, 1637}, and by comparison of gene expression patterns in medulloblastoma to those in the cerebellar EGL {1098}.

The second hypothesis is the basis of the PNET concept and assumes that medulloblastomas are derived from subependymal matrix cells, which reside throughout the embryonal CNS, including the fourth ventricle, and which give rise to neuronal and glial cells. The PNET concept implies that medulloblastomas and supratentorial PNETs originate from a common precursor cell. However, there is evidence that infratentorial PNETs (medulloblastomas) and supratentorial PNETs show different genetic alterations. Unlike medulloblastoma, supratentorial PNETs do not show allelic loss of chromosome arm 17p {264}. Similarly, inactivating mutations of the *PTCH* locus seem not to occur in this entity {2433}. Supratentorial PNETs express the human ACHAETE SCUTE homologue (HASH1) which is absent in medulloblastomas {1940}. Indeed, large scale gene expression analysis shows that medulloblastoma and PNET have distinct profiles {1773}. These findings argue against the hypothesis that PNETs of different locations may derive from closely related progenitor cells by similar genetic mechanisms. Perhaps most likely is a combined theory proposing that medulloblastomas can arise from more than one cell type, a concept supported by a range of expression studies. Calbindin-D, a ventricular matrix-associated calcium binding protein not expressed in the EGL or in granule neurons, was detected in 20 of 49 cerebellar medulloblastoma, primarily those of the classic (non-desmoplastic/nodular) subtype {1060}. Based on this, it was suggested that classic medulloblastoma derive from the ventricular zone, while nodular tumours originate from EGL cells. Others have advanced a similar "dual origin" hypothesis based on the elevated percentage of nodular tumours immunoreactive for the neurotrophin receptor p75, which is highly expressed in the cerebellar EGL but not in the ventricular zone {243}. Wnt activity, in contrast, seems to be associated with non-desmoplastic/nodular tumours, and may represent a signature of some ventricular zone-derived lesions {2244}. OTX1 and OTX2 expression also differentiates medulloblastoma subtypes, with the former associated with desmoplastic/nodular lesions, and the latter found in classic tumours {435}. Our understanding of stem and progenitor cells in the brain continues to evolve, and new candidate cells of origin continue to emerge. One such candidate is a class of CD133 positive stem cells found predominantly in the white matter of the postnatal cerebellum {1271}.

Prognostic and predictive factors

Significant advances have been made in the treatment of childhood medulloblastoma; the 30% 5-year survival in the 1960s has now risen to 60–70%. This improvement has been attributed to improved surgical and anaesthetic techniques, better neuroimaging and perioperative care, and more refined adjuvant therapies, which combine radiotherapeutic and chemotherapeutic regimens {428, 515, 687, 1661, 1662, 1898, 1962}. A similar increase in survival has been achieved in adult patients {210}. Current challenges are finding novel therapies for aggressive disease and the accurate identification of disease risk, which would facilitate the targeted use of adjuvant therapies, intensive regimens for high-risk tumours and reduced long-term adverse effects for patients with relatively responsive tumours {962, 1025}. Since the last edition of this classification, many prognostic indicators have been proposed for the medulloblastoma, but few have been proven to be independent in large cohorts of patients treated in the context of therapeutic trials.

Clinical criteria

The clinical stratification of childhood medulloblastoma currently involves distinguishing high-risk and standard-risk patients. The former group is aged less than 3 years, has an incomplete surgical resection of the tumour (>1.5 cm^2 residuum), or has metastatic disease (Chang stages M1-4) at presentation {962, 1661}.

Histopathology

For some time, distinguishing the histopathological variants of medulloblastoma was not thought to be of particular clinical utility. However, a dismal prognosis has clearly been established for the large cell medulloblastoma {230, 670, 1255, 1435}. This variant is associated with a high frequency of metastatic disease {230, 498, 670}. In addition, several studies have now demonstrated that this variant and classic tumours with anaplastic cytological features form a continuum, and that large cell medulloblastomas and tumours with marked and widespread anaplasia (anaplastic medulloblastoma variant) have a significantly poorer prognosis than other tumours {230, 500, 671, 1435}.

The desmoplastic variant has been associated with a better prognosis than the classic medulloblastoma in some studies, but others report no significant difference in outcome for these two tumour types {82, 322, 1535, 2182}. This discrepancy could relate to the use of different criteria in the diagnosis of desmoplastic medulloblastoma; if diagnosis relies on finding a nodular architecture among reticulin-positive internodular zones, then a better prognosis is often demonstrated for this variant {671, 2182}. A favourable outcome was recognized for

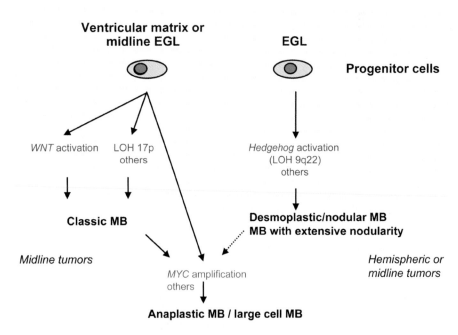

Fig. 8.13 Hypothetical model of the different origin and pathogenetic pathways of medulloblastoma variants. EGL, external granular layer. MB, medulloblastoma.

the desmoplastic/nodular tumours including medulloblastoma with extensive nodularity in a large proportion (47%) of one trial cohort of infants with a medulloblastoma. This tumours were associated with a much better survival than classic medulloblastomas {1963}.

Proliferation and apoptosis

There is no conclusive evidence that measures of proliferation or apoptosis have clinical utility; relevant studies provide conflicting data. However, an association between a simple evaluation of mitotic count or index and survival has been demonstrated for children with medulloblastoma {685, 1435}. Survival analyses do not support the use of PCNA labelling index (LI) or Ki-67/MIB-1 LIs as prognostic indicators {687, 1435, 1484, 1631, 2020}. BrdU LI may be associated with outcome; tumours with a LI of >20% appeared to have a worse prognosis in one study {929}.

Apoptotic indices have not been related to prognosis in a consistent way {780, 1174, 1631, 1756, 2040}. However, the categorization of apoptosis into 'focal', 'diffuse' and 'extensive' produced an association with survival in medulloblastomas with focal apoptosis showing a better prognosis than tumours in the other two categories. This study also found a link between cytological anaplasia and survival {671}. The overall picture is further confounded by studies of markers that have functional roles in the regulation of apoptosis. Thus, although Bcl-2 prevents programmed cell death induced by irradiation, medulloblastomas with immunoreactivity for Bcl-2 do not recur earlier than those lacking Bcl-2 expression {1568}. This result could be related to a lack of correlation between Bcl-2 expression and apoptotic indices {2040}.

Molecular markers

Molecular genetic markers that have been shown to have independent prognostic significance alongside clinical and pathological variables in patients from trial cohorts include isochromosome 17q, loss of 17p, and amplification of the MYCC or MYCN genes {113, 1255, 2015}. These are indicators of an adverse prognosis, as is overexpression of ErbB2 {686}. In contrast, nuclear accumulation of ß-catenin, a marker of activation in the canonical Wnt/Wg pathway, is an independent marker of a good outcome {516}. Medulloblastomas with this immunophenotype generally lack molecular cytogenetic abnormalities, with the exception of monosomy 6 {2244}. Measuring a combination of TrkC expression, which appears to be associated with prolonged survival, and c-MYC expression may be useful in separating biologically distinct groups of medulloblastoma {728}. Abnormally overexpressed PDGF receptor, p53, STK15 and CDK6 may be validated as indicators of a poor prognosis {684, 973, 1371, 1454, 1573, 2440}.

Central nervous system primitive neuroectodermal tumours

R.E. McLendon
A.R. Judkins
C.G. Eberhart
G.N. Fuller
C. Sarkar
H.-K. Ng

Definition

A heterogeneous group of tumours occurring predominantly in children and adolescents. They may arise in the cerebral hemispheres, brain stem, or spinal cord, and are composed of undifferentiated or poorly differentiated neuroepithelial cells which may display divergent differentiation along neuronal, astrocytic and ependymal lines. CNS/ supratentorial PNET is an embryonal tumour composed of undifferentiated or poorly differentiated neuroepithelial cells. Tumours with only neuronal differentiation are termed cerebral neuroblastomas or, if ganglion cells are also present, cerebral ganglioneuroblastomas. Tumours that recreate features of neural tube formation are termed medulloepitheliomas. Tumours with ependymoblastic rosettes are termed ependymoblastomas. Features common to all CNS PNET variants include early onset and aggressive clinical behaviour.

ICD-O codes

CNS PNET, NOS	9473/3
CNS neuroblastoma	9500/3
CNS ganglioneuroblastoma	9490/3
Medulloepithelioma	9501/3
Ependymoblastoma	9392/3

Since the designation of some primitive neuroectodermal tumours of the central nervous system (CNS) is also used for similar, but not identical tumours at extra-cerebral sites, the WHO Working Group proposes to add the prefix CNS to these entities, in order to avoid any confusion. The term CNS PNET, not otherwise specified (NOS) is synonymous with the current ICD-O term supratentorial PNET (9473/3) and used for undifferentiated or poorly differentiated embryonal tumours that occur at any extracerebellar site in the CNS.

Grading

As with other embryonal brain tumours, all CNS PNETs correspond histologically to WHO grade IV.

CNS/supratentorial PNET

Definition

An embryonal tumour composed of undifferentiated or poorly differentiated neuroepithelial cells which have the capacity for, or display, divergent differentiation along neuronal, astrocytic, muscular or melanocytic lines. Tumours with only neuronal differentiation are termed cerebral neuroblastomas or, if ganglion cells are also present, ganglioneuroblastomas.

Incidence

Precise incidence is difficult to determine because of differing viewpoints regarding classification and the rarity of these tumours. One percent of 933 primary paediatric CNS neuroepithelial tumours were found to be located in the cerebrum or suprasellar region; among CNS PNETs, 10 of 178 (5.6%) were located in these regions.

Age and sex distribution

The age range for CNS PNET is 4 weeks to 20 years, with a mean of 5.5 years. The male:female ratio for supratentorial PNETs and cerebral neuroblastomas is 1.2:1.

Localization

These tumours are found most commonly in the cerebrum, but can also be encountered in the spinal cord or suprasellar region.

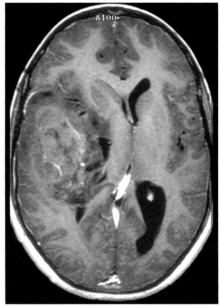

Fig. 8.15 T1-weighted MRI of a large, hemispheric PNET with advanced neuronal differentiation (neuro-blastoma).

Clinical features

Signs and symptoms are related to the site of origin of the tumour. Those arising in the cerebrum often present with seizures, disturbances of consciousness, increased intracranial pressure or motor deficit. The suprasellar lesions produce visual and/or endocrine problems. If the patient is an infant, the head circumference may increase more rapidly than normal.

Neuroimaging

Computed tomographic findings in CNS PNET are similar, regardless of the site of origin of the tumour. They are iso-to-hyperdense, but density increases following injection of contrast material. They may appear as solid masses or may contain cystic or necrotic areas. Between 50 and 70% of all CNS PNET contain calcium. Edema surrounding parenchymal masses is not usually extensive. Appearance of PNET on magnetic resonance imaging may vary with the site of origin. On T1-weighted MRI, the tumours are hypointense relative to cortical grey matter. They look

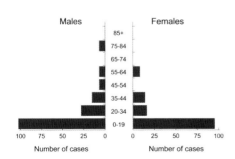

Fig. 8.14 Age and sex distribution of supratentorial PNET and cerebral neuroblastomas, based on 305 cases. Data from CBTRUS 1995-2002 {305}.

similar on T2-weighted imaging, but cystic or necrotic areas are hyperintense. There is contrast enhancement with gadolinium on T1-weighted imaging. If the tumour has bled, the region of haemorrhage is hypointense on T2-weighted imaging.

Macroscopy

The tumours are of variable size at the time of clinical presentation. Those in the suprasellar region tend to be smaller than those in the cerebrum. The parenchymal tumours may be massive growths, with or without cysts or haemorrhages. Demarcation between tumour and brain may range from indistinct to clear-cut. They have a pink-red to purple colour. They are soft unless they contain a prominent desmoplastic component, in which case they are more firm and have a tan colour.

Histopathology

The typical tumour is very poorly differentiated, being composed of cells with round regular nuclei and high nucleus:cytoplasm ratios. Better differentiated tumours may show more clearly neuronal features, with oval to elongated nuclei that have vesicular chromatin and nucleoli; occasionally, processes and even Nissl substance may be encountered in such tumours when more mature populations are evident (ganglioneuroblastomas). Fibrillar cytoplasm may form the background in these tumours. A fibrous stroma can vary from a delicate lobular framework to dense fibrous cords. Homer Wright rosettes are often found but vary in frequency. Tumour cells may occasionally be arranged in parallel streams and palisades, resembling the pattern seen in polar spongioblastoma {868, 1259} or in single file patterns akin to the adrenal neuroblastoma. Populations of more mature round regular neurocytic (granule cell) forms may rarely be found {1865}. Calcification is a relatively constant feature within degenerate regions. Vascular endothelial proliferation may also be seen. Cerebrospinal dissemination can be found in up to one third of patients {868}. Extraneural metastases to bone, liver and cervical lymph nodes have been reported {134}.

An unusual PNET that occurs in the brain stem, cerebellum and cerebrum has been called "embryonal tumour with abundant neuropil and true rosettes" {497}. These are characterized by focal high cellularity, broad bands of neoplastic neuropil, and true rosettes with slit-like or oval lumens that often arise in the fibrillar areas. Tumours with this pattern of growth are associated with extremely poor clinical outcomes, and may eventually be recognized as a unique variant.

Immunohistochemistry

Neuroblastomas express many of the phenotypic markers of neuronal cells, including synaptophysin, class III ß-tubulin, and neurofilament protein {716}. Cerebral neuroblastomas also express S-100, NSE, and Leu-7 (CD-57) {1865}. However, a pure population of phenotypically recognizable neuroblasts is rarely encountered in these neoplasms. Undifferentiated small anaplastic cells, by both light microscopic and ultrastructural methods, typically constitute the majority of the cellular populations of these tumours. Immunohistochemical techniques occasionally reveal GFAP to be expressed among these undifferentiated cells, indicative of divergent cellular phenotypes. Antigen expression is unique for each tumour, making prediction of patterns of expression for one or a group of tumours unreliable.

Electron microscopy

The typical tumour is very poorly differentiated, revealing only a sparse population of cytoplasmic organelles. While microtubules may be found, dense core vesicles, although not always present, are diagnostic of neuroblastoma. With ganglionic differentiation, some processes may terminate as growth cones containing arrays of microtubules. Demonstration of synapses is exceptional {1865}. Compact arrays of cytoplasmic glial filaments supports glial differentiation, although intervening reactive astrocytes must be ruled out {1959}.

Proliferation

PNET at any site show a variable amount of mitotic activity. Proliferation is most accurately measured by use of the immunohistochemical marker Ki-67. The percentage of cells undergoing proliferation is generally high but may vary from 0–85% in any given high-power field.

Genetics

The i(17)q abnormality found in 30 to 50% of medulloblastomas has been found in only one supratentorial PNET

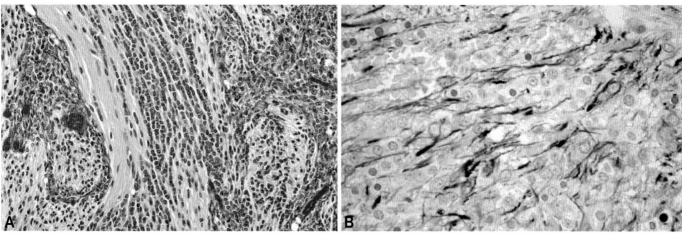

Fig. 8.16 A CNS PNET with advanced neuronal differentiation (cerebral neuroblastoma) exhibiting a nodular architecture with typical streaming of tumour cells. **B** Neurofilament staining predominantly of tumour cell processes.

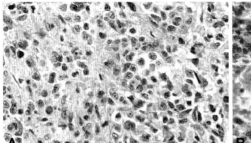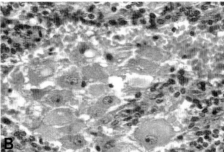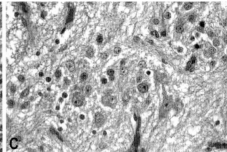

Fig. 8.17 Tumour cells in different stages of neuronal differentiation (**A**) and cluster of mature ganglion cells next to an area of poorly differentiated elements (**B**) in cerebral neuroblastoma. **C** Region of low cellularity in a ganglioneuroblastoma showing some tumour cells with neuronal phenotype.

{1805} and in one neuroblastic tumour with abundant neuropil and true rosettes {627}. Several studies disclosed a variety of non-random cytogenetic gains and losses {264, 152}, but no i(17)q {165}. Scattered reports of other genetic abnormalities in these tumours include identification of *RASSF1A* promoter methylation {318}, expression of the Neuro D family of basic helix-loop-helix transcription factors, and achaete scute, another neurogenic transcription factor with homology to *Neuro D* genes {1940}. This latter gene was actually expressed in 3 of 5 PNET arising outside the cerebellum, but not in medulloblastoma. Thus, although the number of cytogenetic studies is small, it appears that genetic events associated with development of PNET in the supratentorial compartment are different from medulloblastoma {1960, 1425}.

Histogenesis

The histogenesis of PNETs as a group has been a controversial issue for many years, and the only issue upon which consensus has been achieved is that these embryonal tumours arise from primitive neuroepithelial cells {1121, 1921}. The recent identification of neurons derived from haematopoietic stem cells only adds to the controversy {1467A}.

Prognostic and predictive factors

Infants who are less than two years old at the time of diagnosis of a CNS PNET have a bleaker prognosis than older children {663}. Children with CNS PNET have a worse overall 5-year survival rate compared to children with medulloblastoma {662, 2250}. The relationship between survival and various histological features has not been determined in supratentorial PNET.

Medulloepithelioma

Definition

A rare, malignant embryonal brain tumour affecting young children, histologically characterized by papillary, tubular or trabecular arrangements of neoplastic neuroepithelium mimicking the embryonic neural tube.

Age and sex distribution

Medulloepitheliomas are rare tumours that typically affect children between 6 months and 5 years, with half occurring during the first two years {1509}. In 37 published cases the age at presentation ranged from <1 month to 23 years with a mean age of 45 months; cases were equally distributed between males and females (male:female ratio, 1:1) {2068, 1509, 2326, 1606}. Congenital tumours have been described. Rare cases occurring beyond the first decade have also been reported {1509, 2010}.

Localization

Medulloepitheliomas develop in both the supra- and infratentorial compartments {1509, 429, 1606, 1988}. The most common site within the cerebral hemispheres is periventricular, involving in order of frequency: temporal, parietal, occipital and frontal lobes. Occasionally, these tumours may be very large and involve multiple lobes or both cerebral hemispheres {2176}. Medulloepitheliomas may also be intraventricular and have also been described in the sella/parasellar region, cauda equina, and presacral area {578, 1675, 2326}. Outside the central nervous system these tumours may arise along nerve trunks, within the pelvic cavity, and in the eye where they are typically intraorbital {1566, 233, 481}. Intraorbital medulloepitheliomas rarely metastasize, are

effectively treated by enucleation and generally carry a favourable prognosis {1606, 2326}. Medulloepitheliomas may also arise in the optic nerve. Based on a small number of reported cases, these tumours do not appear to carry the favourable prognosis of intraorbital medulloepitheliomas but may be associated with somewhat better long-term survival than intracerebral medulloepitheliomas {720A, 324, 2295, 332}.

Clinical features

The tumour is often large at the time of clinical presentation, with symptoms of increased intracranial pressure such as headaches, nausea and vomiting. All patients have had abnormal neurological examination at clinical presentation. CT and MR imaging characteristics have been variable. At initial presentation, these tumours have been described as well circumscribed and isodense to minimally hypodense on CT and non-enhancing with intravenous contrast; enhancement typically appears with tumour progression {1509}. On T1-weighted MR imaging, medulloepitheliomas have been either hypointense or isointense {431}; however, they are hyperintense on T2-weighted images {1675}. Cysts and calcifications have been reported.

Macroscopy

Medulloepitheliomas are often massive, grayish pink in color and well-circumscribed with areas of haemorrhage and necrosis. Occasionally, there is infiltration of the subarachnoid space at the initial presentation, while diffuse dissemination is frequent at the time of death.

Histopathology

Medulloepitheliomas are malignant neoplasms that mimic the embryonic neural tube and are characterized by papillary,

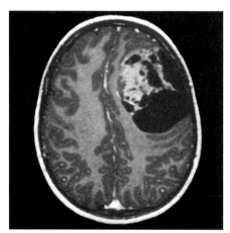
Fig. 8.18 T1-weighted gadolinium-enhanced MRI of a cystic medulloepithelioma in the frontal lobe.

tubular or trabecular arrangements of neoplastic neuroepithelium with an external limiting membrane. These tumours often display multiple lines of differentiation, including neural, glial and mesenchymal elements. The diagnostic feature of medulloepithelioma is the distinctive pseudostratified epithelium arranged in papillary and tubular patterns that resembles the structure of the primitive neural tube {1045}. On the luminal (inner) marginal surface of the tubules there are no cilia or blepharoblasts, but there may be discrete protruding blebs. On the outer surface of the epithelium is an external limiting membrane which stains with PAS and is immunopositive with antiserum to collagen type IV. This basement membrane rests on a delicate network of reticulin. The cells have a columnar to cuboidal shape. The nuclei are oval to piloid, are perpendicular to the inner and outer surfaces, and are characterized by coarse chromatin and multiple nucleoli. Mitotic figures are abundant and tend to be located near the luminal surface similar to the early stages of neural tube development. In areas distinct from the neuroepithelium there are sheets of tumour cells with hyperchromatic nuclei and a high nuclear to cytoplasmic ratio. These cells may show a range of differentiation: neuronal, astrocytic, ependymo-blastic or oligodendroglial {72, 444}. There is also a spectrum in the degree of differentiation from embryonic early differentiated cells to mature neurons and astrocytes. In medulloepitheliomas, ependymoblastomatous rosettes are more common than ependymal rosettes, but both may occur.

Areas of oligodendro-glial differentiation are suggested by round regular nuclei and white halos and negative immunohistochemistry with antiserum for synaptophysin. A primitive neuroectodermal tumour with tubules containing melanin pigment has been described as a pigmented medullo-epithelioma {2068}. Rare tumours may manifest development along mesenchymal lines that range from a prominent vascular and fibrous connective tissue stroma to areas of cartilage, bone and striated muscle {72, 271}.

Immunohistochemistry
The neuroepithelial components of medulloepitheliomas show immunoreactivity for nestin and vimentin. Both of these markers demonstrate an expression gradient with basal greater than luminal labelling; indeed, nestin is largely confined to the basal area {1099, 2254}. Less frequently, tumour cells in some cases may also display focal expression of neurofilament protein, cytokeratins, and epithelial membrane antigen {271, 1099, 2268}. Neuroepithelial areas do not exhibit GFAP, neuron specific enolase or S-100 protein expression. Expression of both basic fibroblast growth factor and insulin-like growth factor I (IGF-I) has been reported in medulloepithelioma {2091}. In areas away from the neuro-epithelium, immunoreactivity reflects the pattern and degree of differentiation of the tumour. Neuron-specific enolase, synaptophysin, neurofilament and microtubule associated proteins reveal an increasing degree of expression commen-surate with the degree of neuronal differentiation {271}. Astrocytic differentiation spans the spectrum, from densely cellular areas with high mitotic activity and variable GFAP expression to areas of low to moderate cellularity with mature differentiation and consistently strong GFAP expression.

Proliferation
Medulloepitheliomas have a high rate of proliferation. The epithelium is also mitotically active, with mitotic figures located predominantly near the luminal surface. Ki-67 labelling may be extremely variable within these tumours with areas of low (1–3%) labelling adjacent to those with extremely high labelling (>50%).

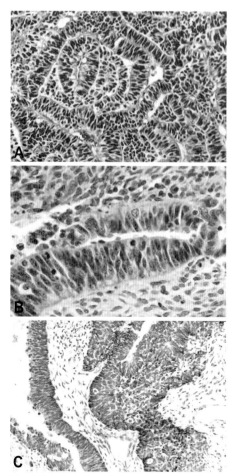
Fig. 8.19 A Typical papillary and trabecular pattern in medulloepithelioma. **B** Immature neuroepithelial cells resting on a basement membrane. Mitotic cells tend to be located towards the luminal surface. **C** Nestin expression predominates on the basal side of neoplastic neuroepithelial cells.

Electron microscopy
Ultrastructural examination of the neuro-epitheliomatous areas reveals extensive primitive lateral cell junctions (zonulae adherentes) and a basal lamina on the outer surface of the epithelial cells, consisting of a distinct, continuous, often folded, basement membrane {1771, 2268}. On the luminal side, there is an amorphous surface coating but no true membrane. Cells appear poorly differentiated with sparse cytoplasmic organelles and absence of cilia or microvilli.

Histogenesis
Microscopy, immunohistochemistry and electron microscopy of medulloepitheliomas demonstrates features that resemble the primitive neural tube {1099, 2254}. It has therefore been proposed that medulloepitheliomas may derive from a primitive

cell population in the subependymal region.

Differential diagnosis
Medulloepitheliomas may show a variety of histologic patterns that can raise a broad differential diagnosis including medulloblastoma, ependymoblastoma, neuroblastoma and choroid plexus carcinoma. However, careful examination of most medulloepitheliomas will reveal the distinctive tubular or trabecular arrangements of neoplastic neuro-epithelium that are unique to this tumour. Where ependymoma and choroid plexus carcinoma may be difficult to eliminate on histologic grounds alone, the distinctive immunohistochemical staining of medullo-epitheliomas will resolve these diagnoses. Immature teratomas are included in the differential diagnosis because they frequently contain primitive medullary epithelium, together with neuroecto-dermal differentiation. The distinction from medulloepithelioma is that immature teratomas contain tissue of foetal appearance from other germ layers.

Genetics
The molecular genetics of medullo-epitheliomas of the central nervous system have not been extensively characterized. However, molecular analysis of two cases demonstrated *hTERT* gene amplification similar to and even exceeding that seen in medulloblastomas. CGH analysis of both the primary and recurrent specimens from one of these tumours was also performed. This showed gains in 3p13-22, 6p21.2-21.3, 14q24-qter, 15q15-25 and 20q in the primary medulloepithelioma. Additional gains were identified in the recurrent tumour including high level gains at 5p15 consistent with *hTERT* gene amplification, as well as losses involving 4p14-q28, 4q34-qter, 5q, 13q and 18q12-qter {549}. Analysis of a single intraocular medullo-epithelioma demonstrated only non-specific cytogenetic changes {146}.

Prognostic and predictive factors
Medulloepitheliomas are rapidly growing tumours that arise at a young age, and their optimal management is unknown. Treatment with gross total resection is a feature of long-term survivors {1509}. Radiation may also provide some benefit. However, most children with medulloepithelioma die within a year of diagnosis, often with cerebrospinal fluid dissemination but rarely with systemic metastases.

Ependymoblastoma

Definition
A rare, malignant, embryonal brain tumour manifesting in neonates and young children, histologically characterized by distinctive multilayered rosettes.

Age and sex distribution
Consistent with the primitive neuroepithelial nature of the tumour, the ependymo-blastoma occurs in young children, including neonates {477, 1393}. Males and females appear to be equally affected.

Localization
These neoplasms are often large and supratentorial and generally relate to the ventricles although they do occur at other sites {1337, 1525}. A sacrococcygeal congenital ependymoblastoma with elevated serum α-fetoprotein {1537} and a primary leptomeningeal ependymo-blastoma have been documented {2354}.

Clinical features
In the first and second year of life, the most common clinical manifestation is increased intracranial pressure and hydrocephalus. Focal neurological signs are more common in older children. Neuroimaging criteria do not allow a distinction from other primitive neuro-ectodermal tumours {484}. CT and MR usually show a contrast-enhancing, large tumour mass surrounded by an extensive area of edema.

Macroscopy
Ependymoblastomas tend to be well circumscribed with a distinct tumour margin, although focal microscopic extension and leptomeningeal invasion are common. Widespread leptomeningeal invasion and extraneural metastases have been described {281}. The unusual extension of a supratentorial ependymo-blastoma through the tentorium into the cerebellum has been documented {1512}.

Histopathology
Diagnostic features are those of a central primitive neuroectodermal tumour with distinctive multilayered rosettes, with cells in the outer rim of the rosette merging with the surrounding undifferentiated neuro-ectodermal cells. The chief histological characteristic of ependymoblastoma is dense cellularity with prominent numbers of distinctive true "ependymoblastomatous" rosettes. These rosettes are multi-layered and form concentric cellular rings around small round central lumina. The nuclei of these cells tend to be pushed away from the lumen towards the outer cell border, and the chromatin is coarse and nuclei distinct. The cells have high mitotic activity. The cells facing the lumen have a defined apical surface beneath which is a faint stippling that corresponds to blepharoplasts. These apical surfaces may form a prominent internal limiting membrane. The outer layer of cells merges with the background of undifferentiated cells with small round-to-oval nuclei and wispy cytoplasmic processes.

Immunohistochemistry
Expression of S-100, vimentin, cytokeratin, GFAP and carbonic anhydrase isoenzyme II has been demonstrated {509, 1393, 400, 1682}. One report describes immuno-reactivity to NF 68, 160 and 200 kDa neurofilaments {1509}.

Electron microscopy
Tumour cells are compactly arranged and poorly differentiated, with large nuclei and a high nuclear to cytoplasmic ratio. Cytoplasm is scanty with few organelles. In rosettes the cells are united by long or short junctional complexes featuring thickened and electron dense membranes. Frequent "abortive" cilia {400} and a few basal bodies oriented toward the lumen of the rosette {1258} have been observed,

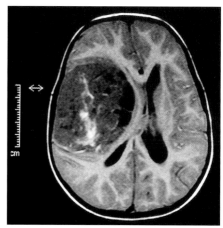

Fig. 8.20 MRI of an ependymoblastoma bordering the lateral ventricle.

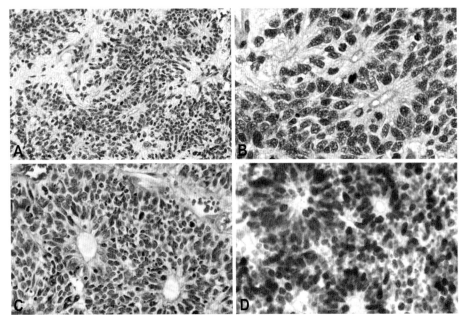

Fig. 8.21 Histological features of ependymoblastoma. **A** and **B** Ependymoblastoma with well-formed true rosettes arising within the background of PNET-like cytology. **C** Ependymoblastoma characterized by ependymal rosette formation. **D** Very high proliferative activity in ependymoblastic rosettes (MIB-1).

as have short bands of glial-like filaments.

Differential diagnosis

Ependymoblastoma must be distinguished from anaplastic ependymoma, which is characterized by prominent perivascular pseudorosettes in which radially-oriented cell processes form nuclei-free zones around blood vessels (perivascular pseudorosettes) and ependymal rosettes that, in contrast to ependymoblastoma-type rosettes, exhibit only a limited, often single, circumferential layering of cells. Medulloepitheliomas may contain ependymoblastoma-type rosettes, but are primarily characterized by distinctive diagnostic neuroepithelium that is based on an outer basement membrane and characteristic architectural features that include long linear tubular, canalicular and papillary patterns. The latter tumours also often display a spectrum of neuro-ectodermal differentiation including ependymal, glial, neuronal and oligo-dendroglial features. Medulloblastomas are characterized by a cerebellar location and frequent presence of Homer Wright (neuroblastoma-type) rosettes that, in contrast to ependymoblastoma-type rosettes, lack a central lumen {396, 1923}. Embryonal tumour with abundant neuropil and true rosettes {497}, discussed previously, should also be considered in this differential.

Histogenesis

These tumours are presumed to arise from periventricular neuroepithelial precursor cells. The term 'ependymoblast' implies an incompletely differentiated phenotype showing glial and ependymal features together with immature characteristics, such as a high nucleus-to-cytoplasmic ratio, dense chromatin and brisk mitotic activity {400, 1948}.

Prognostic and predictive factors

Biological characteristics are similar to other embryonal neuroepithelial tumours {396}. Ependymoblastomas grow rapidly, with craniospinal dissemination and fatal outcome usually within 6 months to one year of diagnosis. Development of effective treatment protocols for ependymoblastomas is limited by the rarity of occurrence, young age of onset and aggressive tumour behaviour. Some studies suggest that gross total resection of ependymoblastoma is a predictor of outcome {1899}. Consistent with the response of other primitive neuroepithelial tumours, post-operative irradiation may prolong survival.

Atypical teratoid/rhabdoid tumour

A.R. Judkins
C.G. Eberhart
P. Wesseling

Definition
A highly malignant CNS tumour predominantly manifesting in young children, typically containing rhabdoid cells, often with primitive neuroectodermal cells and with divergent differentiation along epithelial, mesenchymal, neuronal or glial lines; associated with inactivation of the *INI1/hSNF5* gene in virtually all cases.

ICD-O code   9508/3

Grading
This tumour corresponds to WHO grade IV.

Synonyms and historical annotation
Malignant rhabdoid tumours were initially described in the kidney and subsequently in soft tissues of infants and young children. The first example affecting the CNS was reported in 1985 {1519A} and simply called 'rhabdoid tumour'. These tumours were named 'atypical teratoid/rhabdoid tumours' (AT/RT) when they occurred in the CNS to call attention to the disparate combination of rhabdoid, primitive neuroepithelial, epithelial and mesenchymal components {1924}. The complex histologic pattern resulting from these disparate elements has sometimes resulted in misclassification of these tumours as CNS PNET/medulloblastomas, choroid plexus carcinomas, germ cell tumours and malignant gliomas.

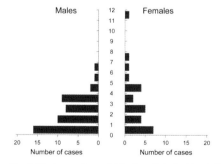

Fig. 8.22 Age and sex distribution of atypical teratoid/rhabdoid tumour, based on 73 patients {823, 2231}.

Incidence
Several large series have established the incidence of AT/RT at 1–2% of paediatric brain tumours {1876, 1922, 2438}. However, due to the preponderance of cases in children under the age of three, AT/RTs are estimated to account for at least 10% of CNS tumours in infants {153}.

Age and sex distribution
AT/RTs are paediatric tumours most often presenting under the age of 3, and rarely in children older than 6 years (mean age, approx 2 years). There is a male predominance ranging from 1.6–2:1 {823, 2231}. AT/RTs occur rarely in adults {1823}.

Localization
In two large series of paediatric cases, the ratio of supratentorial to infratentorial tumours is 1.3:1 {823, 2231}. Supratentorial tumours are often located in the cerebral hemispheres, and less frequently in the ventricular system, suprasellar region or pineal gland. Infratentorial tumours can be located in the cerebellar hemispheres, cerebellopontine angle and brain stem, and are relatively frequent in the first two years of life. Infrequently, AT/RTs arise in the spinal cord. Seeding of AT/RTs via the cerebrospinal fluid pathways is common and may be found in more than 20% of the patients at presentation {823}. Infratentorial localization is relatively rare in adult patients diagnosed with AT/RT {529}.

Clinical features and neuroimaging
Symptoms and signs
Clinical presentation is variable, depending upon the age of the patient, location, and size of the tumour. Infants, in particular, present with non-specific signs of lethargy, vomiting or failure to thrive. More specific problems include head tilt and cranial nerve palsy, most commonly sixth and seventh nerve paresis. Headache and hemiplegia are more commonly reported in children older than three years.

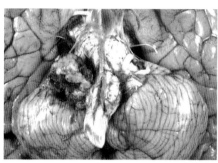

Fig. 8.23 Atypical teratoid/rhabdoid tumour with multiple haemorrhages, arising in the right cerebellopontine angle.

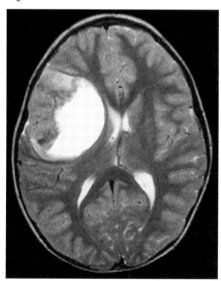

Fig. 8.24 Enhanced, T1-weighted MRI of a large, cystic supratentorial atypical teratoid/rhabdoid tumour.

Neuroimaging
Findings on both CT and MRI are similar to those seen in patients with PNET/medulloblastoma. AT/RTs are iso- to slightly hyperintense by fluid-attenuated inversion-recovery (FLAIR) and show restricted diffusion. Cystic and/or necrotic regions are apparent as zones of heterogeneous signal intensity. Almost all tumours are variably contrast-enhancing, and leptomeningeal dissemination can be seen in up to a quarter of cases at presentation {1466}.

Macroscopy

These tumours (and their deposits along the cerebrospinal fluid pathways) generally have a similar gross appearance to medulloblastoma and other CNS PNET. The tumours tend to be soft, pinkish-red and bulky, and often appear to be demarcated from adjacent parenchyma. They typically contain necrotic foci and may be haemorrhagic. Those with significant amounts of mesenchymal tissue are firm and tan-white in some regions. Tumours arising in the cerebellopontine angle wrap themselves around cranial nerves and vessels and invade the brain stem and cerebellum to a variable extent.

Histopathology

AT/RTs can be heterogeneous lesions that are sometimes difficult to recognize solely using histopathologic criteria {263,1924}. The most striking feature in many cases are cells with classic rhabdoid features: eccentrically placed nuclei containing vesicular chromatin, prominent eosinophilic nucleoli, abundant cytoplasm with an obvious eosinophilic globular cytoplasmic inclusion and well-defined cell borders. In practice, the appearance of these cells typically falls along a spectrum ranging from this classic rhabdoid phenotype to cells with less striking nuclear atypia and large amounts of pale eosinophilic cytoplasm. The cytoplasm of these cells has a fine granular homogeneous character or may contain a poorly defined dense pink 'body' resembling an inclusion. Ultrastructurally, rhabdoid cells typically contain whorled bundles of intermediate filaments filling much of the perikaryon {162, 745}. A frequently encountered artifact in these cells is extensive cytoplasmic vacuolation. Rhabdoid cells may be arranged in nests or sheets and often have a jumbled appearance.

However, it is only the minority of cases in which these cells are the exclusive or predominant histopathologic finding. Most tumours contain variable components with primitive neuroectodermal, mesenchymal and epithelial features. In practice, a small cell embryonal component is the most commonly encountered, in about two thirds of tumours. Mesenchymal differentiation is less common and typically appears as areas with spindle cell features and a basophilic or mucopolysaccharide rich background. Epithelial differentiation is the least common histopathologic feature. When present, however, it can take the form of papillary structures, adenomatous areas or poorly differentiated ribbons and cords. In cases where this is the predominant histopathologic pattern, distinction from choroid plexus carcinoma can be challenging. Mitotic figures are usually abundant. Broad areas of geographic necrosis and haemorrhage are commonly encountered in these tumours.

Immunohistochemistry

AT/RTs demonstrate a broad spectrum of immunohistochemical reactivity that is consistent with their histologic diversity. However, the rhabdoid cells characteristically demonstrate consistent expression of EMA and vimentin, with only slightly less frequent expression of SMA. Expression of GFAP, NFP, synaptophysin and keratins are also commonly observed. By contrast, germ cell markers are not typically expressed. Regions of the tumour showing other histologic patterns may also show expression of these markers, though the pattern and frequency varies. Immunohistochemical staining for expression of the INI1 protein has been shown to be a sensitive and specific marker for AT/RTs. In normal tissue and most neoplasms, INI1 is a constitutively expressed nuclear protein; in AT/RTs, there is loss of nuclear expression of INI1 in tumour cells. Paediatric primitive neuroectodermal CNS tumours without rhabdoid features but with loss of INI1 expression in the biopsy material may very well represent

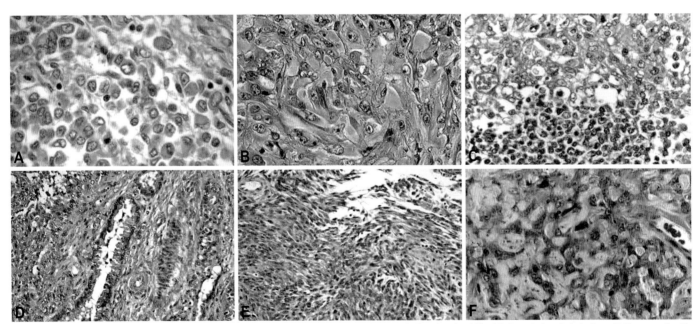

Fig. 8.25 Atypical teratoid/rhabdoid tumours. **A** Rhabdoid cells with vesicular chromatin, prominent nucleoli and eosinophilic globular cytoplasmic inclusions. **B** Tumour cells with abundant pale eosinophilic cytoplasm. **C** Tumour with prominent primitive neuroectodermal component and rhabdoid cells with vacuolar artifact. **D** Tumour with epithelial differentiation exhibiting a glandular component. **E** Tumour with mesenchymal differentiation exhibiting a spindle cell component. **F** Tumour with mesenchymal differentiation exhibiting a mucopolysaccharide-rich background.

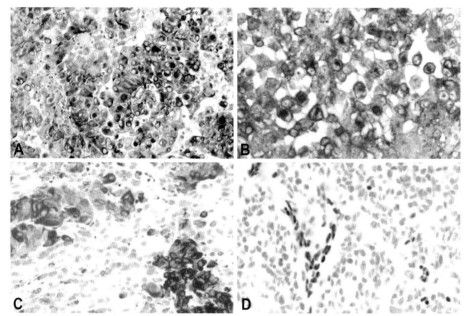

Fig. 8.26 Immunohistochemical features of atypical teratoid/rhabdoid tumours. **A** Strong expression of vimentin. **B** Membranous and cytoplasmic expression of EMA. **C** Expression of GFAP (brown) and NFP (red). **D** Loss of expression of INI1 in nuclei of tumour cells with retained expression in intratumour blood vessels.

AT/RTs {747}. While some authors have reported inactivation of *INI1* in choroid plexus carcinoma, others believe that such lesions have histopathological features justifying a diagnosis of AT/RT and that classic choroid plexus carcinomas do not lose INI1 expression {660,1016}.

Proliferation
AT/RTs in children have marked proliferative activity with Ki-67/MIB-1 labelling indices that are often more than 50%, focally up to 100% {841}. Limited data are available on adult patients, but in some cases the labelling index may be significantly lower {1361}.

Histogenesis
The histogenesis of rhabdoid tumours is unknown. Neural, epithelial, and mesen-

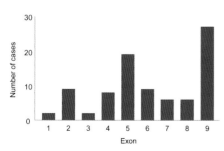

Fig. 8.27 Distribution of mutations in exons 1-9 of the *INI1* gene. Results are representative of 80 patients with brain and spinal cord AT/RTs.

chymal markers can all be expressed and, given their association with young children, it has been suggested that AT/RTs derive from pluripotent fetal cells {204, 1654}. Meningeal, neural crest or germ cell origins have also been proposed {343, 1677, 1924}. In one case, an AT/RT was reported to arise from a ganglioglioma, raising the possibility of progression from other tumour types {44}.

Genetics
AT/RT can occur sporadically or as part of a rhabdoid tumour predisposition syndrome (see Chapter 13) {153}. Mutation or loss of the *INI1(hSNF5/ SMARCB1)* locus at 22q11.2 is the genetic hallmark of AT/RT {156,2322}. The INI1 protein is a component of the mammalian SWI/SNF complex, which functions in an ATP-dependent manner to alter chromatin structure {1897}. The specific function of INI1 and its role in malignant transformation are not entirely clear, but it appears to act at least in part via p16-Rb-E2F and p53-dependent pathways {914, 919}. Loss of INI1 expression at the protein level is seen in almost all AT/RTs, and most (75%) of the tumours have detectable deletions or mutations of *INI1*. Among cases with deletions or mutations, homozygous deletions of the *INI1* locus are detected in 20–24% of tumours {153, 2231}. In

other cases, one *INI1* allele is mutated, and the second allele is lost by deletion or mitotic recombination. Rare tumours demonstrate two coding sequence mutations. Nonsense and frameshift mutations that are predicted to lead to truncations of the protein are identified in the majority of these cases {153}. Localization of mutations within the *INI1* gene appears to vary somewhat between rhabdoid tumours arising at various sites in the body, and exons 5 and 9 are hotspots in CNS AT/RT. No differences in outcome have been identified in patients with mutations in specific *INI1* exons. In familial cases of rhabdoid tumour, both unaffected adult carriers and gonadal mosaicism have been identified {971, 2057}. Because expression of INI1 is sometimes decreased in AT/RT in the absence of genetic alterations, its promoter was analysed in 24 cases, but no evidence of hypermethylation was detected {2492}.

Prognostic and predictive factors
The overall prognosis of AT/RTs is poor. In one study of 55 patients with AT/RT, the mean survival after surgery was only 11 months {263}. A more recent analysis of 42 patients enrolled in a tumour registry found a median survival of 17 months, while an institutional study of 11 cases reported a mean time to death of 24 months {328, 823}. Age older than 3 years appears to be associated with longer survival, perhaps due to the use of more intensive therapies {2231}.

CHAPTER 9

Tumours of the Cranial and Paraspinal Nerves

Schwannoma (WHO grade I)
A benign nerve sheath tumour that is typically encapsulated and composed entirely of well-differentiated Schwann cells. Multiple schwannomas are associated with neurofibromatosis type 2 or schwannomatosis.

Neurofibroma (WHO grade I)
A well-demarcated intraneural or diffusely infiltrative extraneural tumour consisting of a mixture of cell types, including Schwann cells, perineurial-like cells and fibroblasts; multiple and plexiform neurofibromas are typically associated with neurofibromatosis type 1.

Perineurioma (WHO grades I, II or III)
A tumour composed entirely of neoplastic perineurial cells. Intraneural perineuriomas are benign and consist of proliferating perineurial cells within endoneurium, forming characteristic pseudo-onion bulbs. Soft tissue perineuriomas are typically not associated with nerve and are usually benign.

Malignant peripheral nerve sheath tumour (MPNST) (WHO grades II, III or IV)
A malignant tumour arising from a peripheral nerve, or in extra-neural soft tissue if it shows nerve sheath differentiation, excluding tumours originating from epineurial tissue or from peripheral nerve vasculature; somewhat over 50% of malignant peripheral nerve sheath tumours are associated with neurofibromatosis type 1.

Schwannoma

B.W. Scheithauer
D.N. Louis
S. Hunter
J.M. Woodruff
C.R. Antonescu

Definition

A benign nerve sheath tumour that is typically encapsulated and composed entirely of well-differentiated Schwann cells. Multiple schwannomas are associated with neurofibromatosis type 2 or schwannomatosis.

ICD-O code   9560/0

Grading

Conventional, non-melanotic schwannoma corresponds histologically to WHO grade I.

Synonyms

Neurilemoma and neurinoma.

Incidence

Schwannomas represent 8% of intracranial tumours, 85% of cerebellopontine angle tumours and 29% of spinal nerve root tumours {1959}. Approximately 90% of cases are solitary and sporadic, while 4% arise in the setting of neurofibromatosis type 2 (NF2), and 5% are multiple but unassociated with NF2 {56}. Some of the latter are associated with schwannomatosis {1369}.

Age and sex distribution

All ages are affected but paediatric cases are rare. The peak incidence is in the fourth to sixth decade of life. Most studies show no gender predilection, but some series have shown a female

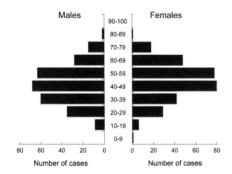

Fig. 9.01 Age and sex distribution of schwannoma based on 582 patients, treated at the University Hospital, Zürich.

predominance among intracranial tumours {415, 1417, 1959}. Cerebral or spinal intra-parenchymal schwannomas are associated with a younger age and a male predominance {293}. Schwannomas of spinal cord parenchyma are too rare to assess their epidemiology {817}.

Localization

The vast majority of schwannomas occur outside the central nervous system. Most often affected is skin and subcutaneous tissue {1682A}. Intracranial schwannomas show a strong predilection for the eighth cranial nerve in the cerebellopontine angle. This is particularly the case in NF2. They arise at the transition zone between central and peripheral myelination and affect the vestibular division. The adjacent cochlear division is almost never their site of origin. This characteristic location, which is not shared by neurofibromas or MPNSTs, results in diagnostically helpful enlargement of the internal auditory meatus by neuroimaging. Intralabyrinthine schwannomas are uncommon {1576}. Intraspinal schwannomas show a strong predilection for sensory nerve roots. Motor and autonomic nerves are far less often affected. Occasional CNS schwannomas are not associated with a recognizable nerve. These include approximately 70 reported cases of spinal intramedullary and 40 of cerebral parenchymal or intra-ventricular schwannomas {293, 416, 817, 1110, 1750, 2388}. Dural examples are rare {58}. Peripheral schwannomas, in contrast with neurofibromas, tend to be attached to nerve trunks, most often involving the head and neck region or flexor surfaces of the extremities. Visceral schwannomas are rare, as are osseous examples {1469, 1801, 2011, 2288}.

Clinical features

Symptoms and signs

Peripherally situated schwannomas may present as asymptomatic paraspinous tumours, as incidental findings on imaging studies, as spinal nerve tumours with radicular pain and signs of nerve root, spinal cord compression, or as eighth

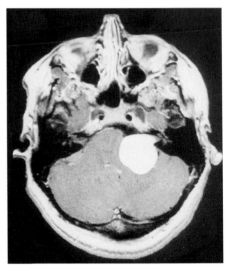

Fig. 9.02 Vestibular schwannoma. MRI showing location in the cerebellopontine angle. Note the tumour protrusion at the upper margin extending into the internal acoustic canal.

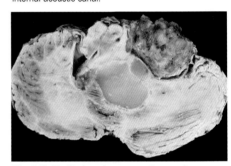

Fig. 9.03 Vestibular schwannoma. Large schwannoma causing compression of and cyst formation in the cerebellum, and displacement of the medulla.

cranial nerve tumours with related symptoms. Motor symptoms are uncommon since schwannomas favour sensory nerve roots. Bilateral vestibular tumours are the sine qua non of NF2. Pain is the most common presentation for schwannomas in patients with schwannomatosis.

Neuroimaging

MRI reveals a well-circumscribed, sometimes cystic and often hetero-geneously enhancing mass. Those in paraspinal and head and neck sites may be associated with bone erosion that is sometimes evident on plain x-rays {293}.

Macroscopy

The majority of schwannomas are globoid masses measuring from a few centimeters to 10 cm in size. With the exception of rare examples arising at intraparenchymal CNS sites, viscera, skin and bone, they usually are encapsulated. In peripheral tumours, a nerve of origin is identified in less than half of cases. The cut surface of the tumour typically reveals light tan glistening tissue interrupted by bright yellow patches with or without cysts and haemorrhage. Infarct-like necrosis related to degenerative vascular changes may be evident in sizable tumours.

Histopathology

Conventional schannoma is a tumour composed entirely of neoplastic Schwann cells and forming two basic patterns in varying proportion: areas of compact, elongated cells with occasional nuclear palisading (Antoni A pattern) and less cellular, loosely textured cells with indistinct processes and variable lipidization (Antoni B). A retiform pattern is very uncommonly seen. The Schwann cells comprising the tumour have moderate quantities of eosinophilic cytoplasm without discernible cell borders. Antoni A tissue features normochromic spindle-shaped or round nuclei approximately the size of those of smooth muscle cells, but tapered instead of blunt-ended. In Antoni B tissue, tumour cells have smaller, often round to ovoid nuclei. Nuclear pleomorphism, including bizarre forms with cytoplasmic-nuclear inclusions ("ancient schwannoma") and the occasional mitotic figure may be seen, but should not be misinterpreted as indicating malignancy. The Antoni A growth pattern consists of closely apposed tumour cells, forming nuclear palisades (Verocay bodies) consisting of alternating, parallel rows of tumour cell nuclei and their

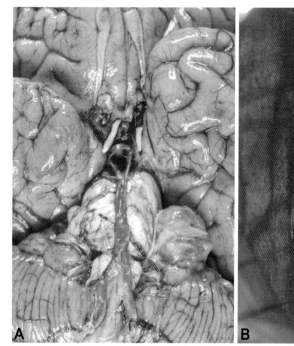

Fig. 9.04 **A** Macroscopic appearance of a vestibular schwannoma in the left cerebellopontine angle and **B** a spinal schwannoma (intraoperative view).

densely packed, aligned cell processes. All schwannoma cells show a pericellular reticulin pattern corresponding to surface basement membranes. In Antoni B areas, tumour cells are loosely arranged. Collections of lipid-laden cells may be present within either Antoni A or B tissue. Schwannoma vasculature is typically thick-walled and hyalinized. In addition, dilated blood vessels surrounded by haemorrhage are common. Eighth cranial nerve schwannomas are known for their infrequent presence of Verocay bodies, predominance of Antoni B tissue, and often clusters of lipid-laden cells. Schwannomas with meningothelial islands are a curiosity and are virtually limited to NF2 {1355}. Malignant transformation, less often microscopic {1436} than exten-

sive and transcapsular, {1436, 2447} rarely occurs in conventional schwannomas. Rhabdomyoblastic differentiation has been reported {1239}.

Cellular schwannoma

This variant is defined as a hypercellular schwannoma composed exclusively or predominantly of Antoni A tissue and devoid of well-formed Verocay bodies {2444}. The most common location of cellular schwannoma is at paravertebral sites in the pelvis, retroperitoneum and mediastinum {2444}. Cranial nerves, especially the fifth and eighth, may be affected {294}. Clinical presentation of cellular schwannoma is similar to that of conventional schwannoma, but the histological features of hypercellularity,

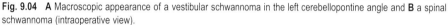

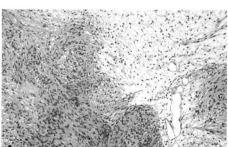
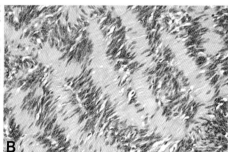
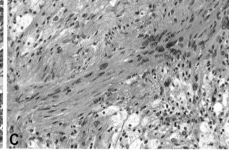

Fig. 9.05 Histological features of schwannoma. **A** Biphasic pattern with cellular Antoni A and hypocellular Antoni B areas. **B** Schwannoma cell nuclei forming palisades. **C** Schwannoma, showing compact fasciles of elongated tumour cells with slight nuclear polymorphism. Note scattered lipid-laden macrophages.

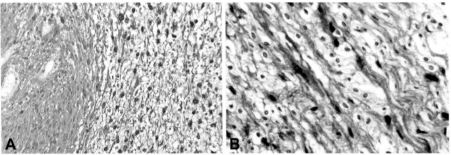

Fig. 9.06 Schwannoma with diffuse S-100 immunoreactivity (**A**). **B** S-100 immunostaining of elongated tumour cells in a predominantly immunonegative Antoni B area.

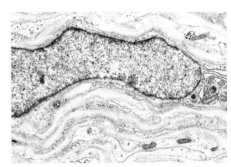

Fig. 9.07 Ultrastructural features of a schwannoma showing a continuous lining of tumour cells by basal lamina.

fascicular growth of cells, occasional nuclear hyperchromasia and atypia, as well as low-level mitotic activity (usually <4/10 HPF) may lead to a mistaken diagnosis of malignancy (MPNST). Again, the reticulin pattern is pericellular. In one series {294}, reported labelling indices for the proliferation markers PCNA and MIB-1 were 5.6% and 6%, respectively, in non-recurring tumours {294}. On flow cytometry, two thirds were diploid, and the rest either tetraploid or aneuploid {294}. p53 immunostaining has been reported in roughly half of cellular schwannomas, but immunolabeled cells are relatively few {294}. Cellular schwannomas are benign. Although recurrences are seen, notably in intracranial, spinal and sacral examples {294}, no cellular schwannoma is known to have metastasized or reportedly followed a clinically malignant, fatal course. Only two examples of cellular schwannoma, one associated with NF2, have been reported to undergo malignant transformation {60}.

Plexiform schwannoma
This variant is defined as schwannoma growing in a plexiform or multinodular manner and can be of either conventional or cellular type {2445}. Presumably involving a nerve plexus, the vast majority

arise in skin or subcutaneous tissue of an extremity, head and neck, or trunk. The tumour has a low association with NF2, but not NF1, and has also been noted in non-NF2 patients with multiple schwannomas (schwannomatosis) {937}. Cranial and spinal nerves are usually spared.

Melanotic schwannoma
This rare, circumscribed but unencapsulated, grossly pigmented tumour is composed of cells having the ultrastructure and immunophenotype of Schwann cells but containing melanosomes and being reactive for melanoma markers. Cytologic atypia is not uncommon, including hyperchromasia and macronucleoli. The reticulin pattern is often poor in this subtype. Its peak incidence is a decade earlier than that of conventional schwannoma. Melanotic schwannomas occur in non-psammomatous {591} and psammomatous {289, 508} varieties. The vast majority of non-psammomatous tumours affect spinal nerves and paraspinal ganglia, whereas the psammomatous lesions also involve autonomic nerves of viscera, such as the intestinal tract and heart. Cranial nerves may also be affected. Distinguishing between these two varieties of melanotic schwannoma is of importance, since about 50% of

patients with psammomatous tumours have Carney complex, an autosomal-dominant disorder {288} characterized by lentiginous facial pigmentation, cardiac myxoma and endocrine over-activity. The latter includes Cushing syndrome associated with multinodular adrenal hyperplasia and acromegaly due to pituitary adenoma {289}. Slightly over 10% of melanotic schwannomas follow a malignant course {2011}.

Immunohistochemistry
Tumour cells strongly and diffusely express S-100 protein {2390}, often express Leu-7 and calretinin {582}, and may focally express GFAP {1448}. All schwannoma cells possess surface basal lamina, so membrane staining for collagen IV and laminin is a regular feature of the tumour. The pattern is rich and most commonly pericellular in all but melanotic schwannomas, where envelopment of cell nests is more frequently seen. Low-level p53 protein immunoreactivity may be seen, particularly in cellular schwannomas {294}. Neurofilament protein-positive axons are generally lacking but small numbers may be encountered within the substance of schwannomas, particularly in NF2 or schwannomatosis-associated tumours {2383}.

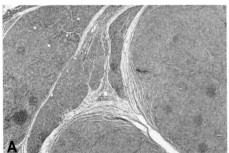
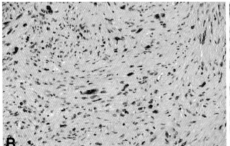
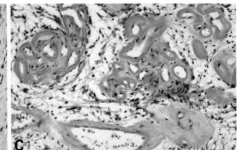

Fig. 9.08 **A** Plexiform schwannoma involving multiple small nerves. **B** Nuclear polymorphism seen in many cellular schwannomas from any site, not to be interpreted as a sign of malignancy. **C** Hyanilized vessels in a Antoni B area of a conventional schwannoma.

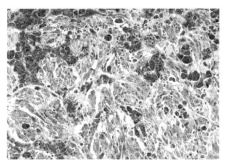

Fig. 9.09 Melanotic schwannoma with clusters of plump, spindled, heavily pigmented tumour cells.

Electron microscopy

Ultrastructural features are diagnostic and consist of cells with convoluted, moderately thin cytoplasmic processes that are nearly devoid of pinocytotic vesicles but are lined by a continuous basal lamina {531}. Stromal long-spacing collagen (Luse body) is a common finding in conventional schwannoma but less so in the cellular variant. Melanotic schwannomas feature true melanosomes and less uniform envelopment of individual cells by basal lamina.

Genetic susceptibility

Although most schwannomas are sporadic in occurrence, multiple schwannomas may occur in the setting of two tumour syndromes. Bilateral vestibular (eighth cranial nerve) schwannomas are pathognomonic of NF2 (see Chapter 13), while multiple peripheral schwannomas in the absence of other NF2 features is characteristic of schwannomatosis (see Chapter 13). Schwannomatosis patients present with multiple, often painful schwannomas, which in some cases are segmental in distribution {613, 644, 1176}. NF2 inactivation has been shown in tumours, but not in non-tumour tissue, suggesting that another gene may be the underlying cause of schwannomatosis {644, 948, 1368}. In addition, psammomatous melanotic schwannoma is a component of Carney complex, in which patients have mutations of the *PRKAR1A* gene on chromosome 17q, encoding the type 1A regulatory subunit of protein kinase A {2161}.

Genetics

Extensive analyses have implicated the *NF2* gene as a tumour suppressor integral to the formation of sporadic schwannomas {950, 2045}. The *NF2* gene and the merlin (schwannomin) protein which it encodes are discussed in detail in the chapter on NF2. Inactivating mutations of the *NF2* gene have been detected in approximately 60% of schwannomas {168, 949, 950, 1941, 2266}. These genetic events are predominantly small frameshift mutations that result in truncated protein products {1352}. Although not been described for exons 16 and 17, mutations occur throughout the coding sequence of the gene and at intronic sites. In most cases, such mutations are accompanied by loss of the remaining wild-type allele on chromosome 22q. Still other cases demonstrate loss of chromosome 22q in the absence of detectable *NF2* gene mutations. Nonetheless, loss of merlin expression, demonstrated by Western blotting or immunohistochemistry, appears to be a universal finding in schwannomas, regardless of their mutation or allelic status {838, 901, 1971}. This suggests that abrogation of merlin function is an essential step in schwannoma tumourigenesis. Loss of chromosome 22 has also been noted in cellular schwannoma {1341}. Other genetic changes are rare in schwannomas, although small numbers of cases with chromosome 1p loss, gain of 9q34 and gain of 17q have been reported {1293, 2367}. Allelic loss of the *PRKAR1A* region on 17q has been noted in tumours from patients with Carney complex, but has not been documented in non-psammomatous melanotic schwannomas {2161}.

Prognostic and predictive factors

Schwannomas are benign, slowly growing tumours that infrequently recur and only very rarely undergo malignant change {2447}. Recurrences are more common (30–40%) for cellular schwannomas of the intracranial, spinal and sacral regions {294}.

Neurofibroma

B.W. Scheithauer
D.N. Louis
S. Hunter
J.M. Woodruff
C.R. Antonescu

Definition

A well-demarcated intraneural or diffusely infiltrative extraneural tumour consisting of a mixture of cell types, including Schwann cells, perineurial-like cells, and fibroblasts; multiple and plexiform neurofibromas are typically associated with neurofibromatosis type 1.

ICD-O codes

Neurofibroma   9540/0
Plexiform neurofibroma 9550/0

Grading

Neurofibroma corresponds histologically to WHO grade I.

Incidence

Neurofibromas are common and occur either as sporadic solitary nodules unrelated to any apparent syndrome or, far less frequently, as solitary, multiple or numerous lesions in individuals with neurofibromatosis type 1 (NF1).

Age and sex distribution

All ages and both sexes are affected.

Localization

Neurofibroma presents most commonly as a cutaneous nodule (localized cutaneous neurofibroma) and less often as a circumscribed mass in a peripheral nerve (localized intraneural neurofibroma) or as a plexiform enlargement of a plexus or major nerve trunk. Less frequent is diffuse but localized involvement of skin

and subcutaneous tissue (diffuse cutaneous neurofibroma), or extensive to massive involvement of soft tissue (localized gigantism and "elephantiasis neuromatosa"). Neurofibromas occasionally involve spinal roots {2049} but are almost unknown on cranial nerves.

Clinical features

Rarely painful, the tumours present as a mass. The presence of multiple neurofibromas is the hallmark of NF1, in which they are associated with pigmented cutaneous macules (café-au-lait spots) as well as 'freckling', often axillary in location (see Chapter 13).

Macroscopy

Cutaneous neurofibromas are either nodular to polypoid and rather circumscribed, or are diffuse and involve skin and subcutaneous tissue. On cut surface, both are firm, glistening and grey-tan. Neurofibromas confined to nerves are fusiform and, in all but their proximal and distal margins, well-circumscribed. Plexiform neurofibromas consist of either multinodular tangles ("bag of worms") when tumour involves multiple trunks of a plexus or rope-like lesions when multiple fascicles of a large, non-branching nerve such as the sciatic are affected {2011, 2441}.

Histopathology

Neurofibromas are composed in large part of Schwann cells with ovoid to thin, curved to elongate nuclei and scant cytoplasm as well as fibroblasts in a matrix of collagen fibers and Alcian blue-positive, myxoid material. The Schwann cells are considerably smaller than those of schwannomas. Cell processes are thin and often not visible on routine light microscopy. Neurofibromas may also exhibit numerous atypical nuclei (atypical neurofibroma) or significantly increased cellularity (cellular neurofibroma). Even in the latter, mitotic figures are rare. Stromal collagen formation varies greatly in abundance and sometimes takes the form of dense, refractile bundles resembling

"shredded carrots." Growth of neurofibroma cells is initially along the course of nerve fibers, which become enmeshed by tumour. When arising from a medium-size or large nerve, neurofibromas often remain confined to the nerve, being encompassed by its thickened epineurium. In contrast, tumours arising in small nerves often spread diffusely into the surrounding dermis and soft tissues. Large diffuse neurofibromas often contain highly characteristic tactile-like structures, specifically pseudo-Meissnerian corpuscles, and may also contain melanotic cells. The multiple fascicles constituting plexiform neurofibromas, although expanded by tumour cells and collagen, commonly demonstrate residual, bundled nerve fibers at their centres. A very small proportion of neurofibromas are thought to exhibit limited perineurial differentiation {2482}. Unlike schwannomas, blood vessels in neurofibromas generally lack hyalinization.

Immunohistochemistry

Staining for S-100 protein is invariably seen, but the proportion of reactive cells is less than in schwannomas. Expression for basement membrane markers is less consistent and more variable than in schwannoma. In contrast to perineurioma, neurofibromas contain only limited numbers of EMA-positive cells {2011, 2482}. In most neurofibromas, EMA reactivity is simply limited to residual perineurium {2011}. Scattered neoplastic cells, presumably the perineurial-like cells seen ultrastructurally (see below) also show glut-1 {834} or claudin positivity {1807}. Axons in varying number, as shown by positivity for neurofilament proteins, are present in neurofibromas, particularly plexiform tumours, within which they are often centrally grouped.

Electron microscopy

Electron microscopy shows a mixture of cell types, the two most diagnostically important being the Schwann cell, either associated or unassociated with axons, and the perineurial-like cell {532, 2011,

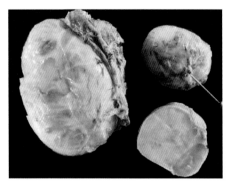

Fig. 9.10 Neurofibroma of a spinal root, with a firm consistency and homogeneous cut surface.

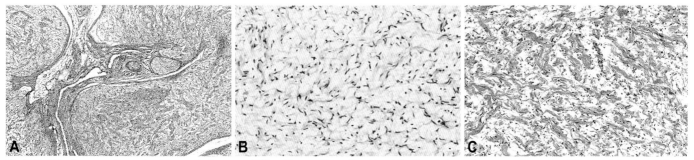

Fig. 9.11 A Plexiform neurofibroma involving small skin nerves. **B** Neurofibroma with small ovoid nuclei lacking obvious cell processes. The eosinophillic curved strans are collagen fibers produced by tumour cells. **C** Extensive collagen formation may cause a 'shredded carrots' appearance.

2441}. The latter features long, very thin cell processes, numerous pinocytotic vesicles, and interrupted basement membrane. Fibroblasts are the least frequent.

Genetic susceptibility

The occurrence of multiple and plexiform neurofibromas is a hallmark of NF1 (see Chapter 13). Neurofibromas are rare in NF2 and schwannomatosis.

Genetics

Given their mixed cellular composition, it has been difficult to determine whether neurofibromas are monoclonal. NF1-associated neurofibromas contain monoclonal neoplastic cells {2110}. As sporadic neurofibromas are histologically identical to those occurring in NF1, it seems likely that they too are monoclonal. Notably, allelic loss of the *NF1* gene region of 17q appears confined to the S-100 protein-immunoreactive Schwann or perhaps

perineurial-like cells in neurofibromas {1730}, suggesting that they are the clonal neoplastic element.

In view of the association of neurofibromas with NF1, investigations of the genetic basis of sporadic tumours have focused on the *NF1* gene. In NF1 patients harbouring germline *NF1* mutations, loss of the remaining wild-type *NF1* allele within their neurofibromas {2052, 2109} confirms the two-hit hypothesis for the genesis of these lesions {370, 1998}. Point mutations affecting *NF1* gene splicing are common {2051}. The situation in sporadic tumours has yet to be elucidated, but the morphologic similarity between sporadic and inherited neurofibromas, as well as the clear involvement of the *NF1* gene in sporadic MPNSTs, suggests that *NF1* alterations are also involved in the genesis of sporadic neurofibromas. This has been documented in rare cases {2158}. Moreover, mitotic recombination events may underlie

biallelic inactivation of *NF1* in neurofibromas {2053}, which would complicate assessment of chromosomal loss in such cases.

Additional chromosomal losses are not common in neurofibromas, but have been noted on 19p, 19q and 22q in NF1-associated neurofibromas and on 19q and 22q in sporadic neurofibromas {1149}.

Prognostic and predictive factors

Plexiform neurofibromas and neurofibromas of major nerves are considered a precursor lesion to the majority of malignant peripheral nerve sheath tumours. Malignant transformation occurs in 5% of sizable plexiform tumours, but is a rare event in diffuse cutaneous and massive soft tissue neurofibromas. Patients with a sizable plexiform neurofibroma are highly likely to have NF1 and must be investigated for other evidence of the disorder.

Perineurioma

B.W. Scheithauer
J.M. Woodruff
C.R. Antonescu

Definition

A tumour composed entirely of neoplastic perineurial cells. Intraneural perineuriomas are benign and consist of proliferating perineurial cells within endoneurium, forming characteristic pseudo-onion bulbs. Soft tissue perineuriomas are typically not associated with nerve and are usually benign.

ICD-O codes

Intraneural and benign soft tissue
    perineurioma   9571/0
Malignant soft tissue perineurioma
                     9571/3

Grading

Intraneural perineuriomas correspond histologically to WHO grade I. In keeping with the FNCLCC approach to grading of soft tissue tumours, soft tissue perineuriomas range from benign (WHO grade I) to variably malignant and corresponding to WHO grades II-III.

Synonyms and historical annotation

Intraneural perineurioma, long mistakenly considered a form of hypertrophic neuropathy, is now recognized as a neoplasm {519}. Soft tissue perineurioma is a morphologically distinct tumour.

Incidence

Both the intraneural and soft tissue variants of perineurioma are rare and represent approximately 1% of nerve sheath and soft tissue neoplasms, respectively. Over 50 cases of intraneural perineurioma have been reported to date, including cranial nerve examples. Well over 100 cases of soft tissue perineurioma have been described {571, 677, 717, 866, 1828}, including a cranial nerve example {107}.

Clinical features

Intraneural perineuriomas typically present in adolescence or early adulthood and show no sex predilection. Progressive muscle weakness with or without obvious atrophy is more frequent than are sensory disturbances. Peripheral nerves of the extremities are primarily affected; cranial nerve lesions are rare {47, 398, 1308}. One example was reportedly associated with Beckwith-Wiedemann syndrome {327}.

Soft tissue perineuriomas occur in adults, predominantly females (2:1), and present with non-specific mass effects. They are deep soft tissue and are, with the rare exception of a cranial nerve example {107}, grossly unassociated with nerve. Visceral involvement is rare {866A, 2298A}. One example involving the central nervous system arose within a lateral ventricle {679}. Malignant examples prone to recurrence and occasional metastasis have been reported {623, 833, 1043, 1927, 2184}, and are apparently unassociated with NF1 {833}.

Macroscopy

Intraneural perineuriomas produce segmental, tubular, several-fold enlargement of the affected nerve. Individual nerve fascicles appear coarse and pale. Most lesions are less than 10 cm in length but one 40 cm long sciatic nerve example has been reported {519}. Although multiple fascicles are often involved, a "bag of worms" plexiform growth is not seen. Involvement of two neighbouring spinal nerves has been reported {519}.

Soft tissue perineuriomas are solitary, generally small (1.5–7 cm) and well-circumscribed but not encapsulated. Rarely, the tumour may be multinodular {60}. Larger examples are exceptional {829, 866}. On cut surface they are firm and grey-white to infrequently focally myxoid. Malignant soft tissue perineuriomas are usually not associated with a nerve and may feature invasive growth as well as variable necrosis.

Histopathology

Intraneural perineurioma consists of neoplastic perineurial cells proliferating throughout the endoneurium, forming concentric layers around nerve fibers, enlargement of fascicles and characteristic pseudo-onion bulbs. This distinctive architectural feature is best seen on cross

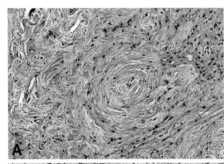

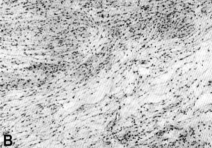

Fig. 9.12 **A** The sclerotic variant of perineurioma features abundant collagen deposition and crude whorls. The latter occasionally center upon nerve fibers. **B** Reticular variant of perineurioma. Tumour cells surround collagen aggregates resulting in a loose-textured tissue pattern.

section, wherein fascicles vary in cellularity. Proliferation of perineurial cells largely takes place within endoneurium but perineurium is often affected as well. Numerous perineurial cells, most of which appear cytologically normal, are concentrically disposed in multiple layers around nerve fibers. Particularly large whorls may envelop numerous nerve fibers. Occasionally, perineurial cells enclosing one or several axons will contribute to an adjacent onion bulb as well. Thus, pseudo-onion bulbs anastomose one with the other, forming a complex endoneurial network. Bielschowsky or Bodian stains often show one or multiple axons at the centre of pseudo-onion bulbs. Luxol-fast blue preparations typically show myelin to be scant or absent. Even within a single fascicle, cell density and the complexity of the lesion may vary. Mitotic activity is rare. In early lesions, axonal density and myelination may be almost normal, whereas in fully developed lesions, when most fibers are surrounded by perineurial cells and therefore widely separated, myelin is often scant or absent on Luxol-fast blue stain. At late stages, only Schwann cells without accompanying axons may remain at the centre of the perineurial whorls. Hyalinization may also be an impressive finding.

Soft tissue perineuriomas are composed of spindled, wavy cells with remarkably thin cytoplasmic processes arranged in lamellae and embedded in collagen fibers. Crude whorls or storiform arrangements are commonly seen. Aggregates of collagen fibers are often encircled by long, remarkably narrow tumour cell processes. Nuclei are elongate with tapered ends and are often curved or wrinkled. Nucleoli are inconspicuous. Granular cells are a very uncommon feature of perineurioma {467}. Mitoses vary in number; in the largest published series {866}, they varied from 0-13/30 high-power (40x) fields (mean, 1), 65% of tumours having none. Degenerative atypia (nuclear pleomorphism, hyperchromasia, cytoplasmic-nuclear inclusions) is seen primarily in long-standing tumours {866}. As a rule, necrosis is lacking. The sclerotic variant of soft tissue perineurioma is characterized by an abundant collagenous stroma has been described occurring mainly in the fingers of young males {571}. This tumour features only crude whorl formation occasionally centred upon a minute nerve. A reticular variant occurring at a variety of anatomic sites and affecting primarily adults, features a lace-like or reticular growth pattern composed of anastomosing cords of fusiform cells {717}. Malignant soft tissue perineuriomas (perineurial MPNSTs) are uncommon and characterized by hypercellularity, hyperchromasia, and variable, often brisk mitotic activity (WHO grade II), necrosis usually being a feature of WHO grade III tumours. Progressive malignant change of WHO grade II to grade III lesions may be seen, but transformation of benign soft tissue pcrineuriomas to malignant examples has yet to be documented.

Immunohistochemistry

All intraneural perineuriomas, like normal perineurial cells, are vimentin and epithelial membrane antigen (EMA)-immunoreactive. The pattern of EMA staining is membranous, as is that for collagen IV and laminin. Axons at the centre of pseudo-onion bulbs and residual Schwann cells stain for neurofilament protein and S-100 protein, respectively. Staining for p53 protein has also been reported {519}.

Soft tissue perineurioma features the same basic immunophenotype as the intraneural variant. Recently, claudin-I {590,1828} and glut-I {834} immunostaining have been applied to perineuriomas. Both have been shown to be diagnostically useful markers of normal and neoplastic perineurial cells. Unlike various other soft tissue tumours, perineuriomas generally lack reactivity for CD34 and particularly S-100 protein. Malignant soft tissue perineuriomas usually show at least some EMA staining and lack S-100 protein reactivity.

Proliferation

Intraneural perineuriomas, despite a paucity of mitoses, may show MIB-1 labelling indices ranging from 5 to 15% {519}. In contrast to the often low mitotic index of benign soft tissue perineuriomas, malignant soft tissue perineuriomas are more proliferative, indices ranging from 1-85/10 high-power fields (median, 16) in the largest reported series {833}.

Electron microscopy

Intraneural perineuriomas feature myelinated nerve fibers circumferentially surrounded by ultrastructurally normal-appearing perineurial cells. The cells have long, thin cytoplasmic processes bearing numerous pinocytotic vesicles and are lined by patchy surface basement membrane. Stromal collagen may be abundant.

Soft tissue perineuriomas typically consist of spindle-shaped cells with long, exceedingly thin cytoplasmic processes embedded in an abundant collagenous stroma. Cytoplasm is scant and contains sparse profiles of rough endoplasmic reticulum, occasional mitochondria and a few randomly distributed intermediate filaments. The processes exhibit numerous pinocytotic vesicles and a patchy lining of basement membrane. Intercellular tight junctions are relatively frequent. One example featuring ribosome-lamella complexes has been reported {462}. Malignant soft tissue perineuriomas show similar ultrastructural features {833, 1927, 2184}, only some being poorly differentiated {833}.

Genetics

Both intraneural and soft tissue perineuriomas feature the same cytogenetic abnormality, monosomy of chromosome 22 {519, 677}. Loss of chromosome 13, an abnormality found in a number of soft tissue tumours, has also been described in soft tissue perineurioma {1530}. Loss of chromosome 10 and a small chromosome 22q deletion involving NF2 have also been reported {224,2044}. No genetic studies of malignant soft tissue perineuriomas have been reported.

Prognosis

Intraneural perineuriomas are benign. Long-term follow-up indicates that they show neither a tendency to recurrence nor metastasis. Biopsy alone is sufficient for diagnosis. Conventional soft tissue perineuriomas are usually amenable to gross total removal; recurrences are very infrequent, even in the face of histologic atypia; none have been reported to metastasize. Neither sclerotic nor reticular tumours are prone to recurrence {571, 717}. Malignant perineuriomas are far less prone to metastasize {623, 833, 1043} than are conventional malignant peripheral nerve sheath tumours {833}.

Malignant peripheral nerve sheath tumour (MPNST)

B.W. Scheithauer
D.N. Louis
S. Hunter
J.M. Woodruff
C.R. Antonescu

Definition

A malignant tumour arising from a peripheral nerve, or in extraneural soft tissue if it shows nerve sheath differentiation, excluding tumours originating from epineurial tissue or from peripheral nerve vasculature; somewhat over 50% of malignant peripheral nerve sheath tumours are associated with neurofibromatosis type 1.

ICD-O code   9540/3

Grading

Histologically, malignant peripheral nerve sheath tumour (MPNST) corresponds to WHO grades II, III or IV, an approach similar to that applied to sarcoma grading {587}.

Synonyms

Once considered equivalent, but misleading and to be avoided, are the terms neurogenic sarcoma, neurofibrosarcoma, and malignant schwannoma.

Incidence

MPNSTs are uncommon, accounting for nearly 5% of malignant tumours of soft tissue {1305}. Approximately one half to two thirds arise from neurofibromas {490, 874, 1178}, often of the plexiform type and in the setting of neurofibromatosis type 1 (NF1). Second in frequency are MPNSTs arising *de novo* from peripheral nerves {2011, 2441}. The remainder are unassociated with a nerve or NF2 and simply resemble invasive soft tissue sarcomas. Only very rare examples develop from conventional schwannoma {2447}, ganglioneuroblastoma/ganglioneuroma {1869, 2011} or phaeochromocytoma {1972}.

Age and sex distribution

MPNSTs primarily affect adults in the third to the sixth decades of life. The mean age of patients with NF1-associated MPNSTs is approximately a decade younger (28–36 years) than that of sporadic cases (40–44 years) {490, 874}. Childhood and adolescent cases are uncommon {489}, children less than six years of age rarely being affected. MPNSTs do not show a strong gender predilection; however, NF1-associated cases are somewhat more common in males, while non-NF1-associated cases may be slightly more common in females, with a M:F ratio of 1.16:1.

Localization

Large and medium-size nerves are distinctly more prone to involvement than are small nerves. Most commonly involved sites include the buttock and thigh, brachial plexus and upper arm, and the paraspinal region. The sciatic nerve is most frequently affected. Cranial nerve MPNSTs are rare {145, 765, 1223, 1434, 1532, 2457}, the vestibular and vagal nerves being most often involved. Cranial nerve examples arise either *de novo* or from schwannoma or neurofibroma {603, 2447}. Primary intraparenchymal MPNST is rare {2072, 2147}.

Clinical features

Symptoms and signs

About half of MPNSTs occur in the clinical setting of NF1. An additional approximately 10% of MPNSTs develop at a site of prior irradiation {487, 589}. The most common presentation of tumours of the extremities is a progressively enlarging mass with or without neurological symptoms {874}. Spinal tumours often present with radicular pain {1178}.

Neuroimaging

Findings correspond to those of a soft tissue sarcoma. Inhomogeneous contrast enhancement and irregularity of contour, a reflection of invasion, are commonly seen. However, some MPNSTs are indistinguishable from benign nerve sheath tumours {2011}.

Macroscopy

The gross appearance of MPNST varies widely. Since a significant proportion arises in neurofibroma, some as focal transformations, the process may be minimally apparent on gross examination.

In contrast, larger, typically high-grade tumours originating in or unassociated with a nerve produce either fusiform, expansile masses or globular soft tissue tumours entirely lacking encapsulation. Both infiltrate surrounding structures. The vast majority of tumours are larger than 5 cm, and examples over 10 cm are common. What appears to be a pseudocapsule is in actuality infiltrated peritumoural soft tissue. Their consistency varies from firm to hard, and the cut surface is typically cream coloured or grey. Foci of necrosis and haemorrhage are common and may be extensive. Both cranial and spinal intradural MPNSTs may show parenchymal invasion {456}. Primary brain or spinal cord examples are rare {2147} as are primary MPNSTs of bone. Metastatic MPNST to the CNS is also very uncommon.

Histopathology

MPNSTs vary greatly in appearance. Many often exhibit a herringbone (fibrosarcoma-like) or interwoven-fasciculated pattern of cell growth. Both feature tightly packed spindle cells with variable quantities of eosinophilic cytoplasm. Nuclei are typically elongate, wavy, and in contrast to those of smooth muscle, have tapered ends. Tumours show either alternating loose and densely cellular areas or a diffuse growth pattern. MPNSTs grow within nerve fascicles but commonly

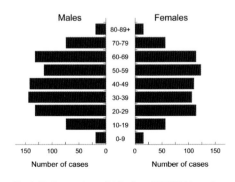

Fig. 9.13 Age and sex distribution of MPNST, based on 1711 histologically confirmed cases. Data from Surveillance Epidemiology and End Result (SEER), National Cancer Institute, Washington DC.

invade through perineurium and epineurium into the adjacent soft tissues. A pseudo-capsule of variable thickness consisting of tumour-invaded soft tissue and reactive fibrous tissue is often present. Three quarters of tumours have geographic necrosis and mitotic activity, often showing more than 4 mitotic figures per high-power field. A distinction is made between WHO grades III and IV based on the presence of necrosis. At the low end of the grading spectrum (WHO grade II), MPNSTs merge with cellular neurofibromas, from which they are distinguished on the basis of increased cellularity, nuclear size (>3x that of neurofibroma cells) and hyperchromasia. An increased mitotic rate is often seen but is not requisite for the diagnosis. Unusual growth patterns may be seen, including haemangiopericytoma-like areas or, rarely, nuclear palisading. Rare MPNST show histologic and ultra-structural features of perineurial differentiation {833}. Standardized routine histologic criteria for distinguishing MPNSTs from high-grade sarcomas are not available; consequently, diagnosis may ultimately rely on demonstration of tumour origin from either a neurofibroma or a peripheral nerve or upon immunohistochemical or ultrastructural features. About 15% of cases exhibit unusual histological

features such as epithelioid morphology or divergent differentiation {488, 2011}. MPNST arising in schwannoma is rare; examples feature either anaplastic small or large, epithelioid cells {1436, 2447}.

Epithelioid MPNST
Fewer than 5% of MPNSTs are either partially or purely epithelioid {469, 1263, 1340}. This variant shows no association with NF1 and can occur in a background of a benign schwannoma. Both superficial (above the fascia) and deep-seated examples are recognized. Superficial tumours carry a better prognosis.

MPNST with mesenchymal differentiation
A variety of mesenchymal tissues may be represented in MPNST. The term "malignant Triton tumour" refers to MPNSTs showing rhabdomyosarcomatous differentiation. Their incidence is nearly four times that of glandular MPNSTs. There are now at least 100 reported cases of this example of divergent mesenchymal differentiation {2446}. Sometimes accompanying the myoid element are areas of chondro- and/or osteosarcoma. Coexistent neoplastic epithelium (pluridirectional differentiation) is less common. Nearly 60% of the patients with malignant Triton tumour have NF1. Few cranial nerve examples have been reported {145,765}.

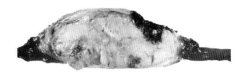

Fig. 9.14 Fusiform MPNST of the sciatic nerve with a partially trimmed pseudocapsule. The cut surface is firm, cream-tan and focally necrotic.

The prognosis of malignant Triton tumours is poor, with 2- and 5-year survival rates of approximately 33 and 12%, respectively {227}. Only one example of MPNST with smooth muscle differentiation has been reported {1903}. Schwannoma with associated angiosarcoma {1953, 2262} or rhabdomyosarcoma {1239} are both exceedingly rare.

Glandular MPNST
This variant is defined as an MPNST containing glandular epithelium that is often histologically benign. The epithelium resembles that of intestine. Neuro-endocrine differentiation is frequently seen, whereas squamous epithelium is far less often encountered. Three quarters of the patients have NF1, and mortality is high (79%) {2443}.

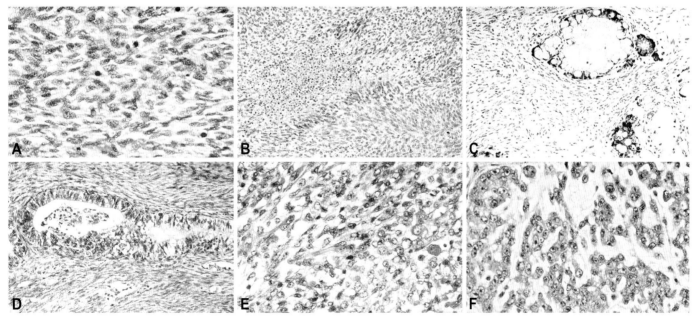

Fig. 9.15 Histological features of MPNST. **A** Brisk mitotic activity. **B** Well-delineated geographic necrosis. **C** Benign glandular MPNST containing neuroendocrine cells immunoreactive to chromogranin. **D** Formation of glands in an MPNST is interpreted as aberrant differentiation and considered as a sign of malignancy. **E** Malignant Triton tumour arising in a plexiform neurofibroma. Note strap-shaped and round rhabdomyoblasts on the background of anaplastic MPNST cells. **F** Epithelioid MPNST. Tumour cells are embedded in a mucinous matrix and show abundant cytoplasm and prominent nucleoli.

Immunohistochemistry

Only 50–70% of MPNSTs exhibit S-100 protein staining. Reactivity is grade-related. In high-grade tumours it is either patchy or found in individual cells, whereas in low-grade examples it may be extensive {2390}. Diffuse S-100 protein expression is more common in the epithelioid variant of MPNST {1263, 1340}. Immunostaining for p53 is present in a majority of tumours, in contrast to the infrequent staining in neurofibromas {758}. Conversely, immunostaining for other selected cell cycle regulatory proteins is common in neurofibromas but uncommon in MPNSTs; these include p27 {1179} and p16 {1591}. Glandular MPNSTs show keratin- and CEA-positive glands and neuroendocrine cells immunoreactive for chromogranin, somato-statin or serotonin.

Electron microscopy

Given the poor differentiation of most MPNSTs, electron microscopy is usually of little diagnostic aid short of excluding histologically similar sarcomas, such as leiomyosarcoma, synovial sarcoma and fibrosarcoma. Glandular MPNSTs show true gland formation with terminal bars and luminal microvilli. Individual cells or cell aggregates featuring dense core granules {346, 2443} may also be seen. Squamous differentiation is less common.

Proliferation

In the majority of MPNSTs, the growth fraction, as determined by Ki-67/MIB-1 immunoreactivity, ranges from 5 to 65%, in contrast to values often below 1% in conventional schwannomas and neurofi-bromas {1115}.

Genetic susceptibility

Approximately one half of MPNSTs manifest in patients with NF1 (see Chapter 13). This association is particularly strong for the malignant Triton tumour and glandular variants of MPNST. NF1 patients with plexiform neurofibromas have the highest likelihood of developing MPNST {2278}.

Genetics

Sporadic and NF1-associated MPNSTs typically have complex karyotypic abnor-malities that are both numerical and structural. Observed abnormalities include near-triploid or hypodiploid chromosome numbers {1462}, chromosomal losses, loss of genetic material related to struc-tural aberrations {998} and recombinations that involve almost all chromosomes {1462}. In one study of 10 tumours, struc-tural abnormalities of chromosome 17 involving the NF1 and TP53 loci were common {998}. Chromosome 22 loss has also been noted {998, 1831}, as have gains of chromosomes 2 and 14 and losses of chromosomes 13, 17 and 18 {1144}. No cytogenetic differences have been noted between sporadic and NF1-associated tumours.

In MPNSTs of NF1 patients, inactivation of both NF1 alleles has occurred {1286}, implicating this gene in MPNST formation (see Chapter 13). Sporadic MPNSTs also show alterations at the NF1 locus, ones which are more likely to be involved in early stages of nerve sheath tumouri-genesis, i.e. in neurofibroma-genesis rather than in malignant progression to MPNST. Instead, the latter is associated with alterations of genes controlling cell cycle regulation. One clearly implicated gene is TP53 {1285, 1349, 1456}. Both TP53 mutations and altered protein expres-sion have been found in MPNSTs. In addition, homozygous deletions of the CDKN2A gene on 9p21, which encodes the p16^{INK4a} and p14^{ARF} cell cycle inhibitory molecules, occur in the progression of neurofibromas to MPNSTs, being found in over 50% of MPNSTs but not in neuro-fibromas {1180, 1591, 1719}. These homo-zygous deletions also inactivate the neigh-bouring CDKN2B gene that encodes the p15 inhibitory molecule {1719}. In combi-nation, these genetic events suggest inactivation of the p53 and pRb regula-tory pathways in approximately 75% of MPNSTs {1719}.

Prognostic and predictive factors

Except those with perineurial cell differ-entiation {833}, MPNSTs are highly aggressive tumours with a poor prognosis. About 60% of patients die of the disease {490}, with an even higher mortality (80%) in individuals with paraspinal lesions {1178} and those (100%) with divergent angiosarcoma {2011}. Overall 5- and 10-year survival rates are 34% and 23% respectively {490}. MPNSTs vary from low-grade lesions to a vast majority of high-grade tumours featuring high cellularity, brisk mitotic activity and necrosis. No firm association has been established between histologic grade and survival, but high (>25%) MIB-1 labelling indices are associated with reduce survival {490, 2375}. The effect of NF1 upon survival is unsettled, in that some report an association with poor survival {490}, whereas others do not {874, 1178}.

CHAPTER 10

Meningeal Tumours

Meningiomas (WHO grades I, II or III)
Meningothelial (arachnoidal) cell neoplasms, typically attached to the inner surface of the dura mater.

Mesenchymal, non-meningothelial tumours
Benign and malignant mesenchymal tumours originating in the CNS and histologically corresponding to tumours of soft tissue or bone.

Haemangiopericytoma (WHO grades II or III)
A highly cellular and vascularized mesenchymal tumour exhibiting a characteristic monotonous low-power appearance and a well-developed, variably thick-walled, branching "staghorn" vasculature; almost always attached to the dura and having a high tendency to recur and to metastasize outside the CNS.

Melanocytic lesions
Primary melanocytic neoplasms of the CNS that arise from leptomeningeal melanocytes and that can be diffuse or circumscribed, benign or malignant. This group includes (1) diffuse melanocytosis and melanomatosis, (2) melanocytoma and (3) malignant melanoma.

Haemangioblastoma (WHO grade I)
A slowly growing, highly vascular tumour of adults, occurring in the cerebellum, brain stem or spinal cord; histologically comprised of stromal cells and small blood vessels; occurring in sporadic forms and in association with von Hippel-Lindau (VHL) syndrome.

Meningiomas

A. Perry
D.N. Louis
B.W. Scheithauer
H. Budka
A. von Deimling

Definition
Meningothelial (arachnoidal) cell neoplasms, typically attached to the inner surface of the dura mater.

ICD-O code
Meningioma   9530/0

Grading
Most meningiomas are benign and correspond to WHO grade I. Certain histological subtypes or meningiomas with specific combinations of morphologic parameters are associated with less favourable clinical outcomes and correspond to WHO grades II (atypical) and III (anaplastic or malignant).

Incidence
Meningiomas account for about 24–30% of primary intracranial tumours occurring in the USA {305, 359}, with an annual incidence rate of up to 13 per 100 000 population in Italy {381}. Many small meningiomas are asymptomatic incidental neuroimaging findings. In Scandinavia,

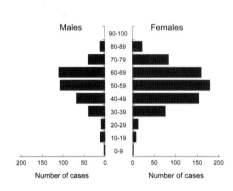

Fig. 10.01 Age and sex distribution of meningioma, based on 1078 cases treated at the University Hospital Zurich.

the incidence has increased between 1968 and 1997 from 2.6 to 4.5 per 100 000 in women, and from 1.4 to 1.9 in men {1119}. In one Italian study, the numbers have remained stable for decades {381}. At autopsy, meningiomas are found incidentally in 1.4% of cases {1836}. Meningiomas are often multiple in patients with neurofibromatosis type 2 (NF2) and in

other, non-NF2 families with a hereditary predisposition to meningioma {1352}. Sporadic meningiomas are multiple in somewhat less than 10% of cases. Atypical meningiomas comprise between 4.7% and 7.2% of meningiomas, although using more current definitions, it has been reported in up to 20%; anaplastic (malignant) meningiomas account for between 1.0% and 2.8% {941, 1384, 1734, 1736, 2413}. An annual incidence of anaplastic (malignant) meningiomas of 0.17 per 100 000 persons has been reported {1911}.

Age and sex distribution
Meningiomas occur most commonly in middle-aged and elderly patients, with a peak during the sixth and seventh decades. Nonetheless, they also occur in children and the elderly. Childhood examples tend to include more aggressive forms of meningioma. Among middle-aged patients, there is a marked female bias, the female:male ratio being approximately 1.7:1 {381}; the ratio peaks at 3.5:1 in the patients 40–44 yeasr of age {1119}. Spinal meningiomas show a marked predominance in women, the frequency approaching 90% in some series. The female:male ratio has increased over time, suggesting the possibility that increasing use of hormonal medications affects meningioma incidence {1119}; however, this hypothesis has not been proven to date. Meningiomas associated with hereditary tumour syndromes generally occur in younger patients, and more equally in men and women. On the other hand, atypical and particularly anaplastic meningiomas show a male predominance {941}. These observations may be related to higher proliferation indices in meningiomas occurring in male patients {1414}.

Etiology
Meningiomas are known to be induced by low-, moderate-, and high-dose radiation, with an average time interval to tumour appearance of 35, 26 and 19–24 years, respectively {1130}. The majority of patients

Table 10.01 Meningiomas grouped by likelihood of recurrence and grade.

Meningiomas with low risk of recurrence and aggressive growth:		
		ICD-O code
Meningothelial meningioma	WHO grade I	9531/0
Fibrous (fibroblastic) meningioma	WHO grade I	9532/0
Transitional (mixed) meningioma	WHO grade I	9537/0
Psammomatous meningioma	WHO grade I	9533/0
Angiomatous meningioma	WHO grade I	9534/0
Microcystic meningioma	WHO grade I	9530/0
Secretory meningioma	WHO grade I	9530/0
Lymphoplasmacyte-rich meningioma	WHO grade I	9530/0
Metaplastic meningioma	WHO grade I	9530/0
Meningiomas with greater likelihood of recurrence and/or aggressive behaviour:		
Chordoid meningioma	WHO grade II	9538/1
Clear cell meningioma (intracranial)	WHO grade II	9538/1
Atypical meningioma	WHO grade II	9539/1
Papillary meningioma	WHO grade III	9538/3
Rhabdoid meningioma	WHO grade III	9538/3
Anaplastic (malignant) meningioma	WHO grade III	9530/3
Meningiomas of any subtype or grade with high proliferation index and/or brain invasion		

with radiation-induced meningiomas have a history of low-dose irradiation (800 rad) to the scalp for tinea capitis. The second largest group of patients with radiation-induced meningiomas received high-dose irradiation (>2000 rad) for primary brain tumours {772}. Radiation-induced meningiomas are more commonly atypical or aggressive, multifocal, highly proliferative, and generally occur in younger age groups {772, 1372, 1540}.

The role of sex hormones in the genesis of meningiomas is less clear. The over-representation of women among meningioma patients suggests an aetiological role for sex hormones. At first operation, 88% of meningiomas have progesterone, 40% have estrogen and 39% have androgen receptors {1168}. In any case, the higher incidence of meningiomas in women cannot be explained by differences of sex hormone expression alone {1168}.

Localization

The vast majority of meningiomas arise in intracranial, intraspinal or orbital locations. Intraventricular and epidural examples are uncommon. Rare meningiomas have been reported in almost all organs. Within the cranial cavity, most meningiomas occur over the cerebral convexities, often para-sagittal in association with the falx and venous sinus. Other common sites include the olfactory grooves, sphenoid ridges,

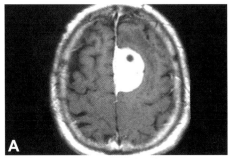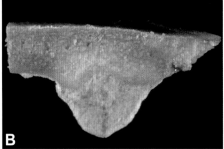

Fig. 10.03 A Large meningioma of the falx, presenting as a contrast-enhanced mass with a central cyst. Note the dural tail at either side of the neoplasm. **B** Ossifying meningioma including hyperostosis in the overlying skull.

para/suprasellar regions, optic nerve sheath, petrous ridges, tentorium and posterior fossa. Most spinal meningiomas occur in the thoracic region. Atypical and anaplastic meningiomas most commonly affect the falx and the lateral convexities {1384}. Among other sites, metastases of malignant meningiomas most often involve lung, pleura, bone and liver.

Clinical features
Symptoms and signs
Meningiomas are generally slowly growing and produce neurological signs and symptoms by compression of adjacent structures; specific deficits depend upon the location of the tumour. Headache and seizures often herald the presence of a meningioma.

Neuroimaging
On MRI, meningiomas are typically iso-dense, contrast-enhancing dural masses. Some, like microcystic meningiomas, may show little enhancement on CT and MRI {2085}. Calcification is best seen on CT scan. A characteristic feature of meningiomas is the so-called 'dural tail' surrounding the dural perimeter of the mass. This familiar imaging sign may or may not indicate dural extension of the tumour or correspond to a rim of reactive fibrovascular tissue. Peritumoural cerebral edema is occasionally prominent, particularly around atypical or anaplastic examples. It has also been described in association with the secretory variant {42} and in meningothelial tumours with so-called pericyte accumulation about vessels {1900}. Cyst formation may occur within or at the periphery of a meningioma. Findings on neuroimaging have not always been reliable in identifying meningiomas, predicting tumour behaviour or excluding differential diagnostic possibilities.

Macroscopy
Most meningiomas are rubbery or firm, well-demarcated, sometimes lobulated, rounded masses that feature broad dural attachment {257, 259, 1261, 1959}. Invasion of underlying dura or of dural sinuses is quite common. Occasional meningiomas invade through dura to involve the skull, where they may induce characteristic hyperostosis: such bony changes are highly indicative of skull invasion. Meningiomas may attach to or encase cerebral arteries, but only rarely do they infiltrate arterial walls. They may also infiltrate the skin and extend to extracranial compartments, such as the orbit. Adjacent brain is often compressed but rarely shows frank parenchymal invasion. In certain sites, particularly along the sphenoid

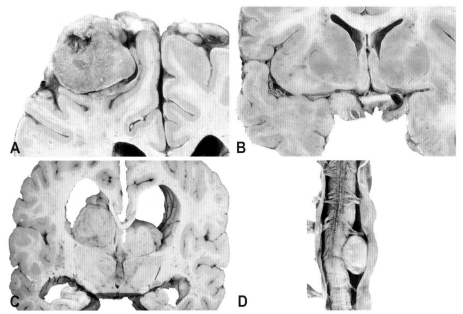

Fig. 10.02 Macroscopic features of meningioma. **A** Large parasaggital meningioma compressing the adjacent parietal lobe. **B** Meningioma of the medial sphenoid wing encasing the carotid artery. **C** Large meningioma of the lateral ventricles and the third ventricle. **D** Spinal meningioma compressing the spinal cord.

wing, meningiomas may grow as a flat, carpet-like mass, a pattern termed "en plaque meningioma." Some meningiomas may appear gritty on gross inspection, implying the presence of numerous psammoma bodies. Bone formation is far less common. Atypical and anaplastic meningiomas tend to be larger than benign examples {1384} and may feature necrosis.

Histopathology

Meningiomas exhibit a wide range of histologic appearances {259, 1079, 1261, 1959}. Of the subtypes in the WHO classification, meningothelial, fibrous and transitional meningiomas are the most common. The majority of subtypes behave in a common clinical manner, but four histologic variants, falling into the grade II and III categories, are far more likely to recur and follow a more aggressive clinical course including metastasis. Pleomorphic nuclei and occasional mitoses may be noted in any of the meningioma variants, without necessarily connoting more aggressive behaviour. Furthermore, the criteria used to diagnose atypical meningiomas are applied independent of specific meningioma subtype.

Meningothelial meningioma

In this classic and common variant, tumour cells form lobules, some partly demarcated by thin collagenous septae. Like normal arachnoidal cap cells, the tumour cells are largely uniform, with oval nuclei with delicate chromatin that on occasion show central clearing, or the

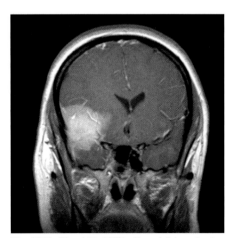

Fig. 10.04 T1-weighted MRI with gadolinium showing large, irregular meningeal mass displaying an indistinct interface with adjacent brain and marked mass effect.

formulation of cytoplasmic-nuclear inclusions. Whorls and psammoma bodies are not common in meningothelial meningioma, but when present tend to be less-well formed than in transitional, fibrous or psammomatous tumour subtypes. Larger lobules should not be confused with the 'sheeting', or loss of architectural pattern seen in atypical meningioma. Within the lobules, tumour cells appear to form a syncytium, as the delicate, intricately interwoven tumour cell processes cannot be discerned at the light microscopic level. Since the tumour cells closely resemble those of the normal arachnoid cap cells, reactive meningothelial hyperplasia may simulate meningioma in small biopsy specimens. The most florid examples are associated with optic nerve gliomas, or adjacent to other tumour types, haemorrhage in the setting of chronic renal disease, advanced patient age, arachnoiditis ossificans, spontaneous intracranial haemorrhage and occasionally in other patients with diffuse dural thickening and contrast enhancement on neuroimaging {1729}.

Fibrous (fibroblastic) meningioma

Uncommon in pure form, this meningioma variant consists of spindle cells forming parallel, storiform and interlacing bundles in a collagen-rich matrix. Whorl formation and psammoma bodies are infrequent. Nuclear features characteristic of meningothelial meningioma are often found focally as well. The tumour cells of fibrous meningioma form wide fascicles, with varying amounts of intercellular collagen. In some cases, collagen deposition may be striking.

Transitional (mixed) meningioma

These common tumours feature the coexistence of meningothelial and fibrous patterns as well as transitions between these patters. Vaguely lobular and fascicular arrangements often appear side by side in association with conspicuous tight whorls and psammoma bodies.

Psammomatous meningioma

This designation is applied to meningiomas containing a predominance of psammoma bodies over that of the tumour cells which give rise to them. They often become confluent, forming irregular calcified masses and occasionally bone.

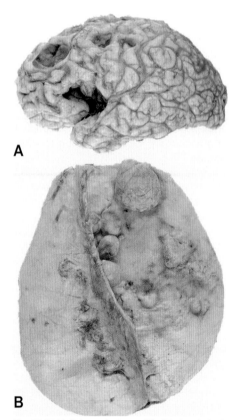

A

B

Fig. 10.05 Multiple meningiomas (**B**) of the hemispheric convexity and (**A**) the impressions caused in the left cerebral hemisphere.

The neoplastic cells of this variant usually have a transitional appearance with whorl formation. Some tumours are almost completely replaced by psammoma bodies, intervening meningothelial cells being hard to find. Psammomatous meningiomas characteristically occur in the thoracic spinal region and usually in middle-aged women.

Angiomatous meningioma

This meningioma variant features a predominance of blood vessels over that of the tumour cells. The vascular channels may be small- or medium-sized, thin-walled or thick. Most are small with markedly hyalinized walls. Moderate to marked degenerative nuclear atypia is common, but the vast majority of such tumours are histologically and clinically benign {783}. The differential diagnosis includes vascular malformations and capillary haemangioblastoma, depending on the prominence of vessels and the occasionally non-meningothelial appearance of the tumour cells. The designation angiomatous should not be equated with the obsolete term 'angioblastic meningioma' (see Haemangiopericytoma). Angiomatous meningiomas do not exhibit aggressive behaviour. Adjacent cerebral edema may be out of proportion to tumour size.

Microcystic meningioma

This variant is characterized by cells with thin, elongate processes encompassing microcysts containing pale, eosinophilic mucinous fluid. Pleomorphic cells may be numerous, but microcystic meningiomas are typically benign. Like the angiomatous variant, accompanying cerebral edema may be seen {1665}.

Secretory meningioma

The hallmark of this tumour variant is the presence of focal epithelial differentiation in the form of intracellular lumina containing PAS-positive, eosinophilic secretion. These structures, known as pseudopsammoma bodies {1076}, show immunoreactivity for carcinoembryonic antigen (CEA) and a variety of other epithelial and secretory markers, while the surrounding tumour cells are both CEA and cytokeratin-positive. Secretory meningiomas may be associated with blood levels of CEA that drop with resection and rise with recurrence {1350}. Mast cells may be numerous. Peritumoural edema may be significant {2251}.

Lymphoplasmacyte-rich meningioma

This meningioma variant features extensive chronic inflammatory infiltrates often over-shadowing the inconspicuous meningothelial component. Lympho-plasmacyte-rich meningioma is among the rarest of variants. Its very existence as a distinct clinicopathologic entity remains controversial, since its behaviour often resembles that of an inflammatory process {235}. Systemic haematologic abnormalities, including hyperglobulinemia and iron refractory anemia have been documented in some cases {665}.

Metaplastic meningioma

A meningioma with striking focal or widespread mesenchymal components including osseous, cartilaginous, lipomatous, myxoid or xanthomatous tissue, singly or in combinations. The clinical significance of these alterations, if any, is unclear. Correlation with intra-operative findings is occasionally needed to distinguish ossified meningiomas from ones exhibiting bone invasion.

Chordoid meningioma

A meningioma variant consisting predominantly of tissue histologically similar to chordoma, featuring cords or trabeculae of eosinophilic, often vacuolated cells in an abundant mucoid matrix background.

Such chordoid areas are often interspersed with more typical meningioma tissue; pure examples are uncommon. Chronic inflammatory infiltrates, often patchy, may be prominent. Chordoid meningiomas are typically large, supratentorial tumours that exhibit a very high rate of recurrence following subtotal resection (WHO grade II) {389}. Infrequently, patients have associated haematological conditions, such as Castleman's disease {1082}.

Clear cell meningioma

An often patternless meningioma composed of polygonal cells with clear, glycogen-rich cytoplasm and prominent blocky perivascular and interstitial collagen. A rare meningioma variant, it shows prominent PAS-positive, diastase-sensitive cytoplasmic clearing due to glycogen accumulation. Classic features of meningioma are few; whorl formation is vague at best and no psammoma bodies are seen. The tumour shows a proclivity for the cerebellopontine angle and cauda equina region. It also tends to affect younger patients, both children and young adults. Clear cell meningiomas are associated with a more aggressive behaviour including frequent recurrence and occasional CSF seeding (WHO grade II) {1655, 2509}.

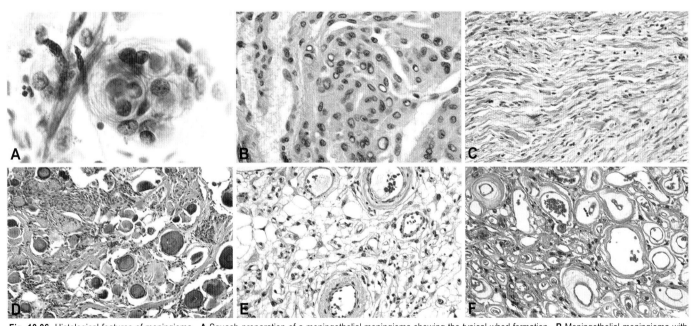

Fig. 10.06 Histological features of meningioma. **A** Squash preparation of a meningothelial meningioma showing the typical whorl formation. **B** Meningothelial meningioma with typical intranuclear inclusions. **C** Fibrous meningioma characterized by parallel fascicles of fibroblastic cells. **D** Psammomatous meningioma with numerous calcified psammoma bodies and inconspicuous meningothelial component. **E** Microcystic meningioma characterized by intercellular microcystic spaces. **F** Angiomatous meningioma dominated by excessive vascularization interspersed with small meningothelial tumour cells.

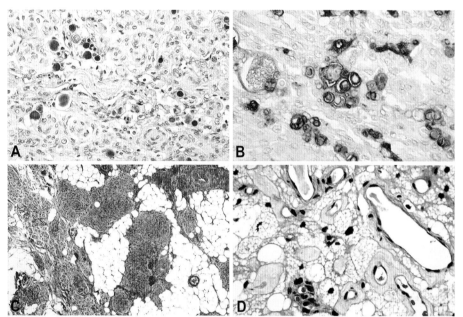

Fig. 10.07 Secretory meningioma with numerous PAS positive pseudopsammoma bodies rich in glycogen (**A**) and marked immunoreactivity for (**B**) epithelial membrane antigen (EMA). **C** Metaplastic/lipomatous meningioma. **D** Metaplastic/xanthomatous meningioma.

Atypical meningioma

A meningioma with increased mitotic activity or three or more of the following histologic features: increased cellularity, small cells with a high nuclear: cytoplasmic ratio, prominent nucleoli, uninterrupted patternless or sheet-like growth, and foci of 'spontaneous' or 'geographic' necrosis. Increased mitotic activity is defined as 4 or more mitoses per 10 high-power (40x) fields (defined as 0.16 mm2) {1736}. The above criteria have been shown to correlate with 8-fold higher recurrence rates {1736}. Alternative grading approaches a) identify individually scored parameters to arrive at a sum {941}, or b) simply combine hypercellularity with 5 or more mitoses per 10 high power fields {1384}. Atypical meningiomas often have moderately high MIB-1 labelling indices and correspond histologically to WHO grade II.

Papillary meningioma

A rare meningioma variant defined by the presence of a perivascular pseudopapillary pattern comprising the majority of the tumour. The pattern frequently increases in extent with recurrences. Papillary meningiomas tend to occur in young patients, including children {1356}. Local invasion and invasion of the brain have been noted in 75% of cases, recurrence in 55%, metastasis in 20% (mostly to lung) and death of disease in roughly half

{1195,1686}. Given their aggressive clinical behaviour {1356}, these tumours have been graded as WHO grade III.

Rhabdoid meningioma

An uncommon tumour predominantly containing sheets of rhabdoid cells, i.e. plump cells with eccentric nuclei, often open chromatin, a prominent nucleolus, and prominent inclusion-like eosinophilic cytoplasm appearing either as discernible whorled fibrils or compact and waxy. Such rhabdoid cells resemble those described in tumours in other sites, particularly kidney and the atypical teratoid/rhabdoid tumour of the brain. Rhabdoid cells may be become increasingly evident with tumour recurrences. Most rhabdoid meningiomas have high proliferative indices and other histological features of malignancy. Some even combine a papillary architecture with rhabdoid cytology. Rhabdoid meningiomas often undergo an aggressive clinical course and correspond to WHO grade III {1085,1733}. A minority of meningiomas with rhabdoid features shows this only focally and lacks other histological features of malignancy; the behaviour of these tumours remains to be determined.

Anaplastic (malignant) meningioma

A meningioma exhibiting histological features of frank malignancy far in excess of the abnormalities present in atypical

meningioma. These include either obviously malignant cytology resembling that of carcinoma, melanoma or high-grade sarcoma, or a markedly elevated mitotic index (20 or more mitoses per ten high-power fields) (defined as 0.16 mm2) {1734}. Tumours that meet the above criteria correspond to WHO grade III and are often fatal, median survival being less than 2 years {1734}. Invasion of the brain alone is not sufficient for a diagnosis of anaplastic meningioma {1734}. Since malignant progression in meningiomas, like that of gliomas, is a continuum of increasing atypia and anaplasia, tumours with features intermediate between atypical and anaplastic meningioma are occasionally encountered.

Other morphologic variations

As a reflection of the wide morphologic spectrum that may be encountered in meningiomas, rare examples are difficult to classify as any of the accepted variants. These include meningiomas with oncocytic, mucinous, sclerosing, whorling-sclerosing, GFAP-expressing and granulofilamentous inclusion-bearing features {41, 139, 277, 746, 861, 863, 1109, 1778, 1914}. There is currently insufficient data to indicate that these tumours represent unique variants. Skepticism is justified in that the majority of tumours once termed "pigmented meningiomas" are now known to be melanocytomas instead. However, recruitment of melanocytes from the adjacent meninges into the substance of a true meningioma accounts for dark pigmentation in rare cases {1580}.

Brain invasion and metastasis

Invasion of the brain by meningioma is characterized by irregular, tongue-like protrusions of tumour cells infiltrating underlying parenchyma, without an intervening layer of leptomeninges. This causes reactive astrocytosis with entrapped islands of GFAP-positive parenchyma at the periphery of the tumour. Brain invasion may occur in histologically benign, atypical or anaplastic (malignant) meningiomas. The presence of brain invasion connotes a greater likelihood of recurrence. Brain-invasive, histologically benign and histologically atypical meningiomas both have recurrence and mortality rates similar to those of atypical meningiomas in general {1736}. As such, they should prognostically be considered

WHO grade II. Whereas the genetic changes that characterize higher-grade meningiomas have generally not been found in brain-invasive, histologically benign meningiomas {1858, 2101, 2378}, one study showed chromosome 1p and 14q deletions in this group, changes similar to those in atypical meningiomas {273}. Anaplastic (malignant) meningiomas are considered WHO grade III whether or not they display brain invasion.

Extracranial metastases are extremely rare, being estimated to occur in roughly 1 in 1000 meningiomas and most often in association with anaplastic tumours. The rare metastases of histologically benign meningiomas typically occur following surgery, but can arise de novo as well.

Immunohistochemistry

The vast majority of meningiomas stain for epithelial membrane antigen (EMA), although EMA immunoreactivity is less consistent in atypical and malignant lesions. Vimentin positivity is found in all meningiomas. Immunohistochemical studies of S-100 protein have found varying positivity in meningiomas, but such staining is not usually prominent. Secretory meningiomas characteristically show strong positive staining for CEA in the pseudopsammoma bodies and in the surrounding cytokeratin-positive cells immediately surrounding the lumina containing them. Claudin-1 has also been found useful in some studies {754, 1825}. Other potentially useful immuno-histochemical markers in selected cases include Ki-67 and progesterone receptor.

Electron microscopy

Diagnostic ultrastructural features of meningiomas include abundance of intermediate filaments (vimentin), complex interdigitating cellular processes (particularly in meningothelial variants), and desmosomal intercellular junctions. These cell surface specializations as well as intermediate filaments are few in fibrous meningiomas, the cells being separated by collagen. Secretory meningiomas feature single or multiple epithelial-like lumina within single meningothelial cells. These cell surfaces show short apical microvilli and surround electron-dense secretions of variable morphology {1230}. Microcystic meningiomas feature long cytoplasmic processes enclosing intercellular electron-lucent matrix and joined by desmosomes. Large cytoplasmic lysosomes may be seen in this tumour variant.

Proliferation

In general, cellular proliferation of tumour cells increases from benign through atypical to anaplastic (malignant) meningioma. Mitotic indices correlate roughly with volume growth rate. There are significant differences in mitotic indices (total counts per ten high-power fields) between tumour grades: 0.08 ± 0.05 in benign, 4.8 ± 0.9 in atypical and 19 ± 4.1 in malignant variants. Similarly, MIB-1/Ki-67 indices show a highly significant increase from benign (mean, 3.8%), through atypical (mean 7.2%), to anaplastic meningiomas (mean 14.7%) {1385}. Other studies have suggested that meningiomas with indices >4% have increased risk of recurrence similar to atypical meningioma, whereas those with indices >20% are associated with death rates analogous to those associated with anaplastic meningioma {1734,1737}. However, significant differences in technique and interpretation make it difficult to apply specific cutoffs that would translate accurately from one laboratory to another.

Flow cytometric studies have demonstrated approximately equal numbers of diploid and aneuploid meningiomas, and have shown significant correlations between aneuploid tumours and features such as recurrence, pleomorphism, high cellular density, mitotic activity and infiltration of brain and soft tissue {401}.

Genetic susceptibility

Meningiomas are a key feature of neurofibromatosis type 2 (see NF2 in Chapter 13). However, a number of families with an increased susceptibility to meningiomas, but without NF2, have also been reported {1352}. In at least one of these families the disease did not show linkage to the NF2 locus on chromosome 22q {1806}, thus suggesting that there may be a second meningioma predisposition locus. The possible relationship of meningioma to other rare, inherited tumour syndromes, such as Gorlin, Werner or Cowden syndromes, is less well-defined {714, 1353}. A familial history of benign brain tumours (meningioma, schwannoma, neurofibroma or neuroma), melanoma and possibly breast cancer may be associated with an increased risk of meningioma development {825}.

Genetics

Meningiomas were among the first solid tumours recognized as having cytogenetic alterations, the most consistent change being deletion of chromosome 22 {2483}. In general, karyotypic abnormalities are

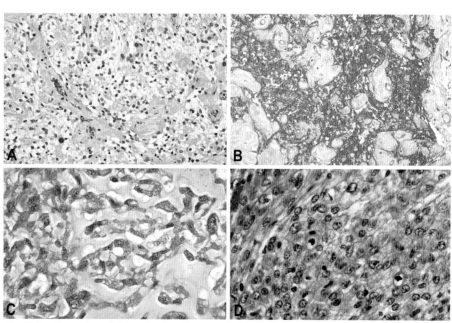

Fig. 10.08 Clear cell meningioma showing (**A**) a patternless neoplasm dominated by clear and (**B**) glycogen-rich cytoplasm (PAS staining). **C** Chordoid meningioma with eosinophilic tumour cells in a mucous-rich matrix. **D** Atypical meningioma with frequent mitoses despite bland cytologic features.

more extensive in atypical and anaplastic (malignant) meningiomas {26, 1727}. Among the other cytogenetic changes associated with meningioma, deletion of the short arm of chromosome 1 {1151} and loss of chromosomes 6, 10, 14, 18 and 19 are the most frequently seen {2483}. Molecular genetic findings indicate that approximately half of meningiomas have allelic losses that involve band q12 on chromosome 22 {494, 1326, 1964}. In addition, atypical meningiomas often show allelic losses of chromosomal arms 1p, 6q, 9q, 10q, 14q, 17p and 18q, suggesting that progression-associated genes may lie at these loci {26, 1457, 1726, 1858, 2101, 2378}. These alterations, with more frequent losses of chromosomes 6q, 9p, 10 and 14q, also occur in anaplastic meningiomas.

Chromosomal gains noted in higher-grade meningiomas include primarily chromosomes 20q, 12q, 15q, 1q, 9q and 17q.

NF2 gene

Mutations in the *NF2* gene are detected in the majority of NF2 associated and in up to 60% of sporadic meningiomas {1288, 2266, 2393}. Most are either small insertions or deletions, or are nonsense mutations that affect splice sites, create stop codons or result in frameshifts occurring mainly in the most 5' two thirds of the gene {1352}. The common predictable effect of these mutations is a truncated and presumably non-functional merlin (schwannomin) protein. The frequency of *NF2* mutations varies among meningioma variants. Fibroblastic, transi-

tional and psammomatous meningiomas often carry *NF2* mutations. In contrast, meningothelial, secretory and micro-cystic meningiomas only rarely harbour *NF2* mutations, suggesting that their genetic origin is largely independent of *NF2* {777, 1193, 2393}. The observation of a close association between allelic loss on 22q and the fibroblastic meningiomas supports this hypothesis {1964}, as does the observation that most non-NF2 meningioma families develop meningothelial tumours {1352}. Furthermore, reduced expression of merlin (schwannomin) has been observed in different histopathological variants of meningiomas, but appears to be rare in meningothelial tumours {1276}. In atypical and anaplastic meningiomas, *NF2* mutations occur in approximately 70% of cases, matching the frequency of *NF2* mutations in benign fibroblastic and transitional meningiomas. In radiation-induced meningiomas, the frequencies of *NF2* mutations and loss of chromosome 22 are lower, whereas structural abnormalities of chromosome 1p are more common than in sporadic tumours. This finding suggests a different molecular pathogenesis for radiation-associated meningiomas {1826, 2094, 2485}.

Other genes

The close association of *NF2* mutations in meningiomas with allelic loss on chromosome 22 suggests that *NF2* is the major meningioma tumour suppressor gene on that chromosome {2393}. Nonetheless, deletion studies of chromosome 22 have detected losses and translocations of genetic material outside the *NF2* region, thus raising the possibility that a second meningioma gene resides on chromosome 22. Candidate genes include *LARGE*, *MN1*, *BAM22*, and *INI1*, although these show only rare alterations {1817, 1889, 2033}. *DAL1* of the protein 4.1 family has also been shown to be deleted in meningiomas, its expression being suppressed in meningiomas {741, 1609}. Although allelic losses of chromosome 17p have been reported to occur in higher-grade meningiomas, studies of the *TP53* gene residing on that chromosome segment have not shown significant gene alterations. Nonetheless, immuno-histochemical positivity for p53 protein occurs in subsets of both benign and atypical meningiomas. Furthermore, rare

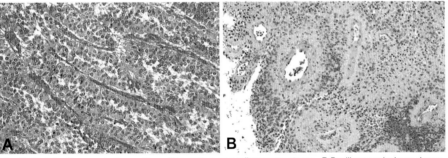

Fig. 10.09 A Papillary meningioma with papillary pattern on a collageneous stroma. **B** Papillary meningioma characterized by discohesive growth with pseudopapillae and perivascular pseudorosettes.

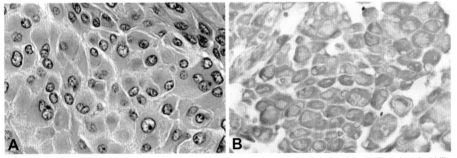

Fig. 10.10 A Rhabdoid meningioma with eccentrically placed vesicular nuclei, prominent nucleoli, and eosinophilic globular/fibrillar paranuclear inclusions (**A**) and cytoplasmic immunoreactivity for vimentin (**B**).

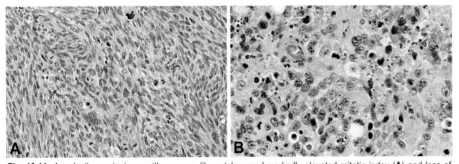

Fig. 10.11 Anaplastic meningioma with sarcoma-like cytology and markedly elevated mitotic index (**A**) and loss of meningiomatous tissue pattern and numerous typical and atypical mitoses (**B**).

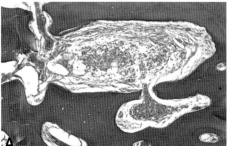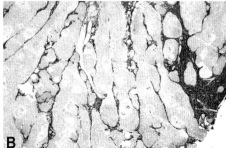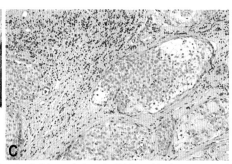

Fig. 10.12 **A** Invasion of bones by meningiomas through osseous canaliculi is not a sign of malignancy. **B** The brain invasion in this meningioma is highlighted by the presence of entrapped GFAP-positive brain parenchyma between tongues of GFAP-negative tumour. **C** Despite otherwise benign histology, this meningioma has breached the pia and has invaded the cerebellum. Brain invasion corresponds to WHO grade II.

anaplastic meningiomas contain *TP53* mutations {2363}. Mutations and deletions of the *CDKN2A* gene are rare in meningiomas, as are alterations of the *PTEN* and *PTCH* genes {1726}. However, deletions of the 9p21 region, which includes the *CDKN2A* gene, are particularly common in the anaplastic meningiomas and are associated with shortened survival {203, 1721}. Other molecular alterations associated with high tumour grade and aggressive clinical behaviour include loss of the *NDRG2* gene on 14q11.2, gains of the *S6K* gene and other loci on the 17q23 amplicon, loss of various *NF2* homologues within the protein 4.1 family, e.g. the *4.1B* gene on chromosome 18p11.3, and loss of the protein 4.1B binding partner TSLC-1 {266, 274, 1359, 1609, 1726, 2181}. In summary, in most of the chromosomal loci commonly gained or lost during meningioma tumour progression, the relevant genes affected have yet to be identified.

Microsatellite instability
This finding is thought to result from mutations in DNA mismatch repair genes. One study reported microsatellite instability in 4 of 16 meningiomas {1810}.

However, other studies have reported low frequencies or absence of microsatellite instability altogether {2100, 2120, 2309}.

Clonality of solitary, recurrent and multiple meningiomas
Studies of X-chromosome inactivation using Southern blot analysis indicate that meningiomas are monoclonal tumours {951}, while PCR-based assays have hinted that a small fraction could be polyclonal {2502}. Nevertheless, both the Southern blot data {951} and the observation that the overwhelming majority of meningiomas with *NF2* mutations only have a single mutation {2393} argue that the origin of this group of lesions is clonal. Similarly, all recurrent meningiomas have been found to be clonal with respect to the primary tumour {2338}. The clonality of multiple meningiomas has also been analysed using studies of X-chromosome inactivation and by mutational analysis of the *NF2* gene in multiple tumours from the same patient {1262, 2141, 2337}. In these, lesions from patients with three or more meningiomas have been shown to have either the same copy of the X-chromosome inactivated, or to carry the same *NF2* mutation. These

data provide strong evidence for a clonal origin of multiple meningiomas in patients with more than two lesions. Furthermore, they suggest that multiple lesions arise through dural spread, a notion also supported by the common finding of peritumoural implants in 10% of meningiomas {201} and of small meningothelial nests in grossly unremarkable dural strips from the convexities of patients with meningiomas {201}. Nevertheless, it remains possible that some cases with multiple meningiomas represent genetic mosaics, with segmental, dural constitutional *NF2* mutations.

Histogenesis
Meningiomas are considered to be derived from meningothelial (arachnoidal) cells.

Prognostic and predictive factors
The major prognostic questions regarding atypical meningiomas involve prediction of recurrence. For malignant variants, the issue is prediction of survival.

Clinical factors. In most cases, meningiomas can be removed entirely according to operative or neuro-radiologic criteria. In one series, 20% of gross-

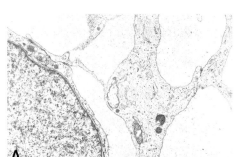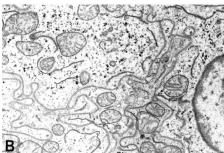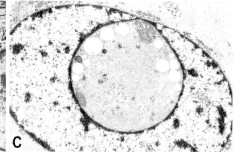

Fig. 10.13 Electron micrographies of meningiomas. **A** Microcystic meningioma characterized by intercellular microcystic spaces. **B** Numerous interdigitated cellular processes and occasional desmosomal junctions. **C** Nucleus containing a pseudoinclusion.

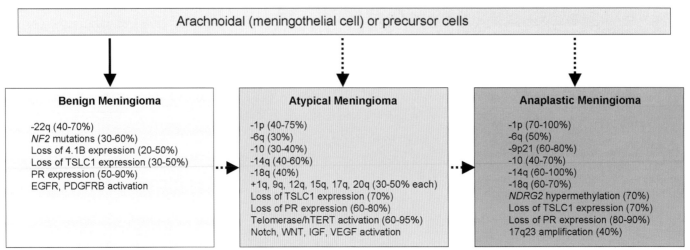

Fig. 10.14 Genetic model of meningioma tumourigenesis and malignant progression.

totally resected, benign meningiomas recurred within 20 years {940}. The major clinical factor in recurrence is extent of resection, which is influenced by tumour site, extent of invasion, attachment to vital intracranial structures, and the skill and experience of the surgeon. Other clinical factors, such as young age and male gender, are less powerful predictors of recurrence. Both are partially explained by the increased frequency of high-grade meningiomas in such patients.

Histopathology and grading. Some histological variants of meningioma are more likely to recur {1726}. Overall, however, histologic grade (WHO I or benign; WHO II or atypical; WHO III or anaplastic) is the most useful morphologic predictor of recurrence. While benign meningiomas have recurrence rates of about 7–25%, atypical meningiomas recur in 29–52% of cases and anaplastic meningiomas at rates of 50–94% {1175, 1384, 1734, 1736}. Malignant histological

features are associated with shorter survival times {1027}, one series reporting a median survival of under 2 years {1734}. Similarly, high proliferation indices correlate with aggressive behaviour.

Progesterone receptor status. The absence of progesterone receptors, and a high mitotic index as well as tumour grade are significant factors in assessing disease-free intervals {1722, 1933}. Multivariate analysis has shown that a three-factor interaction model incorporating a progesterone receptor score of 0, a mitotic index greater than 6, and malignant (WHO III) tumour grade, was a highly significant predictor of poor outcome {212, 875}. Atypical and anaplastic tumours frequently lack progesterone receptors {1722}, thus progesterone-receptor-negative meningiomas tend to be larger than receptor-positive tumours {212}. Since a significant subset of histologically and clinically benign meningiomas also lacks progesterone

receptor expression, the significance of this single immunohistochemical parameter should not be overestimated in the absence of the other features mentioned above.

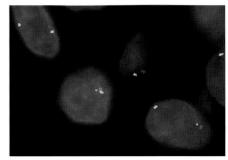

Fig. 10.15 FISH analysis showed hemizygous deletion of the 9p21 (p16^{INK4a}) region (only one red signal in most nuclei) in this anaplastic meningioma, whereas the centromere for chromosome 9 is retained (two green signals in most nuclei). This genetic pattern is associated with decreased survival.

Mesenchymal, non-meningothelial tumours

W. Paulus
B.W. Scheithauer
A. Perry

Definition
Benign and malignant mesenchymal tumours originating in the CNS and histologically corresponding to tumours of soft tissue or bone.

ICD-O codes

Lipoma	8850/0
Liposarcoma	8850/3
Angiolipoma	8861/0
Hibernoma	8880/0
Solitary fibrous tumour	8815/0
Fibrosarcoma	8810/3
Malignant fibrous histiocytoma (MFH)	8830/3
Leiomyoma	8890/0
Leiomyosarcoma	8890/3
Rhabdomyoma	8900/0
Rhabdomyosarcoma	8900/3
Chondroma	9220/0
Osteoma	9180/0
Osteochondroma	9210/0
Chondrosarcoma	9220/3
Osteosarcoma	9180/3
Haemangioma	9120/0
Epithelioid haemangioendothelioma	9133/1
Angiosarcoma	9120/3
Kaposi sarcoma	9140/3
Ewing sarcoma-peripheral primitive neuroectodermal tumour	9364/3

Grading
According to their histological features and clinical behaviour, they range from benign neoplasms (WHO grade I) to highly malignant sarcomas (WHO grade IV).

Terminology and historical annotation
The histological features of mesenchymal tumours affecting the CNS are the same as those of corresponding extracranial soft tissue and bone tumours {258, 527}. Haemangiopericytoma, by far the most common mesenchymal, non-meningothelial neoplasm, is described separately. Antiquated nosologic terms, such as spindle-cell sarcoma, polymorphic cell sarcoma and myxosarcoma have been replaced by designations indicating specific differentiation {527}. The non-specific diagnostic term 'meningeal sarcoma' is also to be avoided since it has been used to denote both malignant meningioma and various types of sarcoma. Some non-mesenchymal tumours were previously classified as sarcomas; examples include CNS lymphoma ('reticulum cell sarcoma'), desmoplastic medulloblastoma ('cerebellar arachnoidal sarcoma') and giant cell glioblastoma ('monstrocellular sarcoma').

Incidence
Whereas the various forms of lipoma represent 0.4% of intracranial tumours, the other benign mesenchymal tumours are rare. Based on two series of 19 and 17 cases, sarcomas represent less than 0.1% to 0.2% of intracranial tumours {1636,1704}. Reported higher values are a reflection of over-diagnosis related to historical classification schemes. The most common tumour types include fibrosarcoma, malignant fibrous histiocytoma (MFH), and undifferentiated sarcoma {1636, 1704}.

Age and sex distribution
Mesenchymal tumours may occur at any age. Rhabdomyosarcoma occurs preferentially in children, while malignant fibrous histiocytoma and chondrosarcoma usually manifest in adults. As a whole, sarcomas show no obvious gender predilection.

Etiology
Intracranial fibrosarcoma, MFH, chondrosarcoma and osteosarcoma may occur several years after cranial irradiation, most commonly for sellar region tumours {257, 1597}. Single cases of intracranial and spinal fibrosarcoma, pleomorphic sarcoma and angiosarcoma have also been related to previous trauma or surgery {845}, an etiology that may be more common to fibromatoses {1490}. The Epstein-Barr virus probably plays a role in the development of intracranial smooth muscle tumours of immunocompromised patients {229}.

Localization
Tumours arising in meninges are more common than ones originating within CNS parenchyma or in choroid plexus. Whereas most mesenchymal tumours are supra- rather than infratentorial or spinal in location, rhabdomyosarcomas are more often infratentorial. Chondrosarcomas involving the CNS arise most often in the skull base. Intracranial lipomas typically occur at midline sites, such as the anterior corpus callosum, quadrigeminal plate, cerebellopontine angle, suprasellar and hypothalamic region as well as the auditory canal. Spinal cord examples involve the conus medullaris–filum terminale as well as occurring at the thoracic level. Intraventricular and tuber cinereum {189} lipomas are rare. Occasional CNS lipomas have a fibrous connection to extend into surrounding soft or subcutaneous tissue. Osteolipomas prefer the suprasellar/interpeduncular regions {189, 2106}. Most spinal lipomas and particularly angiolipomas arise in the epidural space.

Clinical features
Clinical symptoms and signs are variable and non-specific, and depend largely upon tumour location. Spontaneous regression is rare {1228}.
While the neuroradiologic appearance of most mesenchymal tumours is non-specific, the neuroimaging characteristics of lipoma are virtually diagnostic, as T1-weighted MRI images show fat having a high-signal intensity. Speckled calcifications are typical of chondroid and osseous tumours.

Macroscopy
The macroscopic appearance of mesenchymal tumours depends entirely upon their differentiation and is similar to that of the corresponding extracraniospinal soft tissue tumours. Lipomas are bright yellow, lobulated lesions. Whereas epidural lipomas are delicately encapsulated and discrete, intradural examples are often intimately attached to leptomeninges and CNS parenchyma. Lumbosacral lipomas (leptomyelolipomas) are comprised of subcutaneous and intradural

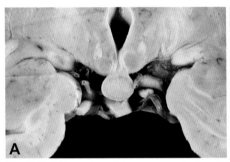
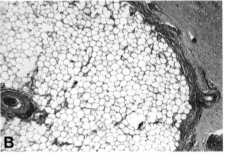

Fig. 10.16 A Lipoma beneath the mammillary bodies. **B** Histology of a cerebral lipoma composed of uniform fat cells sharply delineated from brain tissue.

components, the two being linked by a fibrolipomatous stalk that may attach to the dorsum of the cord, to the filum terminale, or to both. A "tethered cord" commonly results. Chondromas are demarcated, bosselated grey-white, translucent, and typically form large, dural-based masses indenting brain parenchyma. Meningeal sarcomas are firm in texture and tend to invade adjacent brain. Although intracerebral sarcomas appear well delineated, parenchymal invasion is a feature. As a rule, the cut surface of sarcomas is firm and fleshy; high-grade lesions often show necrosis and haemorrhage.

Tumours of adipose tissue
Lipoma
This benign lesion microscopically resembles normal adipose tissue {240}. Most lipomas show lobulation at low magnification. The ample capillary vasculature of even typical encapsulated lipomas is inconspicuous. Patchy hyalinization is a common feature, but calcification and myxoid change are occasionally seen. Osteolipomas are exceedingly rare and may show zonation with central adipose tissue and peripheral bone {2106}.

Angiolipoma
The proportion of adipose cells and vasculature varies in this lipoma variant {1752, 2106}. By definition, vessels are of capillary dimension and generally most prominent beneath the tumour capsule. Fibrin thrombi are a diagnostic finding. With time, interstitial fibrosis may ensue. Angiolipomas may be over-diagnosed since by their nature, ordinary haemangiomas are often accompanied by fat.

Hibernoma
This lipoma variant is rare in the CNS. It

resembles brown fat and is composed of uniform granular or multivacuolated cells with small, centrally placed nuclei {336}.

Complex lipomatous lesions
These vary considerably in terms of their histological composition. For example, lumbosacral lipomas (leptomyelolipomas) {837} consist of lobulated adipose tissue, often in association with fibrous tissue, vascular proliferation, smooth muscle elements, and neuroglial tissue, particularly ependyma ('fibrolipomatous hamartoma'). Lipomas of the cerebellopontine angle {161}, an uncommonly affected off-midline site, may incorporate intradural portions of cranial nerve roots and their ganglia. Many also feature striated muscle or other mesenchymal tissues. It has even been suggested that intracranial lipomas containing various other tissue types represent a transition between lipoma and teratoma {2264}. Whether these various lesions are neoplasms or neomalformative overgrowths remains to be determined.

Epidural lipomatosis
This rare lesion consists of diffuse hypertrophy of spinal epidural adipose tissue. As such, it is not a neoplasm but

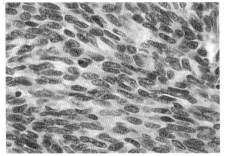

Fig. 10.17 Primary CNS leiomyosarcoma, fascicles of spindle cells showing characteristic cigar-shaped nuclei.

a metabolic response, often to chronic administration of steroids {749}.

Intracranial liposarcoma
This neoplasm is extremely rare. An example associated with subdural haematoma has been described {352}. An example of gliosarcoma with a liposarcomatous element has also been reported {200}.

Fibrous tumours
Fibromatosis
This locally infiltrative but cytologically benign, generally hypocellular lesion is composed of elongate fibroblasts in an abundant collagenous stroma {1490}. The process must be differentiated from pseudotumoural cranial fasciitis of childhood, a process histologically related to nodular fasciitis, featuring rapid growth within the deep scalp, lacking an intradural component and having no malignant potential {1267}. Cranial infantile myofibromatosis also enters into the differential diagnosis {2130}. Another pseudotumoural lesion, hypertrophic intracranial pachymeningitis, entails progressive dural thickening owing to pachymeningeal fibrosis and chronic inflammation often associated with autoimmune disorders {2209}. Myofibroblastomas of the CNS are akin to mammary type myofibroblastoma. They are closely related to benign fibrous proliferation, differing only in their strong smooth muscle actin and desmin immunoreactivity and their myofibroblastic ultrastructure {2089}.

Solitary fibrous tumour
This lesion affects both cranial and spinal meninges, rarely arises in spinal nerve roots, affects mainly adults and may show invasion of CNS parenchyma or nerve roots {287, 964} as well as the skull base {295}. Spinal seeding is rare {1499}. Its spindle cells are disposed in fascicles between prominent, eosinophilic bands of collagen. There is strong immunoreactivity for vimentin, CD34, and Bcl-2, but not EMA or S-100 protein. The relation of solitary fibrous tumour to rare cases of intracranial fibroma {1864} and myxoma {717A} is unclear.

Inflammatory myofibroblastic tumour
Inflammatory myofibroblastic tumour (IMT) is a distinctive neoplastic proliferation once considered synonymous with

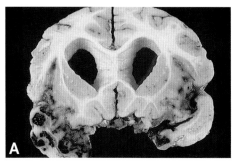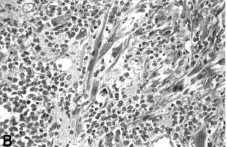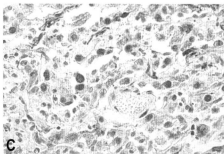

Fig. 10.18 Rhabdomyosarcoma. **A** Bilateral fronto-temporal lesion. **B** Small, undifferentiated cells intermingled with rhabdomyoblasts and strap-like cells. **C** Embryonal rhabdomyosarcoma showing strong desmin immunoreactivity.

inflammatory pseudotumour or plasma cell granuloma and a variant of inflammatory fibrosarcoma {365}. Initially reported to involve the mediastinum and pulmonary parenchyma, IMTs were subsequently found in various other organs. Recent studies demonstrated their neoplastic nature, the demonstration of ALK fusion genes separating IMT from non-neoplastic inflammatory lesions in the "inflammatory pseudotumour" and "plasma cell granuloma" categories.

IMTs of the CNS are rare and can occur at any age. Their radiological characteristics are often similar to meningiomas. Unlike pseudoneoplastic, inflammatory pseudotumours, IMTs appear to be unassociated with immune deficiency or other systemic diseases.

Histologically, IMTs are composed of myofibroblasts in association with stromal lymphoplasmacyte and eosinophil infiltrates. The three different patterns reported in IMTs of soft tissue, including the myxoid-nodular fasciitis-like, fibromatosis-like and scar-like, have all been observed in the CNS. The myofibroblast, the cell comprising the majority component, typically shows significant cytological atypia and mitotic figures. The immunohistochemical stains demonstrate uniform vimentin, smooth muscle actin, and often, but invariably strong, focal or diffuse ALK staining, especially in young patients. Most IMTs have favourable outcomes following gross total resection.

Fibrosarcoma

This rare, malignant tumour shows interlacing bundles of spindle cells disposed in a "herringbone" pattern. Fibrosarcomas are markedly cellular, exhibit brisk mitotic activity, and often feature necrosis {652}. Sclerosing epithelioid fibrosarcoma has also been reported to affect the CNS {169}.

Fibrohistiocytic tumours
Benign fibrous histiocytoma
This lesion, also termed fibrous xanthoma or fibroxanthoma, may involve dura or cranial bone {2292}, is composed of a mixture of spindled (fibroblast-like) and plump (histiocyte-like) cells arranged in a storiform pattern. Scattered giant cells and/or inflammatory cells are commonly seen. Many tumours initially published as fibrous xanthoma were subsequently shown to be GFAP-positive {1078}, and reclassified as pleomorphic xanthoastrocytoma.

Malignant fibrous histiocytoma (MFH)
This neoplasm consists of spindled, plump and pleomorphic giant cells that can be arranged in a storiform or fascicular pattern. Most MFH are obviously malignant, featuring numerous mitoses as well as necrosis. Only isolated cases of the inflammatory variant of MFH have been reported to involve brain {1409}.

Myogenic tumours
Leiomyoma
Most benign smooth muscle tumours are readily recognized by their pattern of intersecting fascicles composed of eosinophilic spindle cells with blunt-ended nuclei {1323}. As a rule, they lack mitotic activity. Occasional examples feature nuclear palisading and should not be mistaken for schwannoma. Diffuse leptomeningeal leiomyomas {967} as well as an angioleiomyomatous variant {1244} have been described. EB virus and AIDS-associated cases have also been reported {1050}.

Leiomyosarcoma
Intracranial leiomyosarcomas {442} correspond histologically to their soft-tissue counterparts, expressing desmin and smooth muscle actin. Most arise in the dura, but the parasellar region and

epidural space may also be affected {1406, 2490}. Parenchymal examples are rare {507}. An association with EB virus and AIDS is established {2490}. One unique example originating in a pineal teratoma has been reported {2108}.

Rhabdomyoma
This lesion consists entirely of mature striated muscle, but one reported example associated with a cranial nerve featured a minor adipose tissue component {2315}. CNS rhabdomyoma must be distinguished from skeletal muscle heterotopias, most of which occur within prepontine leptomeninges {584}.

Rhabdomyosarcoma
Whether meningeal or parenchymal, nearly all CNS rhabdomyosarcomas are of the embryonal type {1827, 2215}, while alveolar rhabdomyosarcoma has not been reported. Strap cells with cross striations may be observed. However, most tumours consist primarily of small cells that show little or no specific differentiation at the H&E level. Thus, immunohistochemistry and/or electron microscopy may be necessary for diagnosis. Immunostains for desmin and myogenin usually confirm the diagnosis. The ultrastructural findings of thick (myosin) and thin (actin) filaments arrayed in sarcomeres is also diagnostic. Rhabdomyosarcoma must be differentiated from other brain tumours that occasionally show skeletal muscle elements, such as medullomyoblastoma, gliosarcoma, germ cell tumours and even a rare meningioma {953}. Malignant ectomesenchymoma, a mixed tumour composed of ganglion cells or neuroblasts and one or more mesenchymal elements, usually rhabdomyosarcoma, may also occur in the brain {1704}.

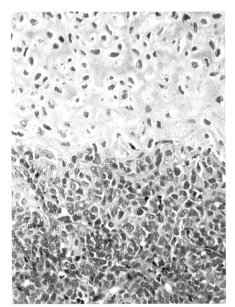

Fig. 10.19 Mesenchymal chondrosarcoma with cellular portion resembling a haemangiopericytoma.

Osteocartilaginous tumours

These benign osteocartilaginous tumours are usually dural-based; outside the CNS, they often develop in the skull and only secondarily displace dura and brain {385, 1235}. Histologically, they correspond to similar tumours arising in bone, but are to be separated from asymptomatic dural calcification, ossification related to metabolic disease or trauma, and neuroectodermal tumours such as astrocytoma and gliosarcoma that occasionally show osseous or chondroid differentiation. Transition of CNS chondroma to chondrosarcoma has rarely been documented {1497}.

Mesenchymal chondrosarcoma

This neoplasm more often arises in bones of the skull or spine than within dura or brain parenchyma {1956, 2009, 2465}. Nonetheless, the CNS is the most common site of extraosseous examples. Some tumours consist primarily of the small-cell component punctuated by scant islands of atypical hyaline cartilage, whereas the cartilage predominates in others. The histological pattern of the small-cell element closely resembles haemangiopericytoma, replete with staghorn vascular spaces and an intercellular pattern of reticulin staining. Although the diagnosis of mesenchymal chondrosarcoma generally poses no problem, in the absence of cartilage, immunohistochemistry is of no particular benefit in distinguishing this lesion from haemangiopericytoma or other small-cell sarcomas {2188}. Even less frequent in the CNS are differentiated chondrosarcoma and myxoid chondrosarcoma {1176, 1704}. Chondrosarcomas arising in the skull base, particularly in the midline, should be distinguished from chondroid chordoma. Unlike chondroid chordoma, chondrosarcomas are non-reactive for keratin and epithelial membrane antigen {1491}. Intracranial, extraosseous chondrosarcomas of the classic type are rare {317, 1650}. The same is true of myxoid chondrosarcoma, which has been reported to arise within brain {321} as well as in the leptomeninges of the brain.

Osteosarcoma

Preferred sites are the skull or spine and, more rarely, the meninges or the brain {115, 283, 1969, 1976, 2055}. Direct formation of bone or osteoid by the proliferating tumour cells is requisite to the diagnosis. Osteosarcomatous elements may exceptionally be encountered as components of germ cell tumour and gliosarcoma {106}.

Vascular tumours

Most vascular lesions of the central nervous system are malformative in nature and include arteriovenous malformation, cavernous angioma, venous angioma and capillary teleangiectasis {984}. Blood vessel tumours are to be differentiated from intravascular papillary endothelial hyperplasia, a tumour-like, reactive papillary proliferation of endothelium associated with thrombosis, which may occur in brain or meninges {1190}. This discussion is limited to vascular neoplasms: benign (haemangioma), intermediate grade (haemangioendothelioma), and malignant (angiosarcoma, Kaposi sarcoma).

Haemangioma

These lesions vary in size from microscopic to massive. Depending upon their histological appearance, haemangiomas are classified as capillary or cavernous. Of those affecting the CNS, most are primary lesions of bone that impinge secondarily upon the CNS. Dural {1, 1072} and parenchymal {2102} haemangiomas are less common.

Epithelioid haemangioendothelioma

Skull base, dura or brain parenchyma are rare locations for this neoplasm {1522, 1604}. Its cells possess relatively abundant eosinophilic cytoplasm and may be vacuolated. In general, nuclei are round or occasionally indented, vesicular, and show only minor atypia. Mitoses and limited necrosis may be seen. Vascular lumens are often small and intracytoplasmic. Their somewhat nodular architecture often features chondroid or myxoid stromal change. Immunohistochemical (factor VIII-related antigen, Ulex europeus lectin, CD31) and ultrastructural studies (Weibel-Palade bodies) confirm the endothelial nature. Conventional haemangioendothelioma {849} and the related epithelioid {80} and polymorphous {1916} variants have all been reported to occur in the central nervous system.

Angiosarcoma

The rare examples originating in brain or meninges {1450} vary in differentiation from patently vascular tumours with anastomosing vascular channels lined by mitotically active, cytologically atypical endothelial cells, to poorly differentiated, often epithelioid lesions in which immunohistochemical and ultrastructural studies are required for a definitive diagnosis. Occasional cytokeratin reactivity complicates distinguishing poorly differentiated

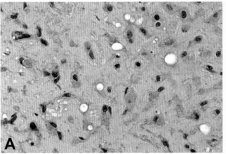
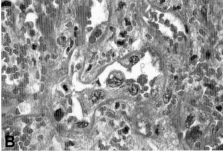

Fig. 10.20 **A** Epithelioid haemangioendothelioma with intracellular lumina and basophilic extracellular matrix. **B** Angiosarcoma showing abnormal vascular channels lined by atypical plump endothelial cells.

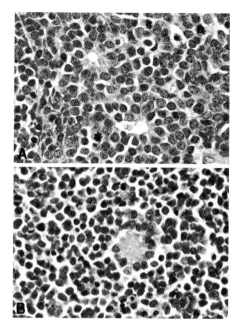

Fig. 10.21 Histological features of EWS-pPNET, showing rare rosettes (**A**) and a rare Homer Wright rosette (**B**).

angiosarcoma from metastatic carcinoma {1893}.

Kaposi sarcoma

This malignant neoplasm is characterized by spindle-shaped cells lining or forming slit-like blood vessels and is only exceptionally encountered as a parenchymal or meningeal tumour in the setting of AIDS {268}. In such instances, it is often difficult to determine whether the lesion is primary or secondary. The tumour is almost always immunopositive for herpesvirus 8 (HHV-8) {1899A}

Meningeal sarcomatosis

Meningeal sarcomatosis is a diffuse leptomeningeal sarcoma lacking circumscribed masses {2287}. Strictly defined as a non-meningothelial mesenchymal tumour, most are poorly differentiated "spindle cell" sarcomas. Re-examination of published cases using immunohistochemistry has revealed that most actually represented carcinoma, lymphoma, glioma or primitive neuroectodermal tumours.

Ewing sarcoma-peripheral primitive neuroectodermal tumour (EWS-pPNET)

EWS-pPNET is a rare small round cell tumour that involves the CNS as either a primary dural neoplasm {450, 1424, 1502, 2097} or by direct extension from contiguous bone or soft tissue (e.g. skull, vertebra, paraspinal soft tissue). Both

spinal and intracranial examples have been encountered and may mimic meningioma radiologically. A wide age range has been reported, although peak incidence is in the second decade. The histology, immunophenotype, and biology is essentially identical to that encountered in bone or soft tissue {587}. The tumour is composed of sheets of small, round, primitive appearing cells with thin rims of PAS-positive, diastase sensitive, glycogen-rich cytoplasm. The latter imparts a variable degree of cytoplasmic clearing. Homer Wright rosettes are occasionally seen, but are usually not prominent. The majority of tumours stain at least focally with neuronal markers, such as synaptophysin and neuron specific enolase, whereas cyto-keratin stains are typically negative or only focally reactive. CD99, the so-called "Ewing sarcoma antigen", shows strong and diffuse membrane immunoreactivity, but can also be expressed by a variety of other tumour types, including haemangiopericytoma and less commonly medulloblastoma/CNS PNET, two potential differential diagnostic considerations. Therefore, it is advisable to confirm the diagnosis of EWS-pPNET genetically via the t(11;22) (q24;q12) either karyotypically or by the presence of an EWS-FLI1 (or other EWS variant) fusion transcript. In paraffin-embedded tissue, FISH may be superior to RT-PCR for demonstrating the latter {223}.

Genetic susceptibility

Several associations with inherited disease are worth noting; intracranial cartilaginous tumours may be associated with Maffucci syndrome and Ollier disease, lipomas with encephalocraniocutaneous lipomatosis, and osteosarcoma with Paget disease.

Genetics

Although the molecular genetic alterations of intracranial sarcomas may be similar to those of corresponding soft tissue lesions {59}, few data are available to date. Nevertheless, examples of meningeal-based EWS-pPNET have shown the typical EWS type rearrangements found in the bone and soft tissue counterparts {450,1424}. One case of MFH showed a complex karyotype, similar to those reported for soft tissue MFH {155}.

Histogenesis

Mesenchymal tumours affecting the CNS are thought to arise from craniospinal

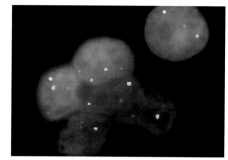

Fig. 10.22 EWS-pPNET with yellow or red-green EWS-FLI1 fusion signals by FISH analysis.

meninges, vasculature and surrounding osseous structures. Osteocartilaginous and myoid tumours may arise: (i) from rarely occurring meningeal heterotopias, (ii) from multipotential mesenchymal cells, (iii) by acquisition of additional lines of mesenchymal differentiation in fibrous or fibrohistiocytic tumours, or (iv) within a teratoma {283}. Since cranial and intracranial mesenchymal structures, such as bone, cartilage and muscle, are in part derived from the neuroectoderm (ectomesenchyme), the development of the corresponding sarcoma types could also represent reversion to a more primitive stage of differentiation. Lipomas arising within the CNS are often associated with developmental anomalies, particularly partial or complete agenesis of the corpus callosum and spinal dysraphism with tethered cord {177, 2466}. Intracranial rhabdomyosarcoma may also be associated with malformations of the CNS {820}.

Prognostic and predictive factors

Whereas most benign mesenchymal tumours can be completely resected and carry a favourable prognosis, primary intracranial sarcomas are aggressive and associated with a poor outcome. Local recurrence and/or distant lepto-meningeal seeding are typical. For example, despite aggressive radiation and chemotherapy, CNS rhabdomyosarcomas have been almost uniformly fatal within two years. Systemic metastases of intracranial sarcomas are relatively common. Nevertheless, primary CNS sarcomas are less aggressive than glioblastomas with 5-year survivals in a series of 18 cases estimated at 28% for high-grade and 83% for low-grade examples {1636}.

Haemangiopericytoma

C. Giannini
E.J. Rushing
J.A. Hainfellner

Definition
A highly cellular and vascularized mesenchymal tumour exhibiting a characteristic monotonous low-power appearance and a well-developed, variably thick-walled, branching "staghorn" vasculature; almost always attached to the dura and having a high tendency to recur and to metastasize outside the CNS.

ICD-O codes
Haemangiopericytoma   9150/1
Anaplastic haemangiopericytoma
                             9150/3

Grading
Haemangiopericytomas correspond histologically to WHO grade II, with anaplastic haemangiopericytomas corresponding to WHO grade III.

Synonyms and historical annotation
Haemangiopericytoma was described as a distinctive soft tissue tumour in 1942 by Stout and Murray {2160}, who postulated its pericytic origin. In 1938, Cushing and Eisenhardt {406} described three variants of 'angioblastic meningiomas'; in retrospect, variant 1 represented haemangiopericytoma {1959}. The 1979 WHO classification {2513} still contained the 'haemangiopericytic' variant of meningioma, but it has now been long accepted that haemangiopericytoma and meningioma are different entities. In soft tissue tumours, the term haemangiopericytoma has evolved to describe a heterogeneous group of tumours, which simply shared a common "haemangiopericytic growth" pattern {586}. The nosological position of CNS haemangiopericytoma remains uncertain, but at present meningeal haemangiopericytoma is still recognized as a clinicopathologically well-characterized malignancy distinct from meningioma. Whereas in most cases it is distinct from solitary fibrous tumour, a spectrum between the two has been suggested {2248}.

Incidence
Meningeal haemangiopericytoma constitutes approximately 0.4% of all primary CNS tumours. In three large series of meningeal tumours, the ratios of meningeal haemangiopericytoma to meningioma were about 1:40 {738}, 1:50 {943} and 1:60 {987}.

Age and sex distribution
Meningeal haemangiopericytomas tend to occur at a younger age than meningiomas, and slightly more often in men than in women. In three large clinical series of 66 men and 47 women (M/F ratio, 1.4:1), the mean age at diagnosis was 43 years {738, 943, 986}.

Localization
Primary haemangiopericytomas of the CNS are almost invariably solitary {2039} and attached to the cranial or spinal dura. In four large series of 153 meningeal haemangiopericytomas, 8% were spinal and two were intraparenchymal {738, 869, 986, 1754}. Rare intraventricular examples have been reported {5, 790, 1543}. Haemangiopericytoma occurs slightly more often in the occipital region, around the confluence of sinuses, and attached to venous sinuses {406, 944, 1754}.

Clinical features
As suggested by their location, the symptoms of meningeal haemangiopericytoma are indistinguishable from those of meningioma.

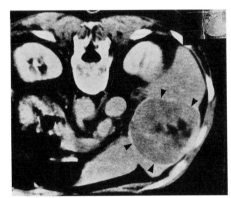

Fig. 10.24 Liver metastasis of a primary intracranial haemangiopericytoma seven and one half years after surgical resection. From Jaaskelainen *et al.* {943}.

Neuroimaging
On plain films, a well-demarcated, lytic lesion of adjacent bone supports haemangiopericytoma, whereas hyperostosis, a typical feature of meningioma, is absent {598, 738, 944}. The hypervascularity seen on angiography explains the tendency to bleed; it typically shows a dual blood supply from meningeal and cortical arteries and corkscrew-like vessels in a densely stained tumour {598, 944}. CT and MRI show a sharply demarcated tumour with dural attachment, smooth or nodular margin and intense contrast enhancement. Significant edema in underlying brain parenchyma is frequently present {598}. Unlike meningiomas, haemangiopericytomas typically lack calcification {40, 598}.

Macroscopy
At surgery, meningeal haemangiopericytoma is a solid, well-demarcated tumour. It has a tendency to bleed during removal, sometimes profusely {943}. The resected tumour specimen is usually globoid, slightly lobulated and rather firm. Cut surfaces are fleshy, greyish to red-brown or frankly hemorrhagic in appearance, often with a number of visible vascular spaces.

Histopathology
Haemangiopericytomas are monomorphous tumours composed of closely

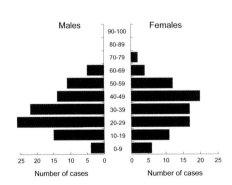

Fig. 10.23 Age and sex distribution of haemangiopericytoma, based on 186 cases.

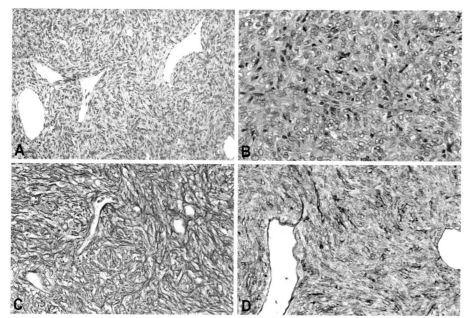

Fig. 10.25 Histological features of haemangiopericytoma. **A** Highly cellular tumour with dilated, staghorn-type vessels. **B** Higher power demonstrates jumbled arrangement of spindle cells. **C** Well developed reticulin fibers. **D** CD34 immunoreactivity in tumour cells and endothelial cells.

packed, randomly oriented tumour cells with little intervening fibrosis. Cytoplasm is scant and cell borders are indistinct. Nuclei are round to oval, occasionally elongated, with moderately dense chromatin and inconspicuous nucleoli, lacking the pseudo-inclusions characteristic of meningiomas {986, 1451}. Nuclear atypia and mitotic activity vary. Anaplastic (grade III) tumours show a high degree of mitotic activity (at least 5 mitoses per 10 HPF) and/or necrosis, plus at least two of the following: haemorrhage, moderate to high nuclear atypia and cellularity {1451}. A rich network of reticulin fibers, typically investing individual cells, is one of the most characteristic but not invariable features of this neoplasm. Haemangiopericytoma is highly vascular, with numerous slit-like vascular channels lined by flattened endothelial cells and frequent gaping, thin-walled and branching vascular spaces, so-called "staghorn sinusoids". The uniform cellularity of the tumour may be interrupted by "geographic" areas of reduced cell density with a corresponding increase in tumour matrix and/or perivascular fibrosis. Necrosis is uncommon. Calcification, including psammoma bodies, are not seen. Despite their gross appearance of forming discrete masses, haemangiopericytomas may invade and destroy adjacent bone, without the

hyperostotic reaction characteristic of meningiomas. Infiltration of adjacent brain parenchyma may be observed.

Immunohistochemistry

Haemangiopericytoma cells are diffusely immunoreactive for vimentin (85%), factor XIIIa (80–100 %) in individual scattered cells, Leu-7 (70%), and, in 33–100% of cases, for CD34 {1732, 1861}. The latter is usually patchy, in contrast to the diffuse pattern typical of solitary fibrous tumour. Focal positivity for desmin, smooth muscle actin, and cytokeratin may be occasionally encountered {986, 1732, 1825, 2418}. Although strong and diffuse immunoreactivity for epithelial membrane antigen and claudin-1 are typical of meningioma {754, 1861}, focal, generally weak immunoreactivity has been reported in haemangiopericytoma {1732, 1825}. Tumour cells are negative for S-100 protein, classical endothelial antigens such as CD31 {1732}, as well as progesterone receptor {492}. Although the immunoreactivity pattern of haemangiopericytoma is diverse and no single antibody is either 100% sensitive or specific, its immunoprofile is generally sufficiently distinctive to permit the exclusion of meningioma and solitary fibrous tumour {1732, 1825, 2248}.

Vascular endothelial growth factor VEGF-A is up-regulated in tumour cells and the

receptors VEGFR-1 and VEGFR-2 (but not VEGFR-3) in endothelial cells, suggesting a paracrine mode of interaction {791}. Endothelial cells also express Tie-1 {791}, a tyrosine kinase receptor associated with enhanced neovascularization.

Electron microscopy

Closely spaced elongated cells with short processes may contain small bundles of intracytoplasmic intermediate filaments and are surrounded by electron-dense, extracellular basement membrane-like material, the ultrastructural equivalent of the reticulin network visible on light microscopy. True desmosomes and gap junctions are absent {414, 986}.

Proliferation

The time to recurrence after complete removal, a rough indicator of the volume growth rate, varies remarkably, but the median time intervals of 40 {738} and 70 months {943} suggest that meningeal haemangiopericytomas grow more rapidly than meningiomas {2039}. In most cases, mitotic activity is prominent. The median Ki-67 (MIB-1) labelling index was 10% (0.6–36%) in a series of 31 tumours {2352} and 5% (1.2–39 %) in another study of 62 tumours {1802}, i.e. values at the level of anaplastic (WHO grade III) meningiomas. The median S-phase fraction was 4% (1.6–15%) in 31 tumours {2352}.

Genetic susceptibility

There is no evidence of familial clustering of meningeal haemangiopericytoma. One report notes the occurrence of peripheral haemangiopericytoma in three members of one family {1763}.

Genetics

Karyotypes of meningeal haemangiopericytomas show abnormalities of chromosome 12, particularly in the region 12q13-15. The second most frequent alterations are abnormalities of chromosome 3 {1407}. Rearrangements of chromosome 12q13, a region that includes a number of oncogenes, are less consistent; alterations on 6p21, 7p15 and 19q13 have been reported in meningeal and/or peripheral haemangiopericytomas {809, 813, 1392}. However, no consistent chromosomal losses or gains were found in 11 peripheral haemangiopericytomas by comparative genomic hybridization (CGH) {1470}. No allelic losses have been reported on 22q, the region harbouring the *NF2* gene. Neither meningeal nor peripheral haemangiopericytomas contain *NF2* mutations (0/38), whereas 32% of meningiomas have such alterations {1009}. Homozygous deletions of the *CDKN2A* gene on 9p were found in about 25% (7/28) of meningeal haemangiopericytomas, but infrequently (1/26) in meningiomas {1647}. No point mutations in *CDKN2A* or *TP53* genes are found {1647}.

Histogenesis

The histogenesis of meningeal haemangiopericytoma is uncertain. The Working Group of the new WHO Classification of Tumours of Soft Tissue and Bone stated that most lesions formerly known as haemangiopericytoma show no evidence of pericytic differentiation and, instead, are fibroblastic in nature and form a morphological continuum with solitary fibrous tumour {586}. This concept may pertain to meningeal haemangiopericytomas as well {657}.

Prognostic and predictive factors

The majority of tumours can be removed in a seemingly complete manner but, unlike meningiomas, local recurrences are almost inevitable. In two series, they occurred in 91% {2352} and 85% of cases {738} after 15 years. In one series, 9 of 17 irradiated haemangiopericytomas recurred with a median of 58 months, but 13 of the 15 non-irradiated tumours

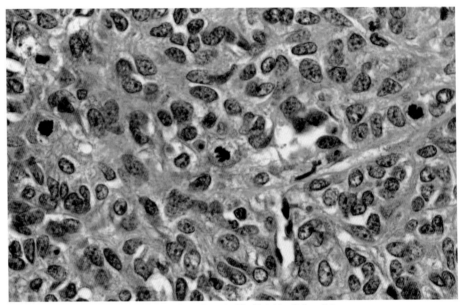

Fig. 10.26 Anaplastic haemangiopericytoma (WHO grade III) with brisk mitotic activity.

recurred with a median of only 29 months {738}. The majority of meningeal haemangiopericytomas eventually metastasize to the bones, lungs and liver. Mean survival time after diagnosis of metastasis was 2 years {738, 2352}. In a series of 28 patients who had survived the primary removal, the probability of tumour-related death was 61% at 15 years {2352}. One study found that the 5-year survival of patients with haemangiopericytoma has improved during the past 10 years and suggested that improved treatment of patients with cancer, a low

intraoperative mortality rate and the use of radiosurgery in the treatment of recurrent disease may all contribute {506}.
The prognostic significance of proliferation is discussed above. Using the criteria noted above {1451} in distinguishing "low-" from "high-" grade tumours, one study found that high-grade tumours recurred 6.7 years earlier than low-grade {506}. Despite the increased recurrence rate for anaplastic examples, no significant survival effect was associated with tumour grade {506}.

Melanocytic lesions

D.J. Brat
A. Perry

Definition
Primary melanocytic neoplasms of the CNS that arise from leptomeningeal melanocytes and that can be diffuse or circumscribed, benign or malignant. This group includes (1) diffuse melanocytosis and melanomatosis, (2) melanocytoma and (3) malignant melanoma.

Incidence
Melanocytomas account for 0.06–0.1% of brain tumours. The annual incidence is approximately 1 per 10 million population {954}. Primary CNS melanomas are also infrequent, with an incidence of 0.005 cases per 100 000 population {804}. The diffuse leptomeningeal melanocytic lesions are rare and population-based incidence is not available {1022}.

Age and sex distribution
Diffuse leptomeningeal melanocytosis and melanomatosis are strongly linked with neurocutaneous melanosis, a rare phakomatosis of childhood that typically presents before age two. Among one series of 39 such cases, ages at presentation ranged from stillbirth to the second decade with an equal gender distribution and no racial predisposition {1022}. Melanocytomas occur in all ages (range 9–73 years), but are most frequent in the fifth decade (45–50 years), with a slight female predominance (female: male 1.5:1) {216, 357}. Primary nodular melanomas arise in patients ranging from 15–71 years old (mean, 43 years).

Localization
Diffuse melanocytosis and melanomatosis involve the supra- and infratentorial leptomeninges and the superficial brain parenchyma. They involve large expanses of the subarachnoid space, with focal or multifocal intensity. Sites of highest frequency include the cerebellum, pons, medulla and temporal lobes. Most melanocytomas arise in the extramedullary, intradural compartment at the cervical and thoracic spinal levels. They can be dural-based or associated with nerve roots or spinal foramina {216, 701}. Less frequently, they arise from the leptomeninges in the posterior fossa and supratentorial compartments. Meckel's cave is a site with a peculiar predilection for primary melanocytic neoplasms and tumours of this site are associated with ipsilateral Ota's nevus {91, 1745}. Nodular melanomas are dura-based and occur throughout the neuroaxis, showing a slight predilection for the spinal cord and posterior fossa.

Clinical features
Symptoms and signs
Melanocytosis and melanomatosis are associated with neurocutaneous melanosis, a rare phakomatosis characterized by large or numerous congenital cutaneous nevi together with benign or malignant diffuse leptomeningeal melanosis {1389}. Neurologic symptoms arise secondary to either hydrocephalus or local effects on the CNS parenchyma. Neuropsychiatric symptoms, bowel and bladder dysfunction, and sensory and motor disturbances are common. Once malignant transformation occurs, symptoms progress rapidly, with increasing intracranial pressure resulting in irritability, vomiting, lethargy and seizures. Melanocytomas and malignant melanomas present with symptoms related to compression of the spinal cord, cerebellum or cerebrum by an extra-axial mass, with focal neurological signs depending on the location {1614}.

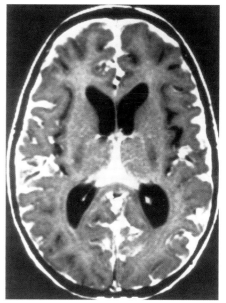

Fig. 10.28 Post-contrast T1-weighted MRI of diffuse melanocytosis, showing contrast enhancement of the infiltrated meninges.

Neuroimaging
CT and MRI of melanocytosis and melanomatosis shows diffuse thickening and enhancement of the leptomeninges, often with focal nodularity. Melanocytomas have characteristic MRI appearance due to the paramagnetic properties of melanin; they are isodense or hyperintense on T1-weighted images and hypointense on T2-weighted images. They also show homogeneous enhancement on post-contrast images {1614}. Primary CNS melanomas show the same general pattern on MRI, depending on the content of melanin. CNS structures adjacent to melanoma are often T2-hyperintense, reflecting vasogenic edema generated in response to rapid tumour growth.

Macroscopy
Diffuse melanocytic lesions appear as a dense black replacement of the subarachnoid space or as dusky clouding of the meninges. Melanocytoma and malignant melanoma are solitary mass lesions, generally extra-axial, that may appear black, red-brown, blue or macroscopically non-pigmented.

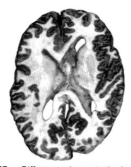

Fig. 10.27 Diffuse melanocytosis involving the subarachnoid space of the cerebral hemisphere and invading the cerebral cortex.

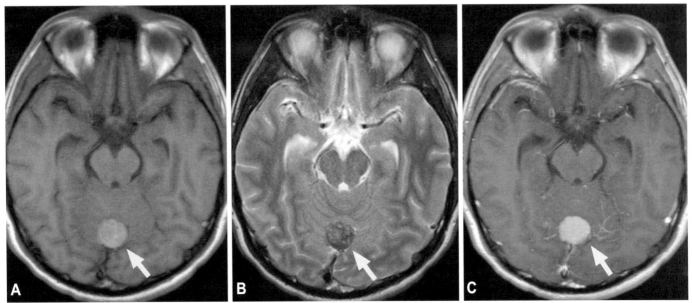

Fig. 10.29 MRI features of melanocytoma. **A** T1-weighted axial images (pre-contrast) reveal a hyperintense, well-circumscribed mass in the midline of the cerebellum arising from the dura. **B** On T2-weighted images, the mass is hypointense. **C** Following the adminstration of contrast agent, the melanocytoma shows homogeneous enhancement.

Histopathology

Diagnosis hinges on the recognition of tumour cells that have melanocytic differentiation. Most benign and malignant melanocytic lesions display melanin pigment finely distributed within tumour cells and coarsely distributed within the tumour stroma and the cytoplasm of tumoural macrophages (melanophages). Rare melanocytomas and occasional primary melanomas will not demonstrate melanin pigment; diagnosis then relies more heavily on electron microscopy and immunohistochemistry. Identification of melanocytic lesions usually requires histopathological examination, yet the diagnosis of diffuse melanosis and melanomatosis has occasionally been made by CSF cytology {307, 468, 1863}.

Diffuse melanocytosis

The pathologic proliferation of lepto-meningeal melanocytes and their production of melanin is the source of melanosis {465, 1022}. Tumour cells diffusely involving the leptomeninges assume a variety of shapes, including spindled, round, oval or cuboidal. In melanocytosis, individual cells are cytologically bland. Melanocytic cells can accumulate within Virchow-Robin spaces without demonstrating overt CNS invasion. In distinction, unequivocal CNS parenchymal invasion should not be seen in melanocytosis, and when identified, must be considered evidence of malignant change to melanomatosis.

Melanocytoma

Melanocytomas are solitary, low-grade tumours that do not invade surrounding structures {216, 1781, 2280}. Slightly spindled or oval tumour cells containing variable melanin often form tight nests with a superficial resemblance to whorls of meningioma. Heavily pigmented tumour cells and tumoural macrophages are seen at the periphery of nests. Other melanocytoma variants demonstrate storiform, vasocentric and sheetlike arrangements. Only rare amelanotic melanocytomas have been described. Nuclei are oval or bean-shaped with small esosinophilic nucleoli. Cytologic atypia and mitoses are generally absent (on average, less 1/10 HPF). It has been suggested that melanocytic tumours with bland cytologic features, such as those of melanocytoma, but showing CNS invasion or elevated mitotic activity, should be classified as intermediate grade melanocytic neoplasms {216}.

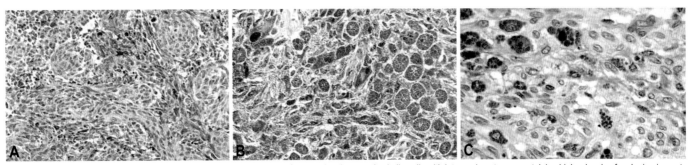

Fig. 10.30 Histological features of melanocytoma. **A** Loose or tight nests of low-grade, pigmented spindle cells with intervening stroma containing higher levels of melanin pigment. **B** Melanin containing macrophages (melanophages). **C** Melanocytoma cells showing clear to eosinophilic cytoplasm with variable fine pigment. Nuclei are bean-shaped and have micronucleoli. Melanin within the cytoplasm of melanophages is typically in larger aggregates.

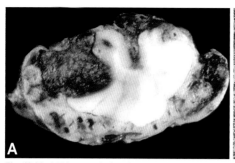 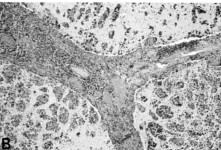 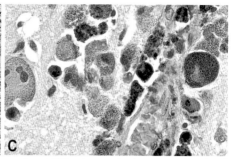

Fig. 10.31 **A** Primary spinal melanoma originating from the spinal cord and invading the subarachnoid space. **B** Primary malignant CNS melanoma showing extensive invasion of the cerebral cortex and subarachnoid space. **C** Highly polymorphic melanin-laden cells of a malignant melanoma invading the cerebral cortex.

Malignant melanoma

Malignant leptomeningeal melanoma is histologically similar to melanomas arising in other sites. Anaplastic spindled or epithelioid cells, arranged in loose nests, fascicles or sheets, display variable cytoplasmic melanin {216, 1863}. Melanomas may contain large cells with bizarre nuclei, numerous typical and atypical mitotic figures, significant pleomorphism, and large, often red nucleoli; others are densely cellular and less pleomorphic, usually consisting of tightly packed spindle cells with high nuclear to cytoplasmic ratios. Melanomas are more pleomorphic, have more anaplastic nuclei and have a higher cell density than melanocytoma, and will often demonstrate unequivocal tissue invasion or coagulative necrosis. Meningeal melanomatosis may arise from diffuse spreading of a primary malignant meningeal melanoma through the subarachnoid space.

Immunohistochemistry

Most tumours react with the anti-melanosomal antibodies HMB-45 or MART-1 (Melan-A), and microphthalmia transcription factor. They also express S-100 protein. Staining for vimentin and neuron-specific enolase are variable.

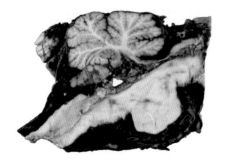

Fig. 10.32 Malignant melanoma infiltrating the meninges around brain stem and cerebellum.

There is no expression of GFAP, neurofilament proteins, cytokeratins and EMA; Ki-67 labelling indices are typically <1–2% in melanocytomas and average around 8% in primary melanomas {216}.

Electron microscopy

The cells of melanocytoma lack junctions and contain melanosomes at varying stages of development. In contrast to Schwann cell tumours, a well-formed pericellular basal lamina is lacking, but groups of melanocytoma cells may be ensheathed {30}. In contrast to meningioma, no desmosomes and no interdigitating cytoplasmic processes are encountered.

Differential diagnosis

Melanocytic lesions of the nervous system are to be distinguished from metastatic malignant melanoma and from histogenetically different nervous system tumours undergoing melanization, such as schwannoma, medulloblastoma, paraganglioma and various gliomas {30, 216}. There is little evidence to support the existence of a true melanotic meningioma, although rare melanocytic colonization of meningiomas has been documented {1580}. Melanotic neuroectodermal tumour of infancy (retinal anlage tumour) has also been reported at intracranial locations {1042}.

Genetic susceptibility

Neurocutaneous melanosis (neurocutaneous melanocytosis) is a combination of diffuse melanocytosis with giant or numerous congenital melanocytic nevi of the skin, usually involving midline, head and neck, and with various malformative lesions, e.g. Dandy Walker malformation, syringomyelia, lipomas, etc. {449, 468}. A genetic trait has not been unequivocally established. Approximately 25% of

patients with diffuse meningeal melanocytosis have significant concomitant cutaneous lesions. On the other hand, about 10–15% of patients with large congenital melanocytic nevi of the skin clinically present with CNS melanocytosis {449}, although radiologic evidence of CNS involvement is noted in up to 23% of asymptomatic children with giant congenital nevi {595}. Diffuse melanocytosis may also be associated with congenital naevus of Ota {91}.

Histogenesis

Melanocytic lesions of the nervous system and its coverings are thought to arise from leptomeningeal melanocytes that are derived from the neural crest. In the normal CNS, melanocytes are preferentially localized at the base of the brain, around the ventral medulla oblongata, and along the upper cervical spinal cord.

Prognostic and predictive factors

Diffuse melanosis carries a poor prognosis even in the absence of histologic malignancy {1863}. Melanocytoma lacks anaplastic features, but a few undergo local recurrences; the intermediate grade melanocytic tumours typically invade the CNS, although too few have been reported to predict the biology of these tumours {216}. A rare example of malignant transformation of a melanocytoma has also been reported {1934}. Malignant melanoma is a highly aggressive and radioresistant tumour with poor prognosis and may metastasize to remote organs. Nevertheless, the prognosis of the primary meningeal melanoma appears to be better than metastatic examples, particularly if localized and complete resection is possible {611}.

Haemangioblastoma

K.D. Aldape
K.H. Plate
A.O. Vortmeyer
D. Zagzag
H.P.H. Neumann

Definition
A slowly growing, highly vascular tumour of adults, occurring in the cerebellum, brain stem or spinal cord; histologically comprised of stromal cells and small blood vessels; occurring in sporadic forms and in association with von Hippel-Lindau (VHL) syndrome.

ICD-O code   9161/1

Grading
Haemangioblastoma corresponds to WHO grade I.

Synonyms and historical annotation
Haemangioblastoma is also referred to as capillary haemangioblastoma. In 1931, Lindau {1325} hypothesized that these tumours may be derived from a "congenital anlage" and that the histological picture revealed an "...embryological type of the tumour cells". Stein *et al.* {2148} suggested an angio-mesenchymal origin of haemangioblastoma, based on original, developmental biologic observations made by Sabin in 1917 {1967}.

Incidence
Haemangioblastomas are uncommon tumours that occur as sporadic as well as familial forms associated with von Hippel-Lindau disease. Accurate incidence rates are not available.

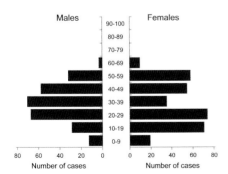

Fig. 10.33 Age and sex distribution of haemangioblastoma, based on 185 patients treated at the Universities of Freiburg (Germany) and Helsinki (Finland).

Age and sex distribution
Haemangioblastomas usually occur in adults. VHL syndrome-associated tumours may present in significantly younger patients than do sporadic tumours {1382}. The male:female ratio is approximately equal.

Localization
Haemangioblastomas may occur in any part of the nervous system. Sporadic tumours occur predominantly in the cerebellum, usually in the hemispheres, whereas VHL-associated haemangioblastomas may be multiple and affect the brain stem, spinal cord and nerve roots in addition to the cerebellum. Supratentorial and peripheral nervous system lesions are rare.

Clinical features
Symptoms generally arise from impaired CSF flow due to a cyst or solid tumour mass, resulting in an increase of intracranial pressure and hydrocephalus. Haemangioblastomas produce erythropoietin, and this may cause secondary polycythaemia.
Imaging studies typically demonstrate a gadolinium-enhancing mass with associated cyst in approximately 75% of cases. The solid component is usually peripheral in location within the cerebellar hemisphere. Flow voids may be seen within the nodule due to enlarged feeding/draining vessels. Angiography is useful to identify small lesions, showing a mass with a dense tangle of vessels, sometimes resembling an arteriovenous malformation. Evidence of calcification on imaging is usually absent. Spinal cord examples are often associated with a syrinx.

Macroscopy
Macroscopically, haemangioblastomas are well-circumscribed, highly vascularized red nodules, often in the wall of large cysts. At places, the tumour may appear yellow owing to its rich lipid content.

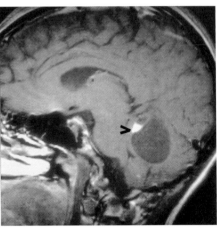

Fig. 10.34 Lateral MRI view of a cerebellar haemangioblastoma showing the hyperdense tumour nodule (arrow) and a large adjacent cyst.

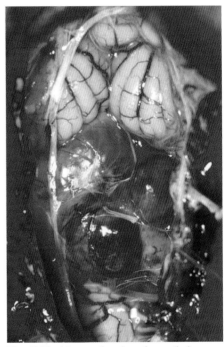

Fig. 10.35 Intraoperative view of a cystic haemangioblastoma in the region of the fourth ventricle and dorsal medulla oblongata.

Histopathology
Haemangioblastomas are characterized histologically by two main components: stromal cells that are characteristically large and vacuolated, but can reveal highly considerable cytologic variation,

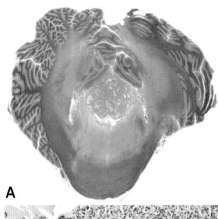

A

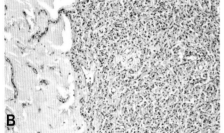

B

Fig. 10.36 Section of a cerebellar haemangioblastoma extending into the fourth ventricle (**A**). Higher magnification shows the typical distribution of tumour cells within a network of small capillaries (**B**). Note the hyalinised vascular stroma (left).

and abundant vascular cells. Cellular and reticular variants are distinguished on the basis of the abundance of the stromal cell component. Numerous thin-walled vessels are apparent and are readily outlined by a reticulin stain. In accordance with the highly vascular nature of haemangioblastoma, intra-tumoural haemorrhage may occur. Some tumours show extensive sclerosis. In adjacent reactive tissues, particularly in cyst and syrinx walls, astrocytic gliosis and Rosenthal fibers are frequently observed. The tumour edge is generally well-demarcated, and infiltration into surrounding neural tissues rarely occurs. Mitotic figures are rare. The stromal cells represent the neoplastic component of the tumour. Their nuclei may vary in size, with occasional atypical and hyper-chromatic nuclei. However, their most characteristic and distinguishing morphological feature is represented by numerous lipid-containing vacuoles, resulting in the typical 'clear cell' morphology of haemangioblastoma, which may resemble metastatic renal cell carcinoma. Adding to the complexity of this differential diagnosis is the fact that patients with VHL syndrome are prone to

renal cell carcinoma. There are also reports of tumour-to-tumour metastasis (renal cell carcinoma metastatic to haemangioblastoma) in this setting {759}.

Immunohistochemistry
The stromal and capillary endothelial cells differ significantly in their expression patterns. Stromal cells lack endothelial cell markers, such as von Willebrand factor and CD34, and do not express endothelium-associated adhesion molecules such as CD31 (PECAM) {191, 2422}. Unlike endothelial cells, stromal cells variably express neuron-specific enolase, neural cell adhesion molecule, S-100, CD56 and ezrin {191, 193, 923}. Vimentin is the major intermediate filament expressed by stromal cells. Stromal cells express a variety of molecules, including CXCR4 {1316, 2477} aquaporin 1 {1344}, several carbonic anhydrase isoenzymes {1803}, as well as EGFR {190}, but do not usually express glial fibrillary acidic protein {2422}. Vascular endothelial growth factor (VEGF), a prime regulator of physiological and pathological angio-genesis, is highly expressed in stromal cells {1187}, with corresponding endo-thelial expression of its receptors VEGFR-1 and -2 {2421}, and the endothelial cell receptor Tie-1 {791}. The endothelial cells of haemangioblastomas also express receptors for other angiogenic growth factors, including platelet-derived growth factors {190}.

Immunohistochemistry is useful to distinguish haemangioblastoma from renal cell carcinoma. Renal cell carci-noma is positive for epithelial markers, such as EMA, while haemangio-blastomas are negative. Additional potentially useful markers include the D2-40 antibody {1945} and inhibin A {847}, which are positive in haemangio-blastoma but generally negative in renal cell carcinoma. CD10 staining, in contrast, shows the opposite results {1018}.

Electron microscopy
Ultrastructurally, the most prominent feature of the stromal cells is an abundant electron-lucent cytoplasm containing lipid droplets. Some studies have demonstrated electron-dense bodies, reminiscent of Weibel-Palade bodies, and small granules, reminiscent of neuroendocrine granules.

Proliferation
Proliferation rates tend to be low, in the range of 0–2%, as measured by the MIB-1 antibody {1493}.

Genetic susceptibility
While most cases of haemangioblastoma are sporadic, a proportion of cases are associated with VHL syndrome (see Chapter 13).

Genetics
Sequencing of constitutional DNA from

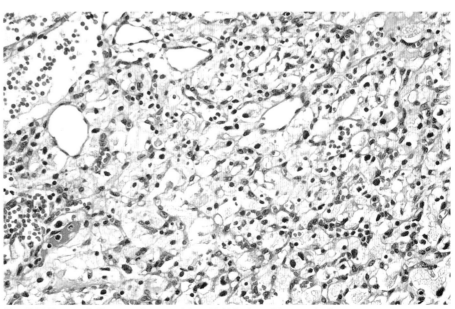

Fig. 10.37 Haemangioblastoma with accumulation of lipid droplets within stromal cells.

patients with haemangioblastoma reveals *VHL* mutations in a proportion of cases, as a recent study identified 5 germline mutations among patients from 16 families {1834}. Among 14 haemangioblastoma patients without evidence of a family history or additional clinical manifestations of VHL syndrome, 2 germline mutations in the *VHL* gene were identified {299}. While biallelic inactivation of the *VHL* gene is a frequent occurrence in familial cases, it is not common in sporadic tumours. Studies on sporadic tumours, including somatic mutation analyses, assessment of allelic loss, and hypermethylation studies have revealed loss or inactivation of the *VHL* gene area only in approximately 20% to 50% of the cases {694, 1277}. One study using comparative genomic hybridization indicated that multiple chromosomal aberrations, including those on 3p and elsewhere, are observed in sporadic tumours {682}. Loss of heterozygosity studies demonstrate allelic imbalance at chromosome 6q in the majority of cases, with a reported minimally deleted region at 6q23-24 {1291}.

Histogenesis

The histogenesis of haemangioblastoma is uncertain. Tissue microdissection, combined with deletion analysis of the *VHL* gene locus, have identified the stromal and not the vascular cells as neoplastic {1277, 2348}. More controversial, however, has been the identification of the nature of the stromal cell. A series of immunohistochemical studies has been performed to elucidate the origin of the stromal cell resulting in identification of markers that are consistently, frequently or only occasionally immunoreactive with the stromal cells.

Neural cell adhesion molecule (NCAM/ CD56) is consistently immunoreactive {192, 923}. Positive immunoreactivity for S-100 protein is frequently but not always observed {856, 1245}. Factor XIIIa has been reported to be expressed by haemangioblastoma stromal cells {1245, 1644}, while other studies found it exclusively expressed by the reactive vascular component {397, 2214}. Similarly, factor VIII has been found in the stromal cells by some authors {1020, 1035, 1644}, whereas others report expression to be limited to vascular cells {2214}. GFAP positivity is variable {923, 963} and it is unclear whether GFAP marks entrapped reactive astrocytes, stromal cells with glial differentiation or stromal cells with intracytoplasmic GFAP from phagocytic activity. It is therefore not surprising that the histogenesis of the stromal cell is controversial. Suggested origins include glial cells {45}, endothelial cells {1020}, arachnoid cells {1501}, embryonic choroid plexus {176}, neuroendocrine cells {123}, fibrohistiocytic cells {1579}, cells of neuroectodermal derivation {12} or heterogeneous cell populations {2214}. It was noted that stromal cells of haemangioblastoma express proteins common to embryonal haemangioblast progenitor cells {696}. It was further noted that one such protein, Scl, has a distribution of expression in the developing nervous system that is similar to the topographical distribution of haemangioblastoma tumours in patients.

Prognostic and predictive factors

The prognosis of CNS haemangioblastoma is excellent if surgical resection can be achieved, which is often possible. Permanent neurological deficits are rare {375} and can be avoided when CNS haemangioblastomas are diagnosed and treated early {695}. Patients with sporadic tumours have an improved outcome compared to patients with VHL syndrome, probably because the latter group tends to develop multiple lesions {1493}.

CHAPTER 11

Tumours of the Haematopoietic System

Malignant lymphomas
Extranodal malignant lymphomas arising in the CNS in the absence of lymphoma outside the nervous system at the time of diagnosis; these tumours need to be differentiated from secondary involvement of the nervous system in systemic lymphomas.

Histiocytic tumours
A heterogeneous group of tumours and tumour-like masses composed of histiocytes that are commonly associated with histologically identical extracranial lesions; Langerhans cell histiocytosis (LCH) shows features of dendritic Langerhans cells whereas most of the various non-LCH show macrophage differentiation.

Malignant lymphomas

M. Deckert
W. Paulus

Definition
Extranodal malignant lymphomas arising in the CNS in the absence of lymphoma outside the nervous system at the time of diagnosis; these tumours need to be differentiated from secondary involvement of the nervous system in systemic lymphomas.

ICD-O code
9590/3

Synonyms and historical annotation
Primary CNS lymphomas (PCNSL) were first described by Bailey in 1929 as "perithelial sarcoma". Until their lymphoid lineage and correct designation as lymphoma were generally accepted, at least 12 synonyms have been used, including adventitial sarcoma, reticulum cell sarcoma and microglioma.

Incidence
The incidence of PCNSL has markedly increased world-wide: from 0.8–1.5% up to 6.6% of primary intracranial neoplasms {1476}, mainly as the consequence of the AIDS epidemic. In immunocompetent patients, the incidence has increased in some but not all series and populations {384}. Prior to the introduction of highly effective antiviral therapy (HAART), the incidence in AIDS patients (4.7 per 1000 person-years) was about 3600-fold higher than in the general population {387}, with 2–12% of AIDS patients developing primary CNS lymphomas,

mainly during late-stage AIDS {280}. HAART has reduced the occurrence of all non-Hodgkin's lymphomas with an incidence rate of 0.4 for primary and secondary brain lymphomas in AIDS patients {1968}. CNS involvement occurs in 22% of post-transplant lymphomas, about 55% being confined to the CNS {1711}.

Age and sex distribution
PCNSL affect all ages, with a peak incidence in immunocompetent subjects during the sixth and seventh decade of life, and a male: female ratio of 3:2. In immunocompromised patients, the age at manifestation is lowest in individuals who have an inherited immunodeficiency (10 years), followed by transplant recipients (37 years) and AIDS patients (39 years, 90% males).

Etiology
Inherited or acquired immunodeficiency predisposes to development of PCNSL. This includes immunodeficiency produced by Wiskott-Aldrich syndrome, AIDS and immunosuppressive therapy following organ transplantation and, to a lesser degree, therapy for Hodgkin disease and autoimmune disorders such as rheumatoid arthritis and Sjögren syndrome.
The Epstein-Barr virus (EBV) plays a major role in immunocompromised patients with PCNSL. The EBV genome is present in tumour cells in more than 95% of immunocompromised patients, but in 0–20% of immunocompetent patients. Lymphoma cells latently infected with EBV variably express EBNA 1–6, LMP1, the major EBV oncoprotein {2493}, 2a, 2b, and EBER1 and EBER2. Expression of these proteins has a wide variety of effects, including activation of the NF-κ-B pathway.
Data on viruses other than EBV are scarce. DNA sequences corresponding to the JCV early genome and the late agnoprotein were present in 22 samples and the JCV late genome encoding the viral capsid proteins in 8 samples of 27 PCNSL investigated {459}. The partial

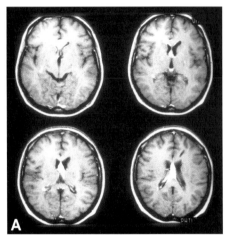

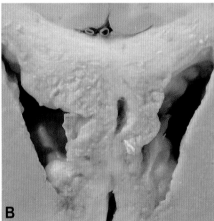

Fig. 11.02 A Malignant lymphoma. T1-weighted MRI and (**B**) macroscopic appearance of malignant lymphoma with diffuse infiltration of the ventricular walls.

co-expression of JCV T antigen with EBV LMP1 suggested JCV to be a cofactor or to provide one of several additional "hits" required for transformation in some PCNSL {459}. The involvement of various other viruses in the pathogenesis of PCNSL has been largely ruled out, including HHV-6 {1700}, HHV-8 {1515}, polyomaviruses SV40 and BKV {1514, 1538}.

Localization
About 60% of PCNSL involve the supra-tentorial space, including the frontal (15%), temporal (8%), parietal (7%) and occipital (3%) lobes, basal ganglia/periventricular regions (10%) and corpus

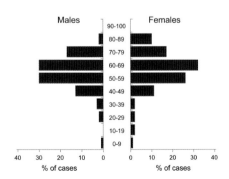

Fig. 11.01 Age and sex distribution of primary CNS lymphomas in immunocompetent patients.

callosum (5%); posterior fossa (13%), and spinal cord (1%) are less commonly involved. Approximately 25–50% are multiple (60–85% in AIDS and post-transplant subjects). Secondary meningeal spread is seen in 30–40% of PCNSL, while primary leptomeningeal lymphoma may account for up to 8% of these tumours {729}. Primary dural and epi-dural malignant lymphomas are very rare {1485}. Ocular disease (which may antedate intracranial lesions) is present in 15–20% of cases, and distant metastases in 6–10% {232}.

Since occult lymphoma has been reported in up to 8% of patients presenting with brain lymphoma, complete systemic staging is recommended {6}. Secondary CNS lymphomas occur preferentially in the dura and leptomeninges, but paren-chymal lesions may also occur. Rare instances of lymphoma restricted to peripheral nerve may be designated as neurolymphomatosis.

Clinical features

Symptoms and signs

Around 50–80% of PCNSL patients present with focal neurological deficits, 20–30% with neuropsychiatric symptoms, 10–30% with signs of increased intracranial pressure, and 5–20% with seizures. Eye symptoms resulting from uveitis or vitrous lymphoma are seen in 5–20% of cases. For PCNSL, the interval between initial symptoms and diagnosis ranges from days to two years, with an average of two months. Angiotropic lymphoma often manifests as rapidly progressing dementia with multifocal neurological deficits {320, 1335}. About 50% of transplantation-associated primary CNS lymphomas appear within a year after transplantation (mean, 32 months) {1711}.

Neuroimaging

MRI is the most sensitive radiologic procedure to detect PCNSL, which is isointense to hyperintense on T2, fluid inversion recovery or diffusion weighted images MRI images, densely enhancing on post-contrast images {112, 1227, 1709}. Bilateral symmetrical subependymal high-signal foci are suggestive of PCNSL. Peritumoural edema is less severe than in malignant gliomas and metastases. FDG-PET scan {852} or Thallium-201-SPECT {57} are helpful in the differential diagnosis of ring-enhancing mass lesions that are frequently seen in AIDS-related

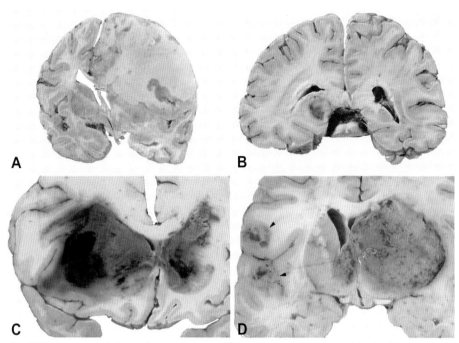

Fig. 11.03 Macroscopic features of primary malignant CNS lymphomas. **A** Large, necrotizing B-cell lymphoma in a HIV-1-infected seven month old infant. **B** B-cell lymphoma involving the medial temporo-occipital lobe. **C,D** Primary malignant CNS lymphomas of the basal ganglia with extension into the contralateral hemisphere. **D** Note the additional foci in the left insular region (arrows).

PCNSL, which are difficult to distinguish from toxoplasmosis and other non-neoplastic conditions by CT or MRI. Meningeal infiltration may present as hyperdense corticomeningeal structures, but CT and MRI can fail to detect meningeal or eye lesions. Steroid-treated lesions may disappear within hours. FDG-PET seems to be suitable for early therapeutic monitoring after chemotherapy {1673}.

CSF cytology

Pleocytosis is found in 35–60% of PCNSL patients, but despite the presence of tumour cells in the CSF, cell counts may be normal. Cytology is of diagnostic value in 5–30% of PCNSL and in 70–95% of metastatic malignant lymphomas, particularly if immunocytochemistry is used to determine monoclonality {581}. The combination of flow cytometry and morphologic examination may enhance the detection of lymphoma cells in the CSF {583}. PCR analysis to identify monoclonal immunoglobulin (IG) heavy chain rearrangement may identify a clonal population in the CSF {700}, but may require repeat puncture {511}. The predictive value of PCR assays for EBV DNA in CSF in AIDS patients is controversial {353, 933}.

Stereotactic biopsy

Surgery is restricted to stereotactic biopsy to establish the histological diagnosis of PCNSL; partial resection is even associ-ated with worse survival {128}. Unless herniation is imminent, corticosteroids should be withheld before biopsy as steroid application may result in non-diagnostic biopsies without detectable tumour cells. The typically dramatic response of primary CNS lymphomas to corticosteroids is usually temporary, but can occasionally be long-term {1753}.

Macroscopy

PCNSL occur as single or multiple masses in the cerebral hemispheres.

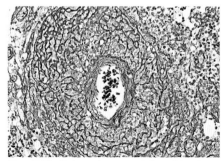

Fig. 11.04 Perivascular accumulation of lymphoma cells embedded in a concentric network of reticulin fibers.

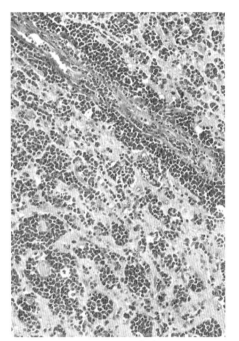

Fig. 11.05 Primary malignant CNS lymphoma, with characteristic perivascular spread of tumour cells.

While they are often deep-seated and adjacent to the ventricular system, superficial tumours may also be encountered. The tumours can be firm, friable, granular, centrally necrotic, focally haemorrhagic, grey-tan, yellow or virtually indistinguishable from the adjacent neuropil. Demarcation from surrounding parenchyma is variable. Some tumours appear well-delineated, like a metastasis. When diffuse borders and architectural effacement are present, the lesions resemble gliomas. Diffusely infiltrating forms without evidence of a cohesive mass lesion have been referred to as "lymphomatosis cerebri" {1912}. AIDS patients tend to have more necrotic areas, which may simulate necrotizing cerebral toxoplasmosis. PSNSL and toxoplasmosis may manifest concomitantly in AIDS patients {2152}. Meningeal lymphoma mimics meningioma or meningitis, or appears macroscopically normal.

Classification systems and their relevance to primary CNS lymphomas

According to the Revised European-American Lymphoma (REAL) classification and the WHO classification {955}, the vast majority of CNS lymphomas is classified as diffuse large B cell lymphoma (DLBCL); however, PCNSL are not specifically included.

Histopathology

Low-power microscopy of PCNSL at the periphery often demonstrates the typical angiocentric infiltration pattern where tumour cells form collars within concentric perivascular reticulin deposits. From these perivascular cuffs, tumour cells invade neural parenchyma, either with compact cellular aggregates and a well-delineated invasion front, or with single diffusely infiltrating tumour cells resembling encephalitis. Virtually all PCNSL show a diffuse growth pattern. Large geographic necroses are common, with perivascular islands of viable tumour cells surrounded by large regions of coagulative necrosis. A focally prominent astrocytic and microglial response, large CD68-positive macrophages, and reactive lymphocytic infiltrates with a predominance of small CD4- as well as CD8-positive T-cells are common.

B-cell lymphoma

B-cell non-Hodgkin lymphomas constitute 92–98% of primary CNS lymphomas. Accordingly, they show immunohistochemical expression of pan-B markers such as CD19, CD20 and CD79a.

Diffuse large B-cell lymphoma

More than 95% of primary CNS B-cell lymphomas are DLBCL. They consist of blastic cells with large pleomorphic nuclei and distinct nucleoli (corresponding to centroblasts or immunoblasts). All morphological variants of DLBCL, i.e. centroblastic, immunoblastic, T-cell/histiocyte-rich and anaplastic, may occur in the CNS. In addition to pan-B markers, the majority of PCNSL express BCL-6, albeit not in all tumour cells {279, 391, 2043}. In 90–100%, tumour cells are MUM-1+. In the majority of tumours, cells express the BCL-2 protein, which is not indicative of a t(14;18) {279, 361, 391, 447}.

Low-grade B-cell lymphoma

Low-grade B-cell lymphomas of the CNS correspond to their systemic counterparts {955}. A retrospective multi-centre series compiled 32 low-grade B-cell lymphomas, the most common type being lymphoplasmacytic lymphoma {959}. While age distribution and perivascular infiltration were similar to the much more frequent DLBCL, low-grade lymphomas differed from DLBCL with respect to better long-term outcome and the common occurrence of atypical neuroimaging features, such as hyperintensity on T2-weighted images,

lack of periventricular localization, absent or inhomogeneous contrast enhancement {959}.

Marginal zone B-cell lymphoma

Intracranial low-grade B-cell lymphoma of mucosa-associated lymphoid tissue (MALT) type or marginal zone B-cell lymphoma (MZBCL), probably representing the most common primary low-grade intracranial lymphoma, usually presents as a dural-based mass mimicking meningioma {2277}. Intracerebral or intraventricular locations are exceptional {1073}. MZBCL is composed of small lymphocytes with clear cytoplasm, an irregular, centrally located nucleus and variable degrees of plasmacytic differentiation. Lymphoid follicles and massive deposition of amyloid may occur. Tumour cells express CD19, CD20 and CD79a but not CD3, CD10 or CD23 and only occasionally CD5. Trisomy 3 is most commonly detected. Female predilection (4:1) and long-term survival following therapy are typical {2277}.

Plasmacytoma

In its purely extraosseous form, intracranial plasmacytoma most often appears as a nodular or plaque-like dural mass, with variable infiltration of the underlying brain. Although rare, exclusively intraparenchymal tumours have also been described. Furthermore, secondary cerebral involvement may be an unusual complication in multiple myeloma {1693}.

Intravascular B-cell lymphoma

This lesion is also termed angiotropic lymphoma and affects multiple organ systems. The CNS, including the entire neuraxis, is involved in more than 30% of cases. Accumulations of large B-cells, exceptionally T-cells, NK cells or histiocytic cells, within small and medium vessels lead to vascular occlusion and disseminated small infarcts {1777}. Cerebral mass lesions may develop on the basis of intravascular B-cell lymphoma {912}.

Other types of B-cell lymphoma

Single cases of a variety of other primary CNS B-cell lymphomas have been reported, such as follicular lymphoma {140}, Burkitt lymphoma {1511}, lymphomatoid granulomatosis {1684}, precursor B-cell lymphoblastic lymphoma {4} and post-transplant lymphoproliferative disorders {296}.

T-cell lymphoma

T-cell lymphomas constitute about 2–5% (Western countries), 8–14% (Japan) and 17% (Korea) of all PCNSL {341}. They are peripheral T-cell lymphomas, and have been seen mainly in the immunocompetent, although single cases in AIDS patients are on record {74}. They occur as solitary or multiple intraparenchymal masses with a higher male: female ratio. The largest study on 45 patients revealed that age distribution, localization and outcome corresponded to those of primary CNS B-cell lymphomas {2076}, while other reviews have noticed a more frequent posterior fossa localization, particularly in the cerebellum, a propensity to arise in the leptomeninges, younger age and an either better or worse prognosis {341}. Molecular genetic demonstration of T-cell monoclonality can be important for excluding T-cell rich B-cell lymphoma and inflammation {1336}.

Anaplastic large-cell lymphoma (ALCL)

ALCL is defined by its composition of large, pleomorphic, CD30 (Ki-1)-positive lymphocytes. In an analysis of 9 primary CNS cases, seven tumours involved the dura or leptomeninges, 7 were T cell, two were null cell, and 5 showed immuno-histochemical expression of the ALK-1 antigen (anaplastic lymphoma kinase), which is highly sensitive and specific for *ALK* translocations, most commonly the (2;5) translocation {659}. Like in systemic ALCL, age less than 18 years and ALK-1 positivity were associated with a better prognosis {659}. Most patients are immunocompetent, while one AIDS patient has been described {1944}.

NK/T-cell lymphoma

Extranodal natural killer (NK)/T-cell lymphomas most commonly involve the nasal cavity. Less than 3% of cases invade or metastasize to the CNS {1360}. A single case of primary cerebral NK / T-cell lymphoma is on record {1029}. The typical immunophenotype is CD2+, CD56+, surface CD3-, CD3ε+ and EBV+.

Hodgkin disease

The diagnosis of Hodgkin disease rests upon the identification of Hodgkin and Reed-Sternberg cells in the appropriate background of non-neoplastic haemato-poietic cells (lymphocytes, plasma cells, histiocytes, eosinophils), where tumour cells are ringed by T-lymphocytes in a rosette-like manner {955}. The entity is rare in the CNS, and is most often seen in the setting of grade III or IV systemic disease, but primary CNS presentation has also been described {446}. Lesions are typically dural-based, but firm and well-demarcated intraparenchymal tumours do occur {819, 1125}.

Proliferation and apoptosis

Proliferative activity in primary CNS lymphoma of the DLBCL type is generally high with Ki-67/MIB-1 labelling indices of 50–70% or even >90% {21, 361, 447}. A variable number of apoptotic cells was detected in the majority (77%) of tumours and may be markedly increased upon corticosteroid treatment {447}.

Genetic susceptibility

With the exception of inherited immuno-deficiency, no genetic predisposition to primary CNS lymphoma has been described to date. A previous or concomitant malignant neoplasm is present in about 8% of immunocompetent primary CNS lymphoma patients, most commonly leukaemia or adenocarcinoma {1860}. Associations of primary CNS lymphoma in individual patients with other brain tumours such as meningioma and glioma {575} or with hereditary tumour syndromes such as neurofibromatosis type 1 {2489} are likely to be coincidental.

Genetics

Classical cytogenetics performed on single cases of primary CNS lymphoma revealed clonal abnormalities of chromosomes 1, 6, 7 and 14, as well as translocations (1;14), (6;14), (13;18) and (14;21) {931}. In contrast to systemic lymphomas, the molecular pathogenesis of primary CNS lymphomas is less well defined. The presence of somatically mutated *IG* genes with evidence for ongoing mutation and the expression of the *BCL6* gene suggested that PCNSL is derived from germinal centre B cells {1516, 2043, 2243}. Further maturation steps of the tumour cells appear to be inhibited as they express IgM without evidence for immunoglobulin class switch due to internal switch micro region deletions {1517}. Recurrent translocations of the *IG* and the *BCL6* gene loci were found in approximately one third of PCNSL {1519, 2043}. For the *BCL6* gene, *IGH*, *IGL*, histone *1H4I*, *GAPD*, *HSPCA* (*HSP90A*), and *LPP* have been identified as translocation partners with subsequent promoter substitution and a block of normal down-regulation of the *BCL6* gene {1513, 1741, 2043}. *TP53* mutations are rare {361}. FISH revealed gains of the

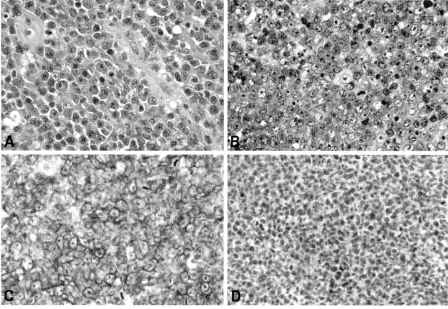

Fig. 11.06 Histological features of primary malignant lymphomas. **A** Malignant, diffuse large B-cell lymphoma. **B** Highly anaplastic malignant lymphoma with numerous mitotic figures and extensive apoptosis. **C** Tumour cells express the pan-B-cell marker CD20. **D** Expression of the BCL6 protein by the tumour cells.

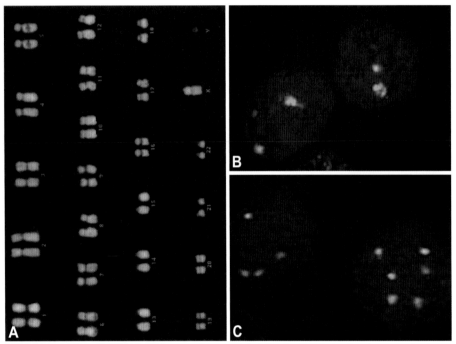

Fig. 11.07 A The fluorescence image of comparative genomic hybridization (CGH), showing chromosomal gains on 1q, 12q, 22q and losses on 5q and 6q. Interphase FISH analyses using differentially labeled probes flanking the IGH (**B**) and MALT (**C**) loci, respectively, demonstrating a breakpoint in the IGH locus (**B**) and multiple co-localized red and green signals indicating amplification of the MALT locus.

MALT1 and *BCL2* in 18q21 as the most common genetic alteration {1519}, which may cause NF-κ-B activation. Genes of the NF-κ-B pathway are expressed {391} and may contribute to the sustained high proliferative activity and the inhibition of apoptosis of the tumour cells. FISH and CGH studies detected gains more frequently than losses of genetic material. Frequently, losses affected 6q21-22 and 6p21, while gains involved 18q, 1q, 9p, 11q, 12p, 12q, 16p, 17q20q and 22q {198, 768, 1519, 1873, 2380}. Loss of chromosome 6q was correlated with shorter survival {1560, 1873}. A candidate gene in 6q22-23 may be *PTPRK* {1560}. The oncogenes *MYC, PAX5, PIM-1,* and *RhoH/TTF* are also targeted by aberrant hypermutation in PCNSL {1518}. Aberrant methylation of *DAPK* (84%), *TSP1* (68%), *CRBP1* (67%), $p16^{INK4a}$ (64%), $p14^{ARF}$ (59%), *MGMT* (52%), *RARbeta2* (50%), *TIMP3* (44%), *TIMP2* (42%), *p15INK4b* (40%), *p73* (28%), *hMLH1* (12%), *RB1* (8%) and *GSTP1* (8%), *HRK* (31%) was observed {348, 361, 708, 1559, 2494}. Reduced folate carrier gene expression by promoter methylation may be of prognostic and therapeutic relevance {569}. Functional polymorphisms of genes regulating the methionine metabolism may either be protective or confer a high risk for therapy-associated white matter changes {1329, 1330}. A cDNA microarray analysis found PCNSL to be distributed among the spectrum of activated B cell-like and germinal centre type DLBCL {1946}. A gene cluster was differentially expressed between CNS and nodal DLBCL including genes involved in apoptosis and proliferation pathways {1946}.

Histogenesis

It is not known whether primary CNS lymphomas arise within or outside the brain. Three hypotheses have been put forward. B-cells may be transformed at a site elsewhere in the body and then develop adhesion molecules specific for cerebral endothelia. However, no adhesion molecules, chemokines or their receptors that would distinguish PCNSL from systemic DLBCL have been identified {958, 1699, 2112}.

Lymphoma cells may be systematically eradicated by an intact immune system but may escape the immune system within the CNS. Astrocyte-derived B cell-activating factor of the tumour necrosis factor family (BAFF) may support survival of the malignant BAFF-receptor expressing B cells {1209}.

A polyclonal intracerebral inflammatory lesion may expand clonally within the brain and progress to the monoclonal neoplastic state. Evidence in support of this idea includes the demonstration in a few patients of transient symptomatic contrast-enhancing brain lesions ('sentinel lesions'), which regress spontaneously or with corticosteroid treatment and ultimately lead to primary CNS lymphoma within one year; histological features are non-specific and include inflammatory T-cell infiltrates, demyelination and gliosis {38}. Possibly, intracerebral antigens or superantigens may stimulate persistence and intracerebral expansion of B-cells. On the other hand, infectious or inflammatory CNS diseases have only exceptionally been described to antedate the development of primary CNS lymphoma {62}.

Prognostic and predictive factors

Radiotherapy alone is insufficient to provide durable remission or cure. Patients developed long-term treatment-related neurotoxicity with combined systemic and intraventricular chemotherapy and whole brain irradiation {7} with severe leukencephalopathy and cortical/subcortical atrophy being more frequent in elderly patients (>60 years) {7}. In the largest polychemotherapy trial including methotrexate as the most efficient cytostatic drug, the Bonn protocol achieved a median overall survival of 50 months, with the best treatment results in patients younger than 61 years (5-year survival: 75%) {1710}. The inclusion of autologous stem cell transplantation may be an option for recurrent tumour in patients less than 60 years and salvage therapy in relapsing or refractory tumour {9, 910, 2126}. The dismal prognosis of HIV-infected patients with primary CNS lymphoma before the era of HAART has improved upon radiotherapy and HAART (median survival: 36 months) {853}.

Histiocytic tumours

W. Paulus
A. Perry

Definition

A heterogeneous group of tumours and tumour-like masses composed of histiocytes that are commonly associated with histologically identical extracranial lesions; Langerhans cell histiocytosis (LCH) shows features of dendritic Langerhans cells whereas most of the various non-LCH show macrophage differentiation.

Synonyms and historical annotation

In 1997, the WHO Committee on Histiocytic/Reticulum Cell Proliferations and the Reclassification Working Group of the Histiocyte Society proposed classifying histiocytic disorders as: (1) dendritic cell-related disorders of varied biological behaviour, such as LCH and juvenile xanthogranuloma; (2) macrophage-related disorders of varied biological behaviour, such as haemophagocytic lymphohistiocytosis and Rosai-Dorfman disease; and (3) malignant histiocytic disorders, such as monocytic leukaemia and histiocytic sarcoma {555}. A minor revision of this classification has more recently been proposed, with group (1) now termed dendritic cell-related disorders, of which LCH is by far the most common.

LCH was previously referred to as histiocytosis X, a term embracing eosinophilic granuloma, Hand-Schüller-Christian disease, Abt-Letterer-Siwe disease and Hashimoto-Pritzker disease, 'X' being the unknown etiological factor {1319}. Because there is much overlap between these subgroups, LCH is currently classified on the basis of extent as unifocal, multifocal (usually polyostotic) and disseminated disease. Historical descriptions of cerebral LCH with principal involvement of the hypothalamus and posterior pituitary were made under terms such as hypothalamic granuloma, Gagel's granuloma and Ayala disease {1078}.

A wide variety of neoplastic and non-neoplastic intracranial masses containing high numbers of macrophages or other foamy ('xanthomatous') cells have previously been referred to as 'xanthogranuloma'

or 'xanthoma', including LCH, dural or osseous masses in hyperlipoproteinaemia and Weber-Christian panniculitis, pleomorphic xanthoastrocytoma ('fibroxanthoma') and inflammatory malignant fibrous histiocytoma ('malignant xanthogranuloma'). Benign and malignant fibrous histiocytomas are mesenchymal tumours and no longer regarded as true histiocytic lesions.

Incidence

In children under 15 years of age, the incidence of LCH is estimated at 0.5 per 100 000 children per year, while non-LCH is even rarer with an incidence of about 1:1 000 000 per year {147}.

LCH typically occurs in children (mean, 12 years), without sex preference. The most common form of LCH (about two third of cases) is a solitary osteolytic lesion of the skull or spine (eosinophilic granuloma). Multifocal LCH lesions of the bone with hypothalamic involvement have been referred to as Hand-Schüller-Christian disease, while Abt-Letterer-Siwe disease involves skin, lymph nodes, viscera and rarely the CNS. Extension from osseous foci to hypothalamus and pituitary gland in multifocal or disseminated LCH is responsible for most cases with CNS involvement, but unifocal or multifocal infiltrates may occur primarily within or even restricted to the hypothalamus, infundibulum, optic chiasm, choroid plexus and cerebral hemispheres {1902}.

Etiology

The etiology of the histiocytic lesions is largely unknown. In most patients with histiocytoses, there is either a mild or no underlying defect in immunologic integrity and the clinical course is benign. Nevertheless, an abnormal immune response is felt to play a potentially important aetiologic role. For example, data suggest defective interactions between T-cells and macrophages in LCH, Erdheim-Chester disease and haemophagocytic lymphohistiocytosis {399, 921, 1253}. In haemophagocytic lymphohistiocytosis, natural killer cell activity is

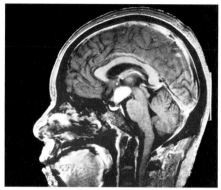

Fig. 11.08 Gadolinium-enhanced MRI of a Langerhans cell histiocytosis in the hypothalamic region (Hand-Schüller-Christian disease).

also diminished {913}. Whether such immune deficits are triggered by genetic predisposition or infectious agents remains unclear in most, although there has been limited support for the latter to date, with one exception: the two major forms of haemophagocytic lymphohistiocytosis include familial and infection-associated, the latter most commonly associated with viruses, especially EBV {1542}. The pathogenesis of the LCH-associated neuro-degenerative disorder is also poorly understood {725, 1492}.

Langerhans cell histiocytosis (LCH)
Clinical features

The most common neurological signs of LCH are diabetes insipidus (25% of children with multifocal or disseminated disease) with or without associated signs of hypothalamic dysfunction (obesity, hypogonadism, growth retardation), signs of raised intracranial pressure, cranial nerve palsies, seizures, visual disturbances (visual field defect, optic atrophy), ataxia and rare progressive tetra- and paraparesis {126}. MRI changes of cranial and intracranial structures include: 1) lesions of the craniofacial bone and skull base (56%) with or without soft-tissue extension; 2) intracranial, extra-axial changes of the hypothalamic-pituitary region (50%), meninges (29%) or choroid plexus (6%); 3) intracranial, intra-axial changes of white matter and gray matter (36%); and 4) cerebral atrophy (8%) {1785}.

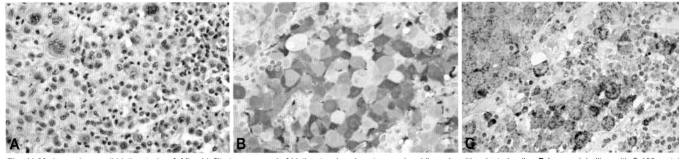

Fig. 11.09 Langerhans cell histiocytosis. **A** Mixed infiltrate composed of histiocytes, lymphocytes, eosinophils and multinucleated cells. **B** Immunolabelling with S-100 protein. **C** Expression of the macrophage marker CD 68.

Macroscopy

Intracranial LCH lesions are often yellow or white and vary from discrete dural-based nodules to granular parenchymal infiltrates. CNS lesions may be well-delineated or ill-defined.

Histopathology

Infiltrates are composed of Langerhans cells, macrophages, lymphocytes, plasma cells and a variable fraction of eosinophils. The nuclei of Langerhans cells are typically slightly eccentric, ovoid, reniform or convoluted with linear grooves and inconspicuous nucleoli. The cytoplasm is large (15–25 μm in diameter) and pale to eosinophilic. Touton giant cells may occur. Abundant deposition of collagen is often seen. LCH occasionally presents with demyelination and no or sparse infiltration of Langerhans cells {724, 1764}. Eosinophils may form into aggregates and undergo necrosis to produce granulomas or abscesses.

Immunohistochemically, Langerhans cells consistently express S-100 protein, vimentin and certain histiocyte markers including CD1a, Langerin (CD207), HLA-DR, ß2-microglobulin and variably CD68, rarely L1 antigen (clone MAC387) and almost never CD45, CD15 and lysozyme {1423}. CD1a expression, being very characteristic but not absolutely specific to LCH, can be demonstrated even on small and routinely processed materials {555, 1423}. The ultrastructural hallmark of Langerhans cells are Birbeck granules (Langerhans cell granules), which are 34-nm wide rod-shaped or tennis-racket-shaped intracytoplasmic pentalaminar structures with cross-striation and a zipper-like central core, possibly originating from the cell membrane and/or Golgi apparatus {530}. Either expression of CD1a or presence of Birbeck granules are currently required for definite diagnosis of LCH.

Neurodegenerative lesions lacking infiltration of CD1a+ cells may also occur. These mainly affect the cerebellum and brain stem, exhibit a profound inflammatory process dominated by CD8-reactive lymphocytes, and are associated with axonal destruction, secondary demyelination, microglial activation and gliosis, resembling paraneoplastic encephalitis {725}.

Proliferation

Immunohistochemical Ki-67/MIB-1 proliferation indices of neoplastic Langerhans cells range from 4% to 16% {752}.

Prognosis and predictive factors

The overall survival rates of all LCH patients at 5, 15, and 20 years are 88%, 88%, and 77%, respectively, with an event-free survival rate of only 30% at 15 years {2412}. While unifocal LCH may spontaneously recover or requires minimal treatment, e.g. surgical resection, multi-systemic disease with organ dysfunction may resist systemic chemotherapy. The mortality rate in this latter subgroup of LCH reaches 20%. Of all patients with LCH, late sequelae are seen in 64%, including skeletal defects in 42%, diabetes insipidus in 25%, growth failure in 20%, hearing loss in 16%, and other CNS dysfunction in 14% {2412}. Concerning histopathologic features of LCH, no prognostic significance of cytologic atypia and mitotic activity was found in most studies {555, 1892}, but it has been suggested that a distinct clinical entity of malignant LCH, characterized morphologically by malignant-appearing Langerhans cells and clinically by male predominance, atypical organ involvement, and an aggressive clinical course, does exist {132}.

Non-Langerhans cell histiocytoses

This group of diseases differs from LCH by the absence of features of dendritic Langerhans cells. Most but not all exhibit macrophage differentiation.

Rosai-Dorfman disease

Rosai-Dorfman disease of lymph nodes is most common in children and young adults, but intracranial disease is usually seen in adults. Intracranially, it typically shows dural-based solitary or multiple masses; parenchymal or intrasellar lesions and intracranial extension from an orbital mass or from nasal and paranasal cavities may also occur. Clinically, the disease most often presents as an intracranial space–occupying mass. The 'classical' signs of cervical lympha-denopathy, fever and weight loss (sinus histiocytosis with massive lympha-denopathy) are absent in 70% of these patients, and 52% have no associated systemic disease {1808}. The radiological appearance of intracranial Rosai-Dorfman disease usually mimics meningioma and carries a favourable prognosis after complete resection or after corticosteroid treatment {1439}. Histopathology shows sheets or nodules of histiocytes with vacuolated or eosinophilic cytoplasm (CD1a-, CD11c+, CD68+, MAC387+, lysozyme -/+, S-100 protein +), foci of lymphocytes and plasma cells, and fibrosis. Emperipolesis, i.e. well-preserved lymphocytes and plasma cells within the cytoplasm of histiocytes, is typical, but may be inconspicuous; it is missing in 30% of leptomeningeal cases {1808}.

Erdheim-Chester disease

The disease typically manifests in adults (mean, 55 years). Intracranial lesions may involve brain (preferentially cerebellum), spinal cord, cerebellopontine angle, choroid plexus, pituitary, meninges and

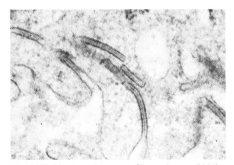

Fig. 11.10 Electron microscopy of Langerhans cell histiocytosis showing several Birbeck granules, apparently originating from cell membrane.

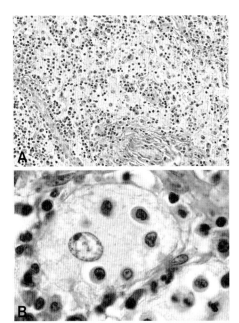

Fig. 11.11 Rosai-Dorfman disease. **A** Heterogeneous dural-based cellular infiltrate composed of lymphocytes, plasma cells, and large pale histiocytic cells with emperipolesis. **B** Histiocyte with emperipolesis of lymphocytes and plasma cells.

orbit {2386}. Retention of MRI gadolinium enhancement for several days may occur {77}. Patients occasionally present with non-specific neurological signs without indication of systemic disease (bones, visceral organs, adipose tissue). Diabetes insipidus and progressive cerebellar dysfunction are common symptoms {2449}. Histopathologically, lesions are composed of lipid-laden histiocytes (CD1a-, CD68+, S-100 protein -) with small nuclei, Touton-like multinucleated giant cells, a scant amount of lymphocytic infiltrates, a minimal number of eosinophils and fibrosis {17}. Elongated, microglia-type cells may be seen in cases with more diffuse brain infiltration.

Haemophagocytic lymphohistiocytosis

This autosomal recessive systemic disease of early infancy (mean, 3 months) diffusely involves leptomeninges and, multifocally, the brain. Neuroimaging is characterized by focal hyperintense lesions in white and grey matter, diffuse abnormal T2 signal intensity in white matter, delayed myelination and paren-chymal atrophy {1152}. Cardinal symptoms are prolonged fever, hepatospleno-megaly and cytopenias. Biochemical markers include elevated triglyceride and ferritin, high levels of the alpha chain of the soluble interleukin-2 receptor and low fibrinogen. Impaired function of natural killer cells and cytotoxic T-cells is characteristic {970}. CNS involvement is seen in almost all patients, in 73% of patients already at time of diagnosis. Isolated CNS involvement has also been reported {2087}. Neurologic symptoms include irritability, bulging fontanelle, neck stiffness, seizures, cranial nerve palsies, ataxia and hemiplegia {812, 1152}. The outcome is lethal without allogeneic stem cell transplantation. Histopathology shows non-malignant diffuse infiltrations of lymphocytes and macrophages with haemophagocytosis. The antigenic profile of the macrophages is CD11c+, CD68+, while staining for CD1a and S-100 protein is variable. Intracranial lesions consist of lympho-histiocytic meningeal and cerebral infiltrations and multifocal cerebral necroses {812}.

Juvenile xanthogranuloma (JXG) and xanthoma disseminatum

Juvenile xanthogranuloma, now classified among the secondary dendritic-cell processes {147}, preferentially manifests in young children as solitary cutaneous nodule, but may arise in the brain or the meninges, either with or without cutaneous lesions; multicentric intracerebral cases have been reported {1294}.
Xanthoma disseminatum occurs preferentially in young adults. Intracranial structures involved typically include hypothalamus, pituitary gland and dura mater {2479}. Pituitary and hypothalamic symptoms are most common (up to 40% of patients), while extracranial signs are related to involvement of skin, eyes, oral and respiratory mucosa.
Both lesions are composed of histiocytes (CD1a-, CD11c+, CD68+, factor XIIIa+, MAC387-/+, lysozyme -, S-100 protein -),

scattered Touton giant cells, lymphocytes and eosinophils {1701}.

Malignant histiocytic disorders

Malignant histiocytic tumours of the nervous system are extremely rare, and only a very few bona fide cases with rigorous immunohistochemical and molecular genetic characterization have been described. Histiocytic sarcoma, a malignant tumour positive for histiocytic markers (CD68, CD163, lysozyme, CD11c, CD14) and negative for myeloid markers, dendritic markers, CD30, ALK1 or other lymphoid markers, may primarily involve brain and meninges {2175}. Intracranial follicular dendritic cell (FDC) sarcoma has also been described {784}. Because vesicular nuclei, whorl formation and positivity for vimentin and EMA may mimic meningioma, immunohistochemistry for follicular dendritic cell markers (CD21, CD23, CD35) is essential.

Genetic susceptibility

Occurrence of multifocal LCH in mono-zygotic twins, in part with simultaneous onset of disease, has been repeatedly reported and suggests genetic sus-ceptibility in at least some cases {1376}. The primary gene responsible for familial haemophagocytic lymphohistiocytosis is the perforin 1 (PRF1) gene on chromo-some 10q22, although other genes have similarly been implicated in smaller subsets {921,1024}.

Genetics

PCR-based X-chromosome inactivation assays of female tissues provided evidence in support of a clonal origin and a neoplastic nature of LCH {2414}, whereas Rosai-Dorfman disease was shown to be polyclonal {1694}. In contrast, clonality studies have yielded mixed

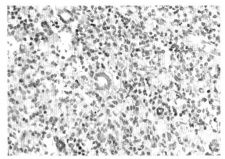

Fig. 11.12 Juvenile xanthogranuloma composed of histiocytes, multinucleated Touton cells and lympho-cytes.

results in Erdheim-Chester disease {27, 329}. Monoclonal rearrangement of T-cell receptor genes was found in haemophagocytic lymphohistiocytosis {1656}, but not in LCH {2414}. *TP53* mutations were not detected in LCH {2389}, while karyotypes and the involvement of oncogenes and tumour suppressor genes are virtually unknown in the histiocytic disorders described in this chapter.

Histogenesis
Data suggest that LCH cells represent immature, partially activated dendritic Langerhans cells {1253}, whereas non-LCH disorders arise from bone marrow derived mononuclear phagocytes (macrophages) at various stages of development and activation. For example, JXG displays a phenotype similar to that of plasmacytoid monocytes {1186}. Microglial cells are the intrinsic histiocytes of the brain, and although single tumours of possible microglial origin are on record {889}, there is no indication that microglia give rise to any one of the histiocytic disorders discussed in this chapter. Nevertheless, they may participate in the genesis of secondary neuronal damage, such as the encephalitis-like neuro-degenerative disorder of the cerebellum and basal ganglia associated with LCH {725}.

CHAPTER 12

Germ Cell Tumours

Morphological and immunophenotypic homologues of gonadal and other extra-neuraxial germ cell tumours.

Germinoma

Mature teratoma

Immature teratoma

Teratoma with malignant transformation

Yolk sac tumour (endodermal sinus tumour)

Embryonal carcinoma

Choriocarcinoma

CNS germ cell tumours

M.K. Rosenblum
Y. Nakazato
M. Matsutani

Definition
Morphological and immunophenotypic homologues of gonadal and other extra-neuraxial germ cell tumours.

ICD-O codes
Germinoma	9064/3
Teratoma	9080/1
Mature teratoma	9080/0
Immature teratoma	9080/3
Teratoma with malignant transformation	9084/3
Yolk sac tumour	9071/3
Embryonal carcinoma	9070/3
Choriocarcinoma	9100/3

Incidence
Geographic incidence varies considerably. Most prevalent in far-east Asia, CNS germ cell tumours accounted for 2–3% of primary intracranial neoplasms, and for 8–15% of specifically paediatric examples, in series from Japan, Taiwan and Korea {842, 1416, 2173}. The highest of these figures emerge from Japan, where one population-based survey revealed an overall, age-adjusted incidence of 0.17 cases per 100 000 person-years (M=0.30, F=0.07) {1232}. In the West, these neoplasms constitute only 0.3–0.6% of primary intracranial tumours and approximately 3–4% of those affecting children {173, 1954, 2030}. An age-adjusted incidence of 0.09 cases per 100 000 person-years (M=0.12, F=0.06) has been reported in the United States {305}.

Age and sex distribution
Approximately 80–90% of CNS germ cell tumours afflict subjects younger than 25 years of age, incidence peaking in 10–14 year-olds, and a clear excess of cases involve males {173, 209, 842, 2000, 2172}. Analysis of the largest registry on record, totalling 1463 Japanese patients, showed that 70% of cases occur in the 10–24 year-old cohort and 73% affect males {209}. Only 2.9% of patients were below 5 years of age and 6.2% were older than 35 years of age in this analysis, but congenital examples (typically teratomas) are well-recognized,

as are exceptional instances of late adult onset. Male:female ratios vary with tumour location and histology. While the great majority of pineal region examples involve boys, an excess of suprasellar germ cell tumours are encountered in girls. All histologic variants exhibit a predilection for males, but this is especially decided with regard to teratomas. In the Japanese registry cited above, 89% of teratomas, 78% of germinomas and 75% of other germ cell tumour types arose in males.

Etiology
The predilection of CNS germ cell tumours for peripubertal subjects, localization to diencephalic centres regulating gonadal activity and increased incidence in the setting of Klinefelter syndrome have been taken as evidence that elevated circulating gonadotropin levels may factor in their pathogenesis. The link to Klinefelter syndrome is presumed also to reflect chromosome X overdosage, a relatively common genetic feature of intracranial germ cell tumours.

Localization
Like other extragonadal germ cell tumours, CNS variants preferentially affect the midline: 80% or more arise in structures about the third ventricle, with the region of the pineal gland being their most common site of origin, followed by the

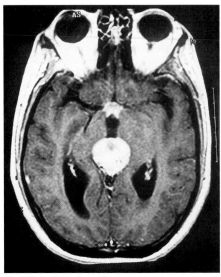

Fig. 12.02 MRI of a solid, contrast-enhancing germinoma of the pineal region, with a smaller CSF-borne metastasis in the suprachiasmatic cistern.

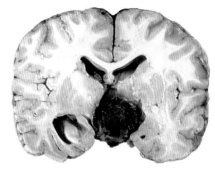

Fig. 12.03 Germinoma of the suprasellar region in a 7-year-old girl.

suprasellar compartment {850, 2000, 2030}. Suprasellar examples originate in the neurohypophyseal axis. Intraventricular, diffuse periventricular, basal ganglionic, thalamic, cerebral hemispheric, cerebellar, bulbar, intramedullary and intrasellar variants may be encountered, as may congenital holocranial examples (usually teratomas) and lesions that involve the brain extensively in complex with the orbit, cervical or cephalic soft tissues. Germinomas are the prevalent tumour type in the suprasellar compartment and basal ganglionic/thalamic regions, with non-germinomatous germ cell tumours dominating at other sites. Multifocal germ

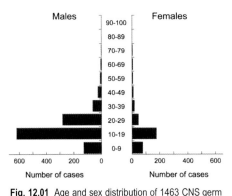

Fig. 12.01 Age and sex distribution of 1463 CNS germ cell tumours. Data from report of Brain Tumour Registry of Japan (1969-1996).

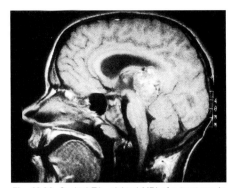

Fig. 12.04 Sagittal T1-weighted MRI of a teratoma in the pineal region, occupying the dorsal aspect of the third ventricle.

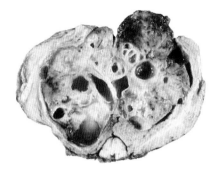

Fig. 12.05 Large teratoma of the cerebellum in a four-week-old infant, with characteristic cysts and chondroid nodules.

cell tumours usually involve the pineal region and suprasellar compartment simultaneously or sequentially. Bilateral basal ganglionic and thalamic lesions are also well recognized. Ventricular endoscopy (neuro-endoscopy) is emerging as especially sensitive in the localization of intracranial germ cell tumours, and can disclose minute tumour nodules on or beneath the ependyma that are not detectable on MRI {2394}.

Clinical features
Symptoms and signs
The presenting clinical manifestations of CNS germ cell tumours and their duration vary with histological type and location. Only the more common signs and symptoms are addressed here. In general, germinomas are associated with a more protracted symptomatic interval than other types. Tumours of the pineal region often compress and obstruct the cerebral aqueduct, resulting in progressive hydrocephalus with intracranial hypertension. Lesions so situated are also prone to compress and invade the tectal plate, producing a characteristic paralysis of upwards gaze and convergence known

as Parinaud syndrome. Neurohypophyseal/suprasellar germ cell tumours typically impinge on the optic chiasm, causing visual field deflects, and often disrupt the hypothalamo-hypophyseal axis as evidenced by the occurrence of diabetes insipidus and manifestations of pituitary failure which include retarded growth and sexual maturation. CNS germ cell tumours may also cause "precocious puberty" by elaborating human chorionic gonadotropin (HCG), a stimulant of testosterone production that is secreted by neoplastic syncytiotrophoblasts. While the latter mechanism would account for cases of precocious sexual development encountered in boys (the overwhelming majority of those encountered in practice), the additional tumour expression of cytochrome P450 aromatase, which catalyses the conversion of C19 steroids to oestrogens, has been suggested to explain rare instances of precocious puberty affecting girls with HCG-producing intracranial germ cell neoplasms {1611}. In the latter context, HCG has also been suggested to have some intrinsic follicle stimulating hormone-like activity {2142}.

Neuroimaging
The neuroradiological profiles of CNS germ cell tumours are largely non-specific, and definitive histological subclassification requires tissue examination. Nevertheless,

a few useful generalizations can be offered {618, 1315}. On CT and MRI, germ cell tumours other than teratomas usually appear as solid masses that are iso- or hyperdense relative to grey matter and show prominent contrast enhancement. Basal ganglia germinomas, which are commonly associated with ipsilateral basal ganglionic atrophy early in their evolution, occasionally exhibit little MRI abnormality in T1-weighted sequences, only ill-defined T2-hyperintensity and no, or faint, contrast enhancement. A diagnosis of teratoma should be considered for a lesion that can be shown to contain intratumoural cysts admixed with calcified regions and foci having the low signal-attenuation characteristics of fat. Intratumoural haemorrhage is particularly characteristic of choriocarcinoma and of mixed neoplasms with choriocarcinomatous elements, but may also be encountered in germinomas associated with HCG elevation (i.e. having syncytiotrophoblastic components). Finally, MRI studies are of considerable value in demonstrating hydrocephalus, invasion of regional structures and CSF-borne metastases, the latter visualized as linear or nodular foci of contrast enhancement along ventricular surfaces or in the craniospinal subarachnoid space.

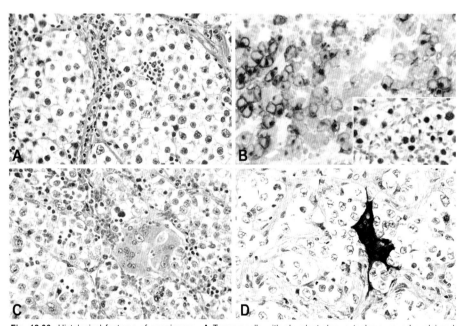

Fig. 12.06 Histological features of germinoma. **A** Tumour cells with abundant clear cytoplasm, round nuclei and prominent nucleoli. Note the lymphocytic infiltrates along fibrovascular septae. **B** Membranous and Golgi region immunolabelling for c-kit and nuclear expression of OCT4 (inset, lower right). **C** Syncytiotrophoblastic giant cell in an otherwise typical germinoma. **D** Immunostaining for human choriogonadotropic hormone (ß-HCG).

Tumour markers in serum and CSF

Assay of serum and CSF for α-fetoprotein (AFP; normally synthesized by yolk sac endoderm, foetal hepatocytes and intestinal epithelium) and ß-HCG (normally secreted by syncytiotrophoblast) is now routine in the presurgical assessment of suspected germ cell tumours. Elevations of either oncoprotein constitute compelling evidence of germ cell neoplasia, the pattern of marker elevation being somewhat predictive of tumour histology {842, 850}. High AFP levels typically signal the presence of yolk sac tumour elements, but modest increases of this marker may result from expression by the enteric components of teratomas. Marked elevations of ß-HCG strongly suggest that components of choriocarcinoma are present, though increases in this oncoprotein may be associated with tumours, including germinomas, that simply harbour syncytiotrophoblastic giant cells. Isolated elevation of placental alkaline phosphatase (PLAP; a cell-surface glycoprotein normally elaborated by syncytiotrophoblast and primordial germ cells) has been correlated with pure germinomatous histology, but this assessment has not been generally employed. Soluble c-kit concentrations in the CSF have been explored as a germinoma marker as well {1498}. Sampling artefact must be presumed to account for the scenario in which tissue morphology and immunohistochemical assays are at odds with serum and CSF profiles.

Macroscopy

Germinoma is generally solid, although it may show small foci of cystic change, and is composed of soft and friable tan-white tissue. Conspicuous necrosis and haemorrhage are usually absent, but when present suggest the presence of more malignant components. Choriocarcinoma is especially prone to extensive haemorrhagic necrosis, while the accumulation of myxoid material lends a gelatinous appearance and consistency to some yolk sac tumours. Teratomatous elements manifest as mucous-laden cysts, fat, chondroid nodules or bony spicules. Rarely, CNS teratomas contain teeth or well-formed hairs.

Histopathology

The accurate histological identification and subclassification of CNS germ cell

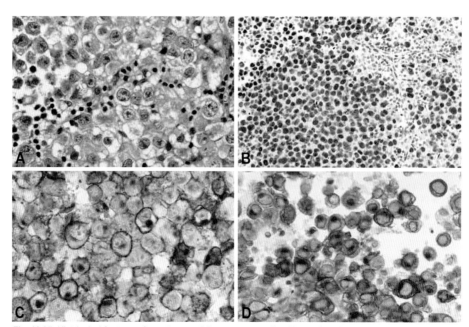

Fig. 12.07 Histological features of germinoma. **A** Large tumour cells with round vesicular nuclei, prominent nucleoli and clear cytoplasm. **B** Germinoma showing OCT4 immunoreactivity. **C** Cytoplasmic and membranous reactivity for PLAP. **D** Expression of c-kit protein in tumour cells.

tumours are critical to current treatment planning and prognostication. While the various entities collected under the generic designation of CNS germ cell tumour are here described in their pure forms, intracranial germinal neoplasms are often of mixed histologic composition. In fact, only the germinoma and teratoma are likely to be encountered as pure tumour types {173, 842, 850, 1954, 2000, 2030}. The pathologist confronted by a mixed CNS germ cell tumour is obliged to specifically enumerate its individual elements and should communicate the relative representation of each component present. Immunohistochemical studies may be required to delineate these entities.

Germinoma

The pure germinoma, the most common CNS germ cell tumour, is populated by large cells that appear undifferentiated and that resemble primordial germinal elements (of which, in theory, they represent the neoplastic counterparts). These are disposed in monomorphous sheets, lobules or, in examples characterized by a desmoplastic stromal response, regimented cords and trabecula. Promptly fixed specimens are typified by round, vesicular and centrally positioned nuclei, prominent nucleoli, discrete cell membranes and relatively abundant

cytoplasm that is often strikingly clear due to glycogen accumulation. These cytological features are basically retained in lumbar puncture or ventricular CSF samples that must be screened for tumour cells. Mitoses are usually identified without difficulty and may be conspicuous, but necrosis is uncommon. Delicate fibrovascular septa variably infiltrated by small lymphocytes—principally T cells of both helper/inducer and cytotoxic/suppressor types—are a usual feature {1999, 2385}. The identification of a biphasic population of mature lymphocytes and larger germinoma cells permits cytological diagnosis of these tumours in smear preparations. Some germinomas show a lymphoid or lymphoplasmacellular reaction so florid as to confound the identification of their neoplastic elements in biopsy material. Germinomas may also masquerade as sarcoidosis or tuberculosis by virtue of an obscuring granulomatous response {1162}. Still other germinomas are extensively overgrown by fibrous tissue.

The most constant immunohistochemical attributes of germinomas are strong cell membrane labelling for c-kit {1556} and nuclear reactivity for OCT4 {789}. Cytoplasmic and cell membrane labelling for PLAP is somewhat less common {173, 562, 789, 842, 1954} and may be particularly difficult to demonstrate in inflammatory-looking examples and in specimens previously frozen. A minority of germinomas show patchy foci of cytoplasmic labelling for cytokeratins {562, 842}. Together with demonstrations of intercellular junctional complex and true lumen formation at the ultrastructural level {1478}, this has been taken as evidence of differentiation along somatic epithelial lines or towards embryonal carcinoma. Such differentiation, to which no clinical significance has yet been attached, would appear to be a more frequent event in the germinoma than in its testicular counterpart, the seminoma. Otherwise typical germinomas may contain syncytiotrophoblastic giant cells that manifest cytoplasmic immunolabelling for β-HCG as well as for human placental lactogen (HPL) and cytokeratins. Germinomas with syncytiotrophoblastic elements certainly do not manifest the virulence of choriocarcinomas and should not be confused with them, but emerge from some studies as more prone to recurrence than pure germinomas following radiation therapy (see below).

Teratoma

Teratomas differentiate along ectodermal, endodermal and mesodermal lines (e.g. they recapitulate somatic development from the three embryonic germ layers). Mature and immature variants require distinction.

Mature teratoma

Mature teratomas are composed exclusively of fully differentiated, 'adult-type' tissue elements. Mitotic activity is low or absent. The more common ectodermal components encountered in such tumours include skin, brain and choroid plexus. Mesodermal representatives include cartilage, bone, fat and muscle (both smooth and striated). Cysts lined by epithelia of respiratory or enteric type are the usual endodermal participants, with some examples also containing pancreatic or hepatic tissue. Not infrequently, gut-like structures are formed, replete with mucosa and muscular coats. Advanced organogenesis and somatic organization may result in the phenomenon of intracranial foetus-in-foetu {1572}, though incorporation of a dizygotic twin via epithelial or neural tube defects that disrupt the amniotic septum has also been suggested to account for some cases of this pathological curiosity {1954}.

Immature teratoma

This teratoma variant contains incompletely differentiated components resembling foetal tissues. Such incompletely differentiated areas mandate classification of the lesion as an immature teratoma even if they constitute only minor elements in an otherwise differentiated tumour. Particularly common are a hypercellular and mitotically active "stroma" reminiscent of embryonic mesenchyme and primitive neuroectodermal elements that may fashion neuroepithelial rosettes and canalicular arrays mimicking the developing neural tube. Clefts lined by melanotic neurepithelium are often encountered, these representing abortive retinal differentiation. Immature intracranial teratomas have been reported to undergo spontaneous differentiation into fully mature somatic-type tissues over time {2059}. However, re-resection

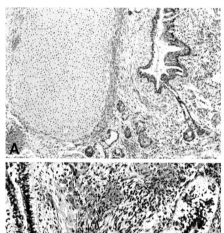

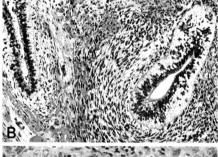

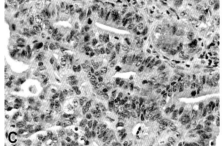

Fig. 12.08 A Mature teratoma with differentiated glands, smooth muscle bundles and a nodule of moderately hypercellular cartilage. B Immature teratoma with foetal-type glands and embryonic mesenchyme-like stroma. C Teratoma with malignant transformation into an enteric-type adenocarcinoma.

specimens composed solely of mature teratoma usually derive from patients whose immature teratomas or mixed germ cell tumours have been subjected to therapy {614}. The apparent tumour "maturation" in such cases presumably reflects the selective radio- or chemoablation of their more actively proliferating components. The enlargement of these residual, differentiated lesions is termed "growing teratoma syndrome" {149, 614}.

Teratoma with malignant transformation

These are generic designations for the occasional teratomatous neoplasm that contains as an additional malignant component a cancer of conventional somatic type. The latter is most often a rhabdomyosarcoma or undifferentiated sarcoma {173, 1954}, less commonly a squamous cell carcinoma or enteric-type adenocarcinoma {173}. Yolk sac tumour elements have also been put forward as the progenitors of select enteric-type adenocarcinomas arising from intracranial germ cell tumours {609}. Curiosities in this setting include the development of erythroleukemia {803}, leiomyosarcoma {2108} and carcinoid {917}. The pathologist detecting evidence of such "malignant transformation" should state the specific histological form that this takes.

On immunohistochemical investigation, the constituent elements of the teratoma can be expected to express those antigens that are appropriate to their native somatic counterparts. Elaboration of AFP by teratomatous glandular epithelium may result in elevated levels of this important marker in the serum and CSF {173, 562, 842, 1954}. Limited immunoexpression of c-kit by included mesenchymal and epithelial elements, as well as increased CSF c-kit levels, has been described {1498}.

Yolk sac tumour

This neoplasm is composed of primitive-appearing epithelial cells—putatively representing yolk sac endoderm—set in a loose, variably cellular and often conspicuously myxoid matrix resembling extra-embryonic mesoblast. The epithelial elements may proliferate in solid sheets but are more commonly disposed about an intervening meshwork of irregular tissue spaces ('reticular' pattern) or line anastomosing sinusoidal channels as a cuboidal epithelium draped, in some cases, over delicate fibrovascular projections to form distinctive papillae known as Schiller-Duval bodies. Yolk sac tumours may also contain eccentrically constricted cysts delimited by flattened epithelial elements ("polyvesicular vitelline" pattern), enteric-type glands lined partially by goblet cells, and foci of apparent hepato-cellular differentiation ("hepatoid" variant). A diagnostic, though inconstant, feature of the yolk sac tumour is the presence of brightly eosinophilic, PAS-positive and diastase resistant hyaline globules that may appear to lie within the cytoplasm of epithelial cells or to be free in the adjoining stroma. Mitotic activity varies considerably and may be conspicuous, but necrosis in uncommon.

Cytoplasmic immunoreactivity for AFP of the epithelial component of the yolk sac tumour is characteristic {173, 562, 842, 1954} and may be of considerable value in distinguishing its solid variant from germinoma and embryonal carcinoma. Furthermore, yolk sac tumours are characteristically non-reactive for c-kit and OCT 4. The hyaline globules of this tumour are also AFP-immunoreactive.

Embryonal carcinoma

The embryonal carcinoma is composed of large cells that proliferate in cohesive nests and sheets, form abortive papillae or line irregular, gland-like spaces. Tumour cells may exceptionally replicate the structure of the early embryo, forming "embryoid bodies" replete with germ discs and miniature amniotic cavities. Markedly enlarged nucleoli, abundant clear to somewhat violet-hued cytoplasm, a high mitotic rate and zones of coagulative necrosis complete the histological picture. The constituent cells uniformly show dense and diffuse cytoplasmic labelling for cytokeratins, attesting to their differentiation along epithelial lines and distinguishing these neoplasms from most germinomas (with which they share PLAP and OCT 4 immunoreactivity) {562, 842}. In addition, c-kit expression is not seen in embryonal carcinoma {1556}.

Choriocarcinoma

The choriocarcinoma is characterized by extra-embryonic differentiation along trophoblastic lines. The diagnosis requires the identification of cytotrophoblastic elements, as well as syncytiotropho-blastic giant cells. The latter may achieve enormous proportions and typically contain multiple, densely hyperchromatic nuclei, often clustered in a knot-like fashion, lying within a large expanse of basophilic or violaceous cytoplasm. The neoplastic syncytiotrophoblast surrounds or partially drapes cohesive masses of large mononucleated cells with vesicular nuclear features and clear or acidophilic cytoplasm, which represent the cytotropho-blastic component. Ectatic stromal vascular channels, blood lakes and extensive haemorrhagic necrosis are the rule. Cytoplasmic immunolabelling of syncytiotrophoblastic giant cells for β-HCG and HPL are characteristic {173, 562, 842, 1954}.

Genetic susceptibility

CNS germ cell tumours typically afflict otherwise healthy individuals. An increased risk of intracranial germ cell neoplasia is associated with Klinefelter syndrome, which is characterized by a 47 XXY genotype and an array of anomalies that includes testicular atrophy, gyneco-mastia, eunuchoid habitus and elevated serum gonadotrophins {1023}. Such patients are also predisposed to media-stinal germ cell tumours. As discussed below, CNS (and other) germ cell tumours commonly exhibit extranumerary X chromosomes. The susceptibility of Klinefelter syndrome patients to such tumours could reflect increased dosage of a chromosome X-associated gene. Noteworthy are descriptions of intracranial germ cell tumours affecting individuals with Down syndrome {334, 779}, which has been associated with an increased risk of testicular germ cell tumourigenesis. Isolated accounts also document CNS germ cell tumours arising in the setting of neurofibromatosis type 1 {2439}, in siblings {61} and in the foetus (intracranial teratoma) of a woman with independent ovarian teratoma {1779}. Rarely, patients with germ cell tumours of the CNS have been reported to develop second gonadal or mediastinal germ cell neoplasms {779, 938, 2374}; one such patient suffered from Down syndrome {779}.

Genetics

The karyotypic and molecular genetic data communicated to date indicate that pure intracranial teratomas presenting as congenital or infantile growths differ fundamentally from the more common CNS germ cell tumours arising beyond early childhood. Whereas the former resemble teratomas of the infant testis in their typically diploid status and general chromosomal integrity, the latter, irrespective of histologic composition, share with their testicular counterparts in young men characteristically aneuploid profiles, complex chromosomal anomalies and clearly overlapping patterns of net genetic imbalance {1633, 1879, 1882, 2034}. These primarily include gains

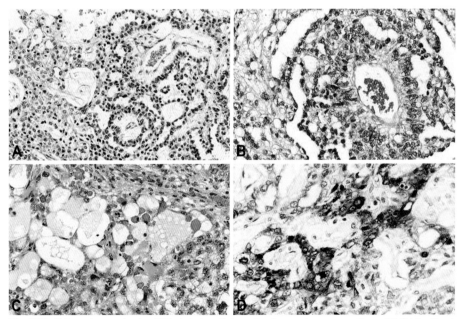

Fig. 12.09 Yolk sac tumour showing (**A**) typical sinusoidal growth pattern and numerous mitoses, (**B**) Schiller-Duval body, (**C**) reticular growth pattern with numerous hyaline globules and (**D**) α-fetoprotein immunolabelling.

involving chromosomes 12p, 8q, 1q and X as well as losses (generally less frequent) of 11q, 13 and 18q {1633, 1882, 2034}. Whether 12p gain and isochromosome 12p formation, especially characteristic of testicular and mediastinal germ cell tumours, occur at comparably high frequency in the CNS setting is debated {1633, 1882, 2034}. Similar considerations apply to the prevalence of X duplication in these locales {1633, 2034}. At the single gene level, there has been limited study of CNS germ cell tumours. The *TP53* and *CDKN2A* genes do not appear to be common targets of mutation in this setting {1607, 1633}. A subset of germinomas share with testicular and mediastinal seminomas mutations involving c-kit {1032}.

Histogenesis

Germ cell tumours of the central neuraxis have long been assumed to represent the neoplastic offspring of primordial germ cells that either migrate in aberrant fashion, or purposefully 'home', to the embryonic CNS rather than the developing genital ridges. In support of a germinal origin for these neoplasms is the fact that they exhibit non-random genetic alterations comparable to those of their morphologic homologues in the gonads. However, studies of the human CNS, including the immunohistochemical screen of foetal pineal glands with antibodies to the primordial germ cell marker PLAP, have never shown it to harbour primitive germ cell elements {562}. Noteworthy in this regard is speculation that germ cells might differentiate into deceptively "somatic" forms

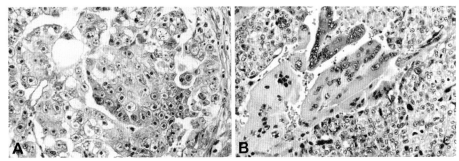

Fig. 12.10 **A** Embryonal carcinoma composed of large epithelial cells forming abortive papillae and glandular structures with macronuclei. **B** Choriocarcinoma with syncytiotrophoblastic giant cells and cytotrophoblasts.

on entering the CNS. Specifically, an enigmatic population of skeletal muscle-like cells native to the developing pineal gland has been proposed as possibly descending from primitive germinal elements attracted to this organ during neuroembryogenesis {1680}. Cited in support of this seemingly far-fetched notion is the fact that striated muscle-type cells of unknown function also populate the thymus, another organ ostensibly devoid of germ cells yet a favoured site of extragonadal germ cell tumourigenesis {1680}.

An alternative to the unifying primordial germ cell hypothesis postulates an origin for CNS germ cell tumours in a variety of displaced embryonic tissues that come to be misincorporated in the developing neural tube {1984}. In this scenario, only the germinoma would derive from misrouted primordial germ cells and so qualify as a true germ cell neoplasm, while intracranial choriocarcinomas would arise from misplaced trophoblast, yolk sac tumours from malpositioned

elements of the secondary yolk sac proper, embryonal carcinomas from primitive constituents of the triploblastic embryo and teratomas from differentiating tissues of the later embryonic period. This theory, too, is based on the existence of ectopic progenitors that have not been detected in the developing human CNS. Furthermore, this scheme must postulate the co-ordinated neoplastic transformation of diverse cell types to account for mixed intracranial germ cell tumours and is difficult to reconcile with the finding of similar genetic abnormalities in neoplasms of different histologic composition. Another speculative proposal would implicate toti- or pluri-potent stem cells in the histogenesis of CNS germ cell tumours {2305}. As such cells are native to all three primitive embryonic layers, defective migration is not requisite to this hypothesis. Implicit in this formulation, however, is the selective genetic programming of uncommitted precursors along the germ cell differentiation pathway, as well as

Table 12.01 Immunohistochemical profiles of CNS germ cell tumours.

	α-Fetoprotein	Human chorionic gonadotropin	Human placental lactogen	Placental alkaline phosphatase	Cytokeratins (CAM 5.2, AE 1/3)	c-kit (CD 117)	OCT4	CD30
Germinoma	-	-[2]	-[2]	+	-[3]	+	+	-
Teratoma	+[1]	-	-	-	+[4]	+/-[6]	-	-
Yolk sac tumour	+	-	-	+/-	+	-	-	-
Embryonal carcinoma	-	-	-	+	+	-	+	+
Choriocarcinoma	-	+	+	+/-	+[5]	-	-	-

[1] α-Fetoprotein is usually restricted to enteric-type glandular components.

[2] Syncytiotrophoblastic giant cells that may be found in otherwise pure germinomas (or in any of the other CNS GCT types) will be immunoreactive for human chorionic gonadotropin and human placental lactogen.

[3] A minority of germinomas exhibit cytokeratin reactivity that is usually distributed in patchy fashion.

[4] Cytokeratin reactivity is a feature of epithelial components.

[5] Immunoreactivity is a regular feature of syncytiotrophoblastic giant cells, while cytotrophoblast is often negative.

[6] Limited immunoexpression by some mesenchymal and epithelioid components may be seen.

their neoplastic transformation. A modified version of this hypothesis suggests a stem cell origin for the pure, diploid teratomas of congenital/infantile onset, reserving a primordial germ cell lineage for the peri- and post-pubertal neoplasms characterized by aneuploidy, over-representation of chromosome 12p and the presence of primitive germ cell-like or mixed histologic components. The differences in these tumour types could, however, reflect the mechanisms of their initiation rather than divergent cellular origins. Also invoked in the histogenesis of CNS teratomas are parthenogenetic mechanisms and the inclusion of blighted twins {1954}. Especially controversial is the nature of teratomatous tumours of the spinal cord. While some have viewed these as complex malformations {1148}, others contend that they are bona fide neoplasms of germ cell origin {29}.

Prognostic and predictive factors

Histological subtype is the single factor most predictive of CNS germ cell tumour outcome {850, 2030}. Mature teratomas are potentially curable by gross total resection. Pure germinomas exhibit a remarkable radiosensitivity foreign to other germ cell tumour types, 10-year survival rates bettering 85% following craniospinal irradiation alone {1616, 2000}. The addition of chemotherapy to germinoma treatment regimes may effect comparable disease control at reduced radiation doses and field volumes {205,1415}. One report excepted {2081}, germinomas harbouring syncytiotrophp-blastic cells or associated with elevated ß-HCG levels have carried an increased risk of local failure and modest decrement in survival compared to their pure counterparts after irradiation alone {2000}. Most virulent are yolk sac tumours,

embryonal carcinomas, choriocarcinomas and mixed lesions in which these subtypes are prominently represented, while immature teratomas and mixed tumours dominated by teratoma or germinoma and containing high-grade non-germinomatous components in relatively limited amounts appear to occupy an intermediate position in terms of biologic potential {1415, 1617, 2000}. The historically dismal prognosis for patients with these malignant, non-germinomatous tumour subtypes has been improved with vigorous adjuvant chemotherapy strategies {1415, 1617} that continue to be investigated. While local recurrence and CSF-borne dissemination are the usual patterns of disease progression, abdominal contamination via ventriculoperitoneal shunts and hematogenous spread (principally to lung and bone) may be encountered.

CHAPTER 13

Familial Tumour Syndromes involving the Nervous System

The elucidation of the molecular basis of inherited cancer syndromes has greatly contributed to the understanding of carcinogenesis in general. The major syndromes with manifestations in the nervous system are listed below.

Syndrome	Gene	Chromosome	Nervous system	Skin	Other tissues
Neurofibromatosis type 1	NF1	17q11	Neurofibroma, MPNST, optic nerve glioma, astrocytoma	Café-au-lait spots, axillary freckling	Iris hamartomas, osseous lesions, phaeochromocytoma, leukaemia
Neurofibromatosis type 2	NF2	22q12	Bilateral vestibular schwannoma, peripheral schwannoma, meningiomas, meningioangiomatosis, spinal ependymoma, astrocytoma, glial hamartias, cerebral calcification	–	Posterior lens opacities, retinal hamartoma
von Hippel-Lindau	VHL	3p25	Haemangioblastoma	–	Retinal haemangioblastoma, renal cell carcinoma, phaeochromocytoma, visceral cysts
Tuberous sclerosis	TSC1 TSC2	9p34 16p13	Subependymal giant cell astrocytoma, cortical tubers	Cutaneous angiofibroma ('adenoma sebaceum'), *peau chagrin*, subungual fibroma	Cardiac rhabdomyoma, adenomatous polyps of the duodenum and the small intestine, cysts of the lung and kidney, lymphangioleiomyomatosis, renal angiomyolipoma
Li-Fraumeni	TP53	17p13	Astrocytomas, PNET	–	Breast carcinoma, bone and soft tissue sarcoma, adrenocortical carcinoma, leukaemia
Cowden	PTEN	10q23	Dysplastic gangliocytoma of the cerebellum (Lhermitte-Duclos), megalencephaly	Multiple trichilemmoma, fibroma	Hamartomatous polyps of the colon, thyroid neoplasms, breast carcinoma
Turcot	APC hMLH1 hPSM2	5q21 3p21 7p22	Medulloblastoma Glioblastoma	Café-au-lait spots	Colorectal polyps Colorectal polyps
Naevoid basal cell carcinoma syndrome (Gorlin)	PTCH	9q31	Medulloblastoma	Multiple basal cell carcinomas, palmar and plantar pits	Jaw cysts, ovarian fibroma, skeletal abnormalities
Rhabdoid tumour predisposition syndrome	INI1	22q11.2	AT/RT	–	Bilateral renal malignant rhabdoid tumours

Neurofibromatosis type 1

A. von Deimling
A. Perry

Definition

An autosomal dominant disorder characterized by neurofibromas, multiple café-au-lait spots, axillary and inguinal freckling, optic gliomas, osseous lesions and iris hamartomas (Lisch nodules); caused by mutations of the *NF1* gene on chromosome 17q11.2.

MIM No.   162200 {1433}.

Synonyms

Von Recklinghausen disease, von Recklinghausen neurofibromatosis, peripheral neurofibromatosis.

Incidence

Although the prevalence in most populations is estimated to be 1:3000 {2360}, higher frequencies have been reported for Arab-Israeli subpopulations {650}.

Diagnostic criteria

The diagnostic criteria for neurofibromatosis type 1 (NF1) are given in Table 13.01.

Nervous system neoplasms

Neurofibromas

The neurofibromas that occur in NF1 patients differ in part from those commonly observed in their sporadic counterparts

Table 13.01 Diagnostic criteria for NF1.

The presence of two or more of the following signs identifies the NF1 patient:
1. Six or more café-au-lait macules (1.5 cm or larger in post-pubertal individuals, 0.5 cm or larger in pre-pubertal individuals)
2. Two or more neurofibromas of any type or one or more plexiform neurofibromas
3. Freckling of armpits or groin
4. Pilocytic astrocytoma of optic pathway ("optic glioma")
5. Two or more Lisch nodules (iris hamartomas)
6. Dysplasia/absence of the sphenoid bone or dysplasia/thinning of long bone cortex
7. First-degree relative with NF1

From Gutmann *et al.* {739}.

(see Chapter 9). Among the major subtypes of neurofibromas, the dermal and plexiform variants are characteristic of NF1.

Dermal neurofibroma is a well-circumscribed, non-encapsulated benign tumour variably composed of Schwann cells and fibroblast-like cells, with an admixture of endothelial cells, lymphocytes, and an unusually large number of mast cells. Deep-seated nodular neurofibromas arise less commonly {897}, have a more solid consistency, and may cause neurological symptoms.

Plexiform neurofibromas produce diffuse enlargement of major nerve trunks and their branches, sometimes yielding a rope-like mass and are almost pathognomonic of NF1. Plexiform neurofibromas may develop during the first one or two years of life as a single subcutaneous swelling with ill-defined margins. They may also cause severe disfigurement later in life, affecting large areas of the body. If these tumours arise in the head or neck region, they can impair vital functions. Plexiform neurofibromas have about a 10% lifetime risk of malignant progression. In contrast, malignant transformation is a very rare event for other neurofibromas.

Malignant peripheral nerve sheath tumours

The malignant peripheral nerve sheath tumours that arise in NF1 patients usually occur at a younger age, may be multiple, and may include rhabdomyoblastic and other heterologous elements. Such lesions, referred to as malignant Triton tumours {2442}, are highly characteristic of NF1. In addition, the glandular variant of malignant peripheral nerve sheath tumour is also a lesion indicative of NF1. Malignant peripheral nerve sheath tumours reduce life expectancy significantly.

Gliomas

The majority of gliomas in NF1 patients are pilocytic astrocytomas that are located within the optic nerve {1306}. Bilateral growth, when present, is characteristic of NF1. Optic nerve gliomas in NF1 patients

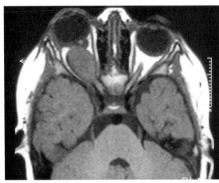

Fig. 13.01 Pilocytic astrocytoma of the optic nerve (optic nerve glioma) in a NF1 patient.

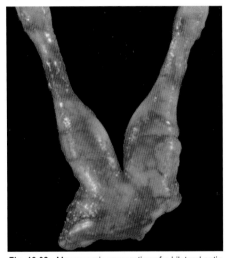

Fig. 13.02 Macroscopic preparation of a bilateral optic nerve glioma in a patient with NF1.

may remain static for many years and some may regress. Other gliomas observed at an increased frequency in NF1 patients include diffuse astrocytomas and glioblastomas {1292A}.

Other CNS manifestations

The following features are more frequent in NF1 patients: macrocephaly {898}, learning disabilities and attention-deficit-hyperactivity disorder {1418}, epilepsy {1868}, hydrocephalus, aquaeductal stenosis and neuropathy {202}.

Extraneural manifestations

Abnormalities of pigmentation

Café-au-lait spots, freckling and Lisch nodules all involve alterations of melanocytes. Café-au-lait spots are often the first manifestation of NF1 in the newborn child. Their number and size increase during infancy, but may remain stable or even decrease in adults. Histopathologically, the ratio of melanocytes to keratinocytes is higher in the unaffected skin of NF1 patients, and this is more marked in the café-au-lait spots {610}. Axillary and/or inguinal freckling occurs

Table 13.02 Manifestations of NF1.

Tumours
Neurofibromas
Dermal
Nodular
Plexiform
Gliomas
Optic glioma
Astrocytoma
Glioblastoma
Sarcomas
Neurofibrosarcoma (MPNST)
Rhabdomyosarcoma
Triton tumour
Gastrointestinal stromal tumour (GIST)
Neuroendocrine/neuroectodermal tumours
Phaeochromocytoma
Carcinoid tumour
Medullary thyroid carcinoma
C-cell hyperplasia
Haematopoietic tumours
Juvenile chronic myeloid leukaemia
Juvenile xanthogranuloma

Other features
Osseous lesions
Scoliosis
Height reduction
Macrocephaly
Pseudoarthrosis
Sphenoid wing dysplasia
Nervous system
Intellectual handicap
Epilepsy
Neuropathy
Hydrocephalus (aqueductal stenosis)
Vascular lesions
Fibromuscular dysplasia/hyperplasia
of renal artery and other arteries
Skin
Café-au-lait spots

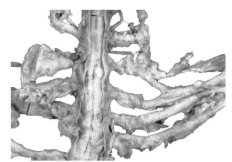

Fig. 13.03 Multiple neurofibromas of the spinal roots and the brachial plexus in a patient with NF1.

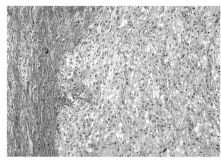

Fig. 13.04 Bilateral optic nerve glioma in a patient with NF1. The histology shows enlargement of the compartments of the optic nerves and collar-like extension into the subarachnoid space.

in about two thirds of NF1 patients, but may have a higher prevalence in young adults {739}. The histopathological features of these freckles are indistinguishable from those of café-au-lait spots. Lisch nodules are small, elevated pigmented hamartomas on the surface of the iris. The presence of Lisch nodules is a particularly useful diagnostic criterion, as they occur in nearly all adults with NF1.

Osseous and vascular lesions
In NF1, the orbits are often affected by sphenoid wing dysplasia. In addition, spinal deformities often result in severe scoliosis that may require surgical intervention. Thinning, bending and pseudoarthrosis may affect the long bones (predominantly tibial), and short stature may also be a component of NF1 {2270}. Fibromuscular dysplasia of the renal and other arteries, including the large cervical vessels, has also been reported as being associated with NF1.

Tumours
NF1 patients have an increased risk of developing rhabdomyosarcomas, juvenile chronic myeloid leukaemia, juvenile xanthogranulomas, gastrointestinal stromal tumours (GIST), duodenal carcinoids, C-cell hyperplasia/medullary thyroid carcinomas, other carcinomas and phaeochromocytomas {2508}.

Genetics
The *NF1* locus is on chromosome 17q11.2 {2046}.

Gene structure
The *NF1* gene is large, containing 59 exons and spanning roughly 350 kb {1947}. One of the two extensive introns, 27b, includes coding sequences for

three embedded genes that are transcribed in a reverse direction: *EVI2A*, *EVI2B* and *OMGP*. There are 12 non-processed *NF1* pseudogenes localized on 8 chromosomes. None of these pseudogenes extends beyond exon 29.

Gene expression
The *NF1* transcript is approximately 13 kb long and includes three alternatively spliced isoforms (exons 9a, 23a, and 48a), variably expressed based on tissue type and differentiation {1947}.

The product of the gene, neurofibromin, is a cytoplasmic protein that can be found in two major isoforms of 2818 amino acids (type 1) and 2839 amino acids (type 2) of 220-250 kD. The protein harbours a GAP-related domain (GRD) and thus belongs to the group of mammalian RasGTPase-activating proteins. In addition to the homology between the GAP domains, it has large segments that show moderate homology to the two Saccharomyces cerevisiae inhibitors of Ras protein, IRA1 and IRA2. While several features of these domains, including alternative splicing and the presence of mutations, suggest that they may be functionally important, their exact role is as yet unknown. Nevertheless, data suggest that neurofibromin loss may selectively activate RAS isoforms, thereby stimulating downstream signalling cascades and mitogenic mediators, such as cAMP, AKT, ERK1/2, RAF, PI3K, mTOR, and S6K {1947}. There is also some evidence for growth-regulatory functions outside of the neurofibromin GRD. Although neurofibromin is expressed almost ubiquitously in most mammalian tissues, the highest levels have been found in the central and peripheral nervous system and in the adrenal gland.

Gene mutations

Mutation screening of the *NF1* gene is difficult due to its large size, the presence of pseudogenes, and the fact that mutations do not appear to cluster in hot spots, perhaps with the exception of exons 10a-10c {1463}. Over 300 mutations have been previously reported (http://www.ncbi.nlm.nih.gov/entrez/disp omim.cgi?id=162200). Using comprehensive screening techniques that may include various strategies, such as long range RT-PCR, protein truncation testing, cDNA sequencing and FISH, up to 95% of mutations may be detected in individuals fulfilling NIH criteria for NF1 {1463}. More than 80% of mutations are predicted to encode truncated proteins or none at all.

Genotype/phenotype correlation

No convincing genotype-phenotype correlations have so far been established, with the exception of the "NF1 microdeletion syndrome"; the latter is encountered in roughly 5–10% of patients and is caused by unequal homologous recombination of *NF1* repeats resulting in the loss of approximately 1.5 Mb of DNA on 17q, including the entire *NF1* gene (http://www.ncbi.nlm.nih.gov/entrez/dispomim.cgi?id=162200). Such patients tend to have a more severe phenotype, including facial dysmorphism, mental retardation, developmental delay, increased burden of neurofibromas and enhanced risk of MPNST development {439}. However, the latter observation was not substantiated by another group studying 30 MPNSTs

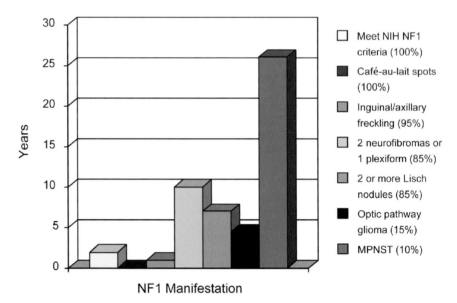

Fig. 13.05 Mean ages of onset for common clinical manifestations in patients with NF1. Estimated frequencies for each manifestation within the NF1 population are given in parentheses.

from NF1 patients {2291}. Genotype-phenotype correlations are also complicated by the unusually high degree of variable expressivity (intrafamilial variability of expression) within NF1 families. Evidence favouring a role for modifying non-allelic genes has been provided by the correlation between clinical manifestations and the degree of relatedness of patients {2191}.

Genetic alterations in NF1-associated tumours

Several observations in sporadic and NF1-associated tumours indicate that neurofibromin acts as a tumour suppressor. Either loss of heterozygosity (LOH) or the presence of a mutation of the second allele has been demonstrated in neurofibromas, MPNSTs, optic gliomas, and other NF1-associated tumours {1286, 1619, 2290}. Only the subpopulation of Schwann cells in neurofibromas exhibited loss of the *NF1* gene {1135}, supporting the hypothesis that Schwann cells are the progenitor cells of neurofibromas. Animal models suggest that a heterozygous state of *NF1* inactivation within adjacent non-neoplastic cells is critical to the formation of both neurofibromas and optic pathway gliomas {88,2504}. MPNSTs contain many other genetic alterations during malignant progression from precursor lesions, such as plexiform

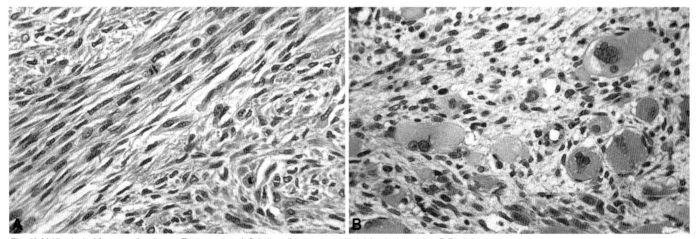

Fig. 13.06 Histological features of malignant Triton tumour. **A** Spindle cell component with brisk mitotic activity. **B** Rhabdomyosarcomatous component.

neurofibroma; commonly reported ones include *TP53* mutation, *CDKN2A* or 9p21 losses, p27 loss, EGFR protein overexpression and occasional gene amplification, topoisomerase II-α (TOP2A) overexpression, and dysregulation of numerous growth factors including neuregulin-1 and the ErbB receptors, as well as hepatocyte growth factor and the c-met receptor {290, 1180, 1591, 1728, 2107}. Karyotypes are often remarkably complex, and there are multiple regions of recurring chromosomal gains and losses for which the target genes are unknown.

NF1 variants

Variants of NF1 that do not co-segregate with the *NF1* gene locus are known {1167, 2450}. Even the autosomal dominant 'café-au-lait-spots only' variant exists as both *NF1*-gene-linked and unlinked entities {3, 234}. Similarly, patients who meet diagnostic criteria for both NF1 and NF2 have occasionally been described, although the vast majority qualify as one or the other and the existence of a 'mixed' form remains controversial. The occurrence of a segmental form of NF1, caused by somatic mosaicism at the *NF1* gene locus, further extends the range of variability {1334,1955}. Such patients often have only pigmentary manifestations within the affected limb or region; however, others develop classic tumours, such as plexiform neurofibromas, optic pathway gliomas, etc.

Although some cell lines derived from malignant peripheral nerve sheath tumours respond to neurofibromin deficiency by dramatically increased levels of RasGTP, their tumourigenicity may depend at least as much on the inactivation of the *TP53* gene as on the loss of function of *NF1* {1456}. The generation of mice deficient in neurofibromin {213, 945} has aided the identification of potential cell-type specific functions of neurofibromin. Loss of the murine *NF1* gene product results in lethality at day 13.5 of embryogenesis due to abnormal cardiac development, a phenotype that has been linked to abnormal regulation of Ras activity {1251}. Mice heterozygous for the *Nf1* knockout allele develop rare tumours associated with human NF1 {945} and display learning and memory defects {2099}. Loss of heterozygosity at the *NF1* locus can be demonstrated in the observed tumours {945}, indicating that the condition in heterozygous mice is similar to the human disease. Schwann cells derived from neurofibromin-deficient embryos are angiogenic, highly invasive and hyperproliferative {1106}. Neurofibromin-deficient sensory neurons survive in the absence of neurotrophins via activation of a Ras-dependent pathway {1131}. Additionally, loss of neurofibromin in fetal liver cells renders the cells hypersensitive to the proliferative effects of multiple haematopoietic cytokines through constitutive activation of Ras signalling {2496}. Several instances in which biological responses to neurofibromin deficiency or overexpression are not accompanied by changes in the level of RasGTP suggest that neurofibromin may have additional functions that are independent of its RasGAP activity, and which may or may not depend on its interaction with the Ras proteins.

Neurofibromatosis type 2

A.O. Stemmer-Rachamimov
O.D. Wiestler
D.N. Louis

Definition

An autosomal dominant disorder characterized by neoplastic and dysplastic lesions that primarily affect the nervous system; bilateral vestibular schwannomas are the hallmark, with other manifestations, including schwannomas of other cranial nerves, spinal and cutaneous schwannomas, intracranial and spinal meningiomas, gliomas, meningioangiomatosis, glial hamartomas, ocular abnormalities and neuropathies, caused by mutations of the *NF2* gene on chromosome 22q12.

MIM No. 101000 {1433}.

Synonyms

Historical terms include central neurofibromatosis and bilateral acoustic neurofibromatosis. The term "von Recklinghausen neurofibromatosis" is associated with NF1 and should not be used for neurofibromatosis type 2 (NF2).

Incidence

The incidence of the disease has been reported as 1 per 40 000 newborns, however recent data suggest that may be an underestimate, and the disorder may be more common (1:25 000) {543}. About half of all cases occur in individuals with

no family history of NF2, and are caused by newly acquired germline mutations.

Diagnostic criteria

The original clinical diagnostic criteria for NF2 (NIH meeting in 1987 {2165}) underwent several revisions. The revised classifications expanded the criteria aiming to identify patients with multiple NF2 features that do not present with bilateral vestibular schwannomas and have no family history of NF2 (NIH Consensus Panel 1991, Man-chester criteria, NNFF criteria) {540, 739}.

Nervous system neoplasms

Schwannoma

NF2-associated schwannomas are WHO grade I tumours that are comprised of neoplastic Schwann cells, but which differ from sporadic schwannomas in a number of ways. NF2 schwannomas present at an earlier age (third decade) than sporadic tumours (sixth decade), and many NF2 patients develop the diagnostic hallmark of the disease, bilateral vestibular schwannomas, by their fourth decade of life {540, 1410}. NF2 vestibular schwannomas may entrap seventh cranial nerve fibres {942} and have higher proliferative activity {55}, although these features do not necessarily connote more aggressive behaviour. In addition to the vestibular

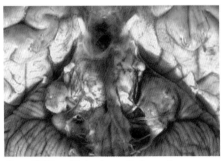

Fig. 13.07 Bilateral vestibular schwannomas, diagnostic for NF2.

division of the eighth cranial nerve, other sensory nerves may be affected, including the fifth cranial nerve and spinal dorsal roots. However, motor nerves such as the twelfth cranial nerve may also be involved {540, 1352}. Cutaneous schwannomas are common and may be plexiform {540, 1410}. NF2 schwannomas may appear multilobular ("cluster of grapes") on both gross and microscopic examination {2403}, and multiple schwannomatous tumourlets may develop along individual nerves, particularly on spinal roots {1352, 2151}.

Meningioma

Multiple meningiomas are the second hallmark of NF2 and occur in half of NF2 patients {1352}. NF2 meningiomas occur earlier in life than sporadic meningiomas

Table 13.03 Diagnostic criteria for NF2.

Definite NF2
1. Bilateral vestibular schwannomas; or

2. First-degree family relative with NF2 and either
  a) Unilateral vestibular schwannoma at <30 years; or
  b) Any two of the following: meningioma, schwannoma, glioma, posterior subcapsular lens opacity.

Probable NF2
1. Unilateral vestibular schwannoma at <30 years and at least one of the following: meningioma, schwannoma, glioma, posterior subcapsular lens opacity; or

2. Multiple meningiomas and either
  a) Unilateral vestibular schwannoma at <30 years; or
  b) One of the following: schwannoma, glioma, posterior lens opacity.

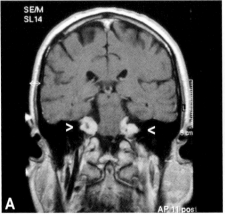
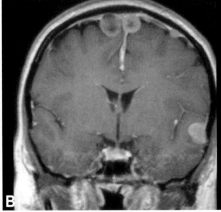

Fig. 13.08 T1-weighted, contrast-enhanced MR images from patients with NF2. **A** Bilateral acoustic schwannomas (arrows), the diagnostic hallmark of NF2. **B** Multiple meningiomas presenting as contrast-enhanced masses.

and may be the presenting feature of NF2, especially in the paediatric population {538, 540, 1410}. Although most of NF2-associated meningiomas are usually WHO grade I tumours, several studies suggest that NF2-associated meningiomas have a higher mitotic index and a more aggressive clinical behaviour than sporadic meningiomas {54, 1724}. All major subtypes of meningioma occur in NF2 patients {54, 1352}.

Glioma

Approximately 80% of gliomas in NF2 patients are spinal intramedullary or cauda equina tumours, with an additional 10% of gliomas occurring in the medulla {1904}. Ependymomas account for approximately 65–75% of all histologically diagnosed gliomas in NF2, and for almost all spinal gliomas {1904, 1959}. In most cases, NF2 spinal ependymomas are multiple intramedullary masses {1904, 1959}. Diffuse and pilocytic astrocytomas also occur in NF2, but are less common.

Neurofibroma

Cutaneous neurofibromas have been reported in NF2. On histological review, however, many 'neurofibromas' prove to be schwannomas, including plexiform schwannomas misdiagnosed as plexiform neurofibromas.

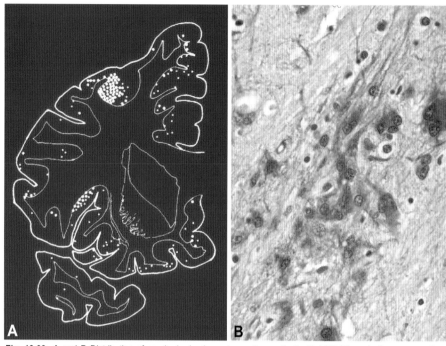

Fig. 13.09 **A** and **B** Distribution of cerebral microhamartomas in a patient with NF2. These lesions are scattered throughout the cortex and basal ganglia and show strong immunoreactivity for S-100 (**B**). Reproduced from Wiestler et al. {2410}.

Other nervous system lesions

Schwannosis This is a proliferation of Schwann cells, sometimes with entangled axons, but without frank tumour formation. In NF2 patients, schwannosis is often found in the spinal dorsal root entry zones, sometimes associated with a schwannoma of the dorsal root, or in the perivascular spaces of the central spinal cord, where the nodules appear more like small traumatic neuromas {1949, 1959}. Less robust, but otherwise identical, schwannosis has been reported in reactive conditions.

Meningioangiomatosis This cortical lesion is characterized by a plaque-like proliferation of meningothelial and fibroblast-like cells surrounding small vessels, and occurs both sporadically and in NF2. Meningioangiomatosis is usually a single, intracortical lesion, although multifocal examples, occur as do non-cortical lesions {1949, 1959}. It may be predominantly vascular, resembling a vascular malformation, or predominantly meningothelial, sometimes with an associated meningioma. Sporadic meningioangiomatosis is a single lesion that usually occurs in young adults or children who present with seizures or persistent headaches. In contrast, NF2-associated meningioangiomatosis may be multifocal and is often asymptomatic and diagnosed only at autopsy {2150}.

Glial hamartia Glial hamartias (or microhamartomas) of the cerebral cortex are circumscribed clusters of cells with medium-to-large atypical nuclei and

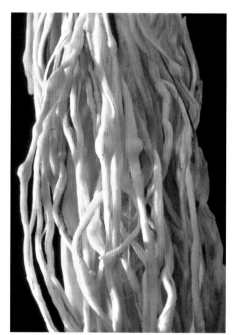

Fig. 13.10 Numerous schwannomas of the cauda equina in a patient with NF2.

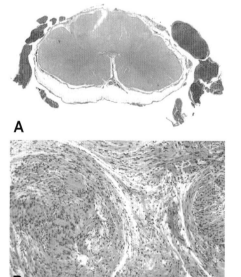

Fig.13.11 **A** Multiple schwannomas of spinal roots. The histology (**B**) shows a nodular schwannoma in NF2 patient.

Table 13.04 Major manifestations of NF2

Schwann cell lesions:
Schwannomas (including bilateral vestibular)
Schwannosis

Meningeal lesions:
Meningiomas
Meningioangiomatosis

Glial lesions:
Spinal ependymomas
Astrocytomas
Glial hamartias

Other lesions:
Posterior lens opacities
Cerebral calcifications

scant, sometimes stellar, eosinophilic cytoplasm. The cells stain strongly for S-100 protein, but only focally for GFAP. Glial hamartias are common in and pathognomonic of NF2 {1949, 2410}, and are not associated with mental retardation or astrocytomas. The hamartias are usually intracortical, with a predilection for the molecular and deeper cortical layers, but have also been observed in the basal ganglia, thalamus and cerebellum {2410}. Merlin expression is retained in glial hamartias, raising the possibility that haplo-insufficiency during development underlies these malformations {2149}.

Cerebral calcification Intracranial calcifications have been noted frequently in neuroimaging studies of patients with NF2. Preferred localizations are the cerebral and cerebellar cortices, periventricular areas and choroid plexus. The histopathological correlates remain unclear.

Peripheral neuropathy Peripheral neuropathies, not related to tumour masses, are increasingly recognized as a common feature of NF2 {385, 1352, 3525}. Mono-neuropathies may be the presenting symptom in children {538}, while progressive polyneuropathies are more common in adults. Sural nerve biopsies from NF2 patients suggest that NF2 neuropathies are mostly axonal and may be secondary to focal nerve compression by tumourlets or onion-bulb-like Schwann cell or perineurial cell proliferations without associated axons {2133, 2242}.

Extraneural manifestations
Posterior lens opacities are common and highly characteristic of NF2. A variety of retinal abnormalities (including hamartomas, tufts and dysplasias) may also be found {314}. Skin lesions other than cutaneous nerve sheath tumours, primarily café-au-lait spots, have been reported.

Genetics
The *NF2* gene is located at chromosome 22q12 {1941, 2266}.

Gene structure
The *NF2* gene {1941, 2266} spans 110 kb, and comprises 17 exons. NF2 mRNA transcripts encode at least two major protein forms generated by alternative splicing at the carboxyl terminus. Isoform 1, encoded by exons 1-15 and 17, has intramolecular interactions similar to the ERM proteins (see below); isoform 2, encoded by exons 1-16, exists only in an unfolded state {737, 2453}.

Gene expression
The *NF2* gene is expressed in most normal human tissues studied, including brain {1941, 2266}. The predicted protein product shows a strong similarity with the highly conserved protein 4.1 family of cytoskeleton-associated proteins, which includes protein 4.1, talin, moesin, ezrin, radixin and protein tyrosine phosphatases.

The similarity of the NF2-encoded protein to moesin, ezrin and radixin (ERM), resulted in the name merlin {2266}; the alternative name schwannomin has also been suggested {1941}. Members of the protein 4.1 family link the cell membrane to the actin cytoskeleton. These proteins consist of a globular amino terminal domain, an α-helical domain containing a praline rich region, and a charged carboxyl terminal domain. The amino terminus interacts with cell membrane proteins such as CD44, CD43, ICAM-1 and ICAM-2, while the carboxy terminal domain contains the actin binding site. The highest degree of structural similarity between merlin and the ERM proteins is in the amino terminal domain. Merlin lacks the actin binding site in the carboxy terminus but may have an alternative actin binding site {2453}. ERM proteins and merlin may be self-regulated by head-to-tail intramolecular associations which result in folded and unfolded states. The folded state of merlin is the functionally active molecule and is inhibited by phosphorylation of the COOH-terminal on serine residues {2075}. Although the precise mechanism of tumour suppression by merlin is still unknown, the structural similarity of merlin to the ERM protein suggests that merlin provides regulated linkage between membrane-associated proteins and the actin cytoskeleton; the tumour suppressor activity may be exerted by regulation of signal transmission from the extracellular environment to the cell {1427}. Many merlin binding partners have been identified {1117, 1539}.

Gene mutations
Numerous germline and somatic *NF2* mutations have been detected, supporting the hypothesis that *NF2* functions as a tumour suppressor gene {736, 1352}.

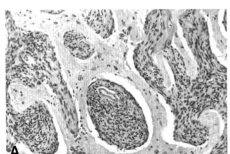
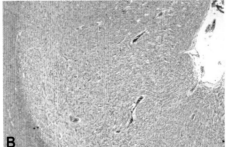
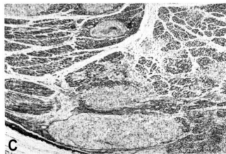

Fig. 13.12 Histological features of lesions associated with NF2. **A** Meningioangiomatosis with predominance of meningothelial cells. **B** Diffuse cortical meningioangiomatosis (trichrome stain). **C** Luxol fast blue staining of a section of the cauda equina with multiple early stages of schwannomas (tumourlets) and characteristic absence of myelin.

Germline *NF2* mutations differ somewhat from somatic mutations identified in sporadic schwannomas (see Chapter 9) and meningiomas (see Chapter 10). The most frequent germline mutations are point mutations that alter splice junctions or create new stop codons {207, 1352, 1367, 1460, 1941, 1970, 2266}. While germline mutations are found in all parts of the gene, with the exception of the alternatively spliced exons, they occur preferentially in exons 1 to 8 {1460}. A possible hot spot for mutations appears to be position 169 in exon 2, in which a C to T transition at a CpG dinucleotide results in a stop at codon 57 {207, 1460}; other CpG dinucleotides are also commonly targets for C to T transitions {1970}.

Prognostic and predictive factors

The clinical course in patients with NF2 varies widely between families and, to a lesser extent, within families {540, 1410}. Some families feature early onset with diverse tumours and high tumour load (Wishart type), while others present later with only vestibular schwannomas (Gardner type). An effect of maternal inheritance on severity has been noted, as have families with genetic anticipation. All families with NF2 show linkage of the disease to chromosome 22 {1570}, implying a single responsible gene, and correlations of genotype with phenotype have therefore attempted to predict clinical course on the basis of the type of the underlying *NF2* mutation. Nonsense

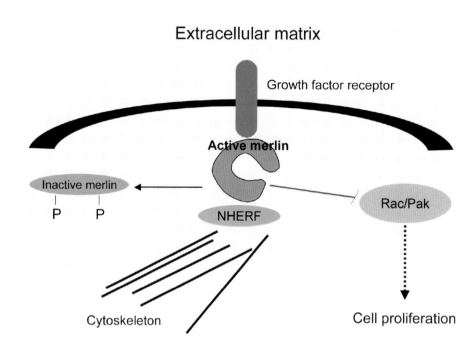

Fig. 13.13 In its active (hypophosphorylated) state merlin suppresses cell proliferation and motility by inhibiting the transmission of growth signals from the extracellular environment to the Pak/Rac signaling system. Inactivated (phosphorylated) merlin dissociates from its protein scaffold thus disinhibiting Rac/Pak signaling and cell proliferation and motility.

and frameshift mutations are often associated with a more severe phenotype, regardless of their position in the gene, while missense mutations that preserve the carboxyl terminus of the protein result in milder phenotypes {1460}. Phenotypic variability is observed in splice site mutations, with more severe phenotypes observed in mutations upstream from exon 7 {1137}. Large deletions and somatic mosaicism have been associated with mild disease {111, 544, 1138}. Clinical predictors associated with increased risk of mortality in NF2 patients include early age at diagnosis, presence of intracranial meningiomas and treatment at non-specialty centres {110}.

Schwannomatosis

Definition

A usually sporadic and sometimes autosomal dominant disorder characterized by multiple spinal, cutaneous and cranial nerve schwannomas, without vestibular schwannomas or other manifestations of neurofibromatosis type 2 (NF2) or neurofibromatosis 1 (NF1); associated with inactivation of the *NF2* gene in tumours but not in the germline.

MIM No.   162091.

Synonyms

Terms used to describe the disorder include "neurilemomatosis", "multiple schwannomas" and "multiple neurilemomas".

Incidence

In several reports, schwannomatosis was found to be almost as common as neurofibromatosis type 2, with an estimated incidence 1:40 000 -1:80 000 {56, 2050}. Familial schwannomatosis is rare; representing only 10–15% of all cases {1369, 2050}.

Diagnostic criteria

Reports of patients with multiple non-vestibular schwannomas date back to 1984 {2090}, but it was long debated whether the condition represents a form of attenuated NF2 or a separate entity. A consensus panel of experts has recently developed standardized clinical diagnostic criteria for schwannomatosis {1366}. Essential for the diagnosis of schwannomatosis is the exclusion of NF2 by clinical criteria and by imaging of the vestibular nerves. The distinction may be particularly challenging in paediatric patients, as vestibular schwannomas may

Table 13.05 Diagnostic criteria for schwannomatosis

> **Definite schwannomatosis**
> - Two or more (pathologically proven) schwannomas and lack of vestibular schwannomas on MRI study at >30 years and no known constitutional *NF2* mutation; or
> - One (pathologically proven) schwannoma and first degree relative with schwannomatosis.
>
> **Probable schwannomatosis**
> - Two or more schwannomas and age under 30 years and no evidence of vestibular schwannomas on MRI scan and no known constitutional *NF2* mutation; or
> - Two or more schwannomas and age over 45 years and no symptoms of cranial nerve VIII dysfunction and no known constitutional *NF2* mutation; or
> - Radiographic evidence of one schwannoma and first-degree relative with schwannomatosis.

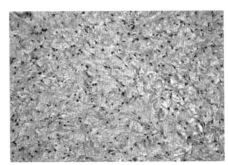

Fig. 13.14 Histopathological features of schwannomas in a schwannomatosis patient. Note a marked myxoid stroma.

develop only later in the course of the disease {542}.

Nervous system neoplasms
Schwannomas
Schwannomatosis patients develop multiple schwannomas. These tumours may develop in spinal roots, cranial nerves and in skin, but not in the vestibular nerves. Cutaneous schwannomas may be plexiform. The tumours have a segmental distribution in 30% of schwannomatosis patients {1066, 1298}. In contrast to NF2 patients, patients with schwannomatosis

often suffer from severe pain from their tumours, whereas neurological deficits and polyneuropathy are rare {1366}. Schwannomatosis tumours may display prominent myxoid stroma and an intraneural growth pattern {1366} and are sometimes misdiagnosed as neurofibromas {542, 1366}.

Other nervous system lesions
There is no association of schwannomatosis with ependymomas or ocular abnormalities, but a rare association with single or multiple meningiomas has been reported {920, 1618, 1918}.

Extraneural manifestations
There are no extraneural manifestation associated with schwannomatosis.

Genetics
NF2 mutations are found in schwannomatosis-associated schwannomas, but are not found in non-tumour tissue, suggesting that *NF2* mutations are somatic rather than germline. In addition, several studies have excluded germline *NF2* mutations in familial schwanno-

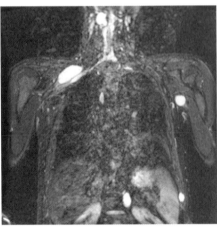

Fig. 13.15 Coronal MRI (STIR) showing multiple, bright, discrete tumours in a schwannomatosis patient.

matosis; analysis of multiple tumours from affected individuals showed no shared *NF2* mutations within the tumours or within families precluding an underlying *NF2* germline mutation {948, 1066, 1368}. This suggests that schwannomatosis is caused by another gene, which remains unknown. Linkage analysis studies suggest that the gene resides on chromosome 22 {1368}.

Von Hippel-Lindau disease and haemangioblastoma

K.H. Plate
A.O. Vortmeyer
D. Zagzag
H.P.H. Neumann

Definition
Von Hippel-Lindau is an autosomal dominant disorder caused by germline mutations of the *VHL* gene on chromosome 3p25–26 and characterized by the development of haemangioblastomas of the nervous system and retina, clear cell renal carcinoma, phaeochromocytoma, epididymal cystadenoma, neuroendocrine tumours and microcystic adenomas of the pancreas and endolymphatic sac tumours.

MIM No.
193300 {1433}.

Synonyms and historical annotation
Lindau {1324} described capillary haemangioblastoma, and also noted its association with retinal vascular tumours, previously described by von Hippel {2343}, and tumours of the visceral organs.

Incidence
Von Hippel-Lindau (VHL) disease is estimated to occur at rates of 1:36 000 {1380} to 1:45 500 population {1375}.

Diagnostic criteria
The clinical diagnosis of VHL disease is based on the presence of capillary haemangioblastoma in the CNS or retina, and the presence of one of the typical VHL-associated tumours, or a previous family history. In VHL disease, germline *VHL* mutations can virtually always be identified {2155}.

Haemangioblastoma
VHL-associated tumours typically occur in young adults, with a mean age of 29 {1382}. Sporadic haemangioblastomas occur predominantly in the cerebellum, whereas VHL-associated haemangioblastomas are localized in the cerebellum, brain stem and spinal cord and nerve roots. Supratentorial and peripheral nervous system lesions are rare. VHL patients often have multiple haemangioblastomas at various sites; multiple tumours are almost exclusively found in VHL patients (See Chapter 10).

Histogenesis
Haemangioblastomas are composed of vascular and stromal cells. Tissue microdissection, combined with deletion analysis of the VHL gene locus, have identified the stromal cells as neoplastic {1277}, but their origin remains enigmatic. Suggested origins include glial cells {45}, endothelial cells {1020}, arachnoid cells {1501}, embryonic choroid plexus {176}, neuroendocrine cells {123}, fibrohistiocytic cells {1579}, cells of neuroectodermal derivation {12, 918, 1086, 2214} or heterogeneous cell populations {2214}. To address this issue, numerous immunohistochemical and ultrastructural studies have been performed. For example, neural cell adhesion molecule (NCAM/CD56) is consistently immunoreactive {190, 192} and there is frequent positive immunoreactivity for S-100 protein {886, 1245, 1579, 1644, 2214}. Factors VIII and XIIIa have been reported in stromal cells {1020, 1035, 1245, 1644}, but some studies have found these molecules exclusively in the vascular component {397, 2214}. GFAP staining of stromal cells has been found only in some reports {923, 963}, and it is unclear whether scattered GFAP-positive cells represent entrapped reactive astrocytes {397, 445, 1579}, stromal cells with glial differentiation {397, 445, 923, 1086} or stromal cells with intracytoplasmic GFAP from phagocytic activity {445, 1020}.

Some ultrastructural studies have found overlapping features between stromal and vascular cells {282, 323, 791, 843, 985, 1020, 1069}, including Weibel-Palade body formation in the cytoplasm of the stromal cells {1245, 2132}, raising the possibility that stromal cells may differentiate into vascular components, but other electron microscopic reports found distinct stromal and vascular cellular constituents {123, 191, 1579, 2214}. In this regard, an intriguing hypothesis is, as originally suggested by Lindau in 1931 {1325}, that these tumours are derived from embryonal cell types with divergent

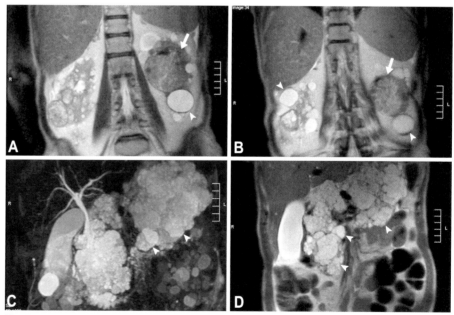

Fig. 13.16 Abdominal MRI in a patient with VHL disease. **A,B** Numerous renal cystic structures (arrowheads) and a solid renal mass (arrows). Coronal T2-weighted MRI images. **C,D** Numerous pancreatic cysts (arrowheads). Coronal T2-weighted MRI images.

Table 13.06 Extracranial manifestations of VHL disease.

Organ	Lesion
Retina	Haemangioblastoma
Peripheral nerve	Haemangioblastoma
Kidney	Cysts Renal cell carcinoma
Pancreas	Cysts Microcystic adenoma Neuroendocrine tumours
Adrenal gland/ paraganglia	Phaeochromocytoma/ paraganglioma
Endolymphatic sac/duct	Endolymphatic sac tumour
Epididymis	Epididymal cystadenoma
Adnexae	Cystadenoma
Other organs	Cysts

differentiation potentials. For example, one ultrastructural study {323} found features characteristic of embryonic cells and concluded that stromal cells and vasoformative elements share a common ancestry, possibly of angioblastic lineage. Decades ago, Stein et al. {2148} had suggested an angiomesenchymal origin of haemangioblastoma, based on original, developmental biologic observations made by Florence Sabin in 1917 {1967}. Haemangioblastomas appear capable of blood island formation with potential extramedullary haematopoiesis analogous to embryonic haemangioblastic stem cells {1943, 2148, 2347, 2488}. Furthermore, haemangioblastomas express the erythropoietin-receptor (EpoR) {2347}, which is also observed during early embryonic blood island formation at mouse embryonic day 8.0–9.5 {1279}; in addition, stromal cells express some proteins that characterize embryonic progenitor cells with haemangioblastic differentiation potential (Scl, brachyury, Csf-1R, Gata-1, Flk-1 and Tie-2) {696}. Furthermore, tumour growth occurs from highly vascularized, VHL-deficient, poorly differentiated precursor structures {2349, 2350}. Therefore, embryonic progenitor cells with haemangioblastic differentiation potential represent a likely cytologic equivalent of the stromal cell. However, the capacity of neuroectodermal cells to differentiate along a haematopoietic lineage remains to be more convincingly demonstrated.

Extraneural manifestations
A variety of neoplasms are known to occur in patients with VHL disease. A common tumour is the retinal von Hippel tumour or angioma, which is histologically identical to capillary haemangioblastoma {1592, 2381}. Many of the other tumours and tumour-like lesions associated with VHL are concentrated in the visceral organs. Of the visceral tumours, clear cell renal carcinomas and phaeochromocytomas are most common {1254, 1328, 1381}. The endolymphatic sac tumour of the inner ear is a hypervascular neoplasm that arises from the temporal petrous region {342, 994, 1381}. Pancreatic involvement with VHL disease includes true cysts, serous cystadenomas, neuro-endocrine tumours, or combined lesions {763}. Cystadenomas of the broad ligament are extremely rare {2395}.

Genetics
The VHL gene is located at chromosome 3p25-26 {1266}. The VHL tumour suppressor gene has three exons and a coding sequence of 639 nucleotides {1266}. It is expressed ubiquitously including in the CNS {382, 1548, 1973}.

Function of the VHL protein
Mutational inactivation of the VHL gene in affected family members is responsible for their genetic susceptibility to capillary haemangioblastoma of the CNS including the retina, renal clear cell carcinoma, phaeochromocytoma, pancreatic islet cell tumour and endolymphatic sac tumour of the inner ear. The mechanisms by which the gene product, the VHL protein (pVHL), causes neoplastic transformation, has remained enigmatic. Several signalling pathways appear to be involved {1628}, one of which points a role of pVHL in protein degradation and angiogenesis. The α domain of pVHL forms a complex with elongin B, elongin C, Cul-2 {1343, 1706, 2144} and Rbx1 {1036} which has ubiquitin ligase activity {935}, thereby targeting cellular proteins for ubiquitination and proteasome-mediated degradation. The domain of the VHL gene involved in the binding to elongin is frequently mutated in VHL-associated neoplasms {2144}.

The β-domain of pVHL interacts with the α subunits of transcription factor, hypoxia-inducible Factor (HIF), which mediates cellular responses to hypoxia. Under normoxic conditions and in the presence of functional pVHL, the α subunits are rapidly degraded. Under hypoxic conditions and in VHL deficient cells, HIFα is stabilised, with a concomitant induction of hypoxia-regulated genes, including vascular endothelial growth factor (VEGF) {1421}. Constitutive overexpression of VEGF through this signalling pathway could explain the extraordinary capillary component of VHL-associated neoplasms {1421}. The capillaries of CNS haemangioblastomas are believed to be under the control of overexpressed VEGF and related angiogenic factors, which are secreted by stromal cells and are considered non-neoplastic.

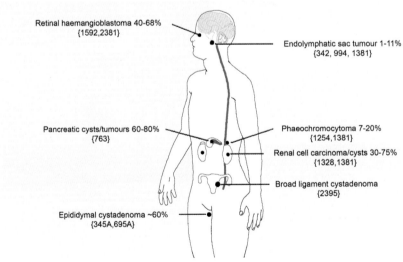

Fig. 13.17 Extraneural manifestations of VHL disease.

Additional functions of the VHL protein may contribute to malignant transformation and the evolution of the phenotype of VHL-associated lesions. Some of these may or may not be mediated by HIF. Studies in renal cell carcinoma cell lines suggest that pVHL is involved in the control of cell cycle exit, i.e. transition from the G2 phase, possibly by preventing accumulation of the cyclin-dependent kinase inhibitor p27 {1705}. Wild-type but not tumour-derived pVHL binds to fibronectin. As a consequence, VHL-deficient renal cell carcinoma cells show a defective assembly of extracellular fibronectin matrix {1629}. Through down-regulation of the response of cells to hepatocyte growth factor/scatter factor and reduced levels of tissue inhibitor of metalloproteinase 2 (TIMP-2), pVHL-deficient tumour cells exhibit a significantly higher capacity for invasion {1164}. Further, inactivated pVHL causes an overexpression of transmembrane carbonic anhydrases that are involved in pH regulation {932} but the biological significance of this dysregulation remains to be assessed.

Based on the discovery of VHL-deficient immature cell deposits in target tissues {2349, 2350}, the capacity of stromal cells to differentiate into red blood cells {2347}, and common protein expression profiles between stromal cells and embryonic progenitor cells with haemangioblastic differentiation potential (Scl, brachyury, Csf-1R, Gata-1, Flk-1, Tie-2) {696}, developmental effects of loss of VHL function have been suggested.

Gene mutations and VHL subtypes

Germline mutations of the *VHL* gene are spread throughout the three exons. Missense mutations are most common, but nonsense mutations, microdeletions/

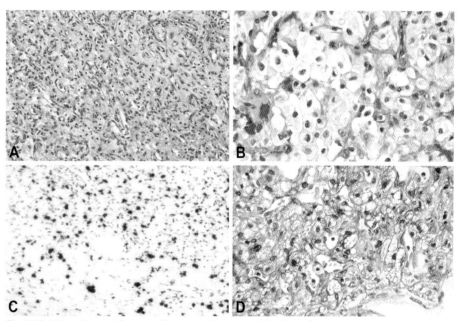

Fig.13.18 Histopathological features of haemangioblastomas. **A** Cellular variant showing many stromal cells. **B** Cellular variant showing densely packed tumour cells. **C** *In situ* hybridization showing expression of VEGF mRNA in stromal cells. **D** Immunostaining for VHL protein in stromal but not endothelial cells.

insertions, splice site mutations and large deletions also occur {1581, 1641, 2487}. The spectrum of clinical manifestations of VHL reflects the type of germline mutation displaying a more or less tight genotype-phenotype correlation. The clinical classification is based on the manifestation of phaeochromocytoma {1346}. Phaeochromocytoma is very rarely found in VHL type 1, whereas this tumour type is the prominent feature in VHL type 2. VHL type 2 is subdivided into type 2A, if both renal cell carcinoma and phaeochromocytoma are present in a given family, and type 2B, if renal cancer is absent or very rare. VHL type 2C has been established for patients who carry a VHL germline mutation but where only phaeochromocytomas occur {71, 325,

698,1582}. VHL types 2B and 2C are usually associated with missense mutations. *VHL* gene mutations are also common in sporadic haemangioblastomas and renal cell carcinomas {1040, 1612}.

Prognostic and predictive factors

While the morbidity and local tumour recurrence rates in sporadic haemangioblastoma are low, many patients with VHL ultimately develop multiple CNS haemangioblastomas. Thus, CNS involvement remains an important cause of morbidity and mortality for VHL patients {1381} in which CNS haemangioblastoma and renal cell carcinoma are the major causes of death {1381, 1872}. The average life expectancy of VHL patients is 40–50 years {1051, 1582, 1592}. In order to detect VHL-associated haemangioblastomas, analysis for germline mutations of the *VHL* gene has been recommended in every patient with CNS haemangioblastoma, particularly those of younger age and with multiple lesions. Yearly lifetime screening of VHL patients by MRI should also start after the age of ten years. This should occur in conjunction with familial screening and counseling {693}.

Table 13.07 Correlation between different VHL phenotypes and *VHL* mutations.

VHL Type	Phenotype	Examples of mutations
Type 1	Predominantly without phaeochromocytoma	*VHL* 75 del Phe *VHL* Arg 161 Stop
Type 2	Predominantly with phaeochromocytoma but not with renal cell carcinoma	*VHL* Arg 161 Pro *VHL* Tyr 98 His
Type 2B	Predominantly with phaeochromocytoma and renal cell carcinoma	*VHL* Arg 167 Trp *VHL* Arg 167 Gln
Type 2C	Predominantly with only phaeochromocytoma	*VHL* Leu 188 Val

Tuberous sclerosis complex and subependymal giant cell astrocytoma

M.B.S. Lopes
O.D. Wiestler
A.O. Stemmer-Rachamimov
M.C. Sharma

Definition

A group of autosomal dominant disorders characterized by hamartomas and benign neoplastic lesions that affect the central nervous system as well as various non-neural tissues; major CNS manifestations include cortical hamartomas (tubers), subcortical glioneuronal hamartomas, subependymal glial nodules and subependymal giant cell astrocytomas; major extraneural manifestations include cutaneous angiofibromas ('adenoma sebaceum'), peau chagrin, subungual fibromas, cardiac rhabdomyomas, intestinal polyps, visceral cysts, pulmonary lymphangioleiomyomatosis and renal angiomyolipomas; caused by a mutation of the *TSC1* gene on 9q or the *TSC2* gene on 16p.

MIM No.

TSC1   191100.
TSC2   191092 {1433}.

Synonyms

Tuberous sclerosis; Bourneville disease; Bourneville-Pringle disease.

Incidence

Variability of clinical manifestations previously led to under diagnosis. Recent data indicate that the disorder affects as many as 25 000 to 40 000 individuals in the United States and about 1 to 2 million individuals worldwide, with an estimated prevalence of 1/6000 newborns.

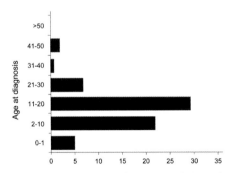

Fig. 13.19 Age distribution of subependymal giant cell astrocytoma (SEGA) at the time of clinical manifestation. Combined data for male and female patients.

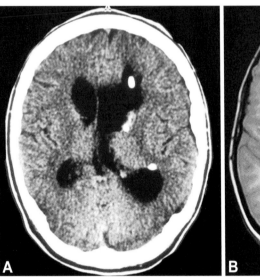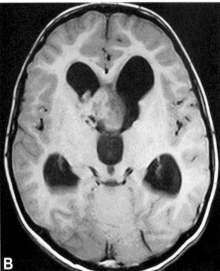

Fig. 13.20 A CT of typical subependymal calcifications in a patient with tuberous sclerosis. **B** A T1-weighted MRI showing mixed iso- and hypodense mass.

(http://www.ninds.nih.gov/disorders/tuberous_sclerosis/detail_tuberous_sclerosis.htm).

Diagnostic criteria

Diagnosis of tuberous sclerosis complex (TSC) is based on clinical features and may be challenging due to great variability of phenotypes. The diagnostic criteria for TSC were revised in 1998 at the Tuberous Sclerosis Consensus Conference {1894, 1895}. Clinical manifestations have been divided into major and minor features and the diagnostic categories defined as Definite, Probable and Suspect {1894}. Most patients have manifestations of TSC before the age of 10 years {20}. Confirmatory testing for *TSC1* and *TSC2* mutations may be helpful when a patient does not meet clinical criteria for definite diagnosis. Prenatal diagnosis by mutation analysis is possible when the mutation in other family members is known.

Clinical features

Neurological symptoms are the most frequent and serious manifestations. Initial signs in a majority of TSC patients tend to be epilepsy and autistic withdrawal {20}. Mental retardation and behavioural abnormalities are usually present {706}. Infantile spasms represent another characteristic neurological manifestation in TSC.

Subependymal giant cell astrocytoma

Definition

Subependymal giant cell astrocytoma (SEGA) is a benign, slowly growing tumour typically arising in the wall of the lateral ventricles and composed of large ganglioid astrocytes.

ICD-O code   9384/1

Grading

Subependymal giant cell astrocytoma corresponds to WHO grade I.

Incidence

Although it is debatable whether SEGA occurs outside TSC, it is the most common CNS neoplasm in TSC patients {20, 706, 2078}. Its incidence ranges from 6%–14% in patients with confirmed TSC {20, 1895, 2078}, and SEGA is one of the major criteria for the diagnosis of TSC {902, 1894}.

Age and sex distribution

This tumour typically occurs during the first two decades of life, although cases involving infants have been reported {1440}. A congenital case diagnosed by antenatal MRI at 24 weeks of gestation has been described {899}.

Clinical features

Most patients show either a worsening of epilepsy or symptoms of increased intracranial pressure. Leptomeningeal dissemination with drop metastases has been described {2233}. Calcifications and signs of previous haemorrhage may also be present. Massive spontaneous haemorrhage has been observed. Some patients of SEGA develop manifestations of TSC in the follow-up period {2064}.

Histopathology

Lesions are circumscribed, often calcified tumours composed mainly of large, plump cells resembling astrocytes. Clustering of tumour cells and perivascular pseudopalisading are common features. The tumour cells show a wide spectrum of astroglial phenotypes. Typical appearances range from polygonal cells with abundant, glassy cytoplasm (resembling gemistocytic astrocytes) to smaller, more elongate elements within a variably fibrillated matrix. Giant pyramidal cells with a ganglionic appearance are common. The nuclei display a finely granular chromatin pattern with distinct nucleoli. Considerable nuclear pleomorphism and multinucleated cells are frequent. SEGA may demonstrate increased mitotic activity. However, these features do not appear to denote an adverse clinical course. Similarly, the occasional presence of endothelial proliferation and necrosis are not indicative of anaplastic progression. The rare examples of SEGA that recur have not been reported to show malignant transformation {2455}. Infiltration of mast cells and lymphocytes, predominantly T-lymphocytes, is a constant feature {2069}.

Proliferation

Proliferative index as measured by Ki-67 (MIB-1) is generally low (mean, 1.5–7.4%), providing further support for the benign nature of these neoplasms {402, 536, 744, 1111, 2064}. Topoisomerase II labelling index is also reportedly low (mean, 2.9%) {2064}. Though extremely uncommon, craniospinal dissemination has been reported in SEGA with increased MIB-1 LI without malignant features {2233}.

Immunohistochemistry

SEGA has been designated as a distinctive well-circumscribed astrocytoma, but due to its usually mixed glioneuronal phenotype, it has also been termed subependymal giant cell tumour {1261}. Tumour cells demonstrate variable immunoreactivity for GFAP and S-100 protein. Neurofilament proteins and neuronal-associated class III ß-tubulin are also demonstrated {1347}. Class III ß-tubulin appears more widespread in its distribution than any other neuronal epitope. Neurofilament is more restricted and mainly highlights cellular processes and a few ganglionic cells. Likewise, SEGA are rarely immunoreactive for synaptophysin in the ganglionic component {2069}. Variable immunoreactivity for neuropeptides has also been detected. These findings suggest cellular lineages with a variable capacity for divergent phenotypes, including glial, neuronal and neuroendocrine differentiation. Ultrastructural features of neuronal differentiation,

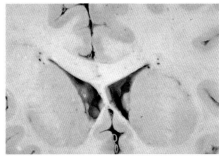

Fig. 13.21 Multiple small subependymal giant cell astrocytomas at the walls of the lateral ventricles.

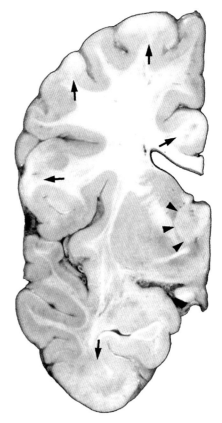

Fig. 13.22 Coronal section of the left hemisphere of a patient with tuberous sclerosis, showing a subependymal giant cell astrocytoma (arrowheads) and multiple cortical tubers.

including microtubules, occasional dense-core granules, and, rarely, synapses may be detectable {830, 1015}.

Other CNS manifestations

CNS lesions include cerebral cortical tubers, white matter heterotopias, and subependymal hamartomatous nodules (candle guttering or drippings).
Cortical tubers in TSC may be detected by either CT or MRI {2077}. These malformative lesions have a strong association with the development of

Table 13.08 Diagnostic criteria for Tuberous Sclerosis Complex. Modified from Roach *et al.* {1894}.

> **Major features**
> Facial angiofibromas or forehead plaque
> Nontraumatic ungual or periungual fibroma
> Hypomelanotic macules (more than 3)
> Shagreen patch (connective tissue nevus)
> Multiple retinal nodular hamartomas
> Cortical tuber
> Subependymal nodule
> Subependymal giant cell astrocytoma
> Cardiac rhabdomyoma, single or multiple
> Lymphangiomatosis
> Renal angiomyolipoma
>
> **Minor features**
> Multiple randomly distributed pits in dental enamel
> Hamartomatous rectal polyps
> Bone cysts
> Cerebral white matter migration lines
> Gingival fibromas
> Nonrenal hamartomas
> Retinal achromic patch
> "Confetti" skin lesions
> Multiple renal cysts
>
> **Definite TSC:** either 2 major features or 1 major feature with 2 minor features
>
> **Probable TSC:** 1 major feature and 1 minor feature
>
> **Possible TSC:** either 1 major feature or 2 or more minor features

epilepsy, especially infantile spasms and generalized tonic-clonic seizures. Microscopically, they consist of giant cells (like those seen in SEGA) and dysmorphic neurons, disrupted cortical lamination, gliosis, calcification of blood-vessel walls and/or parenchyma, and myelin loss. The surrounding cortex usually demonstrates a normal cyto-architecture {900}. Dysmorphic neurons

Table 13.09 Major manifestations of the TSC.

Manifestation	Frequency
Central nervous system	
Cortical tuber	90-100%
Subependymal nodule	90-100%
White matter hamartoma & white matter heterotopias	90-100%
Subependymal giant cell astrocytoma	6-16%
Skin	
Facial angiofibroma (adenoma sebaceum)	80-90%
Hypomelanotic macule	80-90%
Shagreen patch	20-40%
Forehead plaque	20-30%
Peri and subungual fibroma	20-30%
Eyes	
Retinal hamartoma	50%
Retinal giant cell astrocytoma	20-30%
Hypopigmented iris spot	10-20%
Kidney	
Multiple, bilateral angiomyolipomas	50%
Renal cell carcinomas	1.2%
Polycystic kidney disease	2-3%
Isolated renal cysts	10-20%
Heart	
Cardiac rhabdomyoma	50%
Digestive system	
Microhamartomatous rectal polyps	70-80%
Liver hamartoma	40-50%
Hepatic cysts	24%
Adenomatous polyp of the duodenum and small intestine	rare
Lung	
Lymphangioleiomyomatosis	1-2.3%
Pulmonary cysts	40%
Micronodular pulmonary hyperplasias of type 2 pneumocytes	rare
Others	
Gingival fibromas	50-70%
Pitting of dental enamel	30%
Bone cysts	40%
Arterial aneurysms-intracranial arteries, aorta and axillary artery	rare

and giant cells may be seen in all cortical layers and underlying white matter. Dysplastic neurons show altered radial orientation in the cortex, aberrant dendritic arborization and accumulation of perikaryal fibrils, and abnormal somatic morpho-logy with abundant eosinophilic cytoplasm (balloon cells) {568, 830, 900}. Although neurons express neuronal-associated proteins, they display cytoarchitectural features of immature or poorly differenti-ated neurons, such as reduced axonal projections and spine density {830, 900}. Giant cells in cortical tubers show a cellular and molecular heterogeneity similar to that seen in SEGA, and immunohistochemical markers charac-teristic of glial as well as neuronal phenotypes suggest a mixed glioneuronal origin. Many giant cells in tubers express both nestin mRNA and protein {394}. While some giant cells demonstrate immunoreactivity for GFAP {830}, others with an identical morphological phenotype express neuronal markers including connexins 26 and 32, neurofilaments, class III ß-tubulin, MAP2, and α-internexin {394, 830}. Formation of well-defined synapses between giant cells and adjacent neurons is not, however, a consistent finding. Cortical hamartomas morphologically indistinguishable from tubers, may occur in chronic focal epilepsies without clinical evidence for an underlying TSC condition {180}. The pathogenesis of these sporadic lesions is unresolved.

Subependymal hamartomas are elevated, often calcified nodules and are composed of cells indistinguishable from cortical tubers, but are smaller in size.

Extraneural manifestations
Extraneural manifestations of TSC and the frequencies at which they occur are summarized in Table 13.09.

Genetics
Inheritance and genetic heterogeneity
Approximately 50% of TSC patients have a positive family history, indicating a high rate of de novo mutations. In affected kindreds, the disease follows an autosomal dominant pattern of inheritance, with high pene-trance, but considerable phenotypic variability {2093}. Neuroradiological obser-vations suggest that first-degree relatives of affected patients may have minor clinical signs or a forme fruste of the disease.

Molecular genetics
Genetic linkage studies have provided evidence for two distinct TSC loci on chromosome 9q (TSC1), and on chromo-some 16p (TSC2) {371, 1038}. These are likely tumour suppressor genes, as analyses of TSC lesions from affected individuals have demonstrated loss of heterozygosity {284, 720}. It has not been possible to associate TSC1 and TSC2 with distinct clinical phenotypes, suggesting that both genes may be involved in the same regulatory pathway. It has been reported that the two TSC genes products interact within the cell {1759}. Mutations in TSC2 are much more common than those in TSC1 {43}, and TSC1 mutations are significantly underrepresented in sporadic cases {409,1006}. Several studies suggest that patients with TSC1 mutations are less severely affected than patients with TSC2 mutations {409, 1006}. The mildest phenotype is seen in patients in whom mutations were not identified {1980}.

The TSC1 gene
The TSC1 gene maps to chromosome 9q34 {371}, and contains 23 exons, spanning 45kb of genomic DNA {2307}. Of these, 21 appear to carry coding information.

Gene expression. TSC1 encodes an 8.6 kb mRNA. Its gene product, hamartin, has a molecular weight of 130 kD. The protein is located in cytoplasmic vesicles of cultured cells without assigning a specific function to the molecule {1759}. Hamartin is strongly expressed in brain, kidney and heart, all tissues frequently affected in TSC. Immunohistochemically, significant hamartin staining was reported in cortical neurons, kidney epithelia, pancreatic islets, bronchial epithelia and alveolar macrophages {1758}. Its pattern of expression overlaps with that of tuberin, the product of the TSC2 gene. Tuberin and hamartin were shown to directly interact stably in vitro and in vivo {1759}. This may explain the similar clinical manifestations of the two forms of TSC.

Gene mutations. Screening in 225 un-related patients yielded TSC1 mutations in 29 cases (13 %). Virtually all mutations resulted in a truncated gene product, and more than half of the changes affected exons 15 and 17 {2308}. Genotype-phenotype correlations were not apparent.

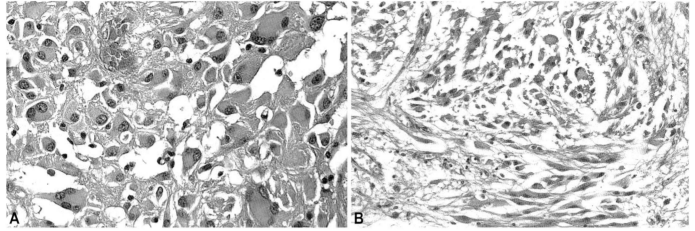

Fig. 13.23 Histological features of subependymal giant cell astrocytoma. **A** Pleomorphic multinucleated eosinophilic tumour cells. **B** Elongated tumour cells forming streams.

The TSC2 gene

The *TSC2* gene maps to chromosome 16p13.3 {1038} and contains 40 exons.

Gene expression. TSC2 encodes a large transcript of 5.5 kb which shows widespread expression in many tissues, including the brain and other organs affected in TSC. Alternatively spliced mRNAs have been reported {2452}. A portion of the 180 kD protein product, tuberin, bears significant homology with the catalytic domain of the GTPase-activating protein, Rap1-GAP, a member of the ras family. Studies in the Eker rat, a strain with hereditary kidney cancer, demonstrated mutations of the rat *TSC2* homologue, providing support for the hypothesis that *TSC2* acts as a tumour suppressor. Immunohistochemical and in situ localization studies of tuberin and TSC2 mRNA revealed expression in normal neurons and glia.

Gene mutations. The mutational spectrum of *TSC2* is wider and includes large deletions, missense, nonsense, frameshift deletions/insertions and splice junction mutations {409, 1006, 1980}; genotype-phenotype correlations have not emerged. Loss of heterozygosity for the *TSC1* or *TSC2* loci has been reported in many types of TSC-associated hamartomas and tumours, but are less common in brain lesions than in kidney tumours {811}, raising the possibility that some lesions in TSC may be due to haploinsufficiency {1594, 2415}. Furthermore, neuroglial lesions that are almost indistinguishable from TSC hamartomas have been observed in the brains of patients with chronic focal epilepsies. A molecular analysis for LOH on chromosomes 9q and 16p failed to detect any involvement of the *TSC1* and *TSC2* loci in these sporadic malformative lesions {2426}. This finding appears to exclude the possibility that some of these patients are afflicted with a forme fruste of TSC.

Signalling pathways involving tuberin and hamartin

The tuberin-hamartin complex integrates and transmits cellular growth factor and stress signals to the PI3K/PKB signalling pathway and negatively regulates mTOR activity in Drosophila and mammalian cells {646, 2230}. Inactivating phosphorylation of tuberin upon insulin or growth factor stimulation causes the disruption of the hamartin/tuberin complex and activation of the mTOR pathway {70}. mTOR signalling increases proliferation and cell growth through two effector molecules: the eukaryotic initiation factor 4E-binding protein 1 (4E-BP1) and ribosomal protein S6 kinase 1 (S6K1) {2230} that are essential for G1 to S phase transition. The mTOR inhibitor, rapamycin, is a logical potential therapeutic agent for TSC. Rapamycin induces apoptosis and reduced proliferation of tuberin null cells, and reduction of tumour size in the Eker rat model of TSC {70}. Oral rapamycin therapy induces regression of astrocytomas associated with TSC {604}. The therapeutic effects of rapamycin and chemical analogs are currently being evaluated in human cancers in preclinical and clinical trials.

Li-Fraumeni syndrome and *TP53* germline mutations

H. Ohgaki
M. Olivier
P. Hainaut

Definition
An autosomal dominant disorder characterized by multiple primary neoplasms in children and young adults, with a predominance of soft tissue sarcomas, osteosarcomas, breast cancer, brain tumours, and adrenocortical carcinoma; most commonly caused by a germline mutation in the *TP53* gene on chromosome 17p13 {606, 1390, 2318}.

MIM No.
Li-Fraumeni syndrome 151623.
TP53 mutations (germline and somatic) 191170 {1433}.

Synonyms
Sarcoma family syndrome of Li and Fraumeni.

Incidence
From 1990 to 2005, a total of 315 families with a *TP53* germline mutation were reported, representing 573 individuals who are confirmed as carriers of a *TP53* germline mutation (IARC *TP53* Database http://www-p53.iarc.fr {1638}).

Diagnostic criteria
The clinical criteria used to identify an affected individual in a Li-Fraumeni family are: (i) occurrence of sarcoma before the age of 45 and (ii) at least one first-degree relative with any tumour before age 45 and (iii) a second (or first) degree relative with cancer before age 45 or a sarcoma at any age {1310}.

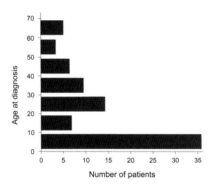

Fig. 13.24 The age distribution of patients with brain tumours associated with *TP53* germline mutations showing bimodal distribution with peaks in children and young adults (n=80, IARC *TP53* database, July 2006).

Criteria for the diagnosis of a LFS variant (Li-Fraumeni like, LFL) have been proposed to better identify *TP53* germline mutation carriers: Criteria of LFL-E2 (2nd definition by Eeles) {1639} are: sarcoma at any age in the proband with two of the following (two of the tumours may be in the same individual), breast cancer at <50 years and/or brain tumour, leukaemia, adrenocortical tumour, melanoma, prostate cancer, pancreatic cancer at <60 years or sarcoma at any age. Criteria of LFL-B (Birch definition) {171} are: proband with any childhood cancer or sarcoma, brain tumour or adrenocortical carcinoma at <45 years, with one first or second degree relative with typical LFS cancer (sarcoma, breast cancer, brain tumour, leukaemia, or adrenocortical carcinoma) at any age, plus one first or

second degree relative in the same lineage with any cancer diagnosed under age 60.

Nervous system neoplasms
In the 573 confirmed individuals carrying a *TP53* germline mutation that are included in the IARC *TP53* Database (July 2006), a total of 708 tumours were reported; 93 of these (13.1%) were located in the nervous system.

Age and sex distribution
Male female ratio of patients with brain tumours associated with *TP53* germline mutation is 1.86, slightly higher than the one of sporadic brain tumours excluding meningiomas (1.6) {1260}.
As with sporadic brain tumours, the age of patients with nervous system neoplasms associated with *TP53* germline mutations shows a bimodal distribution. The first peak of incidence is in children (mainly medulloblastomas and related primitive neuroectodermal and choroid plexus tumours), and the second (mainly astrocytic brain tumours) in the 3rd and 4th decades of life.

Familial clustering
Among 139 families with at least one case of brain tumour, the mean number of CNS tumours per family is 1.55. Several reported families showed a remarkable clustering of brain tumours. This raises the question of whether some mutations carry an organ- or cell-specific risk. A recent analysis of the IARC *TP53* Database of germline mutations showed that brain tumours were more likely to be associated with missense mutations located in the DNA-binding surface of p53 protein that make contact with the minor groove of DNA {1639}. The type of mutation was also associated with the age at onset of brain tumours, truncating mutations being associated with early onset brain tumours {1639}. Familial clustering may also be due to gene-environment interactions, e.g. exposure of families to similar environmental carcinogens or lifestyle factors has been suggested for stomach and breast cancer {1124}.

Table 13.10 Brain tumours associated with *TP53* germline mutations

Histology	No. of tumours	Mean age of patients (years)
Histologically classified (75 cases)		
Astrocytic brain tumour	45 (48%)	34
Medulloblastoma/PNET	10 (11%)	6
Choroid plexus tumour	14 (15%)	3
Ependymoma	3 (3%)	9
Oligodendroglioma	2 (2%)	21
Meningioma	1 (1%)	24
Unclassified (18 cases)	19%	
All (93 cases)	100%	

Histopathology of CNS tumours

Of the 93 brain tumours reported in confirmed carriers of a germline *TP53* mutation, 75 had been classified histologically, and of these, 45 (60%) were of astrocytic origin, including low-grade astrocytoma, anaplastic astrocytoma and glioblastoma. Paediatric brain tumours, including medulloblastoma and related primitive neuroectodermal tumours and choroid plexus tumours were less frequent. This correlates with the occurrence of *TP53* mutations in sporadic brain tumours, which prevail in astrocytoma and are considerably less frequent in medulloblastoma {1621, 1622}. Histopathologically, CNS tumours associated with *TP53* germline mutations are considered indistinguishable from their sporadic counterparts.

Extraneural manifestations

Breast cancer, sarcomas (osteosarcomas and soft tissue sarcomas), and brain tumours are the most frequent manifestations and account for 72% of all tumours in patients carrying a *TP53* germline mutation. The sporadic counterparts of these tumours also show a high frequency of *TP53* mutations, suggesting that in these neoplasms, *TP53* mutations are capable of initiating the process of malignant transformation {1124}. In general, tumours associated with a *TP53* germline mutation develop earlier than their sporadic counterparts, but there are marked organ-specific differences. Adrenocortical carcinoma associated with a *TP53* germline mutation develops almost exclusively in children, in contrast to sporadic adrenocortical carcinoma, which has a broad age distribution with a peak beyond age 40 {109}.

Genetics

In approximately 80% of LFS cases, and 65% of LFL cases, affected family members carry a germline mutation of one allele of the *TP53* tumour suppressor gene (IARC *TP53* Database, July 2006). Conversely, of 244 reported families with *TP53* germline mutations, approximately 45% and 35% meet the criteria of LFS and LFL syndromes respectively. However, the extent of the overlap may be greater, as in some families with *TP53* germline mutations only one tumour was analysed or data were available for only one generation. Two LFS and 3 LFL families have been reported to carry a *CHEK2*

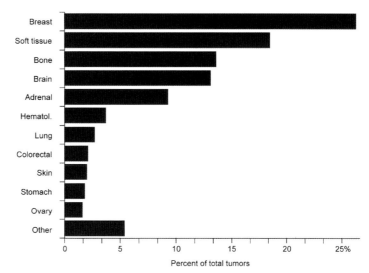

Fig.13.25 Target organs for tumourigenesis in patients carrying a *TP53* germline mutation (n=708, IARC *TP53* Database July 2006). Breast cancer, bone and soft tissue sarcomas, and brain tumours are most frequent neoplasms associated with *TP53* germline mutations.

germline mutation {172, 1280, 2294}. This gene codes for a protein involved in G2 checkpoint control which prevents cells with damaged DNA to enter mitosis {184}. However, it is now considered that *CHEK2* does not predispose to LFS/LFL, but only to the breast cancers that have occurred in the context of these families.

Gene

The *TP53* gene on chromosome 17p13 has 11 exons that span 20 kb. Exon 1 is non-coding, and exons 5 to 8 are highly conserved among vertebrates.

TP53 protein

The *TP53* tumour suppressor gene encodes a 2.8 kb transcript encoding a 393 amino-acid protein which is widely expressed at low levels. This protein is a multi-functional transcription factor involved in the control of cell cycle progression, of DNA integrity and of the survival of cells exposed to DNA-damaging agents as well as several non-genotoxic stimuli such as hypoxia. DNA damage or hypoxia induces a transient nuclear accumulation and activation of the TP53 protein, with transcriptional activation of target genes that are responsible for induction of cell cycle arrest or apoptosis {1143, 1301}. A number of these properties are consistent with a tumour suppressor function. TP53 mutant proteins differ from each other in the extent to which they have lost suppressor function and in their

Table 13.11 Tumour type, age at diagnosis and gender distribution in patients carrying a *TP53* germline mutation.

	Median age at diagnosis (years)		% of male patients	
	TP53 carriers	Sporadic*	*TP53* carriers	Sporadic*
Breast cancer	36	63	0	0.7
Soft tissue sarcoma	18	61	48	53
Bone sarcoma	17	43	49	56
Brain tumour	22	57	65	56
Adrenocortical carcinoma	6	42	25	51
Haematopoietic and lymphoid tumours	24	65	65	55
Lung cancer	44	69	47	66
Colorectal cancer	37	72	50	50
Skin cancer	56	-	10	-
Stomach cancer	37	73	69	62
Ovarian cancer	39	64	0	0
Other tumour	-	-	-	-

* Data based on cancer registries from US, France and UK compiled in Cancer Incidence in Five Continents V.7, 1997 {1680A}.

capacity to inhibit wild-type TP53 in a dominant-negative manner {1054}. In addition, some *TP53* mutants appear to exert an oncogenic activity of their own, but the molecular basis of this gain-of-function phenotype is still unclear {175}. The functional characteristics of each mutant TP53 protein may depend, at least in part, on the degree of structural perturbation that the mutation imposes on the protein.

Distribution of TP53 mutations

TP53 germline mutations associated with the development of brain tumours are located in highly conserved regions of exons 5 to 8, with major hotspots at codons 175, 245, 248 and 273. These codons are also hot spots in sporadic brain tumours as well as other tumours. Mutations observed at these codons are missense mutations that result in mutant proteins with complete loss of function, dominant-negative phenotypes and oncogenic activities.

It is of interest to note that 3 codons (Cys 176, His 179 and Arg 249) that are commonly mutated in tumours with somatic *TP53* mutations have never been reported as germline mutation {1639}. Residues 176 (Cys) and 179 (His) are involved in the co-ordination of a zinc atom that forms a bridge between domain 1 and domain 3, and which is crucial in stabilizing the architecture of the whole DNA-binding domain. Residue 249 (Arg) makes essential contacts with

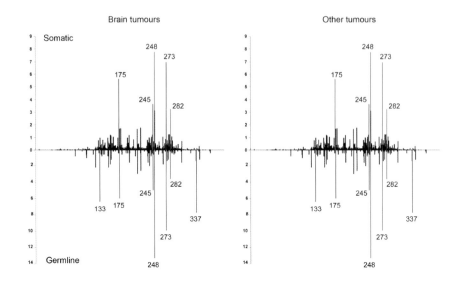

Fig. 13.26 Somatic and germline *TP53* mutations share the major hotspot codons 175, 248 and 273 within the DNA-binding domain (exons 5-8). Germline mutations associated with brain tumours prevail at codons 245 and 248. Based on 82 tumours reported in 77 individuals carrying a single base substitution in *TP53* (http://www-p53.iarc.fr {1638}).

several residues of the scaffold through hydrogen bridges {339}. These substitutions may thus result in mutant TP53 proteins that are not tolerated when present in the germline. Two hot spots (codons 133 and 337) are specific to *TP53* germline mutations, but are not associated with brain tumour development. The mutation at codon 133 (M133T), very rarely observed in sporadic neoplasms, has been found in families with clustering of

early onset breast cancers (3–6 cases by family with a mean age at onset of 34 years; IARC *TP53* Database), whereas a mutation at codon 337 (R337H) has been frequently found in Brazilian children affected by adrenocortical carcinomas {1867} and in Brazilian LFL families {10}.

Type of TP53 mutations

The proportion of G:C->A:T transitions at CpG sites is higher but that of G:C>A:T transitions at non-CpG sites and G:C->T:A transversions is lower in *TP53* germline than in somatic mutations. G:C->A:T transitions at CpG sites are considered to be endogenous, e.g. formed as a result of deamination of 5-methylcytosine, which occurs spontaneously in almost all cell types but which is usually corrected by DNA repair mechanisms. The difference observed may thus be explained by the fact that non-CpG G:C->A:T and G:C->T:A mutations are associated with exogenous carcinogen exposure while germline mutations appear to result mainly from endogenous processes {1640}.

Table 13.12 Type of germline and somatic *TP53* mutations in human neoplasms.

Mutation type	Brain tumours		Other neoplasms	
	Germline[1] (n=96)	Somatic[2] (n=1418)	Germline[3] (n=622)	Somatic[4] (n=19 352)
Missense mutations in DNA binding motifs	55%	56%	45%	49%
Missense mutations outside DNA binding motifs	25%	26%	27%	24%
Deletions/insertions	11%	10%	11%	12%
Nonsense mutations	4%	3%	7%	8%
Other mutations	4%	4%	10%	7%
Point mutations	(n=85)	(n=1259)	(n=542)	(n=16 701)
A:T->C:G	7%	5%	4%	5%
A:T->G:C	8%	14%	13%	13%
A:T->T:A	4%	3%	5%	6%
G:C->A:T not at CpG	15%	20%	12%	22%
G:C->A:T at CpG	48%	44%	55%	28%
G:C->C:G	7%	6%	6%	9%
G:C->T:A	11%	9%	6%	18%

[1] Brain tumours reported in confirmed carriers of a *TP53* germline mutation. [2] Mutations reported in sporadic brain tumours. [3] Tumours other than brain tumours reported in confirmed carriers of a *TP53* germline mutation. [4] Mutations reported in sporadic neoplasms other than brain tumours. Data from IARC *TP53* Database (July 2006).

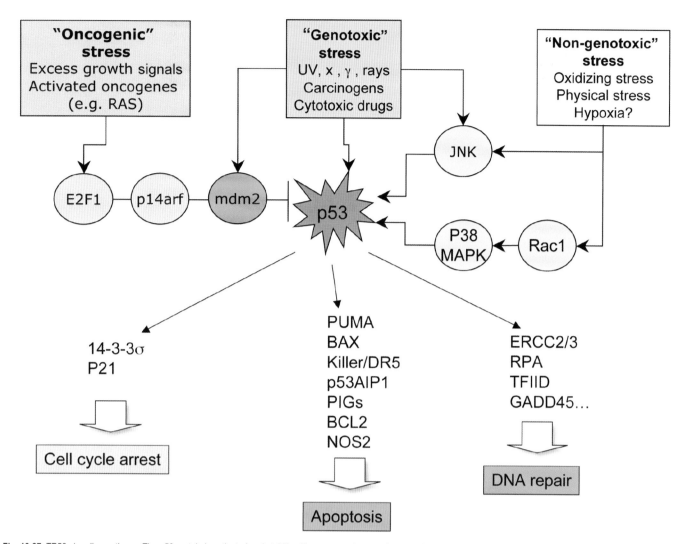

Fig. 13.27 TP53 signaling pathway. The p53 protein is activated and stabilized in response to several genotoxic and non-genotoxic forms of stress. Active p53 acts on downstream effectors through transcriptional repression and protein-protein interactions. Several effectors of p53 are involved in the control of cell cycle progression in G1/S and in G2, in DNA replication, transcription and repair, and in the regulation of apoptosis. Together, this set of cellular responses allows p53 to act as an anti-proliferative agent in cells exposed to various forms of stress. MDM2 is a transcriptional target of p53 involved in a negative, feedback loop to control p53 levels and activity. The extent and consequences of the biological response elicited by p53 vary according to stress and cell type.

Cowden disease and dysplastic gangliocytoma of the cerebellum/ Lhermitte-Duclos disease

C.G. Eberhart
O.D. Wiestler
C. Eng

Definition

An autosomal dominant disorder characterized by multiple hamartomas involving tissues derived from all three germ cell layers and a high risk of breast, non-medullary thyroid and endometrial cancers; the classic hamartoma is the trichilemmoma and is pathognomonic; caused by germline mutations in *PTEN* (Phosphatase and TENsin homologue deleted on chromosome TEN). Adult-onset Lhermitte-Duclos disease (LDD)/dysplastic gangliocytoma of the cerebellum is also considered pathognomonic.

MIM No.   158350 {1433}.

Synonyms and historical annotation

The condition was originally described in 1963 by Lloyd and Dennis in the family of Rachel Cowden {1339}. Weary *et al.* {2376} gave a more detailed description of clinical features and proposed the term multiple hamartoma syndrome.

Incidence

The incidence of Cowden syndrome (CS) before the identification of *PTEN* was estimated to be 1 in a million {1578}. After gene identification, this figure was revised to approximately 1 in 250 000 {1577}. Although the exact proportion of isolated and familial cases is not known, the majority of CS cases appear to be isolated {521, 1405, 2357}. The precise incidence of LDD is unknown although it is viewed as rare {523, 1664}.

Diagnostic criteria and clinical features

A set of operational clinical diagnostic criteria has been established for purposes of identifying families [www.nccn.org] {1748}. Because of a study which found *PTEN* mutations in 15 of 18 unselected patients with the pathologic diagnosis of dysplastic gangliocytoma of the cerebellum {2499}, adult-onset LDD was revised from a major diagnostic criterion to a pathognomonic criterion. Of note, all 15 patients with mutations had adult-onset LDD, while the remaining 3 without

mutations were diagnosed in children less than 12. Thus, the presence of adult-onset LDD, irrespective of other clinical features or family history, can be considered highly predictive of identifying a germline *PTEN* mutation in that patient.

Dysplastic gangliocytoma of the cerebellum (Lhermitte-Duclos disease)

Definition

A benign cerebellar mass composed of dysplastic ganglion cells.

ICD-O code   9493/0

Grading

It is not clear whether this lesion is neoplastic or hamartomatous. If neoplastic, it corresponds histologically to WHO grade I.

Synonyms and historical annotation

Dysplastic gangliocytoma of the cerebellum was first described in 1920 by Lhermitte and Duclos {1307} and by Spiegel {2134}. The disease has also been termed cerebellar granule cell hypertrophy, diffuse hypertrophy of the cerebellar cortex and gangliomatosis of the cerebellum. Over 100 patients have been reported since. However, the association of Cowden disease with dysplastic gangliocytoma of the cerebellum has only recently been recognized {523, 1664, 2327, 2328}.

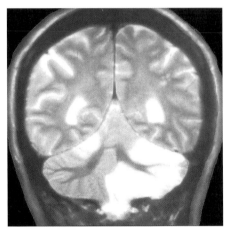

Fig. 13.29 T2-weighted MRI showing the characteristic broadening of the cerebellar cortex (hyperintense signal) on the right side, with a smaller focus in the left cerebellar hemisphere. From Sonier *et al.* {2123A}.

Age distribution

Because of the rarity of LDD, there has not been a systematic study to determine the distribution of age of onset. Most cases have been identified in adults, but a review of the literature reveals that LDD can be diagnosed in infancy, e.g. 3 years old, and as late as in the 70s {523, 1345, 2499}. *PTEN* mutations have been identified in virtually all adult-onset LDD but not in childhood-onset cases {2499}, suggesting the biology of the two is different.

Clinical features

Signs and symptoms. The most common clinical presentations of LDD include dysmetria, other cerebellar signs, and signs and symptoms of mass effect. Macrocephaly and seizures are also often present in LDD patients. Variable periods of preoperative symptoms have been noted, with a mean interval of approximately 40 months {2327}. As cerebellar lesions may develop before the appearance of other features of Cowden disease, patients with Lhermitte-Duclos should be monitored for the development of additional tumours, including breast cancer in females.

Neuroimaging. Neuroradiological studies demonstrate a distorted architecture of

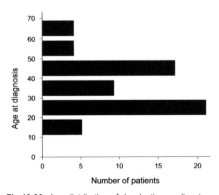

Fig.13.28 Age distribution of dysplastic gangliocytoma of the cerebellum, based on 60 cases.

the affected cerebellar hemisphere with enlarged cerebellar folia and cystic changes in some cases; MRI is particularly sensitive in depicting the enlarged folia {1472}.

Macroscopy

The affected cerebellum displays a discrete region of hypertrophy and a coarse gyral pattern that extends into deeper layers. Usually, the gangliocytoma is confined to one hemisphere, but they can occasionally be multifocal.

Histopathology

The dysplastic gangliocytoma of LDD causes diffuse enlargement of the molecular and internal granular layers of the cerebellum, which are filled by ganglionic cells of varying sizes {2}. An important diagnostic feature is the relative preservation of the cerebellar architecture, in which folia are enlarged and distorted but not obliterated. A layer of abnormally myelinated axon bundles in parallel arrays is often observed in the outer molecular layer. Scattered cells morphologically consistent with granule neurons are also sometimes found under the pia or in the molecular layer. The resulting structure of these dysmorphic cerebellar folia has been referred to as inverted cerebellar cortex. Purkinje cells are reduced in number or absent. Calcification and ectatic vessels are commonly present within the lesion. Vacuoles are sometimes observed in the molecular layer and white matter {2}.

Immunohistochemistry

The dysplastic neuronal cells are immunopositive for synaptophysin. Antibodies to the Purkinje cell antigens Leu-4, L7, PEP19 and calbindin labelled a minor subpopulation of large atypical ganglion cells, but did not react with the majority of the neuronal elements, suggesting that only a small fraction of neurons are derived from a Purkinje cell source {756, 2091}. Immunohistochemistry also demonstrates loss of PTEN protein expression in most dysplastic cells and increased expression of phosphorylated Akt and S6, reflecting aberrant signalling which is predicted to result in increased cell size and lack of apoptosis {2, 2499}.

Proliferation

Undetectable or very low proliferative activity has been reported in the few

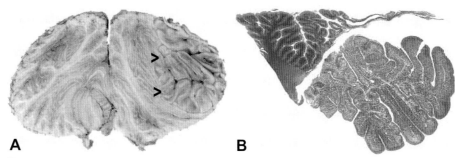

Fig.13.30 A Macroscopic aspect of Lhermitte-Duclos disease (arrows). Note the delineated enlargement and coarsening of the cerebellar folia. **B** Low-power view showing moderate distortion of the cerebellar cortex.

cases analysed with proliferation markers {2, 756}.

Histogenesis

It remains unclear whether Lhermitte-Duclos is hamartomatous or neoplastic in nature. Malformative histopathological features, a very low or absent proliferative activity and the absence of progression support a classification as hamartoma. However, recurrent growth has occasionally been noted and dysplastic gangliocytomas may develop in adult patients with previously normal MRI scans {2, 756, 1395}. It has been suggested that the primary cell of origin is the cerebellar granule neuron {756}, and that a combination of aberrant migration and hypertrophy of granule cells is responsible for formation of the lesions {2}. Murine

transgenic models based on localized PTEN loss support this hypothesis {1241}.

Other CNS manifestations

Additional cerebral manifestations include megalencephaly in 20–70% of cases, as well as heterotopic grey matter, hydrocephalus, mental retardation and seizures {766, 1664}. Although such tumours as meningiomas and glioblastomas have been said to be associated with CS and have been the topic of single case reports {1345, 1391}, there is currently no rigorous epidemiologic evidence that they are true component neoplasias {1748}.

Genetics

Cowden syndrome is an autosomal dominant disorder, with age-related

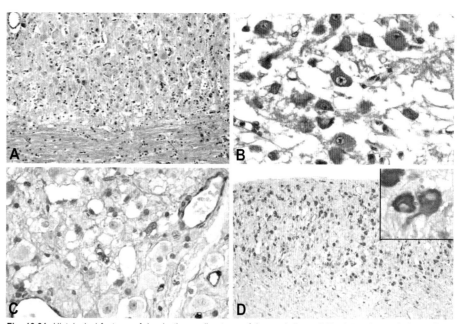

Fig. 13.31 Histological features of dysplastic gangliocytoma of the cerebellum. **A** The internal granule layer of the cerebellum, present at the top of the image, is filled with dysplastic ganglion cells. **B** A higher-power view of ganglion cells. **C** Immunohistochemical stains for PTEN show loss of expression in the enlarged neurons, with preserved staining in vessels. **D** The dysplastic ganglion cells are strongly immunopositive for phosphorylated S6.

penetrance and variable expression {522}. *PTEN* is the susceptibility gene for this syndrome {1318}.

Gene structure and function
PTEN/MMAC1/TEP1 on 10q23, is comprised of 9 exons spanning 120–150 kb of genomic distance and encodes a 1.2 kb transcript and a 403 amino acid lipid dual-specificity phosphatase (it dephosphorylates both protein and lipid substrates), which has homology to the focal adhesion molecules tensin and auxilin {1309, 1312, 2145}. A classic phosphatase core motif is encoded within exon 5, which is the largest exon, constituting 20% of the coding region {1309, 1312}. PTEN is the major 3-phosphatase acting in the phospho-inositol-3-kinase (PI3K)/Akt apoptotic pathway {1377, 2138}. Overexpression of PTEN results, for the most part, in phosphatase-dependent cell cycle arrest at G1 and/or apoptosis, depending on cell type. There is also growing evidence that PTEN can mediate growth arrest independent of the PI3K/Akt pathway and perhaps independent of the lipid phosphatase activity {522, 2357}. Recently, non-traditional means of PTEN inactivation such as nuclear-cytoplasmic partitioning and transcriptional or degradative mechanisms have been found {349, 350, 2212, 2213, 2236}.

Gene mutations
To date, virtually all naturally occurring missense mutations tested abrogate both lipid and protein phosphatase activity, and one mutant, G129E, affects only lipid phosphatase activity {522, 2357}. Approximately 30–40% of germline *PTEN* mutations are found in exon 5, although exon 5 represents only 20% of the coding sequence. Further, approximately 65% of all mutations can be found in one of exons 5, 7 or 8 {522, 1405}. Germline *PTEN* mutations spanning exons 1–9 and the promoter have been found in 85% of all CS probands {2500}. To date, all individuals with adult-onset LDD, irrespective of other features, have *PTEN* mutations {2499}. Although *PTEN* is the major susceptibility gene for CS, one CS family without *PTEN* mutations, was found to have a germline mutation in *BMPR1A*, which is one of the susceptibility genes for juvenile polyposis syndrome {2501}. Whether *BMPR1A* is a minor CS susceptibility gene or whether this family with CS features actually has occult juvenile polyposis is as yet unknown.

Turcot syndrome

W.K. Cavenee
P.C. Burger
S.Y. Leung
E.G. van Meir

Definition

Distinct autosomal dominant disorders having adenomatous colorectal polyps or colon carcinomas and malignant neuro-epithelial tumours, especially medullo-blastomas or glioblastomas. Most cases occur within the setting of hereditary non-polyposis colorectal carcinoma (HNPCC) or familial adenomatous polyposis (FAP); a small proportion of patients have biallelic germline DNA mismatch repair (MMR) gene mutations which augments disease penetrance {92, 1652}.

MIM No.   276300 {1433}.

Incidence

Approximately 170 cases have been reported since it was recognized in 1949.

Diagnostic criteria

There are at least two clinical entities encompassed under the Turcot syndrome (TS) {1676}. The first, Turcot syndrome type 1, consists of glioblastoma in patients without FAP, but often with HNPCC and corresponding germline mutations in the DNA mismatch repair genes PMS2, MLH1 and MSH2. This type can now be distinguished into two subtypes. One occurs in families with classical HNPCC caused by germline mutation of one allele of the MSH2 or MLH1 genes. Another rare form is characterized by homozygous or compound heterozygous mutations, resulting in germline inactivation of both alleles of a MMR gene. The most frequent biallelic germline mutation reported so far involves the PMS2 gene, but mutations involving the MLH1, MSH6 and MSH2 have also been reported. Turcot Syndrome type 2 comprises medulloblastoma in patients with FAP and corresponding mutations in the APC gene. The CNS tumours are similar to their sporadic counterparts except that the medulloblastomas often occur after age 10 and the glioblastomas usually occur before age 30.

Nervous system neoplasms

Medulloblastoma, glioblastoma and anaplastic astrocytoma account for about 95% of brain tumours reported {1676}. Glioblastoma in TS generally occurs in a younger age group than sporadic glioblastoma {2304}. Patients

Table 13.13 Summary of clinical phenotypes and genetic alterations in Turcot cases.

	Turcot syndrome type 1: Glioma-polyposis	Turcot syndrome type 2: Medulloblastoma-polyposis
Intestinal phenotype	Small number of polyps (<100) Large sized polyps (>3cm) No family history of polyposis Colorectal cancer at young age (56%)	Numerous (>100) small polyps Family history of polyposis Colorectal cancer (21%)
Brain tumour types	Astrocytoma or glioblastoma at young age (<20 years)	Medulloblastoma
Skin phenotype	Frequent skin lesions (53%) and café-au-lait spots (38%)	Occasional skin lesions (21%)
Family history	Usually siblings affected No family history of polyposis or brain tumours Finding of glioblastoma at young age might indicate underlying Turcot syndrome type 1 Family history of colorectal cancer	Family history of polyposis
Consanguinity	Frequent (22%)	None
Mode of inheritance	Autosomal dominant with low penetrance behaving like autosomal recessive	Autosomal dominant
Constitutive genetic defect	Mutations in mismatch repair genes: Carry an MLH1 or MSH2 germline mutation or Biallelic germline mutation of PMS2 (occasionally of MLH1, MSH6 and MSH2)	Adenomatous polyposis coli (APC) gene mutations
Related genetic disorder	Hereditary non-polyposis colorectal cancer (HNPCC) Muir-Torre syndrome (sebaceous tumours) Neurofibromatosis type 1 (café-au-lait spots, neurofibromas)	Familial adenomatous polyposis (FAP), Gardner syndrome

with biallelic germline *MMR* gene mutations tend to develop glioma during childhood {92, 1652}, and apart from astrocytomas grades II-IV, oligodendroglioma and supratentorial primitive neuroectodermal tumours have been recorded in some families. It is unclear whether other patients with colonic polyposis and other CNS tumours (lymphoma, pituitary adenoma, meningioma, craniopharyngioma, ependymoma, cervical spinal astrocytoma) are part of the heterogeneity.

Extraneural manifestations
There are two major variants of colorectal manifestations. TS type 1 presents with small numbers of large polyps, and patients develop colorectal cancer at a young age in 56% of cases. Other cancers within the HNPCC spectrum, including cancers arising from the endometrium, stomach, ovary, small intestine, pancreatico-biliary or urinary tracts, as well as sebaceous tumours of Muir-Torre syndrome, may be present in patients or their family members. It has been noted that café-au-lait spots occur in 38% of type 1 patients {1676}. TS patients with café-au-lait spots more likely belong to the group of patients with germline biallelic *MMR* gene mutations {2265}. This syndrome is characterized by very early-onset (usually in the paediatric age group) of colorectal adenomas and cancers, glioblastomas and hematological malignancies (leukaemia and lymphoma). Mild features of neurofibromatosis type 1, especially café-au-lait spots are present in the majority of patients. A minority also have axillary freckles and neurofibromas {92, 1652, 2265}
TS type 2 presents with innumerable adenomatous polyps and 21% of such cases will develop colorectal cancer. Skin lesions occur in approximately 20% of type 2 Turcot patients, usually in forms of epidermoid cysts. Craniofacial exostosis and congenital hypertrophic retinal pigmented epithelium occur in a minority of patients.

Genetics
Genetic heterogeneity
The association of neuroepithelial neoplasms with colorectal polyps was first noted by Crail {393} and genetic predisposition was later suggested by Turcot {2279}. Lewis {1304} proposed three

groups: type (I) those with two or more siblings with multiple colonic polyps and a malignant brain tumour, with neither the parents nor other generations being affected; type (II) affected individuals having an autosomal dominant colonic polyposis and with polyps occurring in several generations of their family; and, type (III) isolated non-familial cases. This led to the proposal that TS was sometimes a variant of the FAP syndrome. Lasser {1265} demonstrated genetic linkage to *APC*, the gene responsible for FAP, in a TS family with medulloblastomas. This was followed by the identification of germline *APC* mutations in three unrelated cases {1523}, two of which presented with medulloblastoma, the other with a malignant astrocytoma. Hamilton and colleagues {762} analysed 14 TS families and found that 10 of the 14 families had germline *APC* mutations and that the predominant tumour was medullo-blastoma.

Mismatch repair associated Turcot syndrome (type 1)
Mismatch repair-associated TS is characterized by an inherited DNA replication error defect that leads to genomic instability.
Gene structure. The major genes involved in *MMR* are: *MLH1* at chromosome 3p21.3, *MSH2* at 2p16, *MSH3* at 5q11-q13, *MSH6/GTBP* at 2p16, *PMS1* at 2q32 and *PMS2* at 7p22. The *PMS2* gene has many paralogous genes with over 90% sequence homology, and these can interfere with mutation detection {441, 1552}.
Gene expression. Recognition and repair of base-pair mismatches in human DNA is mainly mediated by heterodimers of MSH2 and MSH6, which form a sliding clamp on DNA. Cells that are deficient for MSH2 or MSH6 expression are defective in repair of mispaired bases and insertions/deletions of single nucleotides resulting in high mutation rates and microsatellite instability. The carboxy-terminal region of PMS2 interacts with MLH1, and this complex binds to MSH2/MSH6 heterodimers to form a functional strand-specific mispair recognition complex. Most HNPCC families have either *MSH2* or *MLH1* mutations. Replication-error-driven microsatellite instability is rare in adult-on-set brain tumours in the absence of TS but was reported in 27% to 33% of paediatric astrocytoma grades III–IV {49, 1037, 1295}. Overall, a family history of colorectal cancer or other HNPCC-related cancers in young or

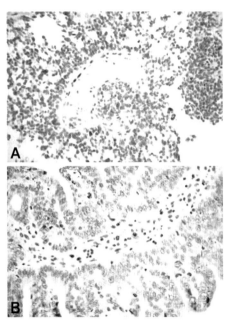

Fig. 13.32 A Turcot patient with heterozygous germline *MSH2* mutation. Immunohistochemical staining shows absence of MSH2 protein expression in the glioblastoma (**A**) and the colonic adenocarcinoma (**B**) arising from the same patient. Note the positive nuclear staining in the endothelial cells and stromal fibroblasts. Modified from Leung *et al.* {1295}.

paediatric glioblastoma patients should raise the suspicion of HNPCC. Screening for lack of expression of mismatch repair genes is possible by immunohistochemistry.
Gene mutations. So far, heterozygous mutations have been found in the germlines of TS families in *MSH2* (4 cases) {1295, 2319} and *MLH1* (two cases) {762, 1037}. These families commonly show a family history of HNPCC with autosomal dominant mode of inheritance. The tumours found in these patients showed evidence of replication errors that lead to genomic instability. This mutator phenotype induces somatic mutations in gatekeeper genes *TP53* and *APC* in the tumours of these patients {1297, 1496}. Notably, these families each had astrocytoma, oligodendroglioma or glioblastoma as the inclusive brain tumour.
The most commonly mutated *MMR* gene reported in TS families is the *PMS2* gene. While the first reported *PMS2* mutation in a TS family affected only one allele, subsequent analysis revealed a mutation in the second allele of the gene {441,762}. Emerging data suggest that most *PMS2* mutations are in forms of homozygous or compound heterozygous

mutations, resulting in replication errors even in the normal tissue of the affected individuals {92,1652}. These families with biallelic germline mutation may manifest an autosomal recessive inheritance pattern, with frequent history of consanguinity in the parents. It is hypothesized that replication errors in normal cells during development may lead to inactivation of the *NF1* gene and lead to the clinical phenotype of mild neurofibromatosis type 1. The lack of cancer history in their parents who are heterozygous *PMS2* mutation carriers suggests that monoallelic germline *PMS2* mutation may confer only a very low risk of cancer. Germline biallelic mutation of *MLH1* (9 families), *MSH2* (3 families) and *MSH6* (3 families) have also been reported in some families with café-au-lait spots and clustering of cancers including gliomas, colon cancers or hematological malignancies. These families usually have more prominent features of HNPCC compared with those with *PMS2* mutation.

FAP-associated Turcot syndrome (type 2)
The APC gene responsible for FAP-associated TS lies on chromosome 5q21.
Gene expression. The *APC* gene encodes an ubiquitously expressed protein of about 300 kDa which interacts with the ß-catenin protein and mediates its degradation. ß-catenin links the cytoplasmic tail of the cell-cell homotypic adhesion molecule cadherin to the actin cytoskeleton. Alteration of APC function may modify the movement/ adhesion of epithelial stem cells in the colonic crypt. It is unclear whether it fulfills a similar function for cerebellar precursor cells, and in the absence of TS, the *APC* gene is rarely mutated in sporadic brain tumours {762, 1265}. About 10% of sporadic medulloblastomas show loss of heterozygosity or mutations in the ß-catenin gene {2517} and *APC* missense point mutations occur in less than 5% of cases {881}. ß-catenin has a role in signalling mediated by the nuclear translocation of transcription factors of

the lymphoid enhancing factor (LEF-1) family. The loss of the *APC* gene product results in increased binding of ß-catenin to LEF-1 and an increase in the transcription of the cell cycle activator cyclin D1 and other genes.
Gene mutations. Truncating germline *APC* mutations are found in most families with FAP-associated TS {1676}. Rare cases show no mutations in the *APC* gene and no evidence for DNA replication errors, suggesting other underlying causes, adding to the aetiological heterogeneity of the syndrome. The association of brain tumours and colon cancer can also occur in the setting of germline *TP53* mutations {1240}.

Prognostic and predictive factors
The median age for occurrence of glioblastoma in TS type 1 was found to be 18 years, while the peak incidence in the general population is 40–70 years of age {2304}. These patients showed an average survival of over 27 months, which is remarkably longer than the 12 month survival for sporadic cases. Although mutation data is not available in most of these families, it is interesting to note that many of the long survivors belong to the group of patients with biallelic germline *PMS2* mutation, some of whom were still alive more than 10 years after treatment of their gliomas {440, 762, 2265}. In Turcot type 2, the median age for occurrence of medulloblastomas was 15 years which is later than the peak occurrence for sporadic medulloblastoma (7 years of age). In FAP families, the appearance of medulloblastoma at young age in patients having no evidence of polyps is of poor prognosis {2304}.

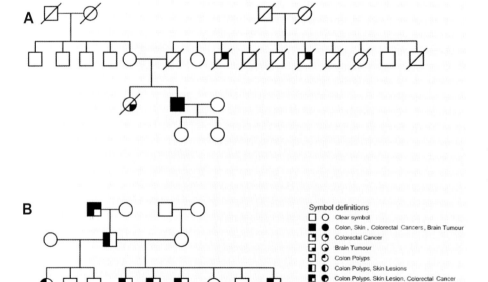

Fig. 13.33 Typical pedigrees of Turcot families. **A** Turcot type 1 (non-polyposis colon cancer and predominantly glioblastomas, frequently associated with mutations in DNA mismatch repair genes). **B** Turcot type 2, characterized by familial adenomatous polyposis, colon carcinomas, and medulloblastomas, caused by an *APC* germline mutation.

Naevoid basal cell carcinoma syndrome

C.G. Eberhart
W.K. Cavenee
T. Pietsch

Definition

An autosomal dominant disease associated with a broad spectrum of developmental disorders and predisposition to benign and malignant tumours, including basal cell carcinomas of the skin, odontogenic keratocysts, palmar and plantar dyskeratotic pits, intracranial calcifications, macrocephaly and medulloblastomas; caused by germline mutations of the *PTCH* gene on 9q22.

MIM No.   109400 {1433}.

Synonyms

Naevoid basal cell carcinoma syndrome (NBCCS) is also known as Gorlin syndrome, Gorlin-Goltz syndrome, basal cell nevus syndrome and fifth phacomatosis.

Incidence

A prevalence of 1 in 57 000 has been reported in a population-based study {539}. Of carriers with germline *PTCH* mutations, about 5% develop medulloblastoma and about 1–2% of medulloblastoma patients carry *PTCH* germline mutation {539}.

Diagnostic criteria and clinical features

The most common manifestations of NBCCS are multiple basal cell carcinomas, as well as odontogenic keratocysts of the jaw, which in one study were found together in more than 90% of affected individuals by the age of 40 {541}. Other major criteria for the syndrome include calcification of the falx cerebri, palmar and plantar pits, bifid or fused ribs, and first degree relatives with NBCCS {1112, 2063}. Minor criteria include medulloblastoma, ovarian fibroma, macrocephaly, congenital facial abnormalities (cleft lip or palate, frontal bossing, hypertelorism), skeletal abnormalities such as digit syndactyly, and radiologic bone abnormalities including bridging of the sella turcica {51, 1112}. A diagnosis of NBCCS is made when two or more major or one major and two or more minor criteria are present {51}. Several other tumour types have been reported in individual NBCCS patients, including meningioma, melanoma, chronic lymphocytic leukaemia, non-Hodgkin lymphoma, ovarian dermoid, as well as breast and lung carcinoma. However, the statistical association of these neoplasms with NBCCS has yet to be shown {2063}. Radiation treatment of NBCCS patients, e.g. craniospinal irradiation for the treatment of cerebellar medulloblastoma, induces multiple basal cell carcinomas of the skin as well as various other tumour types within the radiation field {316, 1610, 2143}.

NBCCS-associated medulloblastoma

In a recent review of 33 medulloblastoma cases associated with NBCCS, all but one tumour developed in a child less than 5 years of age, and 22 cases (66%) presented prior to age 2 {51}. Medulloblastoma associated with NBCCS appear to be exclusively of the desmoplastic/ nodular variant {51, 2035}. It has therefore been proposed that the identification of desmoplastic medulloblastoma in children younger than 2 serve as a major criteria for the diagnosis of NBCCS {51}. The prognosis of NBCCS-associated medulloblastoma appears to be better than that of sporadic cases, and it has been suggested that radiation therapy protocols be altered in NBCCS patients younger than 5 to ameliorate the formation of secondary tumours {51, 2143}.

Other CNS manifestations

There is no statistically proven evidence for an increased risk of other CNS neoplasms in naevoid basal cell carcinoma syndrome. Nevertheless, several instances of meningioma arising in NBCCS patients were reported {35, 2063}. Various malformative changes of the brain and skull including calcification of the falx cerebri and/or tentorium cerebelli at a young age, dysgenesis of the corpus callosum, congenital hydrocephalus, and macrocephaly may occur in affected family members.

Genetics

The condition follows an autosomal dominant pattern of inheritance, with full penetrance but variable clinical phenotypes. The rate of new mutations has not been precisely determined. It has been estimated that a high percentage (14–81%) of the cases represent new mutations {541, 710, 2063, 2408}.

Molecular genetics

NBCCS results from inactivating germline mutations in the human homologue of the Drosophila segment polarity gene patched (*PTCH*) {753, 1005}. The *PTCH* gene maps to chromosome band 9q22.3 {1005}.

Gene structure

The *PTCH* gene spans approximately 50 kb of genomic distance. It has at least 23 exons {753, 1005} with alternative usage

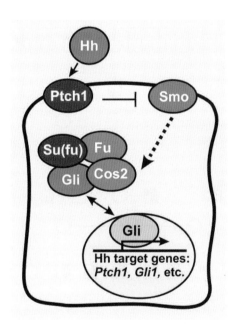

Fig. 13.34 Hedgehog signaling is activated in normal development by interaction of a secreted hedgehog ligand (Hh) with the multipass transmembrane receptor Ptch. Ligand binding relieves the repressive effects of Ptch on Smo, and permits the activation and nuclear translocation of Gli transcription factors. Gli activation is also promoted by Fu, and suppressed by Su(fu). Cos2 proteins are thought to serve as a scaffold for these interactions. Once in the nucleus, Gli factors induce the transcription of various pathway targets, including feedback loops involving Ptch1 and Gli1.

of 5 different first exons {1546}. By extensive splicing events tissue-specific expression pattern of various PTCH isoforms occur, including mRNA species encoding dominant negative forms of PTCH {1545, 1546, 2281}.

Gene function

The *PTCH* gene codes for a 12-trans-membrane protein (Ptch) expressed on many progenitor cell types. It functions as receptor for members of the secreted hedgehog protein family of signalling molecules {1400,2156}. In humans, this family consists of three members designated as Sonic hedgehog, Indian hedgehog, and Desert hedgehog. The *PTCH* gene product has homology to bacterial transporter proteins {2198} and controls another transmembrane protein, Smoothened (Smo) {37, 2156}. In the absence of ligand, Ptch inhibits the activity of Smoh {37,2156}. Binding of hedgehog proteins to Ptch can relieve this inhibition of Smo, which results in signal transduction finally leading to translocation of Gli transcription factors into the cell nucleus and transcription of a set of specific target genes controlling survival, differentiation and proliferation of progenitor cells. In vertebrates, this pathway is critically involved in the development of various tissues and organ systems, such as limbs, gonads, bone, and CNS {709, 916}. Germline mutations in the Sonic hedgehog *(SHH)* and *PTCH* genes were found to cause holoprosencephaly {131, 1483, 1908}.

Gene mutations

So far, 132 different *PTCH* germline mutations associated with NBCCS have been reported {1327}. However, mutations are not detected in all cases {1404}. Mutations are distributed over the entire *PTCH* coding sequence without demonstrating any mutational hot spots, and

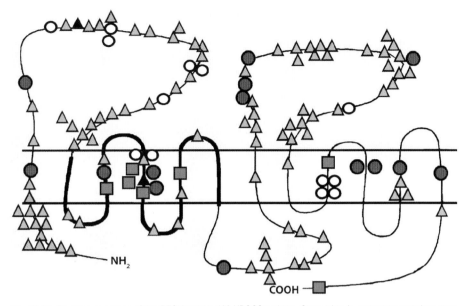

Fig. 13.35 Germline mutations of the *PTCH* gene in 132 NBCCS patients. Green triangle, nonsense mutation; open circle, splice mutation; purple circle, familial missense mutation; black triangle, *de novo* missense mutation; blue square, germline conserved missense mutation. The thick line indicates the location of the sterol sensing domain. Modified from Lindstrom *et al.* {1327}.

there appears to be no clear genotype-phenotype correlation {2409}. Missense mutations cluster in a highly conserved region, the sterol sensing domain, especially in transmembrane domain 4. Somatic mutations of *PTCH* have been demonstrated in various sporadic human tumours (for review see {1327}, including basal cell carcinoma {639, 753, 1005}, trichoepithelioma {2346}, oesophageal squamous cell carcinoma {1378}, invasive transitional cell carcinoma of the bladder {1431}, and medulloblastoma {1327, 1747, 1816, 2345}. Similar to the germline mutations, the vast majority of mutations detected in sporadic tumours result in truncations at the protein level. There is no obvious clustering of mutation sites. One study of 68 sporadic medulloblastomas, *PTCH* mutations were exclusively detected in the desmoplastic

variant, but not in 57 tumours with classical morphology {1747}. In line with these data, LOH analyses of sporadic medulloblastomas demonstrated frequent allelic loss at 9q22.3-q31 in desmoplastic medulloblastomas (up to 50%), but not in classic medulloblastomas {36, 2035}. These data would be consistent with the observation that medulloblastomas associated with NBCCS are predominantly of the desmoplastic variant, indicating a strong association between desmoplastic phenotype and pathological hedgehog pathway activation {51}. However, other studies also reported *PTCH* mutations in classic medulloblastomas {1816, 2345}. *PTCH2*, a *PTCH* homologue located at chromosome band 1p32, can also carry somatic mutations in single cases of medulloblastoma and basal cell carcinomas {2118}.

Rhabdoid tumour predisposition syndrome

P. Wesseling
J.A. Biegel
C.G. Eberhart
A.R. Judkins

Definition

A disorder characterized by a markedly increased risk to develop malignant rhabdoid tumours (MRTs), generally due to constitutional loss or inactivation of one allele of the *INI1* gene.

MIM No.   609322.

Synonyms

Rhabdoid predisposition syndrome; Familial posterior fossa brain tumour syndrome of infancy.

Incidence

Germline *INI1* mutations in patients with atypical teratoid/rhabdoid tumours (AT/RTs), i.e. the central nervous system representative of MRTs, are estimated to occur in up to one third of patients {153}. Because of this risk, it is important to investigate the *INI1* status in all newly diagnosed cases by molecular genetic analysis. Individuals with a germline *INI1* mutation are more likely to present with a tumour in the first year of life. Children with multiple MRTs or with affected siblings or other relatives almost certainly are afflicted by the rhabdoid tumour predisposition syndrome (RTPS). Familial cases have only occasionally been reported {564, 971, 1275, 1364, 1804, 2057, 2225}.

Diagnostic criteria and clinical features

As discussed in the chapter on AT/RTs (see Chapter 8), the histopathological diagnosis of these tumours can be challenging. In most cases, immunohistochemical analysis is very helpful, as the biallelic inactivation of the *INI1* gene in AT/RTs results in lack of INI1 expression in the tumour cell nuclei, while normal cells and almost all other neoplasms show unequivocal nuclear staining {1017}. Demonstration of a germline *INI1* mutation is sufficient for the diagnosis of RTPS. However, a recent study indicates that an alternate locus can cause RTPS as well {616}. As the RTPS was only relatively recently recognized, study of additional affected individuals and families is required to better define this syndrome {971}.

Nervous system neoplasms

Individuals with RTPS frequently present with the central nervous system (CNS) manifestation of MRT, i.e. AT/RT (see Chapter 8). These neoplasms were called "rhabdoid" because of the presence of tumour cells with eccentrically placed nuclei containing vesicular chromatin and prominent nucleoli, as well as abundant cytoplasm with eosinophilic globular cytoplasmic inclusions, features that were originally felt to be reminiscent of skeletal myoblasts. However, the cell of origin of MRTs is not known {153}. Patients with germline mutations or deletions of *INI1* may develop isolated AT/RTs, or an AT/RT with a synchronous renal or extra-renal MRT. AT/RTs generally occur in early childhood, but are occasionally found in adults as well {1823}. Other CNS tumours that have been reported to be associated with the RTPS include choroid plexus carcinoma {660}, medulloblastoma, and supratentorial primitive neuroectodermal tumour {2057}. However, as the histopathological distinction of these tumours from AT/RTs can be challenging, and because the rhabdoid component may be missed due to sampling effects, the occurrence of such other tumours in the context of the RTPS is controversial {747, 1016, 1017, 2289}. Meningiomas may harbour *INI1* mutations {2033}. However, it is not known whether the exon 9 missense mutation described in these tumours is an inactivating mutation. The vast majority of the so-called composite rhabdoid tumours (i.e. meningiomas, gliomas, melanomas, carcinomas with rhabdoid features) retain nuclear INI1 staining {1723}, strongly suggesting they do not contain the same genetic alterations as classic MRT. These composite lesions are therefore unlikely to be part of the RTPS.

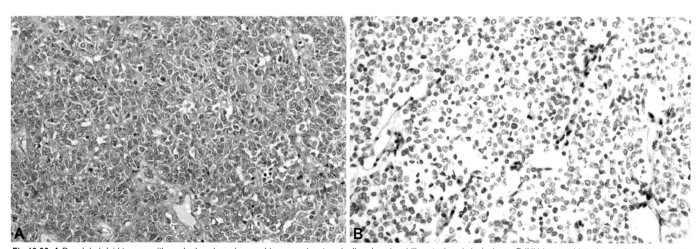

Fig.13.36 A Renal rhabdoid tumour with marked nuclear pleomorphism, prominent nucleoli and eosinophilic cytoplasmic inclusions. **B** INI1 immunohistochemical staining demonstrating loss of expression in neoplastic cells with retained expression in intratumoral blood vessels.

Extraneural manifestations

By far the most frequent extra-CNS location of MRT is the kidney. Bilateral renal MRTs are almost always associated with a germline *INI1* mutation, but infants with an isolated MRT may also carry germline mutations. Occasionally, MRTs have been reported to originate in the head and neck region, paraspinal soft tissues, heart, mediastinum and liver {2402}. Recent reports indicate that *INI1* mutations may occasionally underlie the oncogenesis of other neoplasms such as the proximal type of epithelioid sarcoma {1503}, but to date these sarcomas have not been described in association with the RTPS.

Genetics

Gene

MRTs can occur sporadically or as part of the RTPS {153}. In most cases of both sporadic and RTPS-associated MRTs, *INI1* (*hSNF5*, *SMARCB1*, *BAF47*) can be identified as the causative gene. *INI1* is located at chromosome 22q11.2, has 9 exons and a coding sequence of about 1.2 kb {1028}.

The INI1 protein

The INI1 protein is a member of the ATP-dependent SWI-SNF chromatin-remodelling complex, and is recruited to promotors of genes that regulate the cell cycle, growth, and differentiation. *INI1* functions as a tumour suppressor gene, implying that two successive hits are needed for malignant transformation, and that in familial cancer one hit is inherited {914, 1897}.

Gene mutations

The types of mutations observed in sporadic MRTs are similar to the spectrum of germline mutations reported to date. However, single base deletions in exon 9 appear most often in AT/RTs in patients without detectable germline alterations {153}. The second inactivating event is most frequently a deletion of the wild-type allele, often due to monosomy 22. Prior to the identification of *INI1* as the causative gene, several reports described siblings being affected by AT/RT and/or MRT {1364, 1804}. Subsequently, affected siblings were reported to carry the same germline *INI1* mutation {564, 1275, 2057}. Very few reports exist on involvement of two or more generations of a family {971, 2225}; in these two reported families, germline mutations of *INI1* were transmitted to the affected offspring by a non-affected carrier mother. Alternatively, new mutations can occur during oogenesis/spermatogenesis (gonadal mosaicism), or postzygotically during the early steps of embryogenesis {2057}. For individuals carrying a germline *INI1* mutation, a developmental window seems to exist wherein MRTs occur with sharply increased susceptibility during the first years of life {971}. Such infants generally do not pass the trait to offspring because almost all die before the reproductive age.

Prognostic factors

MRTs are highly aggressive cancers that most frequently occur in young children and are generally lethal within months or a few years. No clear correlation between the type of *INI1* germline alteration and biological behaviour in RTPS patients has been established.

Table13.14 Distribution and nature of *INI1* germline mutations and tumour locations associated with rhabdoid tumour predisposition syndrome.

Exon	Codon	Mutation	Tumour Location
1-9	All	Gene deletion	brain, kidney
1-9	All	Gene deletion	kidney
1-9	All	Gene deletion	brain
1	donor splice site	G -> C	brain
2	47,48	141/4 ins C	kidney
2	51	G152A	brain
2	53	C157T	kidney
2	53	C157T	brain, kidney
2	53	C157T	brain
2	66	C197A	brain, kidney
3	91	271/2 delT	brain, kidney
4	123	C367T	brain
4	*126*	*373 ins 4bp*	*brain*
4	*144*	*430 delG*	*brain*
4	144	430 delG	brain
4	158	C472T	kidney
4	158	C472T	kidney
4	**158**	**C472T**	**brain, soft tissue**
4	**158**	**C472T**	**brain, lung, kidney**
5	**197**	**591 delG**	**brain**
5	198	C592T	brain, kidney
5	198	C592T	brain, kidney
5	201	C601T	brain
5	201	C601T	brain, lung
5	201	C601T	brain, kidney
5	206	G617A	kidney
6	250	750insC	bladder
6	257	C769T	brain, kidney
7	266	797 del 10 bp	kidney
7	297	889 del 7bp	brain, kidney
7	**326**	**C978A**	**brain, kidney**
7	326	C978A	brain
7	326	C978A	epidural
7	*donor splice site*	*G -> A*	*brain*

Data from 34 cases reported in the literature {153, 205A, 564, 622A, 971, 1239A, 1275, 1997A, 2057, 2225, 2409A}. Cases in bold represent families with tumour growth in two or more siblings, cases in italics and bold represent families with tumour development in multiple generations.

CHAPTER 14

Tumours of the Sellar Region

Craniopharyngioma (WHO grade I)
A benign, partly cystic epithelial tumour of the sellar region presumably derived from Rathke pouch epithelium.

Granular cell tumour of the neurohypophysis (WHO grade I)
An intrasellar and/or suprasellar mass arising from the neuro-hypophysis or infundibulum, composed of nests of large cells with granular, eosinophilic cytoplasm due to abundant intra-cytoplasmic lysosomes.

Pituicytoma (WHO grade I)
A rare, circumscribed and generally solid, low-grade, spindle cell, glial neoplasm of adults that originates in the neurohypophysis or infundibulum.

Spindle cell oncocytoma of the adenohypophysis (WHO grade I)
A spindled to epithelioid, oncocytic, non-endocrine neoplasm of the adenohypophysis that manifests in adults and follows a benign clinical course.

Craniopharyngioma

E.J. Rushing
F. Giangaspero
W. Paulus
P.C. Burger

Definition

A benign, partly cystic epithelial tumour of the sellar region presumably derived from Rathke pouch epithelium.

ICD-O codes

Craniopharyngioma 9350/1
Adamantinomatous craniopharyngioma
9351/1
Papillary craniopharyngioma
9352/1

Grading

Craniopharyngiomas correspond histologically to WHO grade I.

Incidence

Craniopharyngiomas account for 1.2–4.6% of all intracranial tumours, corresponding to 0.5–2.5 new cases per million population per year {246}, being more frequent in Nigerian (18% of all CNS tumours) {939} and Japanese children with an annual incidence of 5.25 cases per million in the paediatric population {1231}. They are the most common non-neuroepithelial intracerebral neoplasm in children, accounting for 5–10% of intracranial tumours in this age group {14}.

Age and sex distribution

A bimodal age distribution of adamantino-matous craniopharyngioma is observed {246}, with peaks in children aged 5–15 years and adults aged 45–60 years. Rare neonatal and intrauterine cases have been reported {1150}. Papillary craniopharyngiomas occur virtually exclusively in adults, at a mean age of 40–55 years {14, 395}. Craniopharyngiomas show no obvious sex predilection.

Localization

The most common site is suprasellar with a minor intrasellar component. Unusual locations such as sphenoid sinus have been reported {1166}.

Clinical features

Symptoms and signs

Clinical features are non-specific and essentially include visual disturbances (observed in 62–84% of the patients, more frequently in adults than in children) and endocrine deficiencies (observed in 52–87% of patients, more frequently in children) {2462}. Endocrine deficiencies include those for GH (75%), LH/FSH (40%), ACTH (25%) and TSH (25%). Diabetes insipidus is noted in up to 17% of children and up to 30% of adults. Cognitive impairment and personality changes are observed in about half of patients {2462}. Signs of increased intracranial pressure are frequent, especially in cases with compression or invasion of the third ventricle.

Neuroimaging

For adamantinomatous craniopharyngioma, radiography provides an accurate depiction of the configuration of the sella and the typical calcifications. CTs show contrast enhancement of the solid portions and the cyst capsule, as well as the typical calcifications. On T1-weighted MRI, cystic areas appear as well-delineated homogeneous hyperintense structures, whereas the solid components and mural nodules are isointense, with a

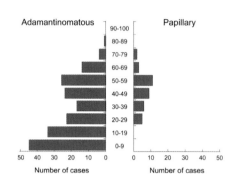

Fig. 14.01 Age distribution of adamantinomatous and papillary craniopharyngioma, based on 224 cases.

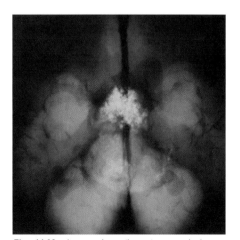

Fig. 14.02 Large adamantinomatous craniopharyngioma extending into the third ventricle. Note the dorsal portion resembling 'machine oil'. Postmortem X-ray showed extensive calcification.

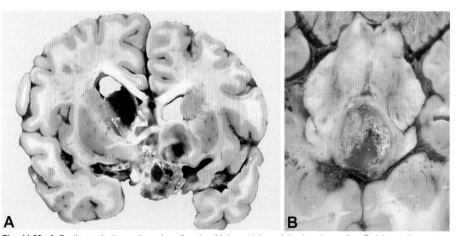

Fig. 14.03 A Cystic craniopharyngioma invading the third ventricle and the basal ganglia. **B** Adamantinomatous craniopharyngioma extending towards the cerebral peduncles. Note the colloid material and calcifications.

slightly heterogeneous quality. In enhanced MRI images, the cystic portion is iso-intense with an enhancing ring, whereas the solid parts are hyperintense {1936}. The papillary craniopharyngioma is non-calcified and has a more uniform appearance in CT and MRI images {395, 1992}.

Macroscopy

Typically a lobulated solid mass, on closer inspection, adamantinomatous cranio-pharyngiomas often demonstrate a spongy quality as a result of a variable cystic component. On sectioning, the cysts may contain dark greenish-brown liquid resembling machinery oil. The gross appearance also reflects the extent of secondary changes such as fibrosis, calcification, ossification and the presence of cholesterol-rich deposits. They often extend beyond their apparent gross confines, superficially penetrating neighbouring brain and adhering to adjacent blood vessels and nerves. By contrast, papillary craniopharyngiomas are well-circumscribed, solid or rarely cystic tumours. An additional distinction from the adamantinomatous variety is the absence of cholesterol-rich machinery oil and calcification.

Histopathology

Adamantinomatous craniopharyngioma is recognized by the presence of squamous epithelium disposed in cords, lobules and irregular trabeculae bordered by palisaded columnar epithelium. These islands of densely packed cells merge with loosely cohesive aggregates of squamous cells known as stellate reticulum. Nodules of "wet keratin" repre-senting remnants of pale nuclei embedded within an eosinophilic kerati-nous mass are found in either the compact or looser areas. Cystic cavities containing squamous debris are lined by flattened epithelium. Granulomatous inflammation associated with cholesterol clefts and giant cells may be seen, but this is more typical of the xanthogranuloma. Piloid gliosis with abundant Rosenthal fibers is often seen at the infiltrative interface of the tumour and should not be mistaken for pilocytic astrocytoma. The question of "malignant transformation" of craniopharyngioma has been raised in the literature {1191}, but this appears to be very rare.

The essential features of papillary cranio-

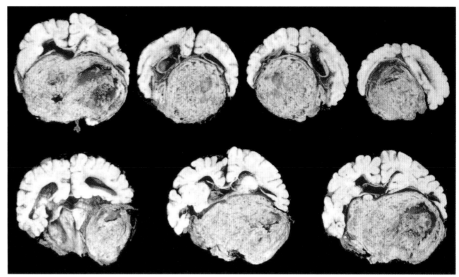

Fig. 14.04 Congenital case of an unusually large, partly cystic craniopharyngioma causing compression and shift of basal brain structures.

pharyngioma include a monomorphous mass of well-differentiated squamous epithelium lacking surface maturation, the picket-fence-like palisades and wet keratin. As noted, another contrasting point is the absence of calcification. Rarely, ciliated epithelium and goblet cells are encountered.

Electron microscopy

Although electron microscopy can serve as a diagnostic adjunct, it is seldom needed given the rather typical features in most cases. In addition to glycogen and the usual organelles, the constituent epithelial cells contain tonofilaments and are joined by desmosomes. Fenestrated capillary endothelium, amorphous ground matrix and collagen fibrils characterize the connective tissue stroma. Mineral precipitates appear to arise in membrane-bound vesicles {1996}.

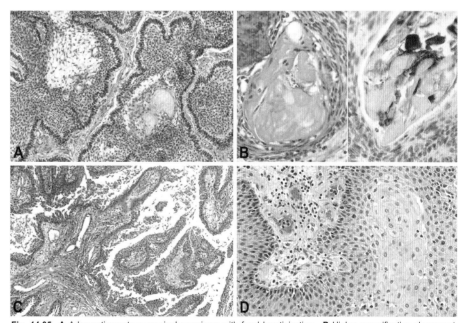

Fig. 14.05 A Adamantinomatous craniopharyngioma with focal keratinization. **B** Higher magnification shows wet keratin structure (left) and immunoreactivity for cytokeratin (right). **C** Papillary craniopharyngioma with well-differentiated epithelium. **D** Well-differentiated squamous epithelium.

Differential diagnosis

Xanthogranuloma of the sellar region {1697} is histologically composed of cholesterol clefts, macrophages (xanthoma cells), chronic inflammatory cellular reaction, necrotic debris and haemosiderin deposits. Although the entity is not yet fully defined and transitional cases do occur, xanthogranuloma of the sellar region is clinico-pathologically distinct from adamantinomatous craniopharyngioma with respect to location, tumour size, age distribution, symptoms and prognosis. Non-adamantinomatous squamous or cuboidal epithelium as well as small tubuli may be focally encountered, while typical adamantinomatous epithelium is usually absent or amounts to less than 10% of tissue {1697}. In contrast to adamantinomatous craniopharyngioma, epithelial cells encountered in xanthogranuloma do not exhibit nuclear accumulation of ß-catenin {267}.

Although the histological appearance of adamantinomatous craniopharyngioma is characteristic, epidermoid and Rathke's cleft cysts are sometimes raised in the differential diagnosis. A reliable distinction of both entities is feasible if attention is paid, in the case of the former, to the presence of a uniloculated cyst lined by squamous epithelium and filled with flaky, "dry keratin". Rathke's cleft cysts rarely pose a significant challenge and only enter into the differential diagnosis when they show extensive squamous metaplasia. More commonly, Rathke's cleft cysts consist of a single layer of flattened, either ciliated or mucin-producing epithelium, occasionally accompanied by a xanthogranulomatous reaction {906}.

Proliferation

MIB-1 immunoreactivity is concentrated in the peripherally palisaded cells in the adamantinomatous type, and is more randomly distributed in the papillary lesions {470, 496}. Reported indices vary considerably from case to case, and, overall, are considerably higher than might be expected given the indolence of the neoplasms {470,496}. No relationship between indices and recurrence has been established.

Genetics

Multiple chromosomal abnormalities have been reported in two cases by classic cytogenetic analysis; both tumours had abnormalities involving chromosomes 2 and 12 {711, 1049}.

More than 70% of craniopharyngiomas of the adamantinomatous type harbour a mutation of the ß-catenin gene {267, 1053, 1632, 2047}. Most of the mutations affect exon 3, which encodes the degradation targeting box of ß-catenin compatible with an accumulation of nuclear ß-catenin protein {267}. In few cases of adamantinomatous craniopharyngiomas, the same ß-catenin mutations occurring in the epithelial cells have been identified in mesenchymal cells. Such observation suggests a biphasic nature of a subgroup of adamantinomatous craniopharyngiomas {2047}. In contrast, no mutations have been demonstrated in papillary craniopharyngiomas. Comparative genomic hybridization (CGH) studies on two large series of craniopharyniogiomas have failed to show significant chromosomal imbalances in adamantinomatous and papillary-type craniopharyngiomas {1880, 2473}. Another CGH study in nine adamantinomatous craniopharyngiomas revealed at least one genomic alteration in 67% of cases {1888}.

Histogenesis

Several observations indicate that craniopharyngiomas arise from neoplastic transformation of ectodermal-derived epithelial cell remants of Rathke's pouch and the craniopharyngeal duct. Epithelial cell rests have been reported to occur between the roof of the pharynx and the floor of the third ventricle, most frequently along the anterior part of the infundibulum and the anterior-superior surface of the adenohypophysis, sites of the previous Rathke's pouch and the involuted duct that links these structures. Metaplasia of cells derived from the tooth promordia gives rise to the adamantinomatous variety, whereas metaplastic changes in cells derived from buccal mucosa promordia gives rise to the squamous papillary variety {1782}.

Further support for the assumption that craniopharyngiomas originate from Rathke's pouch is provided by the occasional occurrence of mixed tumours with characteristics of craniopharyngioma and Rathke's cleft cyst, and by the report of a unique congenital craniopharyngioma {2454} with ameloblastic as well as tooth bud and adenohypophyseal primordia components.

The hypothesis that craniopharyngiomas

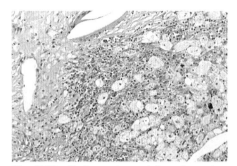

Fig. 14.06 Xanthogranuloma of the sellar region, showing xanthoma cells, lymphocytic infiltrates, haemosiderin deposits, cholesterol clefts and occasional multinucleated giant cells.

contain a neuroendocrine lineage is supported by the finding that scattered tumour cell groups may express one or more pituitary hormones {2190}, chromogranin A {2454} and human chorionic gonadotropin {2193}. Also in support is the observation of a tumour that arose from a Rathke cleft cyst and contained cells that were transitional between squamous, mucus-producing and anterior pituitary lobe secretory cells {1077}.

Prognostic and predictive factors

In large series, 60–93% of patients had a 10-year recurrence-free survival and 64–96% an overall 10-year survival {395, 1824, 2462}. The most significant factor associated with craniopharyngioma recurrence is the extent of surgical resection {1982, 2387, 2462}, with lesions greater than 5 cm in diameter carrying a markedly worse prognosis {2462}. After incomplete surgical resection, the recurrence rate is significantly higher {2387, 2462}. Histological evidence for brain invasion, more frequently documented in the adamantinomatous than in the papillary type, is not correlated with a higher recurrence rate in cases with gross surgical resection {2387}. Some authors have documented a better prognosis for the papillary than for the adamantinomatous type of craniopharyngioma {14, 2224}, while others failed to demonstrate significant differences {395, 2387}. Dissemination in the subarachnoid space {927, 1273} or implantation along the surgical track or path of needle aspiration {100, 1338} is rare. Malignant transformation of craniopharyngioma to squamous carcinoma after irradiation is exceptional {730, 2241}.

Granular cell tumour of the neurohypophysis

G.N. Fuller
P. Wesseling

Definition
An intrasellar and/or suprasellar mass arising from the neurohypophysis or infundibulum, composed of nests of large cells with granular, eosinophilic cytoplasm due to abundant intracytoplasmic lysosomes.

ICD-O code   9582/0

Grading
Granular cell tumours correspond to WHO grade I.

Synonyms
Abrikossoff tumour, choristoma, granular cell myoblastoma, granular cell neuroma, pituicytoma. The term pituicytoma is now reserved for a distinct, circumscribed glial neoplasm originating in the neurohypophysis or infundibulum (see Pituicytoma chapter).

Incidence
Symptomatic granular cell tumours (GCTs) are relatively rare and present in adulthood, with only exceptionally rare childhood cases {133}. There is a clear female predominance of greater than 2:1. The peak incidence is slightly later in men than in women (sixth and fifth decade, respectively). Asymptomatic microscopic clusters of granular cells, termed granular cell tumorettes {2062} or tumorlets {1358}, are more common than the larger, symptomatic tumours, and have been documented at an incidence up to 17% in postmortem series {1358, 2062, 2255}.

Localization
GCTs arise along the anatomic distribution of the neurohypophysis, including the posterior pituitary and pituitary stalk/infundibulum. They exhibit a preference for the pituitary stalk and thus most frequently arise in the suprasellar region, but may also arise from the posterior pituitary and present as an intrasellar mass. GCTs with identical morphologic and immunophenotypic features as those seen in the neurohypophyseal tumours have rarely been reported in other anatomic locations within the central nervous system, including the spinal meninges {1402}, cranial meninges {2316}, third ventricle {2286} and cerebral hemisphere {472}.

Clinical features
Symtoms and signs
The most common presenting symptom is visual field deficit secondary to compression of the optic chiasm {367}.

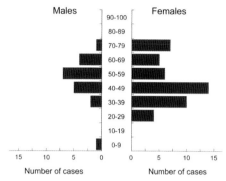

Fig.14.07 Age and sex distribution of neurohypophyseal granular cell tumours based on 66 symptomatic cases published in the literature (M:F = 1:2.3).

Other presenting complaints include panhypopituitarism, galactorrhea, amenorrhea, decreased libido and neuropsychological changes. Diabetes insipidus has been reported, but is relatively uncommon {367}. Symptoms usually develop slowly over a period of years, although acute presentation with sudden-onset diplopia, confusion, headache and vomiting can occur {367}. There are no disease-specific signs or symptoms that reliably distinguish GCT from other suprasellar mass lesions. Several cases have been found in association with pituitary adenoma {105, 367, 1348, 2255}.

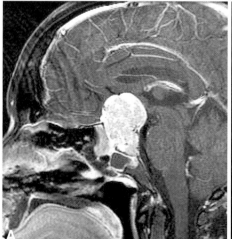
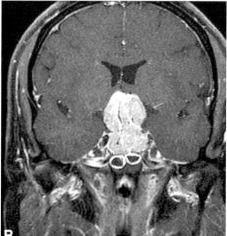
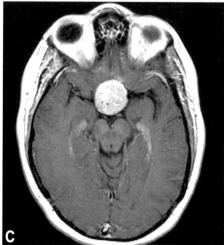

Fig. 14.08 T1-weighted post-contrast MRI of a granular cell tumour in the sagittal (**A**), coronal (**B**), and axial (**C**) planes showing prominent contrast enhancement. Note the characteristic sellar/suprasellar anatomic location.

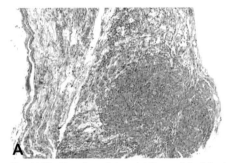 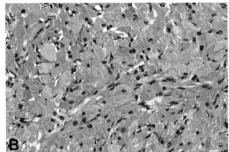

Fig. 14.09 Granular cell tumorlet (tumorette) of the infundibulum. **A** Hematoxylin-eosin whole mount section. **B** High-power magnification showing discrete cellular borders and granular cytoplasm.

Neuroimaging

MRI typically shows a well-circumscribed suprasellar mass that most frequently displays homogeneous or heterogeneous contrast enhancement. Tumour size typically ranges from 1.5 to 6.0 cm {367}. Calcification is unusual and thus helps to distinguish GCT from craniopharyngioma. Similarly, lack of a dural attachment ("dural tail") and the anatomic location centred around the pituitary stalk help to distinguish GCT from most regional meningiomas. Although there are no pathognomonic imaging features, cases in which the tumour can be clearly seen to be separated from the pituitary by the inferior end of the pituitary stalk are suggestive of GCT {63}. Nevertheless, similar to the situation with suprasellar pituicytomas, due to the relative rarity of the tumour, the diagnosis is rarely anticipated prior to surgical resection.

Macroscopy

The tumours are usually lobulated and well-circumscribed, with a soft but rubbery consistency that is firmer than pituitary adenoma. The cut surface is typically grey-to-yellow. Necrosis, cystic degeneration and/or haemorrhage are uncommon. The tumour may infiltrate surrounding structures such as the optic chiasm and cavernous sinus; these features may prevent gross total surgical resection.

Histopathology

GCTs consist of densely packed polygonal cells with abundant granular eosinophilic cytoplasm. The architecture is typically nodular; sheets and/or spindled/fascicular patterns can also be seen. PAS staining of cytoplasmic granules is resistant to diastase digestion. Small foci of foamy cells may be observed. Tumour cell nuclei are small, with inconspicuous nucleoli and evenly distributed chromatin. Perivascular lymphocytic aggregates are common. Mitotic activity is usually inconspicuous, and proliferative activity is usually very low. Some lesions are characterized by nuclear pleomorphism, prominent nucleoli, multinucleated cells and increased mitotic activity (up to 5 mitoses per 10 HPF and Ki-67 labelling index of 7%); these tumours have been referred to as "atypical" GCTs by some authors, although clinical and biological significance is uncertain {1052, 2331}.

Immunohistochemistry

GCTs are variably positive for CD68 (KP1), S-100, α-1-antitrypsin, α-1-antichy-motrypsin and cathepsin B, and negative for neurofilament proteins, cytokeratins, chromogranin A, synaptophysin, desmin, smooth muscle actin and the pituitary hormones. Most tumours are negative for GFAP, although variable immunoreactivity has been noted in a subset of GCTs.

Electron microscopy

The cytoplasm of the granular tumour cells is filled with phagolysosomes containing unevenly distributed electron-dense material and membranous debris. A few other organelles and intracytoplasmic filaments may be observed, but neurose-cretory granules are absent {122}.

Histogenesis

GCT is a descriptive term of a histogeneti-cally heterogeneous group of neoplasms in various anatomic sites throughout the body. Neurohypophyseal GCTs most likely arise from pituicytes, the glial element in the posterior lobe and stalk of the pituitary gland. The conflicting results of immunohis-tochemical studies of these pituitary GCTs may be explained by the presence of different types of pituicytes in the normal neurohypophysis {2203}. GCTs occasion-ally occur in the CNS outside the pituitary gland (meninges, cerebral hemisphere, third ventricle, cranial nerves); these may be derived from glial cells, Schwann cells or macrophages {367, 1878, 2316}.

Genetics

Comparative genomic hybridization analysis of one tumour did not reveal chromosomal imbalances {1878}. In a case of atypical GCT, 95% of the tumour cells showed nuclear accumulation of p53 protein; 15% expressed bcl-2 {2331}.

Prognostic and predictive factors

Most GCTs are clinically benign, with slow progression and lack of invasive growth. Surgical removal is the preferred therapy for larger tumours, but the firm and vascular nature of pituitary GCTs, sometimes combined with absence of an obvious dissection plane from the adjacent brain, may hamper gross total resection.

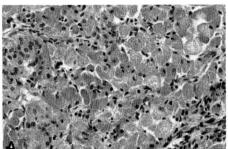 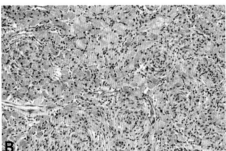 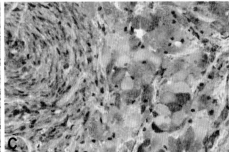

Fig. 14.10 Histological features of granular cell tumour of the neurohypophysis. **A** Characteristic abundant eosinophilic cytoplasm with prominent granularity. **B** Spindled and whorling cellular architecture. **C** S-100 protein expression in granular cell tumour.

Pituicytoma

P. Wesseling
D.J. Brat
G.N. Fuller

Definition

A rare, circumscribed and generally solid, low-grade, spindle cell, glial neoplasm of adults that originates in the neurohypophysis or infundibulum.

ICD-O Code

The provisional code proposed for the fourth edition of ICD-O is *9432/1*.

Grading

Pituicytomas correspond to WHO grade I.

Synonyms and historical annotation

While the term pituicytoma was historically also used for other tumours in the sellar and suprasellar region (granular cell tumours, pilocytic astrocytomas), this term is now reserved for low-grade glial neoplasms that originate in the neurohypophysis or infundibulum and that are distinct from pilocytic astrocytomas. Less preferred terms for pituicytoma include posterior pituitary astrocytoma and, for lesions arising in the pituitary stalk, infundibuloma.

Incidence

Pituicytomas are extremely rare. To date, less than 30 bona fide examples have been described, often as case reports. The largest series reported to date describes 9 tumours pooled from the consultation cases of two large institutions {221}.

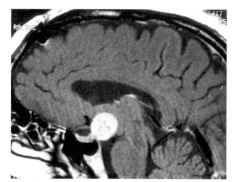

Fig. 14.11 Pituicytoma showing solid, circumscribed growth and diffuse contrast-enhancement on T1-weighted MRI.

Age and sex distribution

All pituicytomas reported to date have occurred in adult patients. In a compiled series of 26 cases, the male to female ratio is 1.6:1 {135, 221, 302, 326, 576, 893, 1065, 1181, 1569, 2041, 2061, 2283, 2285}. Three quarters of these males presented between 40 and 60 years of age; in women, no age peak is observed.

Localization

Pituicytomas arise along the distribution of the neurohypophysis, including the pituitary stalk and posterior pituitary. Accordingly, they may be located within the sella, in the suprasellar region, or occupy both the intrasellar and suprasellar compartments {221, 576, 2061, 2285}.

Clinical features

Symptoms and signs

The most common presenting signs and symptoms of pituicytoma resemble those of other slowly expanding, non-hormonally active primary tumours of the sellar/ suprasellar region that compress the optic chiasm, infundibulum and/or pituitary gland, and include visual disturbance, headache and various features of hypopituitarism such as amenorrhea, decreased libido and mildly elevated serum prolactin ("stalk effect") {221, 2285}. Rarely, asymptomatic cases have been found only at autopsy {2201}.

Neuroimaging

Pituicytomas typically are homogeneous, well-demarcated, uniformly contrast-enhancing masses as seen on preoperative CT or MRI studies. Occasional tumours show heterogeneous contrast enhancement, and rare examples exhibit a cystic component {221}.

Macroscopy

Pituicytomas are solid, well-circumscribed masses that have a firm, rubbery texture and can measure up to several centimeters. Only rarely has a cystic component been reported {221, 2285}. Radiographic studies may give the impression of a smoothly contoured tumour, yet they can be firmly adherent to adjacent structures in the suprasellar space.

Histopathology

Pituicytomas have a solid, compact architecture and consist almost entirely of elongate, bipolar spindle cells arranged in interlacing fascicles or in a storiform pattern {221, 2285}. Tumours can show dense adherence to adjacent structures. Individual tumour cells contain abundant eosinophilic cytoplasm, and cell shapes range from short and plump to elongate and angulated. Cell borders are readily apparent, especially on cross sections of fascicles. There is no significant cytoplasmic granularity or vacuolization, and PAS staining shows only minimal reaction. Nuclei are of moderate size, oval-to-elongate, with little or no atypia. Mitotic figures are rare. Reticulin stain shows a perivascular distribution, intercellular reticulin being sparse. Important for the differential diagnosis with pilocytic astrocytoma and normal neurohypophysis, pituicytomas show no Rosenthal fibers or eosinophilic granular bodies. Herring bodies (axonal dilatations for neuropeptide storage in the histologically similar neurohypophysis) may be seen at the periphery. In contrast to spindle cell oncocytoma, oncocytic change is lacking.

Immunohistochemistry

Pituicytomas are generally positive for vimentin, S-100 protein, and GFAP {221, 576}, although the latter ranges from faint and focal to moderate and patchy. Only rarely is GFAP strongly and diffusely positive. Strong staining is more often seen with S-100 protein and vimentin. Pituicytomas show no reactivity for neuronal or neuroendocrine markers, such as synaptophysin and chromogranin, or for pituitary hormones. Neurofilament protein immunoreactivity is limited to axons in peritumoural neurohypophyseal tissue and is not present within the tumour. Stains for cytokeratins are negative, while those for EMA may show a patchy, cytoplasmic rather than membranous pattern.

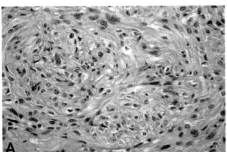 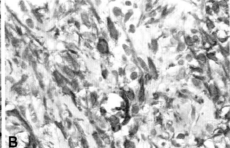 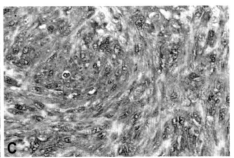

Fig. 14.12 Histological features of pituicytoma. **A** Elongate and plump tumour cells arranged in a fascicular pattern. **B** Patchy staining for GFAP. **C** Diffuse staining for S-100 protein.

Proliferation
Proliferation indices (Ki-67) are low and range from 0.5 to 2.0% {221, 1181}. No correlation of proliferation with outcome has been established.

Histogenesis
Pituicytomas presumably arise from pituicytes, specialized glial cells of the neurohypophysis {221, 988, 1332, 2008}. This origin accounts for the anatomic distribution of pituicytomas and is consistent with the tumour's immunophenotypic characteristics. Although this is widely accepted, an alternative theory of origin from the folliculostellate stromal cells of the adenohypophysis has also been proposed {302}. Another primary neurohypophyseal tumour of presumed pituicyte origin is the granular cell tumour. This may be explained by the possible existence of multiple pituicyte subtypes {2203}.

Prognostic and predictive factors
Pituicytomas are slowly enlarging, localized tumours that are treated by surgical resection. Subtotal resection may be accompanied by gradual regrowth over a period of several years. No instances of malignant transformation or distant metastasis have been reported.

Spindle cell oncocytoma of the adenohypophysis

G.N. Fuller
B.W. Scheithauer
F. Roncaroli
P. Wesseling

Definition

A spindled to epithelioid, oncocytic, non-endocrine neoplasm of the adenohypophysis that manifests in adults and follows a benign clinical course.

ICD-O code

The provisional code proposed for the fourth edition of ICD-O is *8291/0.*

Grading

Spindle cell oncocytoma of the adenohypophysis corresponds to WHO grade I.

Synonyms and historical annotation

Spindle cell oncocytoma (SCO) was reported as a distinct entity by Roncaroli *et al.* in 2002 {1915}. The descriptive term SCO was used instead of one indicating a suspected derivation from folliculo-stellate cells of the anterior pituitary. It is possible that the term folliculo-stellate cell tumour of the pituitary will eventually be applied to this entity.

Incidence

SCO is a rare tumour and its actual incidence is difficult to determine. In the experience of one institution, SCOs represented 0.4% of all sellar tumours {1915}.

Age and sex distribution

Based on the limited number of cases reported, SCO is a tumour of adults. The age of the reported patients ranges between 26 and 71 years (mean 56 years). The distribution is equal between the sexes {410, 1134, 1915, 2298}.

Localization

SCO is a pituitary tumour. At presentation, five lesions showed suprasellar extension and three extended to the cavernous sinus {410, 2298}. One example invaded the sellar floor {1134}.

Clinical features

Symptoms and signs

The clinical presentation and neuroimaging characteristics of patients with SCO are indistinguishable from those with a non-functioning pituitary adenoma. The patients often exhibit pituitary hypofunction and visual field defects, less frequently headache, nausea and vomiting {410, 1134, 1915, 2298}. One patient with a recurrent SCO and involvement of the skull base presented with epistaxis {1134}.

Neuroimaging

On MRI, SCO is generally seen as a sharply demarcated, solid, contrast-enhancing intra- and suprasellar mass with or without sellar or skull base destruction.

Macroscopy

On gross inspection, SCOs are indistinguishable from pituitary adenomas. Most are of macroadenoma dimension, but an exceptional 6.5 cm sellar/parasellar example has been reported {410}. They vary from soft, creamy and easily dissectable lesions to firm tumours that adhere to surrounding structures and infrequently show destruction of the sellar floor {410}. A clear margin with the adjacent normal pituitary is usually absent.

Histopathology

Spindle cell oncocytomas are typically composed of interlacing fascicles of spindled to epithelioid cells with eosinophilic, variably oncocytic cytoplasm. Mild to moderate nuclear atypia and even focal marked pleomorphism may be seen. A minor infiltrate of mature lymphocytes is seen in many lesions. Mitotic counts are typically less than one per 10 HPF. Recurrent lesions may or may not show increased mitotic activity {1134}.

Electron microscopy

Ultrastructural examination is useful in the diagnosis of SCO {1134, 1915}. Neoplastic cells appear spindled or polygonal in configuration and are often filled with mitochondria. Well-formed desmosomes and junctions of intermediate type are encountered and, in addition to a lack of secretory granules, are the hallmarks of this tumour, distinguishing it from pituitary adenoma.

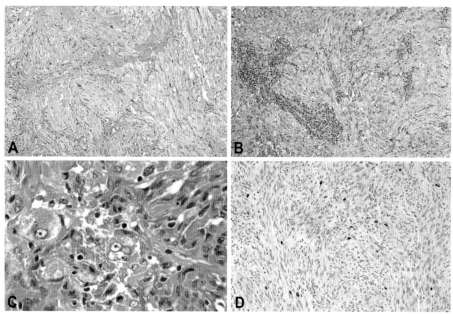

Fig. 14.13 Histological features of spindle cell oncocytoma. **A** The lesion is composed of interlacing fascicles of spindle cells with eosinophilic cytoplasm and mildly to moderately atypical nuclei. **B** Some examples show mild to moderate lymphocytic infiltrates. **C** A minority of tumour cells have pleomorphic nuclei and (**D**) low Ki-67 labelling index.

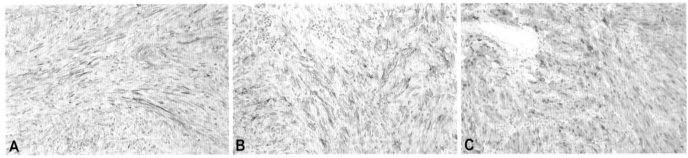

Fig. 14.14 Immunohistochemical features of spindle cell oncocytoma. Neoplastic cells characteristically express vimentin (**A**), EMA (**B**) and S-100 protein (**C**).

Immunohistochemistry

While negative for pituitary hormones, SCOs typically express vimentin, EMA, S-100 protein, and the anti-mitochondrial antibody 113-1. Staining for galectin-3 is seen and, although non-specific, initially suggested a link to the folliculo-stellate cell. A variety of other molecules, including GFAP, cytokeratins, CD34, synaptophysin, chromogranin, bcl-2, smooth muscle actin and desmin have not been shown to be expressed.

Proliferation

The MIB-1 labelling index is usually low. In all but one reported case, labelling has ranged from 1% to 8% (mean 2.8%). One recurrent example featured a MIB-1 labelling index of 20%, no data being available on the proliferation rate of the primary tumour {1134}.

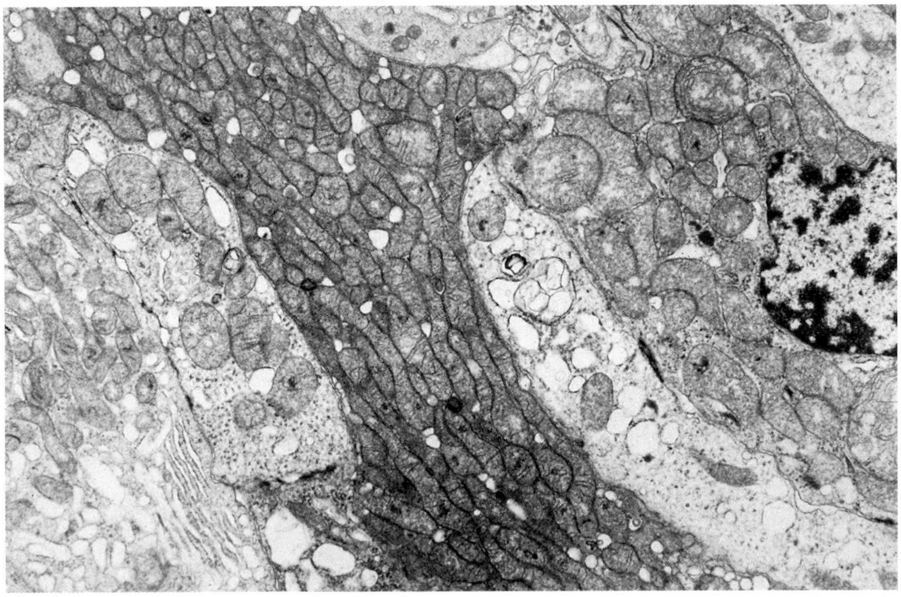

Histogenesis

The cellular origin of SCO is uncertain. The original description {1915} postulated a derivation from folliculo-stellate cells of the anterior hypophysis. This was suggested by similarities between the cells of SCO and folliculo-stellate cells, including the expression of S-100 protein, vimentin and galectin-3, as well as the finding of desmosomes and intermediate junctions.

Prognostic and predictive factors

All five patients in the initial report on SCOs had a benign clinical course after 3 years of follow-up {1915}. Moderate tumour volume and lack of invasion into surrounding structures generally facilitates complete surgical resection. After incomplete removal, some tumours may (after several years) pursue a more aggressive course and show increased MIB-1 labelling indices and necrosis {1134}. Additional clinical follow-up is needed before the prognostic significance of these features can be assessed.

Fig. 14.15 Ultrastructurally, the tumour cells of spindle cell oncocytoma show numerous mitochondria (oncocytic change) as well as several cell-to-cell junctions, mainly short desmosomes.

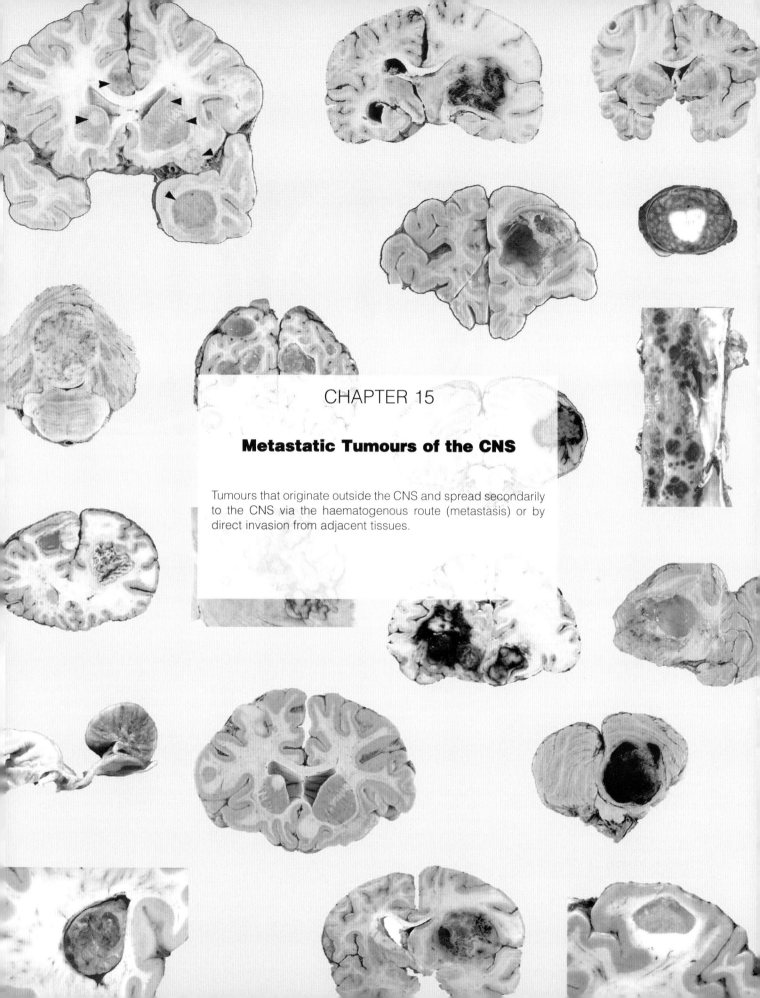

CHAPTER 15

Metastatic Tumours of the CNS

Tumours that originate outside the CNS and spread secondarily to the CNS via the haematogenous route (metastasis) or by direct invasion from adjacent tissues.

Metastatic tumours of the CNS

P. Wesseling
A. von Deimling
K.D. Aldape

Definition
Tumours that originate outside the CNS and spread secondarily to the CNS via the haematogenous route (metastasis) or by direct invasion from adjacent tissues.

Incidence
Metastatic tumours are the most common CNS neoplasms. Due to underdiagnosis and inaccurate reporting, the incidence rates found in the literature for brain metastases (up to 11 per 100 000 population per year) probably underestimate the true incidence {2174}. Autopsy studies revealed that CNS metastases occur in about 25% of patients who die of cancer {654}. Leptomeningeal metastases occur in 4–15% of patients with solid tumours {2197} and dural metastases in 8–9% of cancer patients with advanced cancer {1250}. Spinal epidural metastases are found in 5–10% of all patients with cancer and are much more frequent than spinal leptomeningeal or intramedullary metastases {1541}. Direct intracranial extension from local primary tumours is rare {1129}.

Age and sex distribution
The incidence of CNS metastases increases from less than one per 100 000 below 25 years of age to greater than 30 per 100 000 at age 60 years {2174}. Up

Table 15.01 Origin of brain metastases.

Primary tumour site	% of brain metastases
Respiratory tract	50%
Breast	15%
Skin/melanoma	11%
Unknown primary site	11%

Table 15.02 Origin of metastases causing epidural spinal cord compression.

Primary tumour site	Percentage
Breast	22%
Lung	15%
Prostate	10%
Malignant lymphoma	10%

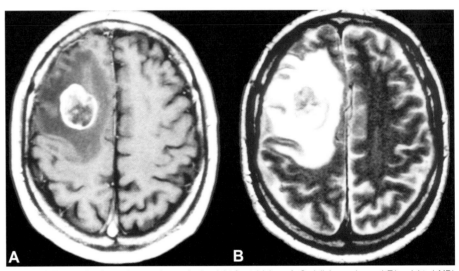

Fig. 15.01 Metastasis of an adenocarcinoma in the right frontal lobe. **A** Gadolinium-enhanced T1-weighted MRI showing a large area of hyperintensity corresponding to a perifocal edema that (**B**) shows bright hyperintensity on T2-weighted MRI.

to 30% of adults and 6–10% of children with cancer will develop brain metastases {1096}. The relative proportions of various primary tumours are different for the two sexes, but for most tumours gender lacks a significant independent effect on the occurrence of CNS metastasis {104, 2174}.

Origin of CNS metastases
The most common sources of brain metastases in adults are, in descending order, lung cancer (especially small cell and adenocarcinoma), breast cancer, melanoma, renal cancer and colon cancer; in children, in descending order, leukaemia, lymphoma, osteogenic sarcoma, rhabdomyosarcoma and Ewing sarcoma {2174}. Prostate, breast and lung cancer are the most common origin of spinal epidural metastasis, followed by non-Hodgkin lymphoma, multiple myeloma and renal cancer {1541}. Tumours vary in their propensity to metastazise to the CNS {104, 404, 2036}. In up to 10% of the patients with brain metastases no primary tumour is found at presentation {1096}. Primary neoplasms in the head and neck region (e.g. squamous cell carcinoma, esthesioneuroblastoma) may extend intracranially by direct invasion

and occasionally present as an intracranial tumour {257}.

Localization
More than 80% of brain metastases are located in the cerebral hemispheres, especially in arterial border zones and at the junction of cerebral cortex and white matter. Approximately 15% are found in the cerebellum. Of the brain metastases, less than half are single (i.e. the only metastasis in the brain), and very few are solitary (i.e. the only metastasis detected in the body) {654}. Other intracranial sites include the dura and leptomeninges; in these sites, extension from or to other compartments is common {1128, 1250}. The vast majority of metastases affecting the spinal cord expand from the vertebral body or paravertebral tissues into the epidural space {1541}. Occasionally, metastatic CNS tumours seed along the walls of the ventricles or are located in the pituitary gland, choroid plexus, or a pre-existing lesion like a meningioma. The posterior fossa is relatively frequently involved in patients with colorectal and renal carcinoma and tumours of the pelvic organs. Dural metastases are relatively common in cancer of the

prostate, breast, lung, and in haematologic malignancies {1250}; leptomeningeal metastasis in patients with lung and breast cancer, melanoma, and haematopoietic tumours {2174, 2197}; spinal epidural metastasis in cancer of prostate, breast, lung, kidney, non-Hodgkin lymphoma and multiple myeloma; and intramedullary spinal cord metastasis in small cell lung carcinoma {1541}.

Clinical features
Symptoms and signs
The neurological signs and symptoms of intracranial metastases are generally caused by increased intracranial pressure or local effect of the tumour on the adjacent brain tissue. They may progress gradually and include headache, altered mental status, paresis, ataxia, visual complaints, nausea or sensory disturbances. Some patients present acutely with seizure, infarct or haemorrhage {1096}. Many patients with leptomeningeal metastasis have multiple, varied neurological symptoms and signs at presentation, including headache, mental alteration, ataxia, cranial nerve dysfunction and radiculopathy. Cytological examination reveals malignant cells in the initial CSF sample in about 50% of such patients; this figure may increase to 90% when CSF sampling is repeated and adequate volumes (10 mL) are available for cytological analysis {699}. Spinal metastases generally result in compression of the spinal cord or nerve roots and may cause back pain, weakness of the extremities, sensory disturbances, and incontinence in the course of hours, days or weeks {2017}.

Neuroimaging
On MRI, intraparenchymal metastases are generally circumscribed and show mild T1-hypointensity, T2-hyperintensity, and diffuse or ring-like contrast-enhancement with a surrounding zone of parenchymal edema. Haemorrhagic metastases and metastatic melanomas containing melanin-pigment may demonstrate hyperintensity on non-contrast MRI or CT {2475}. In patients with leptomeningeal metastasis, MRI can reveal focal or diffuse leptomeningeal thickening and contrast-enhancement (sometimes with dispersed tumour nodules in the subarachnoid space); in addition, enhancement and enlargement of the cranial nerves and communicating hydrocephalus may be

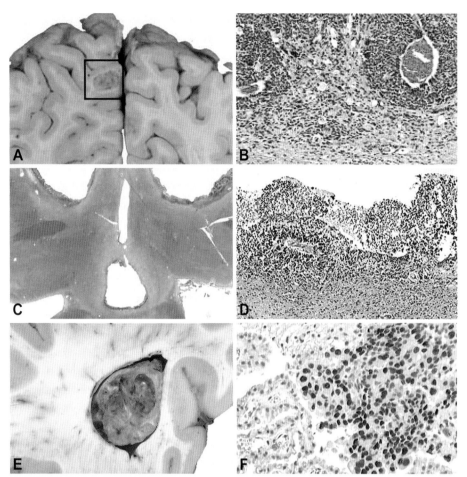

Fig. 15.02 **A,B** Intracerebral subcortical metastasis of small cell lung carcinoma. **C**, **D** Extensive spread of small cell lung carcinoma cells along the walls of both lateral ventricles and the third ventricle. **D** Higher magnification of ventricular wall. **E,F** Intraventricular/choroid plexus metastasis of lung adenocarcinoma. Note the TTF1 staining of tumour cell nuclei (**F**).

found {699, 1541}. MRI can depict dural metastases as nodular masses or dural thickening along the bone structures, while metastases in vertebral bodies are visualised as discrete, confluent or diffuse areas of low signal intensity. CT scan may be useful for detection of bone involvement {1250}.

Macroscopy
Metastases in the brain and spinal cord

parenchyma often form grossly circumscribed and rounded, grey white or tan masses with variable central necrosis and peritumoural edema. Metastases of adenocarcinomas may contain collections of mucoid material. Haemorrhage is relatively frequent in metastases of choriocarcinoma, melanoma and renal cell carcinoma. Melanoma metastases with abundant melanin-pigment have a brown to black colour. Leptomeningeal

Table 15.03 Cumulative incidence of brain metastasis from the most common primary sites.

Primary tumour site	Cumulative incidence of brain metastasis with interval after diagnosis of primary tumour		
	< 1 month	< 1 year	< 5 years
Lung	7.8%	14.8%	16.3%
Breast	0.4%	1.0%	5.0%
Melanoma	0.7%	4.0%	7.4%
Renal	1.7%	5.2%	9.8%
Colorectal	0.1%	0.6%	1.2%

Adapted from Schouten et al. {2036}.

metastasis may produce diffuse opacification of the membranes or present as multiple nodules {1866}. Dural metastases can grow as localized plaques or nodules and as diffuse lesions {1128}. Primary neoplasms in the head and neck region that extend intracranially by direct invasion generally cause significant destruction of the skull bones. In some cases, however, the skull is penetrated by relatively subtle perivascular or perineural invasion without major bone destruction {257}.

Histopathology

The histological, ultrastructural, and immunohistochemical features of secondary CNS tumours are as diverse as in the primary tumours from which they arise. Most intraparenchymal metastases are histologically relatively well demarcated. Rather than by infiltration of single cells in the neuropil, these tumours often expand by growth of groups of tumour cells in the Virchow-Robin spaces, ultimately resulting in destruction of the neuroglial tissue and a variety of reactive changes including gliosis, inflammation and florid microvascular proliferation. Tumour necrosis may be extensive, leaving recognizable tumour tissue only at the periphery of the lesion and around blood vessels {1866}. Metastases of some carcinomas, particularly small cell carcinomas of the lung, may show relatively

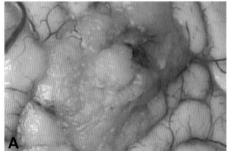
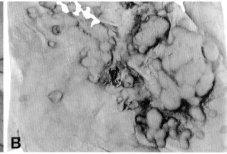

Fig. 15.03 A Leptomeningeal metastasis of non-Hodgkin lymphoma. B Dural metastasis of mammary carcinoma.

diffuse ("pseudogliomatous") infiltration in the neuropil {116, 1583}. In leptomeningeal metastasis, the tumour cells are dispersed in the subarachnoid and Virchow-Robin spaces and may invade the adjacent CNS parenchyma and nerve roots {2197}.

Immunohistochemistry

The immunohistochemical characteristics in secondary CNS tumours are generally similar to those in the tumours from which they originate. Immunohistochemical analysis is often helpful for distinguishing primary from secondary CNS tumours and, in case of an unknown primary tumour, for assessment of the exact nature and origin of the metastatic neoplasm {118, 143A, 485}.

Proliferation

Metastatic CNS tumours show variable

and often marked mitotic activity. The proliferation index may be higher than in the primary neoplasm {338}.

Pathogenesis

Before they present as haematogenous metastases in the CNS, tumour cells must successfully complete a series of steps: escape from the primary tumour, entry and survival in the blood stream, arrest and extravasation in the CNS, and survival and growth in the CNS microenvironment {1571}. Secondary CNS tumours may also develop by direct extension from primary tumours in adjacent anatomic structures (e.g. paranasal sinuses, bone), but such tumours are not considered metastases in a strict sense because they remain in continuity with the primary neoplasm. Once in contact with the CSF containing compartments, cells of those tumours may disseminate ("seed") around the CNS {2168}.

Genetics

Using comparative genomic hybridization, a high degree of conformity was found between brain metastases and the corresponding primary tumours outside the CNS {1740}. Detailed information on genes that are crucial in the metastatic process {1571} is not yet used for diagnostic, prognostic or therapeutic purposes.

Prognostic and predictive factors

Based on the data of Radiation Therapy Oncology Group (RTOG) trials, three classes for predicting outcome in patients with brain metastases were suggested: class 1, with the best outcomes (median survival after whole brain radiotherapy 7.1 months), includes patients with Karnofsky performance status (KPS) of 70 or higher, of age younger than 65, and with controlled

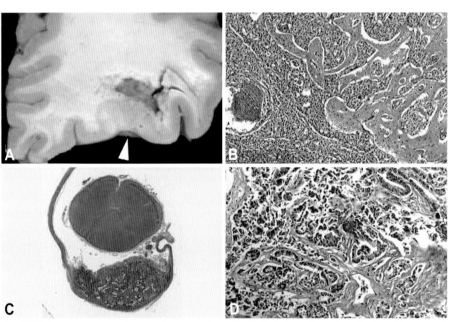

Fig. 15.04 Leptomeningeal metastasis of colon carcinoma (A,B). Note the perivascular infiltration of the cerebral cortex (B). Intraspinal dural metastasis of lung adenocarcinoma (C,D).

primary tumour and no extracranial metastases; class 3 (median survival 2.3 months) includes patients with KPS < 70; class 2 (median survival 4.2 months) encompasses all other patients. Other prognostic factors include the sensitivity of the tumour to therapy and the number and location of CNS metastases. In general, patients with one brain metastasis have improved quality of life and probable survival benefit from surgical resection or radiosurgery of the lesion {651, 1100, 2330}.

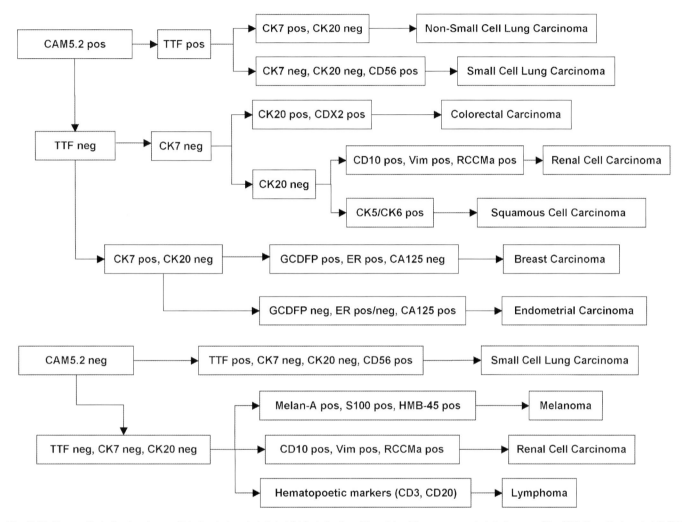

Fig. 15.05 Diagram illustrating how immunohistochemical analysis is helpful for indication of the origin of the common metastatic tumours of the CNS. From Becher *et al.* {143A}, reproduced with permission of the *Journal of Neuropathology and Experimental Neurology*. CDX2, caudal type homeobox transcription factor 2; GCDFP, gross cystic disease fluid protein; RCCMa, renal cell carcinoma marker; TTF, thyroid transcription factor.

Contributors

Dr. Kenneth D. ALDAPE*
Department of Pathology
MD Anderson Cancer Center
Box 85, 1515 Holcombe Blvd.
Houston, TX 77030
USA
Tel. +1 713 792 7935
Fax. +1 713 745 1105
kaldape@mdanderson.org

Dr. Cristina R. ANTONESCU
Department of Pathology
Memorial Sloan Kettering Cancer Center
1275 York Avenue
New York, NY 10021
USA
Tel. +1 212 639 5905
Fax. +1 212 717 3203
antonesc@mskcc.org

Dr. Albert J. BECKER
Department of Neuropathology
Bonn University Medical Center
Sigmund-Freud Strasse 25
53105 Bonn
GERMANY
Tel. +49 228 287 11352
Fax. +49 228 287 14331
albert_becker@uni-bonn.de

Dr. Jacklyn A. BIEGEL
Division of Human Genetics
Department of Pediatrics
University of Pennsylvania School of Medicine
Philadelphia, PA 19104
USA
Tel. +1 215 590 3856
Fax. +1 215 590 3764
biegel@mail.med.upenn.edu

Dr. Wojciech BIERNAT
Department of Neuropathology
and Molecular Pathology
Medical University Gdansk
80-210 Gdansk
POLAND
Tel. +48 58 349 1650
Fax. +48 58 349 1650
biernat@amg.gda.pl

Dr. Darell D. BIGNER
Department of Pathology
Duke University Medical Center, Box 3156
Research Drive 177 MSRB
Durham, NC 27710
USA
Tel. +1 919 684 5018
Fax. +1 919 684 458
bigne001@mc.duke.edu

Dr. Ingmar BLÜMCKE
Department of Neuropathology
Friedrich-Alexander University of
Erlangen-Nuremberg
91054 Erlangen
GERMANY
Tel. +49 9131 85 26031
Fax. +49 9131 85 26033
Ingmar.bluemcke@neuropatho.med.uni-erlangen.de

Dr. Fredrik T. BOSMAN*
Institute of Pathology
University of Lausanne Medical School
Rue du Bugnon 25
1011 Lausanne
SWITZERLAND
Tel. +41 21 314 7202
Fax. +41 21 314 7205
fred.bosman@chuv.hospvd.ch

Dr. Sebastian BRANDNER
Division of Neuropathology and
Department of Neurodegenerative Disease
Institute of Neurology, Queen Square
London WC1N 3BG,
UK
Tel. +44 20 7676 2188
Fax. +44 20 7676 2157
s.brandner@ion.ucl.ac.uk

Dr. Daniel J. BRAT*
Department of Pathology and Lab. Medicine
Emory University Hospital, H-176
1364 Clifton Rd. NE
Atlanta, GA 30322,
USA
Tel. +1 404 712 1266
Fax. +1 404 712 0148
dbrat@emory.edu

Dr. Herbert BUDKA
Institute of Neurology
University of Vienna
Währinger Gürtel 18-20, Postfach 48
1097 Vienna
AUSTRIA
Tel. +43 1 40400 5501
Fax. +43 1 40400 5511
herbert.budka@meduniwien.ac.at

Dr. Peter C. BURGER*
Pathology Building, Room 706
Johns Hopkins University
36 Whitfield Road
Baltimore, MD 21210
USA
Tel. +1 410 955 8378
Fax. +1 410 614 9310
pburger@jhmi.edu

Dr. Webster K. CAVENEE*
Ludwig Institute for Cancer Research
University of California, San Diego
9500 Gilman Drive
La Jolla, CA 92093-0660
USA
Tel. +1 858 552 4920 ext. 7805
Fax. +1 858 534 7750
wcavenee@ucsd.edu

Dr. Leila CHIMELLI
Department of Pathology
University Hospital CFF - UFRJ
Ilha de Fundao,
CEP 21941 590 Rio de Janeiro RJ,
BRAZIL
Tel. +55 21 2562 2450
Fax. +55 21 2562 2450
chimelli@hucff.ufrj.br

Dr. V. Peter COLLINS*
Department of Pathology
University of Cambridge
Tennis Court Road
Cambridge CB2 1QP
UK
Tel. +44 1223 336072 / 217164
Fax. +44 1223 216980
vpc20@cam.ac.uk

*The asterisk indicates participation in the Working Group Meeting on the WHO Classification of Tumours of the Nervous System that was held in Heidelberg, Germany, November 17-18, 2006

Dr. Catherine DAUMAS-DUPORT
Pathology Departement
Saint-Anne Hospital Center
1 rue Cabanis
75014 Paris
FRANCE
Tel. +33 1 45 65 82 05
Fax. +33 1 45 65 87 28
c.daumas@ch-sainte-anne.fr

Dr. Martina DECKERT
Department of Neuropathology
University of Cologne
Kerpener Strasse 62
50324 Köln
GERMANY
Tel. +49 221 478 5265
Fax. +49 221 478 7237
martina.deckert@uni-koeln.de

Dr. Charles G. EBERHART*
Department of Pathology
Johns Hopkins University
720 Rutland Avenue, Ross Bldg 558
Baltimore, MD 21205
USA
Tel. +1 410 502 5185
Fax. +1 410 955 9777
ceberha@jhmi.edu

Dr. David W. ELLISON
Dept. Pathology
St.Jude Children's Research Hospital
332 N. Lauderdale St.
Memphis, TN 38105
USA
Tel. +1 901 495 5438
Fax. +1 901 495 3100
david.ellison@stjude.org

Dr. Charis ENG
Genomic Medicine Institute
Cleveland Clinic Lerner Research Institute
9500 Euclid Avenue, Mailstop NE-50
Cleveland, OH 44195
USA
Tel. +1 216 444 3440
Fax. +1 216 636 0655
engc@ccf.org

Dr. Dominique FIGARELLA-BRANGER*
Department of Pathology and Neuropathology
La Timone Hospital
13385 Marseille cedex 05
FRANCE
Tel. +33 4 91 32 44 43 / 45 88
Fax. +33 4 91 25 42 32
Dominique.Figarella-
Branger@medecine.univ-mrs.fr

Dr. Gregory N. FULLER*
Department of Pathology
MD Anderson Cancer Center
Unit 085, 1515 Holcombe Blvd.
Houston, TX 77030
USA
Tel. +1 713 792 2042
Fax. +1 713 792 3696
gfuller@mdanderson.org

Dr. Felice GIANGASPERO*
Department of Experimental Medicine
University of Rome La Sapienza
& IRCCS Neuromed, Pozzilli (IS)
Viale del Policlinico 155
00161 Roma,
ITALY
Tel. +39 0649 979 175
Fax. +39 0649 979 175
felice.giangaspero@uniroma1.it

Dr. Caterina GIANNINI
Anatomic Pathology
Mayo Clinic College of Medicine
200 1st Street SW
Rochester, MN 55905
USA
Tel. +1 507 538 1181
Fax. +1 507 284 1599
giannini.caterina@mayo.edu

Dr. Hannu HAAPASALO
Department of Pathology
Tampere University Hospital
POB 2000
SF-33521 Tampere
FINLAND
Tel. +358 3 247 6560
Fax. +358 3 247 5503
hannu.haapasalo@pshp.fi

Dr. Pierre HAINAUT
International Agency for
Research on Cancer (IARC)
69008 Lyon,
FRANCE
Tel. +33 4 72 73 85 32
Fax. +33 4 72 73 83 22
hainaut@iarc.fr

Dr. Johannes A. HAINFELLNER*
Institute of Neurology
Medical University of Vienna
Waehringer Guertel 18-20
1097 Vienna
AUSTRIA
Tel. +43 1 40400 5507
Fax. +43 1 40400 5511
Johannes.Hainfellner@meduniwien.ac.at

Dr. Volkmar H. HANS
Institute of Neuropathology
Evangelisches Krankenhaus Bielefeld
Remterweg 2
33617 Bielefeld
GERMANY
Tel. +49 521 772 790 10
Fax. +49 521 772 790 14
Volkmar.Hans@evkb.de

Dr. Cynthia HAWKINS
Division of Pathology
Department of Paediatric Laboratory Medicine
The Hospital for Sick Children
Toronto, Ontario M5G 1X8
CANADA
Tel. +1 416 813 5938
Fax. +1 416 813 5974
cynthia.hawkins@sickkids.ca

Dr. Stephen HUNTER
Department of Pathology
Emory University School of Medicine
1364 Clifton Road, N.E.
Atlanta, GA 30322
USA
Tel. +1 404 712 4278
Fax. +1 404 712 0714
stephen_hunter@emory.org

Dr. Anne JOUVET*
Laboratory of Neuropathology
Neurology Hospital
59 boulevard Pinel
69003 Lyon
FRANCE
Tel. +33 4 72 35 76 34
Fax. +33 4 72 35 70 67
jouvet@laennec.univ-lyon1.fr

Dr. Alexander R. JUDKINS
Department of Pathology
University of Pennsylvania School of
Medicine and Children's Hospital of
Philadelphia
Philadelphia, PA 19104
USA
Tel. +1 215 590 1728
Fax. +1 215 590 1605
judkins@mail.med.upenn.edu

Dr. Paul KLEIHUES*
Department of Pathology
University Hospital
Schmelzbergstr. 12
8091 Zurich
SWITZERLAND
Tel. +41 44 255 3516
Fax. +41 44 255 2525
Kleihues@pathol.unizh.ch

Dr. Andrey KORSHUNOV
Department of Neuropathology
NN Burdenko Neurosurgical Institute
Fadeeva Str. 5
125047 Moscow
RUSSIAN FEDERATION
Tel. +7 495 972 85 60
Fax. +7 495 250 29 44
akorshunov@nsi.ru

Dr. Johan M. KROS*
Division of Pathology/Neuropathology
Erasmus Medical Center
Dr. Molewaterplein 50
3015 Rotterdam
THE NETHERLANDS
Tel. +31 10 4087905
Fax. +31 10 4087905
j.m.kros@erasmusmc.nl

Dr. Arielle LELLOUCH-TUBIANA
Department of Neuropathology
René Descartes-Paris 5 University
Necker Hospital for Sick Children
149 rue de Sèvres, 75015 Paris,
FRANCE
Tel. +33 1 44 49 49 92
Fax. +33 1 44 49 49 99
arielle.lellouch@orange.fr

Dr. Suet Yi LEUNG
Department of Pathology
The University of Hong Kong
Queen Mary Hospital
Pokfulam Road
Hong Kong,
SAR CHINA
Tel. +852 285 54401
Fax. +852 287 25197
suetyi@hkucc.hku.hk

Dr. Pawel LIBERSKI
Department of Molecular Pathology
and Neuropathology
Medical University of Lodz
ul. Czechoslowacka 8/10
92-216 Lodz
POLAND
Tel. +48 42 679 1477
Fax. +48 42 679 1477
ppliber@csk.am.lodz.pl

Dr. M. Beatriz S. LOPES
Department of Pathology
Box 800214 - HSC
University of Virginia Health System
Charlottesville, VA 22908-0214
USA
Tel. +1 434 924 9175
Fax. +1 434 924 9177
msl2e@virginia.edu

Dr. David N. LOUIS*
James Homer Wright Pathology Laboratories,
Massachusetts General Hospital and
Harvard Medical School
55 Fruit Street, WRN225
Boston, MA 02114,
USA
Tel. +1 617 726 2966
Fax. +1 617 726 7533
dlouis@partners.org

Dr. Masao MATSUTANI
Department of Neurosurgery
Saitama Medical School
Moroyamamachi Morohongo 38
350-04 Saitama
JAPAN
Tel. +81 492 76 1551
Fax. +81 492 76 1551
matutani@saitama-med.ac.jp

Dr. Roger E. MCLENDON*
Department of Pathology
Duke University Medical Center
Box 3712
Durham, NC 27710
USA
Tel. +1 919 684 6940
Fax. +1 919 681 7634
mclen001@mc.duke.edu

Dr. Yoichi NAKAZATO*
Department of Human Pathology
Gunma University Graduate School of
Medicine
3-39-22 Showamachi,
Maebashi Gunma 371-5811
JAPAN
Tel. +81 27 220 7970
Fax. +81 27 220 7978
nakazato@med.gunma-u.ac.jp

Dr. Hartmut P.H. NEUMANN
Department of Nephrology and Hypertension
Albert-Ludwigs University
Hugstetterstr. 55, 79106 Freiburg
GERMANY
Tel. +49 761 270 3578
Fax. +49 761 270 3778
hartmut.neumann@uniklinik-freiburg.de

Dr. Ho-Keung NG*
Department of Anatomical and Cellular
Pathology
Prince of Wales Hospital
The Chinese University of Hong Kong
Shatin, Hong Kong
SAR CHINA
Tel. +852 2632 3337
Fax. +852 2637 6274
hkng@cuhk.edu.hk

Dr. Hiroko OHGAKI*
International Agency for
Research on Cancer (IARC)
150, cours Albert Thomas
69008 Lyon
FRANCE
Tel. +33 4 72 73 85 34
Fax. +33 4 72 73 86 98
ohgaki@iarc.fr

Dr. Magali OLIVIER
International Agency for
Research on Cancer (IARC)
150, cours Albert Thomas
69008 Lyon
FRANCE
Tel. +33 4 72 73 86 69
Fax. +33 4 72 73 83 22
molivier@iarc.fr

Dr. Werner PAULUS*
Institute of Neuropathology
University Hospital Münster
Domagkstr. 19
48129 Münster
GERMANY
Tel. +49 251 83 56966
Fax. +49 251 83 56971
werner.paulus@uni-muenster.de

Dr. Arie PERRY*
Division of Neuropathology
Washington University School of Medicine
Campus Box 8118, 660 South Euclid Ave.
St Louis, MO 63110
USA
Tel. +1 314 362 7426
Fax. +1 314 362 7765
aperry@wustl.edu

Dr. Torsten PIETSCH*
Department of Neuropathology
University of Bonn Medical Center
Sigmund-Freud Str. 25
53105 Bonn
GERMANY
Tel. +49 228 287 16606
Fax. +49 228 287 14331
t.pietsch@uni-bonn.de

Dr. Karl H. PLATE
Neurology Institute (Edinger Institute)
Johann Wolfgang Goethe-University
Deutschordenstr. 46
60528 Frankfurt/Main
GERMANY
Tel. +49 69 63016042
Fax. +49 69 679487
karl-heinz.plate@kgu.de

Dr. Matthias PREUSSER
Institute of Neurology and Department of
Internal Medicine
Medical University of Vienna
Waehringer Guertel 18-20
1097 Vienna
AUSTRIA
Tel. +43 1 40400 4457
Fax. +43 1 40400 6088
matthias.preusser@meduniwien.ac.at

Dr. Guido REIFENBERGER*
Department of Neuropathology
Heinrich-Heine University
Moorenstrasse 5
NRW 40225 Düsseldorf
GERMANY
Tel. +49 211 8 11 86 60
Fax. +49 211 8 11 78 04
reifenberger@med.uni-duesseldorf.de

Dr. Federico RONCAROLI
Department of Neuropathology
Imperial College of London
Faculty of Medicine, Charing Cross Campus
London W6 8RP
UK
Tel. +44 20 8846 7178
Fax. +44 20 8846 7794
f.roncaroli@imperial.ac.uk

Dr. Marc K. ROSENBLUM
Department of Pathology
Memorial Sloan Kettering Cancer Center
1275 York Avenue
New York, NY 10021
USA
Tel. +1 212 639 8410
Fax. +1 212 772 8521
rosenbl1@mskcc.org

Dr. Elisabeth J. RUSHING
Department of Neuropathology and
Ophthalmic Pathology
Armed Forces Institute of Pathology
Washington, DC 20306-6000
USA
Tel. +1 202 782 3603
Fax. +1 202 782 4099
elisabeth.rushing@gmail.com

Dr. Chitra SARKAR
Department of Pathology
All India Institute of Medical Sciences
110029 New Delhi
INDIA
Tel. +91 11 26593371
Fax. +91 11 26588663 / 26588641
drchitrasarkar@yahoo.com

Dr. Bernd W. SCHEITHAUER*
Department of Laboratory Medicine and
Pathology
Mayo Clinic
200 First St. SW, Rochester, MN 55905
USA
Tel. +1 507 284 8350
Fax. +1 507 284 1599
scheithauer.bernd@mayo.edu

Dr. Davide SCHIFFER
Foundation Policlinico di Monza
University of Turin
Via Cherasco 15
C.so Massimo D'Azeglio 51
PIEM 10126 Turin,
ITALY
Tel. +39 011 663 62 66
Fax. +39 011 696 34 87
davide.schiffer@unito.it

Dr. Sursala K. SHANKAR
Department of Neuropathology
National Institute of Mental Health and
Neurosciences
560 029 Bangalore
INDIA
Tel. +91 80 2699 5130
Fax. +91 80 0265 64830
shankar@nimhans.kar.nic.in

Dr. Mehar C. SHARMA
Department of Pathology
All India Institute of Medical Sciences
Ansari Nagar
110029 New Delhi
INDIA
Tel. +91 11 2659 3371
Fax. +91 11 2658 8663
sharmamehar@yahoo.co.in

Dr. Dov SOFFER
Department of Pathology
Hadassah University Hospital
Kiryat Hadassah, POB 12000
IL-91120 Jerusalem
ISRAEL
Tel. +972 2 675 8207
Fax. +972 2 642 6268
soffer@cc.huji.ac.il

Dr. Figen SÖYLEMEZOGLU
Department of Pathology
Haceteppe University
Tip Fakultesi, Patoloji Anabilim Dali
06100 Ankara
TURKEY
Tel. +90 312 241 9951
Fax. +90 312 212 9006
figensoylemez@yahoo.com

Dr. Anat O. STEMMER-RACHAMIMOV
Molecular Neuro-Oncology Laboratory, CNY6
Massachusetts General Hospital
Building 149
Charlestown, MA 02129
USA
Tel. +1 617 726 5510
Fax. +1 617 726 5079
astemmerrachamimov@partners.org

Dr. Ana Lia TARATUTO
Department of Neuropathology/FLENI
Referral Center for CJD and other TSEs
Institute for Neurological Research
C1428AQK Buenos Aires
ARGENTINA
Tel. +54 11 5777 3200 / 2325
Fax. +54 11 5777 3209
ataratuto@fleni.org.ar

Dr. Tarik TIHAN
Department of Pathology
University of California at San Francisco
Brain Tumor Research Center
M551, 505 Parnassus Avenue
San Francisco, CA 94143-0102
USA
Tel. +1 415 476 5236
Fax. +1 415 476 7963
tarik.tihan@ucsf.edu

Dr. Erwin G. VAN MEIR
Winship Cancer Institute
Emory University School of Medicine
1365-C Clifton Rd., N.E,. Suite C 5078
Atlanta, GA 30322
USA
Tel. +1 404 778 5563
Fax. +1 404 778 5550
evanmei@emory.edu

Dr. Scott R. VANDENBERG
University of California San Francisco
513 Parnassus Avenue
HSW 408
San Francisco, CA 94143-0511
USA
Tel. +1 415 502 7796
Fax. +1 415 476 7963
scott.vandenberg@ucsf.edu

Dr. Andreas VON DEIMLING*
Departement of Neuropathology
Institute of Pathology
Im Neuenheimer Feld 220/221
69120 Heidelberg
GERMANY
Tel. +49 6221 56 2603 / 2604
Fax. +49 6221 56 4566
Andreas.vonDeimling@med.uni-heidelberg.de

Dr. Alexander O. VORTMEYER
Surgical Neurology Branch
National Institute for Neurological Disorders
and Stroke (NINDS)
Bldg. 10, Rm. 5D37, Bethesda, MD 20892
USA
Tel. +1 301 594 29 14
Fax. +1 301 402 03 80
vortmeyera@mail.nih.gov

Dr. Pieter WESSELING
Department of Pathology
Radboud University Nijmegen Medical Center
6500 HB Nijmegen
THE NETHERLANDS
Tel. +31 24 3614323
Fax. +31 24 3668750
p.wesseling@pathol.umcn.nl

Dr. Otmar D. WIESTLER*
German Cancer Research Center
Im Neuenheimer Feld 280
69120 Heidelberg
GERMANY
Tel. +49 6221 42 28 50
Fax. +49 6221 42 28 40
o.wiestler@dkfz.de

Dr. James M. WOODRUFF
P.O. Box 1200
73 North Longyard Rd
Southwick, MA 01077
USA
Tel. +1 413 569 6878
woodrufj@earthlink.net

Dr. David ZAGZAG
Department of Pathology
NYU Medical Center and School of Medicine
550 First Avenue, New York, NY 10016
USA
Tel. +1 212 263 6449
Fax. +1 212 263 8994
dz4@nyu.edu

Source of charts and photographs

1.01	Kleihues P.		Dept. of Pathology,	3.06	Wiestler O.D.
1.02A-D	Burger P.C.		University of Kansas	3.07A,B	Wiestler O.D.
1.03	Westphal M.M.		Medical Center, USA	3.08	Schiffer D.
	Neurosurgical Clinic	1.34B	Iwasaki Y.	3.09	Westphal M.M.
	University of Hamburg		Miyagi National Hospital	3.10A-C	Kleihues P.
1.04	Paulus W.		Miyagi, Japan	3.11A	Schiffer D.
1.05A,B	Burger P.C.	1.34C	Kleihues P.	3.11B	Louis D.N.
1.05C,D	Kleihues P.	1.34D	Iwasaki Y.	3.11C	Schiffer D.
1.06A,B	Nakazato Y.	1.35A,B	Kleihues P.	3.11D	Kleihues P.
1.06C,D	Burger P.C.	1.35C	Acker T.	3.11E,F	Nakazato Y.
1.06E	Rorke L.B.		Edinger Institut, Frankfurt,	3.12A	Perry A.
	Dept. of Pathology and		Germany	3.12B,C	Nakazato Y.
	Lab. Medicine,	1.35D	Ohgaki H.	3.12D	Rosenblum M.K.
	The Childrens Hospital	1.36	Ohgaki H.	3.13	Rosenblum M.K.
	of Philadelphia, USA	1.37	Perry A.	3.14	Westphal M.M.
1.06F	Burger P.C.	1.38	Ichimura K. & Collins V.P.	3.15	Jellinger K.
1.07A-D	Tihan T.	1.39	Ohgaki H.		Ludwig Boltzmann Inst.
1.08	Tihan T.	1.40	Burger P.C.		Clin. Neurobiology
1.09	Giannini C.	1.41A-C	Nakazato Y.		Vienna, Austria
1.10	Giannini C.	1.41D,E	Kleihues P.	3.16A	Rosenblum M.K.
1.11	Kros J.M.	1.41F	Nakazato Y.	3.16B	Schiffer D.
1.12A,B	Giannini C.	1.42A,B	Kleihues P.	3.16C	Nakazato Y.
1.12C	Paulus W.	1.42C	Nakazato Y.	3.16D	Kleihues P.
1.12D	Kros J.M.	1.43	Fuller G.N.		
1.12E,F	Giannini C.	1.44	Kleihues P.		
1.13	Liberski P.	1.45	Jennings M.T.		
1.14	Kleihues P.	1.46A,B	Nakazato Y.	4.01	Vital A.
1.15A-C	Westphal M.M.				Lab. of Neuropathology
1.16	Westphal M.M.				Victor Segalen
1.17	Kleihues P.				University, Bordeaux,
1.18A	Kleihues P.	2.01	Reifenberger G.		France
1.18B-D	Nakazato Y.	2.02A,B	Kleihues P.	4.02A	Rorke L.B.
1.19A,B	Fuller G.N.	2.03A,B	Kleihues P.	4.02B	Rosenblum M.K.
1.19C,D	Ohgaki H.	2.04A-D	Nakazato Y.	4.03	Paulus W.
1.20	Kros J.M.	2.05A	Nakazato Y.	4.04	Louis D.N.
1.21	Ohgaki H.	2.05B	Kros J.M.	4.05A	Paulus W.
1.22	Kleihues P.	2.06	Kros J.M.	4.05B,C	Aguzzi A.
1.23A-C	Kleihues P.	2.07	Reifenberger G.		Inst. of Neuropathology
1.24A,B	Perry A.	2.08A,B	Nakazato Y.		University of Zurich,
1.24C	Kleihues P.	2.08C	Reifenberger G.		Switzerland
1.25A,B	Rosenblum M.K.	2.08D	Nakazato Y.	4.06A	Nakazato Y.
1.26	Ohgaki H.	2.09A	Nakazato Y.	4.06B,C	Fuller G.N.
1.27	Valavanis A.	2.09B	Reifenberger G.	4.07A	Nakazato Y.
	Institute of	2.10A	Wiestler O.D.	4.07B	Paulus W.
	Neuroradiololgy	2.10B	Perry A.		
	University Hospital,	2.11	Reifenberger G.		
	Zurich, Switzerland	2.12A-D	Reifenberger G.		
1.28	Plate K.H.			5.01	Rosenblum M.K.
1.29	Kleihues P.			5.02A	Rosenblum M.K.
1.30	Ohgaki H.			5.02B	Aldape K.D.
1.31A,B	Ohgaki H.	3.01	McLendon R.E.	5.02C	Rosenblum M.K.
1.32A	Nakazato Y.	3.02A,B	Kleihues P.	5.03A,B	Rosenblum M.K.
1.32B	Kleihues P.	3.03A,B	Fuller G.N.	5.04	Brat D.J.
1.32C	Reifenberger G.	3.03C	Paulus W.	5.05	Brat D.J.
1.32D	Perry A.	3.03D-F	Fuller G.N.	5.06A-C	Brat D.J.
1.33A,B	Kleihues P.	3.04	McLendon R.E.	5.07	Burger P.C.
1.34A	Kepes J.J.	3.05	Nakazato Y.	5.08A	Figarella-Branger D.

5.08B	Fuller G.N.	7.01	Jouvet A.	8.19B,C	Becker L.E.
5.08C	Figarella-Branger D.	7.02	Mena H.	8.20	Kros J.M.
5.08D-F	Burger P.C.		Dept. of Neuropathology,	8.21A,B	Perry A.
			Armed Forces Institute of	8.21C	McLendon R.E.
			Pathology, USA	8.21D	Paulus W.
6.01	Brat D.J.	7.03A	Nakazato Y.	8.22	Judkins A.R.
6.02A	Zimmerman R.A.	7.03B,C	Mena H.	8.23	Rorke L.B.
	Neuroradiology	7.04	Scheithauer B.W.	8.24	Zimmerman R.A.
	Department	7.05	Jouvet A.	8.25A	Judkins A.R.
	The Childrens Hospital	7.06A	Mena H.	8.25B	Wesseling P.
	of Philadelphia, USA	7.06B	Jouvet A.	8.25C-F	Judkins A.R.
6.02B	Taratuto A.L.	7.06C	Nakazato Y.	8.26A	Wesseling P.
6.03A	Taratuto A.L.	7.07	Jouvet A.	8.26B-D	Judkins A.R.
6.03B	Nakazato Y.	7.08	Mena H.	8.27	Biegel J.A.
6.03C,D	Rorke L.B.	7.09A	Taratuto A.L.		
6.04A	Nakazato Y.	7.09B	Rosenblum M.K.		
6.04B	Taratuto A.L.	7.10A	Rosenblum M.K.		
6.05A,B	Brat D.J.	7.10B	Mena H.	9.01	Kleihues P.
6.06	Daumas-Duport C.	7.10C	Kros J.M.	9.02	Soffer D.
6.07	Daumas-Duport C.	7.10D	Nakazato Y.	9.03	Kleihues P.
6.08	Daumas-Duport C.	7.11	Nakazato Y.	9.04A	Kleihues P.
6.09	Daumas-Duport C.	7.12A,B	Fevre-Montange M.	9.04B	Soffer D.
6.10A,B	Daumas-Duport C.		Lab of Neuropathology	9.05A-C	Nakazato Y.
6.11A	Daumas-Duport C.		Neurology Hospital, Lyon,	9.06A	Nakazato Y.
6.11B	Nakazato Y.		France	9.06B	Kleihues P.
6.11C	Daumas-Duport C.	7.12C	Nakazato Y.	9.07	Nakazato Y.
6.12	Daumas-Duport C.			9.08A-C	Woodruff J.M.
6.13A-D	Daumas-Duport C.			9.09	Woodruff J.M.
6.14	Blümcke I.			9.10	Budka H.
6.15	Wiestler O.D.	8.01	Pietsch T.	9.11A-C	Woodruff J.M.
6.16	Kleihues P.	8.02	Kleihues P.	9.12A,B	Scheithauer B.W.
6.17	Blümcke I.	8.03A	Tortori P.	9.13	Scheithauer B.W.
6.18A,B	Kleihues P.		Gaslini Hospital,	9.14	Woodruff J.M.
6.19A-D	Blümcke I.		Genua, Italy	9.15A-F	Woodruff J.M.
6.20	Söylemezoglu F.	8.03B	Giangaspero F.		
6.21A	Nakazato Y.	8.04A	Giangaspero F.		
6.21B	Burger P.C.	8.04B,C	Kleihues P.		
6.22A,B	Kleihues P.	8.05A,B	Kleihues P.	10.01	Kleihues P.
6.23A	Burger P.C.	8.05C	Rorke L.B.	10.02A,B	Kleihues P.
6.23B	Söylemezoglu F.	8.06A	Nakazato Y.	10.02C,D	Budka H.
6.24A,B	Nakazato Y.	8.06B	Kalimo H.	10.03A	Schaefer P.W.
6.25A	Figarella-Branger D.		Dept. of Pathology		Dept. of Radiology,
6.25B	Liberski P.		Turku University Central		Massachusetts General
6.26A,B	Nakazato Y.		Hospital, Turku, Finland		Hospital, Boston, USA
6.27	Ohgaki H.	8.06C	Wiestler O.D.	10.03B	Louis D.N.
6.28	Brandner S.	8.07	Garcia-Bragado F.	10.04	Perry A.
6.29	Ohgaki H.		Dept. of Pathology,	10.05A,B	Kleihues P.
6.30A	Giangaspero F.		Hospital Virgen del	10.06A	Budka H.
6.30B,C	Kleihues P.		Camino, Pamplona, Spain	10.06B-D	Louis D.N.
6.31	Ohgaki H.	8.08A-D	Pietsch T.	10.06E,F	Nakazato Y.
6.32	Nakazato Y.	8.09A,B	Giangaspero F.	10.07A	Kleihues P.
6.33	Nakazato Y.	8.10A	Perry A.	10.07B-D	Nakazato Y.
6.34A-C	Nakazato Y.	8.10B	Burger P.C.	10.08A-D	Nakazato Y.
6.34D	Figarella-Branger D.	8.10C	Pietsch T.	10.09A	Nakazato Y.
6.35	Hainfellner J.A.	8.10D	Perry A.	10.09B	Perry A.
6.36A,B	Hainfellner J.A.	8.11A,B	Ellison D.W.	10.10A	Perry A.
6.37	Hainfellner J.A.	8.12	Kleihues P.	10.10B	Bleggy-Torres L.F.
6.38A	Louis D.N.	8.13	Pietsch T.		Dept. of Pathology,
6.38B-D	Hainfellner J.A.	8.14	McLendon R.E.		Federal University of
6.39	Soffer D.	8.15	McLendon R.E.		Parana, Curitiba, Brazil
6.40	Soffer D.	8.16A,B	Nakazato Y.	10.11A	Perry A.
6.41A	Soffer D.	8.17A	McLendon R.E.	10.11B	Kros J.M.
6.41B	Brandner S.	8.17B	Kleihues P.	10.12A	Kleihues P.
6.41C	Soffer D.	8.17C	Nakazato Y.	10.12B,C	Perry A.
6.41D	Kleihues P.	8.18	Becker L.E.	10.13A	Nakazato Y.
6.42	Brandner S.	8.19A	Fuller G.N.	10.13B	Budka H.

10.13C	Liberski P.	University of Erlangen	
10.14	Perry A.	Medical School, Erlangen,	
10.15	Perry A.	Germany	
10.16A,B	Paulus W.	11.11A	Perry A.
10.17	Louis D.N.	11.11B	Jones R.V.
10.18A	Kleihues P.		Dept. of Neuropathology,
10.18B	Scheithauer B.W.		Armed Forces institute of
10.18C	Paulus W.		Pathology,Washington,
10.19	Scheithauer B.W.		USA
10.20A	Scheithauer B.W.	11.12	Paulus W.
10.20B	Haltia M.J.		

13.23A Paulus W.
13.23B Kleihues P.
13.24 Ohgaki H.
13.25 Ohgaki H.
13.26 Olivier M.
13.27 Olivier M.
13.28 Eberhart C.G.
13.29 Sonier C.B.
Neuroradiology, Laennec
Hospital, Nantes, France
13.30A Reifenberger G.
13.30B Nakazato Y.
13.31A Eberhart C.G.
13.31B Nakazato Y.
13.31C,D Eberhart C.G.
13.32A,B Leung S.Y.
13.33 Cavenee W.K.
13.34 Eberhart C.G.
13.35 Pietsch T.
13.36A Judkins A.R.
13.36B Eberhart C.G.

10.20B Haltia M.J.
Dept. of Pathology,
University of Helsinki,
Finland
10.21A,B Perry A.
10.22 Perry A.
10.23 Giannini C.
10.24 Jääskeläinen J.
Department of
Neurosurgery, Helsinki
University Hospital,
Finland
10.25A Haltia M.J.
10.25B Giannini C.
10.25C,D Nakazato Y.
10.26 Fuller G.N.
10.27 Nakazato Y.
10.28 Jellinger K.
10.29 Wesseling P.
10.30A-C Brat D.J.
10.31A Louis D.N.
10.31B,C Rorke L.B.
10.32 Nakazato Y.
10.33 Böhling T.
Dept of Pathology,
University of Helsinki,
Finland
10.34 Plate K.H.
10.35 Westphal M.M.
10.36 Kleihues P.
10.37 Nakazato Y.

12.01 Matsutani M.
12.02 Rosenblum M.K.
12.03 Nakazato Y.
12.04 Westphal M.M.
12.05 Olvera-Rabiela J.E.
Dept. of Pathology,
Memorial Sloan-Kettering
Cancer Center, New York
USA
12.06A-D Rosenblum M.K.
12.07A-D Nakazato Y.
12.08A-C Rosenblum M.K.
12.09A-D Rosenblum M.K.
12.10A,B Rosenblum M.K.

14.01 Paulus W.
14.02 Kleihues P.
14.03A,B Kleihues P.
14.04 Pizzolato G.P.
Dept. of Pathology,
University Hospital,
Geneva, Switzerland
14.05A Burger P.C.
14.05B,C Giangaspero F.
14.05D Burger P.C.
14.06 Paulus W.
14.07 Fuller G.N.
14.08A-C Fuller G.N.
14.09A,B Fuller G.N.
14.10A-C Fuller G.N.
14.11 Brat D.J.
14.12A-C Brat D.J.
14.13A-D Roncaroli F.
14.14A-C Roncaroli F.
14.15 Roncaroli F.

13.01 Kros J.M.
13.02 Nelson J.S.
Dept. of Pathology,
Louisiana State University
Medical Center,
New Orleans, USA
13.03 Kleihues P.
13.04 Burger P.C.
13.05 Perry A.
13.06A,B Louis D.N.
13.07 Wiestler O.D.
13.08A Plate K.H.
13.08B Schaefer P.W.
13.09A,B Wiestler O.D.
13.10 Wiestler O.D.
13.11A Wiestler O.D.
13.11B Louis D.N.
13.12A,B Louis D.N.
13.12C Wiestler O.D.
13.13 Stemmer-Rachamimov A.O.
13.14 Stemmer-Rachamimov A.O.
13.15 Salamipour H.
13.16A-D Zagzag D.
13.17 Zagzag D.
13.18A Wiestler O.D.
13.18B Vortmeyer A.O.
13.18C,D Plate K.H.
13.19 Wiestler O.D.
13.20A Westphal M.M.
13.20B Sharma M.C.
13.21 Paulus W.
13.22 Vonsattel J.-P.
Dept. of Neuropathology
and Neurosurgery,
Massachusettes General
Hospital, Boston, USA

11.01 Paulus W.
11.02A Huk W.J.
Neuroradiology,
University of Erlangen
Medical School, Erlangen,
Germany
11.02B Kleihues P.
11.03A-D Kleihues P.
11.04 Nakazato Y.
11.05 Haltia M.J.
11.06A,B Nakazato Y.
11.06C,D Deckert M.
11.07A Rickert C.H.
Inst. of Neuropathology
University of Münster
Münster, Germany
11.07B,C Siebert R. and Deckert M.
11.08 Nakazato Y.
11.09A Peiffer J.
11.09B,C Nakazato Y.
11.10 Fartasch M.
Dept. of Dermatology,

15.01A,B Westphal M.M.
15.02A-D Wesseling P.
15.02E Kleihues P.
15.02F Wesseling P.
15.03A Wesseling P.
15.03B Kleihues P.
15.04A-D Wesseling P.
15.05 Becher M.
Dept. of Pathology
Vanderbilt University
School of Medicine,
Nashville, USA

References

1. Abe M, Tabuchi K, Tanaka S, Hodozuka A, Kunishio K, Kubo N, Nishimura Y (2004). Capillary hemangioma of the central nervous system. J Neurosurg 101: 73-81.

2. Abel TW, Baker SJ, Fraser MM, Tihan T, Nelson JS, Yachnis AT, Bouffard JP, Mena H, Burger PC, Eberhart CG (2005). Lhermitte-Duclos disease: a report of 31 cases with immunohistochemical analysis of the PTEN/AKT/mTOR pathway. J Neuropathol Exp Neurol 64: 341-349.

3. Abeliovich D, Gelman K, Silverstein S, Lerer I, Chemke J, Merin S, Zlotogora J (1995). Familial cafe au lait spots: a variant of neurofibromatosis type. J Med Genet 32: 985-986.

4. Abla O, Naqvi A, Ye C, Bhattacharjee R, Shago M, Abdelhaleem M, Weitzman S (2004). Leptomeningeal precursor B-cell lymphoblastic lymphoma in a child with minimal bone marrow involvement. J Pediatr Hematol Oncol 26: 469-472.

5. Abrahams JM, Forman MS, Lavi E, Goldberg H, Flamm ES (1999). Hemangiopericytoma of the third ventricle. Case report. J Neurosurg 90: 359-362.

6. Abrey LE, Batchelor TT, Ferreri AJ, Gospodarowicz M, Pulczynski EJ, Zucca E, Smith JR, Korfel A, Soussain C, DeAngelis LM, Neuwelt EA, O'Neill BP, Thiel E, Shenkier T, Graus F, van den BM, Seymour JF, Poortmans P, Armitage JO, Cavalli F (2005). Report of an international workshop to standardize baseline evaluation and response criteria for primary CNS lymphoma. J Clin Oncol 23: 5034-5043.

7. Abrey LE, DeAngelis LM, Yahalom J (1998). Long-term survival in primary CNS lymphoma. J Clin Oncol 16: 859-863.

8. Abrey LE, Louis DN, Paleologos N, Lassman AB, Raizer JJ, Mason W, Finlay J, Weaver S, Forsyth P, Macdonald DR, Lieberman F, Rosenfeld S, DeAngelis LM, Cairncross JG (2007). for the Oligodendroglioma Study Group: Survey of practice patterns for anaplastic oligodendroglioma. Neuro-oncol. In Press.

9. Abrey LE, Moskowitz CH, Mason WP, Crump M, Stewart D, Forsyth P, Paleologos N, Correa DD, Anderson ND, Caron D, Zelenetz A, Nimer SD, DeAngelis LM (2003). Intensive methotrexate and cytarabine followed by high-dose chemotherapy with autologous stem-cell rescue in patients with newly diagnosed primary CNS lymphoma: an intent-to-treat analysis. J Clin Oncol 21: 4151-4156.

10. Achatz MI, Olivier M, Calvez FL, Martel-Planche G, Lopes A, Rossi BM, Ashton-Prolla P, Giugliani R, Palmero EI, Vargas FR, Rocha JC, Vettore AL, Hainaut P (2007). The TP53 mutation, R337H, is associated with Li-Fraumeni and Li-Fraumeni-like syndromes in Brazilian families. Cancer Lett 245:96-102.

10A. Acker T, Plate KH (2004). Hypoxia and hypxia inducible factors (HIF) as important regulators of tumor physiology. Cancer Treat Res. 117:219-48.

11. Actor B, Cobbers JM, Buschges R, Wolter M, Knobbe CB, Lichter P, Reifenberger G, Weber RG (2002). Comprehensive analysis of genomic alterations in gliosarcoma and its two tissue components. Genes Chromosomes Cancer 34: 416-427.

12. Adams SA, Hilton DA (2002). Recurrent haemangioblastoma with glial differentiation. Neuropathol Appl Neurobiol 28: 142-146.

13. Adamson DC, Cummings TJ, Friedman AH (2005). Myxopapillary ependymoma and fatty filum in an adult with tethered cord syndrome: a shared embryological lesion? Case report. Neurosurgery 57: E373

14. Adamson TE, Wiestler OD, Kleihues P, Yasargil MG (1990). Correlation of clinical and pathological features in surgically treated craniopharyngiomas. J Neurosurg 73: 12-17.

15. Addo-Yobo SO, Straessle J, Anwar A, Donson AM, Kleinschmidt-DeMasters BK, Foreman NK (2006). Paired overexpression of ErbB3 and Sox10 in pilocytic astrocytoma. J Neuropathol Exp Neurol 65: 769-775.

16. Adesina AM, Nalbantoglu J, Cavenee WK (1994). p53 gene mutation and mdm2 gene amplification are uncommon in medulloblastoma. Cancer Res 54: 5649-5651.

17. Adle-Biassette H, Chetritt J, Bergemer-Fouquet AM, Wechsler J, Mussini JM, Gray F (1997). Pathology of the central nervous system in Chester-Erdheim disease: report of three cases. J Neuropathol Exp Neurol 56: 1207-1216.

18. Aerts I, Pacquement H, Doz F, Mosseri V, Desjardins L, Sastre X, Michon J, Rodriguez J, Schlienger P, Zucker JM, Quintana E (2004). Outcome of second malignancies after retinoblastoma: a retrospective analysis of 25 patients treated at the Institut Curie. Eur J Cancer 40: 1522-1529.

19. Agamanolis DP, Malone JM (1995). Chromosomal abnormalities in 47 pediatric brain tumors. Cancer Genet Cytogenet 81: 125-134.

20. Ahlsen G, Gillberg IC, Lindblom R, Gillberg C (1994). Tuberous sclerosis in Western Sweden. A population study of cases with early childhood onset. Arch Neurol 51: 76-81.

21. Aho R, Haapasalo H, Alanen K, Haltia M, Paetau A, Kalimo H (1995). Proliferative activity and DNA index do not significantly predict survival in primary central nervous system lymphoma. J Neuropathol Exp Neurol 54: 826-832.

22. Aicardi J (2005). Aicardi syndrome. Brain Dev 27: 164-171.

23. Aker FV, Ozkara S, Eren P, Peker O, Armagan S, Hakan T (2005). Cerebellar liponeurocytoma/lipidized medulloblastoma. J Neurooncol 71: 53-59.

24. Akhaddar A, Zrara I, Gazzaz M, El Moustarchid B, Benomar S, Boucetta M (2003). Cerebellar liponeurocytoma (lipomatous medulloblastoma). J Neuroradiol 30: 121-126.

25. Akyurek S, Chang EL, Yu TK, Little D, Allen PK, McCutcheon I, Mahajan A, Maor MH, Woo SY (2006). Spinal myxopapillary ependymoma outcomes in patients treated with surgery and radiotherapy at M.D. Anderson Cancer Center. J Neurooncol 80: 177-183.

26. Al Mefty O, Kadri PA, Pravdenkova S, Sawyer JR, Stangeby C, Husain M (2004). Malignant progression in meningioma: documentation of a series and analysis of cytogenetic findings. J Neurosurg 101: 210-218.

27. Al Quran S, Reith J, Bradley J, Rimsza L (2002). Erdheim-Chester disease: case report, PCR-based analysis of clonality, and review of literature. Mod Pathol 15: 666-672.

28. Al Sarraj S, King A, Martin AJ, Jarosz J, Lantos PL (2001). Ultrastructural examination is essential for diagnosis of papillary meningioma. Histopathology 38: 318-324.

29. Al Sarraj ST, Parmar D, Dean AF, Phookun G, Bridges LR (1998). Clinicopathological study of seven cases of spinal cord teratoma: a possible germ cell origin. Histopathology 32: 51-56.

30. Alameda F, Lloreta J, Galito E, Roquer J, Serrano S (1998). Meningeal melanocytoma: a case report and literature review. Ultrastruct Pathol 22: 349-356.

31. Alaminos M, Davalos V, Ropero S, Setien F, Paz MF, Herranz M, Fraga MF, Mora J, Cheung NK, Gerald WL, Esteller M (2005). EMP3, a myelin-related gene located in the critical 19q13.3 region, is epigenetically silenced and exhibits features of a candidate tumor suppressor in glioma and neuroblastoma. Cancer Res 65: 2565-2571.

32. Alatakis S, Stuckey S, Siu K, McLean C (2004). Gliosarcoma with osteosarcomatous differentiation: review of radiological and pathological features. J Clin Neurosci 11: 650-656.

33. Albanese A, Mangiola A, Pompucci A, Sabatino G, Gessi M, Lauriola L, Anile C (2005). Rosette-forming glioneuronal tumour of the fourth ventricle: report of a case with clinical and surgical implications. J Neurooncol 71: 195-197.

34. Albrecht S, Connelly JH, Bruner JM (1993). Distribution of p53 protein expression in gliosarcomas: an immunohistochemical study. Acta Neuropathol 85: 222-226.

35. Albrecht S, Goodman JC, Rajagopalan S, Levy M, Cech DA, Cooley LD (1994). Malignant meningioma in Gorlin's syndrome: cytogenetic and p53 gene analysis. Case report. J Neurosurg 81: 466-471.

36. Albrecht S, von Deimling A, Pietsch T, Giangaspero F, Brandner S, Kleihues P, Wiestler OD (1994). Microsatellite analysis of loss of heterozygosity on chromosomes 9q, 11p and 17p in medulloblastomas. Neuropathol Appl Neurobiol 20: 74-81.

37. Alcedo J, Noll M (1997). Hedgehog and its patched-smoothened receptor complex: a novel signalling mechanism at the cell surface. Biol Chem 378: 583-590.

38. Alderson L, Fetell MR, Sisti M, Hochberg F, Cohen M, Louis DN (1996). Sentinel lesions of primary CNS lymphoma. J Neurol Neurosurg Psychiatry 60: 102-105.

39. Aldosari N, Bigner SH, Burger PC, Becker L, Kepner JL, Friedman HS, McLendon RE (2002). MYCC and MYCN oncogene amplification in medulloblastoma. A fluorescence in situ hybridization study on paraffin sections from the Children's Oncology Group. Arch Pathol Lab Med 126: 540-544.

40. Alen JF, Lobato RD, Gomez PA, Boto GR, Lagares A, Ramos A, Ricoy JR (2001). Intracranial hemangiopericytoma: study of 12 cases. Acta Neurochir 143: 575-586.

41. Alexander RT, McLendon RE, Cummings TJ (2004). Meningioma with eosinophilic granular inclusions. Clin Neuropathol 23: 292-297.

42. Alguacil G, Pettigrew NM, Sima AA (1986). Secretory meningioma. A distinct subtype of meningioma. Am J Surg Pathol 10: 102-111.

43. Ali JBM, Sepp T, Ward S, Green AJ, Yates JRW (1998). Mutations in the TSC1 gene account for a minority of patients with sclerosis. J Med Genet 35: 969-972.

44. Allen JC, Judkins AR, Rosenblum MK, Biegel JA (2006). Atypical teratoid/rhabdoid tumor evolving from an optic pathway ganglioglioma: case study. Neuro-oncol 8: 79-82.

45. Alles JU, Bosslet K, Schachenmayr W (1986). Hemangioblastoma of the cerebellum - an immunocytochemical study. Clin Neuropathol 5: 238-241.

46. Alleyne CH, Jr., Hunter S, Olson JJ, Barrow DL (1998). Lipomatous glioneurocytoma of the posterior fossa with divergent differentiation: case report. Neurosurgery 42: 639-643.

47. Almefty R, Webber BL, Arnautovic KI (2006). Intraneural perineurioma of the third cranial nerve: occurrence and identification. Case report. J Neurosurg 104: 824-827.

48. Almqvist PM, Mah R, Lendahl U, Jacobsson B, Hendson G (2002). Immunohistochemical detection of nestin in pediatric brain tumors. J Histochem Cytochem 50: 147-158.

49. Alonso M, Hamelin R, Kim M, Porwancher K, Sung T, Parhar P, Miller DC, Newcomb EW (2001). Microsatellite instability occurs in distinct subtypes of pediatric but not adult central nervous system tumors. Cancer Res 61: 2124-2128.

50. Alvarez JA, Cohen ML, Hlavin ML (1996). Primary intrinsic brainstem oligodroglioma in an adult. Case report and review of the literature. J Neurosurg 85: 1165-1169.

51. Amlashi SF, Riffaud L, Brassier G, Morandi X (2003). Nevoid basal cell carcinoma syndrome: relation with desmoplastic medulloblastoma in infancy. A population-based study and review of the literature. Cancer 98: 618-624.

52. Ammerlaan AC, de Bustos C, Ararou A, Buckley PG, Mantripragada KK, Verstegen MJ, Hulsebos TJ, Dumanski JP (2005). Localization of a putative low-penetrance ependymoma susceptibility locus to 22q11 using a chromosome 22 tiling-path genomic microarray. Genes Chromosomes Cancer 43: 329-338.

53. Amoaku WM, Willshaw HE, Parkes SE, Shah KJ, Mann JR (1996). Trilateral retinoblastoma. A report of five patients. Cancer 78: 858-863.

54. Antinheimo J, Haapasalo H, Haltia M, Tatagiba M, Thomas S, Brandis A, Sainio M, Carpen O, Samii M, Jaaskelainen J (1997). Proliferation potential and histological features in neurofibromatosis 2-associated and sporadic meningiomas. J Neurosurg 87: 610-614.

55. Antinheimo J, Haapasalo H, Seppala M, Sainio M, Carpen O, Jaaskelainen J (1995). Proliferative potential of sporadic and neurofibromatosis 2- associated meningiomas as studied by MIB-1 (Ki-67) and PCNA labeling. J Neuropathol Exp Neurol 54: 776-782.

56. Antinheimo J, Sankila R, Carpen O, Pukkala E, Sainio M, Jaaskelainen J (2000). Population-based analysis of sporadic and type 2 neurofibromatosis-associated meningiomas and schwannomas. Neurology 54: 71-76.

57.   Antinori A, De Rossi G, Ammassari A, Cingolani A, Murri R, Di Giuda D, De Luca A, Pierconti F, Tartaglione T, Scerrati M, Larocca LM, Ortona L (1999). Value of combined approach with thallium-201 single-photon emission computed tomography and Epstein-Barr virus DNA polymerase chain reaction in CSF for the diagnosis of AIDS-related primary CNS lymphoma. J Clin Oncol 17: 554-560.

58.   Anton T, Guttierez J, Rock J (2006). Tentorial schwannoma: a case report and review of the literature. J Neurooncol 76: 307-311.

59.   Antonescu CR (2006). The role of genetic testing in soft tissue sarcoma. Histopathology 48: 13-21.

60.   Antonescu CR, Woodruff JM (2006). Primary Tumors and Cranial, Spinal and Peripheral Nerves. In: Russel and Rubinstein's Pathology of the Nervous System. McLendon RE, Rosenblum MK, Bigner DD, eds. Hoder Arnold: 787-835.

61.   Aoyama I, Kondo A, Ogawa H, Ikai Y (1994). Germinoma in siblings: case reports. Surg Neurol 41: 313-317.

62.   Aozasa K, Saeki K, Horiuchi K, Yoshimine T, Ikeda H, Nakao K, Hayakawa T (1993). Primary lymphoma of the brain developing in a boy after a 5-year history of encephalitis: polymerase chain reaction and in situ hybridization analyses for Epstein-Barr virus. Hum Pathol 24: 802-805.

63.   Aquilina K, Kamel M, Kalimuthu SG, Marks JC, Keohane C (2006). Granular cell tumour of the neurohypophysis: a rare sellar tumour with specific radiological and operative features. Br J Neurosurg 20: 51-54.

64.   Aquilina K, Nanra JS, Allcutt DA, Farrell M (2005). Choroid plexus adenoma: case report and review of the literature. Childs Nerv Syst 21: 410-415.

65.   Argenti B, Gallo R, Di Marcotullio L, Ferretti E, Napolitano M, Canterini S, De Smaele E, Greco A, Fiorenza MT, Maroder M, Screpanti I, Alesse E, Gulino A (2005). Hedgehog antagonist REN(KCTD11) regulates proliferation and apoptosis of developing granule cell progenitors. J Neurosci 25: 8338-8346.

66.   Aronica E, Leenstra S, van Veelen CW, van Rijen PC, Hulsebos TJ, Tersmette AC, Yankaya B, Troost D (2001). Glioneuronal tumors and medically intractable epilepsy: a clinical study with long-term follow-up of seizure outcome after surgery. Epilepsy Res 43: 179-191.

67.   Arseni C, Ciurea AV (1981). Statistical survey of 276 cases of medulloblastoma (1935—1978). Acta Neurochir 57: 159-162.

68.   Arslanoglu A, Cirak B, Horska A, Okoh J, Tihan T, Aronson L, Avellino AM, Burger PC, Yousem DM (2003). MR imaging characteristics of pilomyxoid astrocytomas. AJNR Am J Neuroradiol 24: 1906-1908.

69.   Artigas J, Cervos N, Iglesias JR, Ebhardt G (1985). Gliomatosis cerebri: clinical and histological findings. Clin Neuropathol 4: 135-148.

70.   Astrinidis A, Henske EP (2005). Tuberous sclerosis complex: linking growth and energy signaling pathways with human disease. Oncogene 24: 7475-7481.

71.   Atuk NO, Stolle C, Owen JA, Carpenter JT, Vance ML (1998). Pheochromocytoma in von Hippel-Lindau disease: clinical presentation and mutation analysis in a large multigenerational kindred. J Clin Endocrinol Metab 83: 117-120.

72.   Auer RN, Becker LE (1983). Cerebral medulloepithelioma with bone, cartilage, and striated muscle. Light microscopic and immunohistochemical study. J Neuropathol Exp Neurol 42: 256-267.

73.   Auguste KI, Gupta N (2006). Pediatric intramedullary spinal cord tumors. Neurosurg Clin N Am 17: 51-61.

74.   Aydin F, Bartholomew PM, Vinson DG (1998). Primary T-cell lymphoma of the brain in a patient at advanced stage of acquired immunodeficiency syndrome. Arch Pathol Lab Med 122: 361-365.

75.   Aydin F, Ghatak NR, Salvant J, Muizelaar P (1993). Desmoplastic cerebral astrocytoma of infancy. A case report with immunohistochemical, ultrastructural and proliferation studies. Acta Neuropathol 86: 666-670.

76.   Azzarelli B, Rekate HL, Roessmann U (1977). Subependymoma: a case report with ultrastructural study. Acta Neuropathol 40: 279-282.

77.   Babu R, Lansen T, Chadburn A, Kasoff S (1997). Erdheim-Chester disease of the central nervous system. J Neurosurg 86: 888-892.

78.   Backlund LM, Nilsson BR, Goike HM, Schmidt EE, Liu L, Ichimura K, Collins VP (2003). Short postoperative survival for glioblastoma patients with a dysfunctional Rb1 pathway in combination with no wild-type PTEN. Clin Cancer Res 9: 4151-4158.

79.   Badiali M, Pession A, Basso G, Andreini L, Rigobello L, Galassi E, Giangaspero F (1991). N-myc and c-myc oncogenes amplification in medulloblastomas. Evidence of particularly aggressive behavior of a tumor with c-myc amplification. Tumori 77: 118-121.

80.   Baehring JM, Dickey PS, Bannykh SI (2004). Epithelioid hemangioendothelioma of the suprasellar area: a case report and review of the literature. Arch Pathol Lab Med 128: 1289-1293.

81.   Baeza N, Masuoka J, Kleihues P, Ohgaki H (2003). AXIN1 mutations but not deletions in cerebellar medulloblastomas. Oncogene 22: 632-636.

82.   Bailey CC, Gnekow A, Wellek S, Jones M, Round C, Brown J, Phillips A, Neidhardt MK (1995). Prospective randomised trial of chemotherapy given before radiotherapy in childhood medulloblastoma. International Society of Paediatric Oncology (SIOP) and the (German) Society of Paediatric Oncology (GPO): SIOP II. Med Pediatr Oncol 25: 166-178.

83.   Bailey P, Bucy PC (1929). Oligodendrogliomas of the brain. J Path Bact 32: 735-751.

84.   Bailey P, Bucy PC (1930). Astroblastomas of the brain. Acta Psychiatr Neurol 5: 439-461.

85.   Bailey P, Cushing H (1925). Medulloblastoma cerebelli: a common type of mid-cerebellar glioma of childhood. Arch Neurol Psychiatry 14: 192-224.

86.   Bailey P, Cushing H (1926). A classification of tumors of the glioma group on a histogenetic basis with a correlation study of prognosis. Lippincott: Philadelphia.

87.   Baisden BL, Brat DJ, Melhem ER, Rosenblum MK, King AP, Burger PC (2001). Dysembryoplastic neuroepithelial tumor-like neoplasm of the septum pellucidum: a lesion often misdiagnosed as glioma: report of 10 cases. Am J Surg Pathol 25: 494-499.

88.   Bajenaru ML, Hernandez MR, Perry A, Zhu Y, Parada LF, Garbow JR, Gutmann DH (2003). Optic nerve glioma in mice requires astrocyte Nf1 gene inactivation and Nf1 brain heterozygosity. Cancer Res 63: 8573-8577.

89.   Balesaria S, Brock C, Bower M, Clark J, Nicholson SK, Lewis P, de Sanctis S, Evans H, Peterson D, Mendoza N, Glaser MG, Newlands ES, Fisher RA (1999). Loss of chromosome 10 is an independent prognostic factor in high-grade gliomas. Br J Cancer 81: 1371-1377.

90.   Balko MG, Blisard KS, Samaha FJ (1992). Oligodendroglial gliomatosis cerebri. Hum Pathol 23: 706-707.

91.   Balmaceda CM, Fetell MR, O'Brien JL, Housepian EH (1993). Nevus of Ota and leptomeningeal melanocytic lesions. Neurology 43: 381-386.

92.   Bandipalliam P (2005). Syndrome of early onset colon cancers, hematologic malignancies & features of neurofibromatosis in HNPCC families with homozygous mismatch repair gene mutations. Fam Cancer 4: 323-333.

93.   Banerjee AK, Sharma BS, Kak VK, Ghatak NR (1989). Gliosarcoma with cartilage formation. Cancer 63: 518-523.

94.   Bannykh S, Strugar J, Baehring J (2005). Paraganglioma of the lumbar spinal canal. J Neurooncol 75: 119.

95.   Bannykh SI, Stolt CC, Kim J, Perry A, Wegner M (2006). Oligodendroglial-specific transcriptional factor SOX10 is ubiquitously expressed in human gliomas. J Neurooncol 76: 115-127.

96.   Bao S, Wu Q, McLendon RE, Hao Y, Shi Q, Hjelmeland AB, Dewhirst MW, Bigner DD, Rich JN (2006). Glioma stem cells promote radioresistance by preferential activation of the DNA damage response. Nature 444: 756-760.

97.   Barak Y, Gottlieb E, Juven G, Oren M (1994). Regulation of mdm2 expression by p53: alternative promoters produce transcripts with nonidentical translation potential. Genes Dev 8: 1739-1749.

98.   Barbashina V, Salazar P, Holland EC, Rosenblum MK, Ladanyi M (2005). Allelic losses at 1p36 and 19q13 in gliomas: correlation with histologic classification, definition of a 150-kb minimal deleted region on 1p36, and evaluation of CAMTA1 as a candidate tumor suppressor gene. Clin Cancer Res 11: 1119-1128.

99.   Barbashina V, Salazar PA, Ladanyi M, Rosenblum MK (2007). Glioneuronal tumour with neuropil-like islands GTNI). A report of 8 cases with chromosome 1p/19q deletion analysis. Am J Surg Pathol. In Press.

100.   Barloon TJ, Yuh WT, Sato Y, Sickels WJ (1988). Frontal lobe implantation of craniopharyngioma by repeated needle aspirations. AJNR Am J Neuroradiol 9: 406-407.

101.   Barnard RO, Bradford TS, Thomas DGT (1986). Gliomyosarcoma: Report of a case of rhabdomyosarcoma arising in malignant glioma. Acta Neuropathol 69: 23-27.

102.   Barnard RO, Geddes JF (1987). The incidence of multifocal cerebral gliomas. A histologic study of large hemisphere sections. Cancer 60: 1519-1531.

103.   Barnes NP, Pollock JR, Harding B, Hayward RD (2002). Papillary glioneuronal tumour in a 4-year-old. Pediatr Neurosurg 36: 266-270.

104.   Barnholtz-Sloan JS, Sloan AE, Davis FG, Vigneau FD, Lai P, Sawaya RE (2004). Incidence proportions of brain metastases in patients diagnosed (1973 to 2001) in the Metropolitan Detroit Cancer Surveillance System. J Clin Oncol 22: 2865-2872.

105.   Barrande G, Kujas M, Gancel A, Turpin G, Bruckert E, Kuhn JM, Luton JP (1995). [Granular cell tumors. Rare tumors of the neurohypophysis]. Presse Med 24: 1376-1380.

106.   Barresi V, Cerasoli S, Morigi F, Cremonini AM, Volpini M, Tuccari G (2006). Gliosarcoma with features of osteoblastic osteosarcoma: a review. Arch Pathol Lab Med 130: 1208-1211.

107.   Barrett AW, Hopper C, Landon G (2002). Intra-osseous soft tissue perineurioma of the inferior alveolar nerve. Oral Oncol 38: 793-796.

108.   Bartolomei JC, Christopher S, Vives K, Spencer DD, Piepmeier JM (1997). Low-grade gliomas of chronic epilepsy: a distinct clinical and pathological entity. J Neurooncol 34: 79-84.

109.   Barzilay JI, Pazianos AG (1989). Adrenocortical carcinoma. Urologenic Clincs N America 16: 457-468.

110.   Baser ME, Friedman JM, Aeschliman D, Joe H, Wallace AJ, Ramsden RT, Evans DG (2002). Predictors of the risk of mortality in neurofibromatosis 2. Am J Hum Genet 71: 715-723.

111.   Baser ME, Kuramoto L, Joe H, Friedman JM, Wallace AJ, Gillespie JE, Ramsden RT, Evans DG (2004). Genotype-phenotype correlations for nervous system tumors in neurofibromatosis 2: a population-based study. Am J Hum Genet 75: 231-239.

112.   Batchelor T, Loeffler JS (2006). Primary CNS lymphoma. J Clin Oncol 24: 1281-1288.

113.   Batra SK, McLendon RE, Koo JS, Castelino P, Fuchs HE, Krischer JP, Friedman HS, Bigner DD, Bigner SH (1995). Prognostic implications of chromosome 17p deletions in human medulloblastomas. J Neurooncol 24: 39-45.

114.   Batzdorf U, Malamud U (1963). The problem of multicentric gliomas. J Neurosurg 20: 122-136.

115.   Bauman GS, Wara WM, Ciricillo SF, Davis RL, Zoger S, Edwards MSB (1997). Primary intracerebral osteosarcoma: a case report. J Neurooncol 32: 209-213.

116.   Baumert BG, Rutten I, Dehing-Oberije C, Twijnstra A, Dirx MJ, Debougnoux-Huppertz RM, Lambin P, Kubat B (2006). A pathology-based substrate for target definition in radiosurgery of brain metastases. Int J Radiat Oncol Biol Phys 66: 187-194.

117.   Baylac F, Martinoli A, Marie B, Bracard S, Marchal JC, Sommelet D, Hassoun J, Plenat F (1997). Une variete exceptionelle de medulloblastome: le medulloblastome melanotique. Ann Pathol 17: 403-405.

118.   Becher MW, Abel TW, Thompson RC, Weaver KD, Davis LE (2006). Immunohistochemical analysis of metastatic neoplasms of the central nervous system. J Neuropathol Exp Neurol 65: 935-944.

119.   Bechtel JT, Patton JM, Takei Y (1978). Mixed mesenchymal and neuroectodermal tumor of the cerebellum. Acta Neuropathol 41: 261-263.

120.   Becker AJ, Klein H, Baden T, Aigner L, Normann S, Elger CE, Schramm J, Wiestler OD, Blumcke I (2002). Mutational and expression analysis of the reelin pathway components CDK5 and doublecortin in gangliogliomas. Acta Neuropathol 104: 403-408.

121.   Becker AJ, Lobach M, Klein H, Normann S, Nothen MM, von Deimling A, Mizuguchi M, Elger CE, Schramm J, Wiestler OD, Blumcke I (2001). Mutational analysis of TSC1 and TSC2 genes in gangliogliomas. Neuropathol Appl Neurobiol 27: 105-114.

122.   Becker DH, Wilson CB (1981). Symptomatic parasellar granular cell tumors. Neurosurgery 8: 173-180.

123.   Becker I, Paulus W, Roggendorf W (1989). Histogenesis of stromal cells in cerebellar hemangioblastomas. An immunohistochemical study. Am J Pathol 134: 271-275.

124.   Becker RL, Becker AD, Sobel DF (1995). Adult medulloblastoma: review of 13 cases with emphasis on MRI. Neuroradiology 37: 104-108.

125.   Beckmann MJ, Prayson RA (1997). A clinicopathologic study of 30 cases of oligoastrocytoma including p53 immunohistochemistry. Pathology 29: 159-164.

126.   Belen D, Colak A, Ozcan O (1996). CNS involvement of Langerhans cell histiocytosis. report of 23 surgically treated cases. Neurosurg Rev 19: 247-252.

127.   Bell DA, Woodruff JM, Scully RE (1984). Ependymoma of the broad ligament. A report of two cases. Am J Surg Pathol 8: 203-209.

128. Bellinzona M, Roser F, Ostertag H, Gaab RM, Saini M (2005). Surgical removal of primary central nervous system lymphomas (PCNSL) presenting as space occupying lesions: a series of 33 cases. Eur J Surg Oncol 31: 100-105.

129. Bello MJ, Alonso ME, Aminoso C, Anselmo NP, Arjona D, Gonzalez-Gomez P, Lopez-Marin I, de Campos JM, Gutierrez M, Isla A, Kusak ME, Lassaletta L, Sarasa JL, Vaquero J, Casartelli C, Rey JA (2004). Hypermethylation of the DNA repair gene MGMT: association with TP53 G:C to A:T transitions in a series of 469 nervous system tumors. Mutat Res 554: 23-32.

130. Bello MJ, Rey JA, de Campos JM, Kusak ME (1993). Chromosomal abnormalities in a pineocytoma [letter]. Cancer Genet Cytogenet 71: 185-186.

131. Belloni E, Muenke M, Roessler E, Traverso G, Siegel B, Frumkin A, Mitchell HF, Donis K, Helms C, Hing AV, Heng HH, Koop B, Martindale D, Rommens JM, Tsui LC, Scherer SW (1996). Identification of Sonic hedgehog as a candidate gene responsible for holoprosencephaly. Nat Genet 14: 353-356.

132. Ben-Ezra J, Bailey A, Azumi N, Delsol G, Stroup R, Sheibani K, Rappaport H (19991). Malignant histiocytosis X. A distinct clinicopathologic entity. Cancer 68: 1050-1060.

133. Benites Filho PR, Sakamoto D, Machuca TN, Serapiao MJ, Ditzel L, Bleggi Torres LF (2005). Granular cell tumor of the neurohypophysis: report of a case with unusual age presentation. Virchows Arch 447: 649-652.

134. Bennett JP, Jr., Rubinstein LJ (1984). The biological behavior of primary cerebral neuroblastoma: a reappraisal of the clinical course in a series of 70 cases. Ann Neurol 16: 21-27.

135. Benveniste RJ, Purohit D, Byun H (2006). Pituicytoma presenting with spontaneous hemorrhage. Pituitary 9: 53-58.

136. Berens ME, Giese A (1999). "...those left behind." Biology and oncology of invasive glioma cells. Neoplasia 1: 208-219.

137. Bergmann M, Pietsch T, Herms J, Janus J, Spaar HJ, Terwey B (1998). Medullomyoblastoma: a histological, immunohistochemical, ultrastructural and molecular genetic study. Acta Neuropathol 95: 205-212.

138. Bergsagel DJ, Finegold MJ, Butel JS, Kupsky WJ, Garcea RL (1992). DNA sequences similar to those of simian virus 40 in ependymomas and choroid plexus tumors of childhood. N Engl J Med 326: 988-993.

139. Berho M, Suster S (1994). Mucinous meningioma. Report of an unusual variant of meningioma that may mimic metastatic mucin-producing carcinoma. Am J Surg Pathol 18: 100-106.

140. Beriwal S, Hou JS, Miyamoto C, Garcia-Young JA (2003). Primary dural low grade BCL-2 negative follicular lymphoma: a case report. J Neurooncol 61: 23-25.

141. Berkman RA, Clark WC, Saxena A, Robertson JT, Oldfield EH, Ali IU (1992). Clonal composition of glioblastoma multiforme. J Neurosurg 77: 432-437.

142. Bernstein JJ, Woodard CA (1995). Glioblastoma cells do not intravasate into blood vessels. Neurosurgery 36: 124-132.

143. Beschorner R, Schittenhelm J, Schimmel H, Iglesias-Rozas JR, Herberts T, Schlaszus H, Meyermann R, Wehrmann M (2006). Choroid plexus tumors differ from metastatic carcinomas by expression of the excitatory amino acid transporter-1. Hum Pathol 37: 854-860.

143A. Becher MW, Abel TW, Thompson RC, Weaver KD, Davis LE (2006). Immunohistochemical analysis of metastatic neoplasms of the central nervous system. J Neuropathol Exp Neurol 65: 935-9444.

144. Best PV (1973). A medulloblastoma-like tumour with melanin formation. J Pathol 110: 109-111.

145. Best PV (1987). Malignant triton tumour in the cerebellopontine angle. Report of a case. Acta Neuropathol 74: 92-96.

146. Betts DR, Leibundgut KE, Niggli FK (1996). Cytogenetic analysis in a case of intraocular medulloepithelioma. Cancer Genet Cytogenet 92: 144-146.

147. Beverley PC, Egeler RM, Arceci RJ, Pritchard J (2005). The Nikolas Symposia and histiocytosis. Nat Rev Cancer 5: 488-494.

148. Bhattacharjee MB, Armstrong DD, Vogel H, Cooley LD (1997). Cytogenetic analysis of 120 primary pediatric brain tumors and literature review. Cancer Genet Cytogenet 97: 39-53.

149. Bi WL, Bannykh SI, Baehring J (2005). The growing teratoma syndrome after subtotal resection of an intracranial nongerminomatous germ cell tumor in an adult: case report. Neurosurgery 56: 188

150. Bickerstaff ER, Connolly RC, Woolf AL (1967). Cerebellar medulloblastoma occurring in brothers. Acta Neuropathol 8: 104-107.

151. Biegel JA (1997). Genetics of pediatric central nervous system tumors. J Pediatr Hematol Oncol 19: 492-501.

152. Biegel JA (1999). Neuro-oncology [serial on line], Doc. 98-30. URL<neuro-oncology mc duke edu>

153. Biegel JA (2006). Molecular genetics of atypical teratoid/rhabdoid tumor. Neurosurg Focus 20: E11.

154. Biegel JA, Fogelgren B, Zhou JY, James CD, Janss AJ, Allen JC, Zagzag D, Raffel C, Rorke LB (2000). Mutations of the INI1 rhabdoid tumor suppressor gene in medulloblastomas and primitive neuroectodermal tumors of the central nervous system. Clin Cancer Res 6: 2759-2763.

155. Biegel JA, Perilongo G, Rorke LB, Parmiter AH, Emanuel BS (1992). Malignant fibrous histiocytoma of the brain in a six-year-old girl. Genes Chromosomes Cancer 4: 309-313.

156. Biegel JA, Zhou JY, Rorke LB, Stenstrom C, Wainwright LM, Fogelgren B (1999). Germ-line and acquired mutations of INI1 in atypical teratoid and rhabdoid tumors. Cancer Res 59: 74-79.

157. Biernat W, Aguzzi A, Sure U, Grant JW, Kleihues P, Hegi ME (1995). Identical mutations of the p53 tumor suppressor gene in the gliomatous and the sarcomatous components of gliosarcomas suggest a common origin from glial cells. J Neuropathol Exp Neurol 54: 651-656.

158. Biernat W, Huang H, Yokoo H, Kleihues P, Ohgaki H (2004). Predominant expression of mutant EGFR (EGFRvIII) is rare in primary glioblastomas. Brain Pathol 14: 131-136.

159. Biernat W, Kleihues P, Yonekawa Y, Ohgaki H (1997). Amplification and overexpression of MDM2 in primary (de novo) glioblastomas. J Neuropathol Exp Neurol 56: 180-185.

160. Biernat W, Tohma Y, Yonekawa Y, Kleihues P, Ohgaki H (1997). Alterations of cell cycle regulatory genes in primary (de novo) and secondary glioblastomas. Acta Neuropathol 94: 303-309.

161. Bigelow DC, Eisen MD, Smith PG, Yousem DM, Levine RS, Jackler RK, Kennedy DW, Kotapka MJ (1998). Lipomas of the internal auditory canal and cerebellopontine angle. Laryngoscope 108: 1459-1469.

162. Biggs PJ, Garen PD, Powers JM, Garvin AJ (1987). Malignant rhabdoid tumor of the central nervous system. Hum Pathol 18: 332-337.

163. Bigner SH, Friedman HS, Vogelstein B, Oakes WJ, Bigner DD (1990). Amplification of the c-myc gene in human medulloblastoma cell lines and xenografts. Cancer Res 50: 2347-2350.

164. Bigner SH, Mark J, Friedman HS, Biegel JA, Bigner DD (1988). Structural chromosomal abnormalities in human medulloblastoma. Cancer Genet Cytogenet 30: 91-101.

165. Bigner SH, McLendon RE, Fuchs HE, McKeever PE, Friedman HS (1997). Chromosomal characteristics of childhood brain tumors. Cancer Genet Cytogenet 97: 125-134.

166. Bigner SH, Rasheed BK, Wiltshire R, McLendon RE (1999). Morphologic and molecular genetic aspects of oligodendroglial neoplasms. Neuro-Oncology 1: 52-60.

167. Bigner SH, Vogelstein B (1990). Cytogenetics and molecular genetics of malignant gliomas and medulloblastoma. Brain Pathol 1: 12-18.

168. Bijlsma EK, Merel P, Bosch DA, Westerveld A, Delattre O, Thomas G, Hulsebos TJ (1994). Analysis of mutations in the SCH gene in schwannomas. Genes Chromosomes Cancer 11: 7-14.

169. Bilsky MH, Schefler AC, Sandberg DI, Dunkel IJ, Rosenblum MK (2000). Sclerosing epithelioid fibrosarcomas involving the neuraxis: report of three cases. Neurosurgery 47: 956-959.

170. Birch BD, Johnson JP, Parsa A, Desai RD, Yoon JT, Lycette CA, Li YM, Bruce JN (1996). Frequent type 2 neurofibromatosis gene transcript mutations in sporadic intramedullary spinal cord ependymomas. Neurosurgery 39: 135-140.

171. Birch JM, Blair V, Kelsey AM, Evans DG, Harris M, Tricker KJ, Varley JM (1998). Cancer phenotype correlates with constitutional TP53 genotype in families with the Li-Fraumeni syndrome. Oncogene 17: 1061-1068.

172. Birch JM, Hartley AL, Tricker KJ, Prosser J, Condie A, Kelsey AM, Harris M, Jones PH, Binchy A, Crowther D (1994). Prevalence and diversity of constitutional mutations in the p53 gene among 21 Li-Fraumeni families. Cancer Res 54: 1298-1304.

173. Bjornsson J, Scheithauer BW, Okazaki H, Leech RW (1985). Intracranial germ cell tumors: pathobiological and immunohistochemical aspects of 70 cases. J Neuropathol Exp Neurol 44: 32-46.

174. Blades DA, Hardy RW, Cohen M (1991). Cervical paraganglioma with subsequent intracranial and intraspinal metastases. Case report. J Neurosurg 75: 320-323.

175. Blandino G, Levine AJ, Oren M (1999). Mutant p53 gain of function: differential effects of different p53 mutants on resistance of cultured cells to chemotherapy. Oncogene 18: 477-485.

176. Bleistein M, Geiger K, Franz K, Stoldt P, Schlote W (2000). Transthyretin and transferrin in hemangioblastoma stromal cells. Pathol Res Pract 196: 675-681.

177. Blount JP, Elton S (2001). Spinal lipomas. Neurosurg Focus 10: E3.

178. Blumcke I, Giencke K, Wardelmann E, Beyenburg S, Kral T, Sarioglu N, Pietsch T, Wolf HK, Schramm J, Elger CE, Wiestler OD (1999). The CD34 epitope is expressed in neoplastic and malformative lesions associated with chronic, focal epilepsia. Acta Neuropathol 97: 481-490.

179. Blumcke I, Becker AJ, Normann S, Hans V, Riederer BM, Krajewski S, Wiestler OD, Reifenberger G (2001). Distinct expression pattern of microtubule-associated protein-2 in human oligodendrogliomas and glial precursor cells. J Neuropathol Exp Neurol 60: 984-993.

180. Blumcke I, Lobach M, Wolf HK, Wiestler OD (1999). Evidence for developmental precursor lesions in epilepsy-associated glioneuronal tumors. Micros Res Techn 46:53-8.

181. Blumcke I, Luyken C, Urbach H, Schramm J, Wiestler OD (2004). An isomorphic subtype of long-term epilepsy-associated astrocytomas associated with benign prognosis. Acta Neuropathol 107: 381-388.

182. Blumcke I, Muller S, Buslei R, Riederer BM, Wiestler OD (2004). Microtubule-associated protein-2 immunoreactivity: a useful tool in the differential diagnosis of low-grade neuroepithelial tumors. Acta Neuropathol 108: 89-96.

183. Blumcke I, Wiestler OD (2002). Gangliogliomas: an intriguing tumor entity associated with focal epilepsies. J Neuropathol Exp Neurol 61: 575-584.

184. Boddy MN, Russell P (1999). DNA replication checkpoint control. Front Biosci 4: D841-D848.

185. Bodey B, Bodey B, Jr., Siegel SE (1995). Immunophenotypic characterization of infiltrating polynuclear and mononuclear cells in childhood brain tumors. Mod Pathol 8: 333-338.

186. Bodey B, Bodey V, Siegel SE, Kaiser HE (2004). Survivin expression in childhood medulloblastomas: a possible diagnostic and prognostic marker. In Vivo 18: 713-718.

187. Boesel CP, Suhan JP, Sayers MP (1978). Melanotic medulloblastoma. Report of a case with ultrastructural findings. J Neuropathol Exp Neurol 37: 531-543.

188. Bogler O, Huang HJ, Kleihues P, Cavenee WK (1995). The p53 gene and its role in human brain tumors. Glia 15: 308-327.

189. Bognar L, Balint K, Bardoczy Z (2002). Symptomatic osteolipoma of the tuber cinereum. Case report. J Neurosurg 96: 361-363.

190. Bohling T, Hatva E, Kujala M, Claesson Welsh L, Alitalo K, Haltia M (1996). Expression of growth factors and growth factor receptors in capillary hemangioblastoma. J Neuropathol Exp Neurol 55: 522-527.

191. Bohling T, Maenpaa A, Timonen T, Vantunen L, Paetau A, Haltia M (1996). Different expression of adhesion molecules in stromal cells and endothelial cells of capillary hemangioblastoma. Acta Neuropathol 92: 461-466.

192. Bohling T, Plate KH, Haltia MJ, Alitalo K, Neumann HPH (2000). Von Hippel-Lindau disease and capillary haemangioblastoma. In: Tumours of the Nervous System. Kleihues P, Cavenee WK, eds. IARC Press: Lyon, pp. 223-226.

193. Bohling T, Turunen O, Jaaskelainen J, Carpen O, Sainio M, Wahlstrom T, Vaheri A, Haltia M (1996). Ezrin expression in stromal cells of capillary hemangioblastoma. An immunohistochemical survey of brain tumors. Am J Pathol 148: 367-373.

194. Bohner G, Masuhr F, Distl R, Katchanov J, Klingebiel R, Zschenderlein R, von Deimling A, van Landeghem FK (2005). Pilocytic astrocytoma presenting as primary diffuse leptomeningeal gliomatosis: report of a unique case and review of the literature. Acta Neuropathol 110: 306-311.

195. Bonnin JM, Rubinstein LJ (1989). Astroblastomas: a pathological study of 23 tumors, with a postoperative follow-up in 13 patients. Neurosurgery 25: 6-13.

196. Bonnin JM, Rubinstein LJ, Palmer NF, Beckwith JB (1984). The association of embryonal tumors originating in the kidney and in the brain. A report of seven cases. Cancer 54: 2137-2146.

197. Boon K, Eberhart CG, Riggins GJ (2005). Genomic amplification of orthodenticle homologue 2 in medulloblastomas. Cancer Res 65: 703-707.

198. Boonstra R, Koning A, Mastik M, van den BA, Poppema S (2003). Analysis of chromosomal copy number changes and oncoprotein expression in primary central nervous system lymphomas: frequent loss of chromosome arm 6q. Virchows Arch 443: 164-169.

199. Borit A, Blackwood W, Mair WG (1980). The separation of pineocytoma from pineoblastoma. Cancer 45: 1408-1418.

200. Borota OC, Scheie D, Bjerkhagen B, Jacobsen EA, Skullerud K (2006). Gliosarcoma with liposarcomatous component, bone infiltration and extracranial growth. Clin Neuropathol 25: 200-203.

201. Borovich B, Doron Y (1986). Recurrence of intracranial meningiomas: the role played by regional multicentricity. J Neurosurg 64: 58-63.

202. Bosch EP, Murphy MJ, Cancilla PA (1981). Peripheral neurofibromatosis and peroneal muscular atrophy. Neurology 31: 1408-1414.

203. Bostrom J, Meyer-Puttlitz B, Wolter M, Blaschke B, Weber RG, Lichter P, Ichimura K, Collins VP, Reifenberger G (2001). Alterations of the tumor suppressor genes CDKN2A (p16(INK4a)), p14(ARF), CDKN2B (p15 (INK4b)), and CDKN2C (p18(INK4c)) in atypical and anaplastic meningiomas. Am J Pathol 159: 661-669.

204. Bouffard JP, Sandberg GD, Golden JA, Rorke LB (2004). Double immunolabeling of central nervous system atypical teratoid/rhabdoid tumors. Mod Pathol 17: 679-683.

205. Bouffet E, Baranzelli MC, Patte C, Portas M, Edan C, Chastagner P, Mechinaud-Lacroix F, Kalifa C (1999). Combined treatment modality for intracranial germinomas: results of a multicentre SFOP experience. Societe Francaise d'Oncologie Pediatrique. Br J Cancer 79: 1199-1204.

205A. Bourdeaut F, Freneaux P, Thuille B, Lellouch-Tubiana A, Nicolas A, Couturier J, Pierron G, Sainte-Rose C, Bergeron C, Bouvier R, Rialland X, Laurence V, Michon J, Sastre-Garau X, Delattre O (2007). hSNF5/INI1-deficient tumours and rhabdoid tumours are convergent but not fully overlapping entities. J Pathol 323-30.

206. Bourgeois M, Sainte-Rose C, Lellouch-Tubiana A, Malucci C, Brunelle F, Maixner W, Cinalli G, Pierre-Kahn A, Renier D, Zerah M, Hirsch JF, Goutieres F, Aicardi J (1999). Surgery of epilepsy associated with focal lesions in childhood. J Neurosurg 90: 833-842.

207. Bourn D, Carter SA, Mason S, Gareth D, Evans R, Strachan T (1994). Germline mutations in the neurofibromatosis type 2 tumour suppressor gene. Hum Mol Genet 3: 813-816.

208. Bouvier-Labit C, Daniel L, Dufour H, Grisoli F, Figarella-Branger D (2000). Papillary glioneuronal tumour: clinicopathological and biochemical study of one case with 7-year follow up. Acta Neuropathol 99: 321-326.

209. Brain Tumor Registry of Japan (2003). Report of Brain Tumor Registry of Japan (1969-1996). Neurol Med Chir (Tokyo) 43 Suppl:i-vii, 1-111.: i-111.

210. Brandes AA, Palmisano V, Monfardini S (1999). Medulloblastoma in adults: clinical characteristics and treatment. Cancer Treat Rev 25: 3-12.

211. Brandis A, Heyer R, Hori A, Walter GF (1997). Cerebellar neurocytoma in an infant: an important differential diagnosis from cerebellar neuroblastoma and medulloblastoma? Neuropediatrics 28: 235-238.

212. Brandis A, Mirzai S, Tatagiba M, Walter GF, Samii M, Ostertag H (1993). Immunohistochemical detection of female sex hormone receptors in meningiomas: correlation with clinical and histological features. Neurosurgery 33: 212-217.

213. Brannan CI, Perkins AS, Vogel KS, Ratner N, Nordlund ML, Reid SW, Buchberg AM, Jenkins NA, Parada LF, Copeland NG

(1994). Targeted disruption of the neurofibromatosis type-1 gene leads to developmental abnormalities in heart and various neural crest-derived tissues. Genes Dev 8: 1019-1029.

214. Brat DJ, Castellano-Sanchez AA, Hunter SB, Pecot M, Cohen C, Hammond EH, Devi SN, Kaur B, Van Meir EG (2004). Pseudopalisades in glioblastoma are hypoxic, express extracellular matrix proteases, and are formed by an actively migrating cell population. Cancer Res 64: 920-927.

215. Brat DJ, cohen KJ, Sanders JM, Feuerstein BG, Burger PC (1999). Clinicopathologic features of astroblastoma. J Neuropathol Exp Neurol 58: 509-509.

216. Brat DJ, Giannini C, Scheithauer BW, Burger PC (1999). Primary melanocytic neoplasms of the central nervous systems. Am J Surg Pathol 23: 745-754.

217. Brat DJ, Hirose Y, cohen KJ, Feuerstein BG, Burger PC (2000). Astroblastoma: clinicopathologic features and chromosomal abnormalities defined by comparative genomic hybridization. Brain Pathol 10: 342-352.

218. Brat DJ, Scheithauer BW, Eberhart CG, Burger PC (2001). Extraventricular neurocytomas: pathologic features and clinical outcome. Am J Surg Pathol 25: 1252-1260.

219. Brat DJ, Scheithauer BW, Medina-Flores R, Rosenblum MK, Burger PC (2002). Infiltrative astrocytomas with granular cell features (granular cell astrocytomas): a study of histopathologic features, grading, and outcome. Am J Surg Pathol 26: 750-757.

220. Brat DJ, Scheithauer BW, Staugaitis SM, Cortez SC, Brecher K, Burger PC (1998). Third ventricular chordoid glioma: a distinct clinicopathologic entity. J Neuropathol Exp Neurol 57: 283-290.

221. Brat DJ, Scheithauer BW, Staugaitis SM, Holtzman RN, Morgello S, Burger PC (2000). Pituicytoma: a distinctive low-grade glioma of the neurohypophysis. Am J Surg Pathol 24: 362-368.

222. Brat DJ, Seiferheld WF, Perry A, Hammond EH, Murray KJ, Schulsinger AR, Mehta MP, Curran WJ (2004). Analysis of 1p, 19q, 9p, and 10q as prognostic markers for high-grade astrocytomas using fluorescence in situ hybridization on tissue microarrays from Radiation Therapy Oncology Group trials. Neuro-oncol 6: 96-103.

223. Bridge RS, Rajaram V, Dehner LP, Pfeifer JD, Perry A (2006). Molecular diagnosis of Ewing sarcoma/primitive neuroectodermal tumor in routinely processed tissue: a comparison of two FISH strategies and RT-PCR in malignant round cell tumors. Mod Pathol 19: 1-8.

224. Brock JE, Perez-Atayde AR, Kozakewich HP, Richkind KE, Fletcher JA, Vargas SO (2005). Cytogenetic aberrations in perineurioma: variation with subtype. Am J Surg Pathol 29: 1164-1169.

225. Broderick DK, Di C, Parrett TJ, Samuels YR, Cummins JM, McLendon RE, Fults DW, Velculescu VE, Bigner DD, Yan H (2004). Mutations of PIK3CA in anaplastic oligodendrogliomas, high-grade astrocytomas, and medulloblastomas. Cancer Res 64: 5048-5050.

226. Broholm H, Madsen FF, Wagner AA, Laursen H (2002). Papillary glioneuronal tumor—a new tumor entity. Clin Neuropathol 21: 1-4.

227. Brooks JS, Freeman M, Enterline HT (1985). Malignant "Triton" tumors. Natural history and immunohistochemistry of nine new cases with literature review. Cancer 55: 2543-2549.

228. Brooks WH, Markesbery WR, Gupta GD, Roszman TL (1978). Relationship of lymphocyte invasion and survival of brain tumor

patients. Ann Neurol 4: 219-224.

229. Brown HG, Burger PC, Olivi A, Sills AK, Barditch-Crovo PA, Lee RR (1999). Intracranial leiomyosarcoma in a patient with AIDS. Neuroradiology 41: 35-39.

230. Brown HG, Kepner JL, Perlman EJ, Friedman HS, Strother DR, Duffner PK, Kun LE, Goldthwaite PT, Burger PC (2000). "Large cell/anaplastic" medulloblastomas. A pediatric oncology group study. J Neuropathol Exp Neurol 59: 857-865.

231. Brown HM, Komorowski RA, Wilson SD, Demeure MJ, Zhu YR (1999). Predicting metastasis of pheochromocytomas using DNA flow cytometry and immunohistochemical markers of cell proliferation: A positive correlation between MIB-1 staining and malignant tumor behavior. Cancer 86: 1583-1589.

232. Brown MT, McClendon RE, Gockerman JP (1995). Primary central nervous system lymphoma with systemic metastasis: case report and review. J Neurooncol 23: 207-221.

233. Bruggers CS, Welsh CT, Boyer RS, Byrne JL, Pysher TJ (1999). Successful therapy in a child with a congenital peripheral medulloepithelioma and disruption of hindquarter development. J Pediatr Hematol Oncol 21: 161-164.

234. Brunner HG, Hulsebos T, Steijlen PM, der K, Steen A, Hamel BC (1993). Exclusion of the neurofibromatosis 1 locus in a family with inherited cafe-au-lait spots. Am J Med Genet 46: 472-474.

235. Bruno MC, Ginguene C, Santangelo M, Panagiotopoulos K, Piscopo GA, Tortora F, Elefante A, De Caro ML, Cerillo A (2004). Lymphoplasmacyte rich meningioma. A case report and review of the literature. J Neurosurg Sci 48: 117-124.

236. Buccoliero AM, Bacci S, Mennonna P, Taddei GL (2004). Pathologic quiz case: infratentorial tumor in a middle-aged woman. Oncocytic variant of choroid plexus papilloma. Arch Pathol Lab Med 128: 1448-1450.

237. Buccoliero AM, Caldarella A, Bacci S, Gallina P, Taddei A, Di Lorenzo N, Romagnoli P, Taddei GL (2005). Cerebellar liponeurocytoma: morphological, immunohistochemical, and ultrastructural study of a relapsed case. Neuropathology 25: 77-83.

238. Buccoliero AM, Giordano F, Mussa F, Taddei A, Genitori L, Taddei GL (2006). Papillary glioneuronal tumor radiologically mimicking a cavernous hemangioma with hemorrhagic onset. Neuropathology 26: 206-211.

239. Buczynski J, Jesionek-Kupnicka D, Kordek R, Zakrzewski K, Polis L, Liberski PP (2002). Apoptosis in non-astrocytic brain tumours in children. Folia Neuropathol 40: 155-159.

240. Budka H (1974). Intracranial lipomatous hamartomas (intracranial "lipomas"). A study of 13 cases including combinations with medulloblastoma, colloid and epidermoid cysts, angiomatosis and other malformations. Acta Neuropathol 28: 205-222.

241. Budka H, Chimelli L (1994). Lipomatous medulloblastoma in adults: a new tumor type with possible favorable prognosis [letter]. Hum Pathol 25: 730-731.

242. Buhl R, Barth H, Hugo HH, Hutzelmann A, Mehdorn HM (1998). Spinal drop metastases in recurrent glioblastoma multiforme. Acta Neurochir 140: 1001-1005.

243. Buhren J, Christoph AH, Buslei R, Albrecht S, Wiestler OD, Pietsch T (2000). Expression of the neurotrophin receptor p75NTR in medulloblastomas is correlated with distinct histological and clinical features: evidence for a medulloblastoma subtype derived from the external granule cell layer. J Neuropathol Exp Neurol 59: 229-240.

244. Bunin GR, Kuijten RR, Buckley JD, Rorke LB, Meadows AT (1993). Relation

between maternal diet and subsequent primitive neuroectodermal brain tumors in young children. N Engl J Med. 19;329: 536-541.

245. Bunin GR, Kushi LH, Gallagher PR, Rorke-Adams LB, McBride ML, Cnaan A (2005). Maternal diet during pregnancy and its association with medulloblastoma in children: a children's oncology group study (United States). Cancer Causes Control 16: 877-891.

246. Bunin GR, Surawicz TS, Witman PA, Preston-Martin S, Davis F, Bruner JM (1998). The descriptive epidemiology of craniopharyngioma. J Neurosurg 89: 547-551.

247. Burger PC (1996). Pathology of brain stem astrocytomas. Pediatr Neurosurg 24: 35-40.

248. Burger PC (2002). What is an oligodendroglioma? Brain Pathol 12: 257-259.

249. Burger PC, Breiter SN, Fisher PG (1996). Pilocytic and fibrillary astrocytomas of the brain stem - a comparative clinical, radiological and pathological study. J Neuropathol Exp Neurol 55: 640.

250. Burger PC, Dubois PJ, Schold SC, Jr., Smith KR, Jr., Odom GL, Crafts DC, Giangaspero F (1983). Computerized tomographic and pathologic studies of the untreated, quiescent, and recurrent glioblastoma multiforme. J Neurosurg 58: 159-169.

251. Burger PC, Grahmann FC, Bliestle A, Kleihues P (1987). Differentiation in the medulloblastoma. A histological and immunohistochemical study. Acta Neuropathol 73: 115-123.

252. Burger PC, Green SB (1987). Patient age, histologic features, and length of survival in patients with glioblastoma multiforme. Cancer 59: 1617-1625.

253. Burger PC, Heinz ER, Shibata T, Kleihues P (1988). Topographic anatomy and CT correlations in the untreated glioblastoma multiforme. J Neurosurg 68: 698-704.

254. Burger PC, Kleihues P (1989). Cytologic composition of the untreated glioblastoma with implications for evaluation of needle biopsies. Cancer 63: 2014-2023.

255. Burger PC, Pearl DK, Aldape K, Yates AJ, Scheithauer BW, Passe SM, Jenkins RB, James CD (2001). Small cell architecture—a histological equivalent of EGFR amplification in glioblastoma multiforme? J Neuropathol Exp Neurol 60: 1099-1104.

256. Burger PC, Scheithauer BW (1994). Tumors of paraganglionic tissue. In: Tumors of the Central Nervous System. Atlas of Tumor Pathology. Tumors of the Central Nervous System. Atlas of Tumor Pathology. Armed Forces Institute of Pathology: Washington D.C., pp. 317-320.

257. Burger PC, Scheithauer BW (1994). Tumors of the Central Nervous System. Armed Forces Institute of Pathology: Washington.

258. Burger PC, Scheithauer BW (2006). Tumors of the Central Nervous System. In: Atlas of Tumor Pathology. Atlas of Tumor Pathology. Armed Forces Institute of Pathology: Washington

259. Burger PC, Scheithauer BW, Vogel FS (1991). Surgical pathology of the nervous system and its coverings. Churchill Livingstone: London.

260. Burger PC, Shibata T, Kleihues P (1986). The use of the monoclonal antibody Ki-67 in the identification of proliferating cells: application to surgical neuropathology. Am J Surg Pathol 10: 611-617.

261. Burger PC, Vogel FS, Green SB, Strike TA (1985). Glioblastoma multiforme and anaplastic astrocytoma. Pathologic criteria and prognostic implications. Cancer 56: 1106-1111.

262. Burger PC, Vollmer RT (1980). Histologic factors of prognostic significance in the glioblastoma multiforme. Cancer 46: 1179-1186.

263. Burger PC, Yu IT, Tihan T, Friedman HS, Strother DR, Kepner JL, Duffner PK, Kun LE, Perlman EJ (1998). Atypical teratoid/rhabdoid tumor of the central nervous system: a highly malignant tumor of infancy and childhood frequently mistaken for medulloblastoma: a Pediatric Oncology Group study. Am J Surg Pathol 22: 1083-1092.
263A. Burkhard C, Di-Patre P-L, Schuler D, Schuler G, Yasargil MG, Yonekawa Y, Lutolf UM, Kleihues P, Ohgaki H (2003). A population-based study of the incidence and survival rates in patients with pilocytic astrocytoma. J Neurosurg 98:1170-1174.
264. Burnett ME, White EC, Sih S, von Haken MS, Cogen PH (1997). Chromosome arm 17p deletion analysis reveals molecular genetic heterogeneity in supratentorial and infratentorial primitive neuroectodermal tumors of the central nervous system. Cancer Genet Cytogenet 97: 25-31.
265. Burns KL, Ueki K, Jhung SL, Koh J, Louis DN (1998). Molecular genetic correlates of p16, cdk4, and pRb immunohistochemistry in glioblastomas. J Neuropathol Exp Neurol 57: 122-130.
266. Buschges R, Ichimura K, Weber RG, Reifenberger G, Collins VP (2002). Allelic gain and amplification on the long arm of chromosome 17 in anaplastic meningiomas. Brain Pathol 12: 145-153.
267. Buslei R, Nolde M, Hofmann B, Meissner S, Eyupoglu IY, Siebzehnrubl F, Hahnen E, Kreutzer J, Fahlbusch R (2005). Common mutations of beta-catenin in adamantinomatous craniopharyngiomas but not in other tumours originating from the sellar region. Acta Neuropathol 109: 589-597.
268. Buttner A, Marquart KH, Mehraein P, Weis S (1997). Kaposi's sarcoma in the cerebellum of a patient with AIDS. Clin Neuropathol 16: 185-189.
269. Buzanska L, Spassky N, Belin MF, Giangrande A, Guillemot F, Klambt C, Labouesse M, Thomas JL, Domanska-Janik K, Zalc B (2001). Human medulloblastoma cell line DEV is a potent tool to screen for factors influencing differentiation of neural stem cells. J Neurosci Res 65: 17-23.
270. Cabello A, Madero S, Castresana A, Diaz L (1991). Astroblastoma: electron microscopy and immunohistochemical findings: case report. Surg Neurol 35: 116-121.
271. Caccamo DV, Herman MM, Rubinstein LJ (1989). An immunohistochemical study of the primitive and maturing elements of human cerebral medulloepitheliomas. Acta Neuropathol 79: 248-254.
272. Caccamo DV, Ho KL, Garcia JH (1992). Cauda equina tumor with ependymal and paraganglionic differentiation. Hum Pathol 23: 835-838.
273. Cai DX, Banerjee R, Scheithauer BW, Lohse CM, Kleinschmidt-DeMasters BK, Perry A (2001). Chromosome 1p and 14q FISH analysis in clinicopathologic subsets of meningioma: diagnostic and prognostic implications. J Neuropathol Exp Neurol 60: 628-636.
274. Cai DX, James CD, Scheithauer BW, Couch FJ, Perry A (2001). PS6K amplification characterizes a small subset of anaplastic meningiomas. Am J Clin Pathol 115: 213-218.
275. Cairncross G, Berkey B, Shaw E, Jenkins R, Scheithauer B, Brachman D, Buckner J, Fink K, Souhami L, Laperierre N, Mehta M, Curran W (2006). Phase III trial of chemotherapy plus radiotherapy compared with radiotherapy alone for pure and mixed anaplastic oligodendroglioma: Intergroup Radiation Therapy Oncology Group Trial 9402. J Clin Oncol 24: 2707-2714.
276. Cairncross JG, Ueki K, Zlatescu MC, Lisle DK, Finkelstein DM, Hammond RR, Silver JS, Stark PC, Macdonald DR, Ino Y, Ramsay DA, Louis DN (1998). Specific genetic predictors of chemotherapeutic response and survival in patients with anaplastic oligodendrogliomas. J Natl Cancer Inst 90: 1473-1479.
277. Caldarella A, Buccoliero AM, Marini M, Taddei A, Mennonna P, Taddei GL (2002). Oncocytic meningioma: a case report. Pathol Res Pract 198: 109-113.
278. Caldemeyer KS, Zimmerman RA, Azzarelli B, Smith RR, Moran CC (1995). Gliofibroma: CT and MRI. Neuroradiology 37: 481-485.
279. Camilleri-Broet S, Criniere E, Broet P, Delwail V, Mokhtari K, Moreau A, Kujas M, Raphael M, Iraqi W, Sautes-Fridman C, Colombat P, Hoang-Xuan K, Martin A (2006). A uniform activated B-cell-like immunophenotype might explain the poor prognosis of primary central nervous system lymphomas: analysis of 83 cases. Blood 107: 190-196.
280. Camilleri-Broet S, Davi F, Feuillard J, Seilhean D, Michiels JF, Brousset P, Epardeau B, Navratil E, Mokhtari K, Bourgeois C, Marelle L, Raphael M, Hauw JJ (1997). AIDS-related primary brain lymphomas: histopathologic and immunohisochemical study of 51 cases. The French study group for HIV-associated tumors. Hum Pathol 28: 367-374.
281. Campbell AN, Chan HS, Becker LE, Daneman A, Park TS, Hoffman HJ (1984). Extracranial metastases in childhood primary intracranial tumors. A report of 21 cases and review of the literature. Cancer 53: 974-981.
282. Cancilla PA, Zimmerman HM (1965). The fine structure of a cerebellar hemangioblastoma. J Neuropathol Exp Neurol 24: 621-628.
283. Cannon TC, Bane BL, Kistler D, Schoenhals GW, Hahn M, Leech RW, Brumback RA (1998). Primary intracerebellar osteosarcoma arising within an epidermoid cyst. Arch Pathol Lab Med 122: 737-739.
284. Carbonara C, Longa L, Grosso E, Mazzucco G, Borrone C, Garre ML, Brisigotti M, Filippi G, Scabar A, Giannotti A, Falzoni P, Monga G, Garini G, Gabrielli M, Riegler P, Danesino C, Ruggieri M, Magro G, Migone N (1996). Apparent preferential loss of heterozygosity at TSC2 over TSC1 chromosomal region in tuberous sclerosis hamartomas. Genes Chromosomes Cancer 15: 18-25.
285. Carlotti CG, Jr., Salhia B, Weitzman S, Greenberg M, Dirks PB, Mason W, Becker LE, Rutka JT (2002). Evaluation of proliferative index and cell cycle protein expression in choroid plexus tumors in children. Acta Neuropathol 103: 1-10.
286. Carlsson B, Havel G, Kindblom LG, Knutson F, Mark J (1989). Ependymoma of the ovary. A clinico-pathologic, ultrastructural and immunohistochemical investigation. A case report. APMIS 97: 1007-1012.
287. Carneiro SS, Scheithauer BW, Nascimento AG, Hirose T, Davis DH (1996). Solitary fibrous tumor of the meninges: a lesion distinct from fibrous meningioma. A clinicopathologic and immunohistochemical study. Am J Clin Pathol 106: 217-224.
288. Carney JA (1990). Psammomatous melanotic schwannoma. A distinctive, heritable tumor with special associations, including cardiac myxoma and the Cushing syndrome. Am J Surg Pathol 14: 206-222.
289. Carney JA, Gordon H, Carpenter PC, Shenoy BV, Go VL (1985). The complex of myxomas, spotty pigmentation, and endocrine overactivity. Medicine Baltimore 64: 270-283.
290. Carroll SL, Stonecypher MS (2005). Tumor suppressor mutations and growth factor signaling in the pathogenesis of NF1-associated peripheral nerve sheath tumors: II. The role of dysregulated growth factor signaling. J Neuropathol Exp Neurol 64: 1-9.
291. Carstens PH, Johnson GS, Jelsma LF (1995). Spinal gliosarcoma: a light, immunohistochemical and ultrastructural study. Ann Clin Lab Sci 25: 241-246.
292. Carter M, Nicholson J, Ross F, Crolla J, Allibone R, Balaji V, Perry R, Walker D, Gilbertson R, Ellison DW (2002). Genetic abnormalities detected in ependymomas by comparative genomic hybridisation. Br J Cancer 86: 929-939.
293. Casadei GP, Komori T, Scheithauer BW, Miller GM, Parisi JE, Kelly PJ (1993). Intracranial parenchymal schwannoma. A clinicopathological and neuroimaging study of nine cases. J Neurosurg 79: 217-222.
294. Casadei GP, Scheithauer BW, Hirose T, Manfrini M, Van Houton C, Wood MB (1995). Cellular schwannoma. A clinicopathologic, DNA flow cytometric, and proliferation marker study of 70 patients. Cancer 75: 1109-1119.
295. Cassarino DS, Auerbach A, Rushing EJ (2003). Widely invasive solitary fibrous tumor of the sphenoid sinus, cavernous sinus, and pituitary fossa. Ann Diagn Pathol 7: 169-173.
296. Castellano-Sanchez AA, Li S, Qian J, Lagoo A, Weir E, Brat DJ (2004). Primary central nervous system posttransplant lymphoproliferative disorders. Am J Clin Pathol 121: 246-253.
297. Castellano-Sanchez AA, Schemankewitz E, Mazewski C, Brat DJ (2001). Pediatric chordoid glioma with chondroid metaplasia. Pediatr Dev Pathol 4: 564-567.
298. Cataltepe O, Turanli G, Yalnizoglu D, Topcu M, Akalan N (2005). Surgical management of temporal lobe tumor-related epilepsy in children. J Neurosurg 102: 280-287.
299. Catapano D, Muscarella LA, Guarnieri V, Zelante L, D'Angelo VA, D'Agruma L (2005). Hemangioblastomas of central nervous system: molecular genetic analysis and clinical management. Neurosurgery 56: 1215-1221.
300. Cenacchi G, Giangaspero A, Cerasoli S, Manetto V, Martinelli GN (1996). Ultrastructural characterization of oligodendroglial-like cells in central nervous system tumors. Ultrastruct Pathol 20: 537-547.
301. Cenacchi G, Giangaspero F (2004). Emerging tumor entities and variants of CNS neoplasms. J Neuropathol Exp Neurol 63: 185-192.
302. Cenacchi G, Giovenali P, Castrioto C, Giangaspero F (2001). Pituicytoma: ultrastructural evidence of a possible origin from folliculostellate cells of the adenohypophysis. Ultrastruct Pathol 25: 309-312.
303. Cenacchi G, Roncaroli F, Cerasoli S, Ficarra G, Merli GA, Giangaspero F (2001). Chordoid glioma of the third ventricle: an ultrastructural study of three cases with a histogenetic hypothesis. Am J Surg Pathol 25: 401-405.
304. Central Brain Tumor Registry of the United States (1995). First annual report.
305. Central Brain Tumor Registry of the United States (2006). http://www.cbtrus.org.
306. Ceppa EP, Bouffet E, Griebel R, Robinson C, Tihan T (2007). The Pilomyxoid Astrocytoma and its Relationship to Pilocytic Astrocytoma: Report of a Case and a Critical Review of the Entity. J Neurooncol 81: 191-196.
307. Cerda-Nicolas M, Kepes JJ (1993). Gliofibromas (including malignant forms), and gliosarcomas: a comparative study and review of the literature. Acta Neuropathol 85: 349-361.
308. Cerda-Nicolas M, Lopez-Gines C, Gil-Benso R, Donat J, Fernandez-Delgado R, Pellin A, Lopez-Guerrero JA, Roldan P, Barbera J (2006). Desmoplastic infantile ganglioglioma. Morphological, immunohistochemical and genetic features. Histopathology 48: 617-621.
309. Cerda-Nicolas M, Lopez-Gines C, Peydro O, Llombart-Bosch A (1993). Central neurocytoma: a cytogenetic case study. Cancer Genet Cytogenet 65: 173-174.
310. Cervera-Pierot P, Varlet P, Chodkiewicz JP, Daumas D (1997). Dysembryoplastic neuroepithelial tumors located in the caudate nucleus area: report of four cases. Neurosurg 40: 1065-1069.
311. Cervoni L, Celli P, Caruso R, Gagliardi FM, Cantore GP (1997). [Neurinomas and ependymomas of the cauda equina. A review of the clinical characteristics]. Minerva Chir 52: 629-633.
312. Challa VR, Goodman HO, Davis CH, Jr. (1983). Familial brain tumors: studies of two families and review of recent literature. Neurosurgery 12: 18-23.
313. Chan AS, Leung SY, Wong MP, Yuen ST, Cheung N, Fan YW, Chung LP (1998). Expression of vascular endothelial growth factor and its receptors in the anaplastic progression of astrocytoma, oligodendroglioma, and ependymoma. Am J Surg Pathol 22: 816-826.
314. Chan CC, Koch CA, Kaiser-Kupfer MI, Parry DM, Gutmann DH, Zhuang Z, Vortmeyer AO (2002). Loss of heterozygosity for the NF2 gene in retinal and optic nerve lesions of patients with neurofibromatosis 2. J Pathol 198: 14-20.
315. Chan CH, Bittar RG, Davis GA, Kalnins RM, Fabinyi GC (2006). Long-term seizure outcome following surgery for dysembryoplastic neuroepithelial tumor. J Neurosurg 104: 62-69.
316. Chan GL, Little JB (1983). Cultured diploid fibroblasts from patients with the nevoid basal cell carcinoma syndrome are hypersensitive to ionizing radiation. Am J Pathol 111: 50-55.
317. Chandler JP, Yashar P, Laskin WB, Russell EJ (2004). Intracranial chondrosarcoma: a case report and review of the literature. J Neurooncol 68: 33-39.
318. Chang Q, Pang JC, Li KK, Poon WS, Zhou L, Ng HK (2005). Promoter hypermethylation profile of RASSF1A, FHIT, and sFRP1 in intracranial primitive neuroectodermal tumors. Hum Pathol 36: 1265-1272.
319. Chang S, Prados MD (1994). Identical twins with Ollier's disease and intracranial gliomas: case report. Neurosurgery 34: 903-906.
320. Chapin JE, Davis LE, Kornfeld M, Mandler RN (1995). Neurologic manifestations of intravascular lymphomatosis. Acta Neurol Scand 91: 494-499.
321. Chaskis C, Michotte A, Goossens A, Stadnik T, Koerts G, D'Haens J (2002). Primary intracerebral myxoid chondrosarcoma. Case illustration. J Neurosurg 97: 228.
322. Chatty EM, Earle KM (1971). Medulloblastoma. A report of 201 cases with emphasis on the relationship of histologic variants to survival. Cancer 28: 977-983.
323. Chaudhry AP, Montes M, Cohn GA (1978). Ultrastructure of cerebellar hemangioblastoma. Cancer 42: 1834-1850.
324. Chavez M, Mafee MF, Castillo B, Kaufman LM, Johnstone H, Edward DP (2004). Medulloepithelioma of the optic nerve. J Pediatr Ophthalmol Strabismus 41: 48-52.
325. Chen F, Slife L, Kishida T, Mulvihill J, Tisherman SE, Zbar B (1996). Genotype-phenotype correlation in von Hippel-Lindau disease: identification of a mutation associated with VHL type 2A. J Med Genet 33: 716-717.
326. Chen KT (2005). Crush cytology of pituicytoma. Diagn Cytopathol 33: 255-257.
327. Chen L, Li Y, Lin JH (2005). Intraneural perineurioma in a child with Beckwith-Wiedemann syndrome. J Pediatr Surg 40: E12-E14.
328. Chen ML, McComb JG, Krieger MD (2005). Atypical teratoid/rhabdoid tumors of the central nervous system: management and out-

comes. Neurosurg Focus 18: E8.
329. Chetritt J, Paradis V, Dargere D, Adle-Biassette H, Maurage CA, Mussini JM, Vital A, Wechsler J, Bedossa P (1999). Chester-Erdheim disease: a neoplastic disorder. Hum Pathol 30: 1093-1096.
330. Chetty R (1999). Cytokeratin expression in cauda equina paragangliomas [letter]. Am J Surg Pathol 23: 491.
331. Chidambaram B, Santhosh V, Shankar SK (1998). Identical twins with medulloblastoma occurring in infancy. Childs Nerv Syst 14: 421-425.
332. Chidambaram B, Santosh V, Balasubramaniam V (2000). Medulloepithelioma of the optic nerve with intradural extension—report of two cases and a review of the literature. Childs Nerv Syst 16: 329-333.
333. Chiechi MV, Smirniotopoulos JG, Mena H (1995). Pineal parenchymal tumors: CT and MR features. J Comput Assist Tomogr 19: 509-517.
334. Chik K, Li C, Shing MM, Leung T, Yuen PM (1999). Intracranial germ cell tumors in children with and without Down syndrome. J Pediatr Hematol Oncol 21: 149-151.
335. Chikai K, Ohnishi A, Kato T, Ikeda J, Sawamura Y, Iwasaki Y, Itoh T, Sawa H, Nagashima K (2004). Clinico-pathological features of pilomyxoid astrocytoma of the optic pathway. Acta Neuropathol 108: 109-114.
336. Chitoku S, Kawai S, Watabe Y, Nishitani M, Fujimoto K, Otsuka H, Fushimi H, Kotoh K, Fuji T (1998). Intradural spinal hibernoma: case report. Surg Neurol 49: 509-512.
337. Cho BK, Wang KC, Nam DH, Kim DG, Jung HW, Kim HJ, Han DH, Choi KS (1998). Pineal tumors: experience with 48 cases over 10 years. Childs Nerv Syst 14: 53-58.
338. Cho KG, Hoshino T, Pitts LH, Nomura K, Shimosato Y (1988). Proliferative potential of brain metastases. Cancer 62: 512-515.
339. Cho Y, Gorina S, Jeffrey PD, Pavletich NP (1994). Crystal structure of a p53 tumor suppressor-DNA complex: understanding tumorigenic mutations. Science 265: 346-355.
340. Choi BH, Kim RC (1984). Expression of glial fibrillary acidic protein in immature oligodendroglia. Science 223: 407-409.
341. Choi JS, Nam DH, Ko YH, Seo JW, Choi YL, Suh YL, Ree HJ (2003). Primary central nervous system lymphoma in Korea: comparison of B- and T-cell lymphomas. Am J Surg Pathol 27: 919-928.
342. Choo D, Shotland L, Mastroianni M, Glenn G, van Waes C, Linehan WM, Oldfield EH (2004). Endolymphatic sac tumors in von Hippel-Lindau disease. J Neurosurg 100: 480-487.
343. Chou SM, Anderson JS (1991). Primary CNS malignant rhabdoid tumor (MRT): report of two cases and review of literature. Clin Neuropathol 10: 1-10.
344. Chow E, Jenkins JJ, Burger PC, Reardon DA, Langston JW, Sanford RA, Heideman RL, Kun LE, Merchant TE (1999). Malignant evolution of choroid plexus papilloma. Pediatr Neurosurg 31: 127-130.
345. Chowdhury C, Roy S, Mahapatra AK, Bhatia R (1985). Medullomyoblastoma. A teratoma. Cancer 55: 1495-1500.
345A. Choyke PL, Glenn GM, Wagner JP, Lubensky IA, Thakore K, Zbar B, Linehan WM, Walther MM (1997). Epididymal cystadenomas in von Hippel-Lindau disease. Urology 49: 926-931.
346. Christensen WN, Strong EW, Bains MS, Woodruff JM (1988). Neuroendocrine differentiation in the glandular peripheral nerve sheath tumor. Pathologic distinction from the biphasic synovial sarcoma with glands. Am J Surg Pathol 12: 417-426.
347. Christov C, Adle-Biassette H, Le Guerinel C, Natchev S, Gherardi RK (1998). Immunohistochemical detection of vascular endothelial growth factor (VEGF) in the vasculature of oligodendrogliomas. Neuropathol Appl Neurobiol 24: 29-35.
348. Chu LC, Eberhart CG, Grossman SA, Herman JG (2006). Epigenetic silencing of multiple genes in primary CNS lymphoma. Int J Cancer 119: 2487-2491.
349. Chung JH, Eng C (2005). Nuclear-cytoplasmic partitioning of phosphatase and tensin homologue deleted on chromosome 10 (PTEN) differentially regulates the cell cycle and apoptosis. Cancer Res 65: 8096-8100.
350. Chung JH, Ginn-Pease ME, Eng C (2005). Phosphatase and tensin homologue deleted on chromosome 10 (PTEN) has nuclear localization signal-like sequences for nuclear import mediated by major vault protein. Cancer Res 65: 4108-4116.
351. Ciardiello F, Tortora G (2001). A novel approach in the treatment of cancer: targeting the epidermal growth factor receptor. Clin Cancer Res 7: 2958-2970.
352. Cinalli G, Zerah M, Carteret M, Doz F, Vinikoff L, Lellouch T, Husson B, Pierre K (1997). Subdural sarcoma associated with chronic subdural hematoma. Report of two cases and review of the literature. J Neurosurg 86: 553-557.
353. Cingolani A, De Luca A, Larocca LM, Ammassari A, Scerrati M, Antinori A, Ortona L (1998). Minimally invasive diagnosis of acquired immunodeficiency syndrome- related primary central nervous system lymphoma. J Natl Cancer Inst 90: 364-369.
354. Cirak B, Horska A, Barker PB, Burger PC, Carson BS, Avellino AM (2005). Proton magnetic resonance spectroscopic imaging in pediatric pilomyxoid astrocytoma. Childs Nerv Syst 21: 404-409.
355. Clarenbach P, Kleihues P, Metzel E, Dichgans J (1979). Simultaneous clinical manifestation of subependymoma of the fourth ventricle in identical twins. Case report. J Neurosurg 50: 655-659.
356. Clark GB, Henry JM, McKeever PE (1985). Cerebral pilocytic astrocytoma. Cancer 56: 1128-1133.
357. Clarke DB, Leblanc R, Bertrand G, Quartey GR, Snipes GJ (1998). Meningeal melanocytoma. Report of a case and a historical comparison. J Neurosurg 88: 116-121.
358. Clarke MR, Weyant RJ, Watson CG, Carty SE (1998). Prognostic markers in pheochromocytoma. Hum Pathol 29: 522-526.
359. Claus EB, Bondy ML, Schildkraut JM, Wiemels JL, Wrensch M, Black PM (2005). Epidemiology of intracranial meningioma. Neurosurgery 57: 1088-1095.
360. Clusmann H, Kral T, Fackeldey E, Blumcke I, Helmstaedter C, von Oertzen J, Urbach H, Schramm J (2004). Lesional mesial temporal lobe epilepsy and limited resections: prognostic factors and outcome. J Neurol Neurosurg Psychiatry 75: 1589-1596.
361. Cobbers JM, Wolter M, Reifenberger J, Ring GU, Jessen F, An HX, Niederacher D, Schmidt EE, Ichimura K, Floeth F, Kirsch L, Borchard F, Louis DN, Collins VP, Reifenberger G (1998). Frequent inactivation of CDKN2A and rare mutation of TP53 in PCNSL. Brain Pathol 8: 263-276.
362. Coca S, Moreno M, Martos JA, Rodriguez J, Barcena A, Vaquero J (1994). Neurocytoma of spinal cord. Acta Neuropathol 87: 537-540.
363. Coca S, Vaquero J, Escandon J, Moreno M, Peralba J, Rodriguez J (1992). Immunohistochemical characterization of pineocytomas. Clin Neuropathol 11: 298-303.
364. Coffin CM, Braun JT, Wick MR, Dehner LP (1990). A clinicopathologic and immunohistochemical analysis of 53 cases of medulloblastoma with emphasis on synaptophysin expression. Mod Pathol 3: 164-170.
365. Coffin CM, Fletcher JA (2002). Inflammatory myofibroblastic tumour. In: Pathology and Genetics of Tumours of Soft Tissue and Bone. Fletcher CDM, Unni KK, Mertens F, eds. IARC Press: Lyon, pp. 91-93.
366. Coffin CM, Swanson PE, Wick MR, Dehner LP (1993). An immunohistochemical comparison of chordoma with renal cell carcinoma, colorectal adenocarcinoma, and myxopapillary ependymoma: a potential diagnostic dilemma in the diminutive biopsy. Mod Pathol 6: 531-538.
367. Cohen-Gadol AA, Pichelmann MA, Link MJ, Scheithauer BW, Krecke KN, Young WF, Jr., Hardy J, Giannini C (2003). Granular cell tumor of the sellar and suprasellar region: clinicopathologic study of 11 cases and literature review. Mayo Clin Proc 78: 567-573.
368. Colin C, Baeza N, Bartoli C, Fina F, Eudes N, Nanni I, Martin PM, Ouafik L, Figarella-Branger D (2006). Identification of genes differentially expressed in glioblastoma versus pilocytic astrocytoma using Suppression Subtractive Hybridization. Oncogene 25: 2818-2826.
369. Colin C, Baeza N, Tong S, Bouvier C, Quilichini B, Durbec P, Figarella-Branger D (2006). In vitro identification and functional characterization of glial precursor cells in human gliomas. Neuropathol Appl Neurobiol 32: 189-202.
370. Colman SD, Williams CA, Wallace MR (1995). Benign neurofibromas in type 1 neurofibromatosis (NF1) show somatic deletions of the NF1 gene. Nat Genet 11: 90-92.
371. Connor JM, Pirrit LA, Yates JR, Fryer AE, Ferguson-Smith MA (1987). Linkage of the tuberous sclerosis locus to a DNA polymorphism detected by v-abl. J Med Genet 24: 544-546.
372. Constantine C, Miller DC, Gardner S, Balmaceda C, Finlay J (2005). Osseous metastasis of pineoblastoma: a case report and review of the literature. J Neurooncol 74: 53-57.
373. Constantini S, Soffer D, Siegel T, Shalit MN (1989). Paraganglioma of the thoracic spinal cord with cerebrospinal fluid metastasis. Spine 14: 643-645.
374. Conti P, Mouchaty H, Spacca B, Buccoliero AM, Conti R (2006). Thoracic extradural paragangliomas: a case report and review of the literature. Spinal Cord 44: 120-125.
375. Conway JE, Chou D, Clatterbuck RE, Brem H, Long DM, Rigamonti D (2001). Hemangioblastomas of the central nervous system in von Hippel-Lindau syndrome and sporadic disease. Neurosurgery 48: 55-62.
376. Coons SW, Johnson PC (1993). Regional heterogeneity in the proliferative activity of human gliomas as measured by the Ki-67 labeling index. J Neuropathol Exp Neurol 52: 609-618.
377. Coons SW, Johnson PC, Pearl DK (1997). The prognostic significance of Ki-67 labeling indices for oligodendrogliomas. Neurosurgery 41: 878-884.
378. Coons SW, Johnson PC, Scheithauer BW, Yates AJ, Pearl DK (1997). Improving diagnostic accuracy and interobserver concordance in the classification and grading of primary gliomas. Cancer 79: 1381-1393.
379. Cooper ERA (1935). The relation of oligodendrocytes and astrocytes in cerebral tumours. J Path Bact 41: 259-266.
380. Corapcioglu F, Memet OM, Sav A, Uren D (2006). Congenital pineoblastoma and parameningeal rhabdomyosarcoma: concurrent two embryonal tumors in a young infant. Childs Nerv Syst 22: 533-538.
381. Cordera S, Bottacchi E, D'Alessandro G, Machado D, De Gonda F, Corso G (2002). Epidemiology of primary intracranial tumours in NW Italy, a population based study: stable incidence in the last two decades. J Neurol 249: 281-284.
382. Corless CL, Kibel AS, Iliopoulos O, Kaelin WG, Jr. (1997). Immunostaining of the von Hippel-Lindau gene product in normal and neoplastic human tissues. Hum Pathol 28: 459-464.
383. Corn B, Curtis MT, Lynch D, Gomori JM (1994). Malignant oligodendroglioma arising after radiation therapy for lymphoma [clinical conference]. Med Pediatr Oncol 22: 45-52.
384. Corn BW, Marcus SM, Topham A, Hauck W, Curran WJ, Jr. (1997). Will primary central nervous system lymphoma be the most frequent brain tumor diagnosed in the year 2000? Cancer 79: 2409-2413.
385. Cosar M, Iplikcioglu AC, Bek S, Gokduman CA (2005). Intracranial falcine and convexity chondromas: two case reports. Br J Neurosurg 19: 241-243.
386. Costello JF, Plass C, Arap W, Chapman VM, Held WA, Berger MS, Huang HJS, Cavenee WK (1997). Cyclin-dependent kinase 6 (CDK6) amplification in human gliomas identified using two-dimensional separation of genomic DNA. Cancer Res 57: 1250-1254.
387. Cote TR, Manns A, Hardy CR, Yellin FJ, Hartge P (1996). Epidemiology of brain lymphoma among people with or without acquired immunodeficiency syndrome. AIDS/Cancer Study Group. J Natl Cancer Inst 88: 675-679.
388. Cottingham SL, Boesel CP, Yates AJ (1996). Pilocytic astrocytoma in infants: a distinctive histologic pattern. J Neuropathol Exp Neurol 55: 654.
389. Couce ME, Aker FV, Scheithauer BW (2000). Chordoid meningioma: a clinicopathologic study of 42 cases. Am J Surg Pathol 24: 899-905.
390. Couce ME, Perry A, Webb P, Kepes JJ, Scheithauer BW (1999). Fibrous meningioma with tyrosine-rich crystals. Ultrastruct Pathol 23: 341-345.
391. Courts C, Montesinos-Rongen M, Martin-Subero JI, Brunn A, Siemer D, Zühlke-Jenisch R, Pels H, Jürgens A, Schlegel U, Schmidt-Wolf IG, Schaller C, Reifenberger G, Sabel M, Warnecke-Ebertz U, Wiestler OD, Küppers R, Siebert R, Deckert M (2007). Transcriptional profiling of the NF-κB pathway identifies a subgroup of primary lymphoma of the central nervous system with low BCL10 expression. J Neuropathol Exp Neurol 66: 230-237.
392. Courville CB, Broussalian SL (1961). Plastic ependymomas of the lateral recess. Report of eight verified cases. J Neurosurg 18:792-799.
393. Crail HW (1949). Multiple primary malignancies arising in the rectum, brain and thyroid. US Nav Bull 49: 123-128.
394. Crino PB, Trojanowski JQ, Dichter MA, Eberwine J (1996). Embryonic neuronal markers in tuberous sclerosis: single-cell molecular pathology. Proc Natl Acad Sci USA 93: 14152-14157.
395. Crotty TB, Scheithauer BW, Young WF, Jr., Davis DH, Shaw EG, Miller GM, Burger PC (1995). Papillary craniopharyngioma: a clinicopathological study of 48 cases. J Neurosurg 83: 206-214.
396. Cruz-Sanchez FF, Rossi ML, Hughes JT, Moss TH (1991). Differentiation in embryonal neuroepithelial tumors of the central nervous system. Cancer 67: 965-976.
397. Cruz-Sanchez FF, Rossi ML, Rodriguez-Prados S, Nakamura N, Hughes JT,

Coakham HB (1990). Haemangioblastoma: histological and immunohistological study of an enigmatic cerebellar tumour. Histol Histopathol 5: 407-413.
398. Cruz Perez DE, Amanajas de Aguiar FC Jr, Leon JE, Graner E, Paes dA, Vargas PA (2006). Intraneural perineurioma of the tongue: a case report. J Oral Maxillofac Surg 64: 1140-1142.
399. Cruz AA, de Alencar VM, Falcao MF, Elias J, Jr., Chahud F (2006). Association between Erdheim-Chester disease, Hashimoto thyroiditis, and familial thrombocytopenia. Ophthal Plast Reconstr Surg 22: 60-62.
400. Cruz S, Haustein J, Rossie ML, Cervos N, Hughs JT (1988). Ependymoblastoma: a histological, immunohistological and ultrastructural study of five cases. Histopathology 12: 17-27.
401. Cruz S, Miquel R, Rossi ML, Figols J, Palacin A, Cardesa A (1993). Clinico-pathological correlations in meningiomas: a DNA and immunohistochemical study. Histol Histopathol 8: 1-8.
402. Cuccia V, Zuccaro G, Sosa F, Monges J, Lubienieky F, Taratuto AL (2003). Subependymal giant cell astrocytoma in children with tuberous sclerosis. Childs Nerv Syst 19: 232-243.
403. Cummings TJ, Hulette CM, Longee DC, Bottom KS, McLendon RE, Chu CT (1999). Gliomatosis cerebri: cytologic and autopsy findings in a case involving the entire neuraxis. Clin Neuropathol 18: 190-197.
404. Curless RG, Toledano SR, Ragheb J, Cleveland WW, Falcone S (2002). Hematogenous brain metastasis in children. Pediatr Neurol 26: 219-221.
405. Cushing H (1931). Experiences with the cerebellar astrocytomas. A critical review of seventy-six cases. Surg Gynecol Obstet 52: 1129-1204.
406. Cushing H, Eisenhardt L (1938). Meningiomas, their classification, regional behaviour, life history, and end surgical results. Meningiomas, their classification, regional behaviour, life history, and end surgical results. Charles C. Thomas: Springfield, pp. 42-47.
407. Czerwionka M, Korf HW, Hoffmann O, Busch H, Schachenmayr W (1989). Differentiation in medulloblastomas: correlation between the immunocytochemical demonstration of photoreceptor markers (S- antigen, rod-opsin) and the survival rate in 66 patients. Acta Neuropathol 78: 629-636.
408. D'Ambrosio AL, O'Toole JE, Connolly ES, Jr., Feldstein NA (2003). Villous hypertrophy versus choroid plexus papilloma: a case report demonstrating a diagnostic role for the proliferation index. Pediatr Neurosurg 39: 91-96.
409. Dabora SL, Jozwiak S, Franz DN, Roberts PS, Nieto A, Chung J, Choy YS, Reeve MP, Thiele E, Egelhoff JC, Kasprzyk-Obara J, Domanska-Pakiela D, Kwiatkowski DJ (2001). Mutational analysis in a cohort of 224 tuberous sclerosis patients indicates increased severity of TSC2, compared with TSC1, disease in multiple organs. Am J Hum Genet 68: 64-80.
410. Dahiya S, Sarkar C, Hedley-Whyte ET, Sharma MC, Zervas NT, Sridhar E, Louis DN (2005). Spindle cell oncocytoma of the adenohypophysis: report of two cases. Acta Neuropathol 110: 97-99.
411. Dahmen RP, Koch A, Denkhaus D, Tonn JC, Sorensen N, Berthold F, Behrens J, Birchmeier W, Wiestler OD, Pietsch T (2001). Deletions of AXIN1, a component of the WNT/wingless pathway, in sporadic medulloblastomas. Cancer Res 61: 7039-7043.
411A. Dal Cin P, Van den Berghe H, Buonamici L, Losi L, Roncaroli F, Calbucci F (1999). Cytogenetic investigation in subependymoma. Cancer Genet Cytogenet 108: 84.
412. Dang L, Fan X, Chaudhry A, Wang M, Gaiano N, Eberhart CG (2006). Notch3 signaling initiates choroid plexus tumor formation. Oncogene 25: 487-491.
413. Danks RA, Chopra G, Gonzales MF, Orian JM, Kaye AH (1995). Aberrant p53 expression does not correlate with the prognosis in anaplastic astrocytoma. Neurosurgery 37: 246-254.
414. Dardick I, Hammar SP, Scheithauer BW (1989). Ultrastructural spectrum of hemangiopericytoma: a comparative study of fetal, adult, and neoplastic pericytes. Ultrastruct Pathol 13: 111-154.
415. Darrouzet V, Martel J, Enee V, Bebear JP, Guerin J (2004). Vestibular schwannoma surgery outcomes: our multidisciplinary experience in 400 cases over 17 years. Laryngoscope 114: 681-688.
416. Darwish BS, Balakrishnan V, Maitra R (2002). Intramedullary ancient schwannoma of the cervical spinal cord: case report and review of literature. J Clin Neurosci 9: 321-323.
417. Dasgupta B, Yi Y, Chen DY, Weber JD, Gutmann DH (2005). Proteomic analysis reveals hyperactivation of the mammalian target of rapamycin pathway in neurofibromatosis 1-associated human and mouse brain tumors. Cancer Res 65: 2755-2760.
418. Dasgupta B, Yi Y, Hegedus B, Weber JD, Gutmann DH (2005). Cerebrospinal fluid proteomic analysis reveals dysregulation of methionine aminopeptidase-2 expression in human and mouse neurofibromatosis 1-associated glioma. Cancer Res 65: 9843-9850.
419. Daumas-Duport C (1993). Dysembryoplastic neuroepithelial tumours. Brain Pathol 3: 283-295.
420. Daumas-Duport C (1995). Dysembryoplastic neuroepithelial tumours in epilepsy surgery. In: Dysplasia of Cerebral Cortex and Epilepsy. Guerrini R, ed. Raven Press: New York, pp. 125-147.
421. Daumas-Duport C, Scheithauer B, O'Fallon J, Kelly P (1988). Grading of astrocytomas. A simple and reproducible method. Cancer 62: 2152-2165.
422. Daumas-Duport C, Scheithauer BW, Chodkiewicz JP, Laws ER, Jr., Vedrenne C (1988). Dysembryoplastic neuroepithelial tumor: a surgically curable tumor of young patients with intractable partial seizures. Report of thirty-nine cases. Neurosurgery 23: 545-556.
423. Daumas-Duport C, Scheithauer BW, Kelly PJ (1987). A histologic and cytologic method for the spatial definition of gliomas. Mayo Clin Proc 62: 435-449.
424. Daumas-Duport C, Tucker ML, Kolles H, Cervera P, Beuvon F, Varlet P, Udo N, Koziak M, Chodkiewicz JP (1997). Oligodendrogliomas. Part II: A new grading system based on morphological and imaging criteria. J Neurooncol 34: 61-78.
425. Daumas-Duport C, Varlet P (2003). [Dysembryoplastic neuroepithelial tumors]. Rev Neurol (Paris) 159: 622-636.
426. Daumas-Duport C, Varlet P, Bacha S, Beuvon F, Cervera-Pierot P, Chodkiewicz JP (1999). Dysembryoplastic neuroepithelial tumors: nonspecific histological forms — a study of 40 cases. J Neurooncol 41: 267-280.
427. Daumas Duport C (1995). Patterns of tumor growth and problems associated with histological typing of low-grade gliomas. In: Benign Cerebral Gliomas. Apuzzo LJ, ed. AANS: Park Ridge, pp. 125-147.
428. David KM, Casey ATH, Hayward RD, Harkness WFJ, Phipps K, Wade AM (1997). Medulloblastoma: is the 5-year survival rate improving? J Neurosurg 86: 13-21.
429. Davidson A, Desai F, Stannard C, Ivey A, Solomon R, Sinclair-Smith C (2006). Intraocular rhabdomyosarcoma in the sibling of a patient with a cerebellar medulloepithelioma. J Pediatr Hematol Oncol 28: 476-478.
430. Davies MP, Gibbs FE, Halliwell N, Joyce KA, Roebuck MM, Rossi ML, Salisbury J, Sibson DR, Tacconi L, Walker C (1999). Mutation in the PTEN/MMAC1 gene in archival low grade and high grade gliomas. Br J Cancer 79: 1542-1548.
431. Davies RP, Lee CS (1988). Medulloepithelioma: MRI appearances. Australas Radiol 32: 503-505.
432. Davis FG, Preston-Martin S (1998). Epidemiology. Incidence and survival. In: Russell and Rubinstein's Pathology of Tumors of the Nervous System. Bigner DD, McLendon RE, Bruner JM, eds. Arnold: London, pp. 5-45.
433. de Chadarevian JP, Montes JL, O'Gorman AM, Freeman CR (1987). Maturation of cerebellar neuroblastoma into ganglioneuroma with melanosis. A histologic, immunocytochemical, and ultrastructural study. Cancer 59: 69-76.
434. de Chadarevian JP, Pattisapu JV, Faerber EN (1990). Desmoplastic cerebral astrocytoma of infancy. Light microscopy, immunocytochemistry, and ultrastructure. Cancer 66: 173-179.
435. de Haas T, Oussoren E, Grajkowska W, Perek-Polnik M, Popovic M, Zadravec-Zaletel L, Perera M, Corte G, Wirths O, van Sluis P, Pietsch T, Troost D, Baas F, Versteeg R, Kool M (2006). OTX1 and OTX2 expression correlates with the clinicopathologic classification of medulloblastomas. J Neuropathol Exp Neurol 65: 176-186.
436. De Jesus O, Rifkinson N (1995). Pleomorphic xanthoastrocytoma with invasion of the tentorium and falx. Surg Neurol 43: 77-79.
437. De Munnynck K, Van Gool S, Van Calenbergh F, Demaerel P, Uyttebroeck A, Buyse G, Sciot R (2002). Desmoplastic infantile ganglioglioma: a potentially malignant tumor? Am J Surg Pathol 26: 1515-1522.
438. De Potter P, Shields CL, Shields JA (1994). Clinical variations of trilateral retinoblastoma: a report of 13 cases. J Pediatr Ophthalmol Strabismus 31: 26-31.
439. De Raedt T, Brems H, Wolkenstein P, Vidaud D, Pilotti S, Perrone F, Mautner V, Frahm S, Sciot R, Legius E (2003). Elevated risk for MPNST in NF1 microdeletion patients. Am J Hum Genet 72: 1288-1292.
440. De Vos M, Hayward BE, Charlton R, Taylor GR, Glaser AW, Picton S, Cole TR, Maher ER, McKeown CM, Mann JR, Yates JR, Baralle D, Rankin J, Bonthron DT, Sheridan E (2006). PMS2 mutations in childhood cancer. J Natl Cancer Inst 98: 358-361.
441. De Vos M, Hayward BE, Picton S, Sheridan E, Bonthron DT (2004). Novel PMS2 pseudogenes can conceal recessive mutations causing a distinctive childhood cancer syndrome. Am J Hum Genet 74: 954-964.
442. de Vries J, Scheremet R, Altmannsberger M, Michilli R, Lindemann A, Hinkelbein W (1993). Primary leiomyosarcoma of the spinal leptomeninges. J Neurooncol 18: 25-31.
443. Deb P, Sharma MC, Gaikwad S, Gupta A, Mehta VS, Sarkar C (2005). Cerebellopontine angle paraganglioma - report of a case and review of literature. J Neurooncol 74: 65-69.
444. Deck JH (1969). Cerebral medulloepithelioma with maturation into ependymal cells and ganglion cells. J Neuropathol Exp Neurol 28: 442-454.
445. Deck JH, Rubinstein LJ (1981). Glial fibrillary acidic protein in stromal cells of some capillary hemangioblastomas: significance and possible implications of an immunoperoxidase study. Acta Neuropathol 54: 173-181.
446. Deckert-Schluter M, Marek J, Setlik M, Markova J, Pakos E, Fischer R, Wiestler OD (1998). Primary manifestation of Hodgkin's disease in the central nervous system. Virchows Arch 432: 477-481.
447. Deckert-Schluter M, Rang A, Wiestler OD (1998). Apoptosis and apoptosis-related gene products in primary non-Hodgkin's lymphoma of the central nervous system. Acta Neuropathol 96: 157-162.
448. Deckert M, Reifenberger G, Wechsler W (1989). Determination of the proliferative potential of human brain tumors using the monoclonal antibody Ki-67. J Cancer Res Clin Oncol 115: 179-188.
449. DeDavid M, Orlow SJ, Provost N, Marghoob AA, Rao BK, Wasti Q, Huang CL, Kopf AW, Bart RS (1996). Neurocutaneous melanosis: clinical features of large congenital melanocytic nevi in patients with manifest central nervous system melanosis. J Am Acad Dermatol 35: 529-538.
450. Dedeurwaerdere F, Giannini C, Sciot R, Rubin BP, Perilongo G, Borghi L, Ballotta ML, Cornips E, Demunter A, Maes B, Dei Tos AP (2002). Primary peripheral PNET/Ewing's sarcoma of the dura: a clinicopathologic entity distinct from central PNET. Mod Pathol 15: 673-678.
451. Degen R, Ebner A, Lahl R, Leonhardt S, Pannek HW, Tuxhorn I (2002). Various findings in surgically treated epilepsy patients with dysembryoplastic neuroepithelial tumors in comparison with those of patients with other low-grade brain tumors and other neuronal migration disorders. Epilepsia 43: 1379-1384.
452. DeGirolami U, Schmidek H (1973). Clinicopathological study of 53 tumors of the pineal region. J Neurosurg 39: 455-462.
453. DeGirolami U, Zvaigzne O (1973). Modification of the Achucarro-Hortega pineal stain for paraffin- embedded formalin-fixed tissue. Stain Technol 48: 48-50.
454. Dehghani F, Maronde E, Schachenmayr W, Korf HW (2000). Neurofilament H immunoreaction in oligodendrogliomas as demonstrated by a new polyclonal antibody. Acta Neuropathol 100: 122-130.
455. Dehghani F, Schachenmayr W, Laun A, Korf HW (1998). Prognostic implication of histopathological, immunohistochemical and clinical features of oligodendrogliomas: a study of 89 cases. Acta Neuropathol 95: 493-504.
456. Deinsberger W, Kastner S, Schachenmayr W, Boker DK (2000). Malignant peripheral nerve sheath tumour infiltrating the spinal cord. Acta Neurochir 142: 1071-1072.
457. Del Bigio MR, Deck JH (1993). Rosenthal fibers producing a granular cell appearance in a glioblastoma. Acta Neuropathol 86: 100-104.
458. del Carpio-O'Donovan R, Korah I, Salazar A, Melancon D (1996). Gliomatosis cerebri. Radiology 198: 831-835.
459. Del Valle L, Enam S, Lara C, Miklossy J, Khalili K, Gordon J (2004). Primary central nervous system lymphoma expressing the human neurotropic polyomavirus, JC virus, genome. J Virol 78: 3462-3469.
460. Del Valle L, Enam S, Lara C, Ortiz-Hidalgo C, Katsetos CD, Khalili K (2002). Detection of JC polyomavirus DNA sequences and cellular localization of T-antigen and agnoprotein in oligodendrogliomas. Clin Cancer Res 8: 3332-3340.
461. Del Valle L, Gordon J, Enam S, Delbue S, Croul S, Abraham S, Radhakrishnan S, Assimakopoulou M, Katsetos CD, Khalili K (2002). Expression of human neurotropic polyomavirus JCV late gene product agnoprotein in human medulloblastoma. J Natl Cancer Inst

94: 267-273.

462. Dhimes P, Martinez-Gonzalez MA, Carabias E, Perez-Espejo G (1996). Ultrastructural study of a perineurioma with ribosome-lamella complexes. Ultrastruct Pathol 20: 167-172.

463. Di Marcotullio L, Ferretti E, De Smaele E, Argenti B, Mincione C, Zazzeroni F, Gallo R, Masuelli L, Napolitano M, Maroder M, Modesti A, Giangaspero F, Screpanti I, Alesse E, Gulino A (2004). REN(KCTD11) is a suppressor of Hedgehog signaling and is deleted in human medulloblastoma. Proc Natl Acad Sci U S A 101: 10833-10838.

464. Di Rocco F, Carroll RS, Zhang J, Black PM (1998). Platelet-derived growth factor and its receptor expression in human oligodendrogliomas. Neurosurgery 42: 341-346.

465. Di Rocco F, Sabatino G, Koutzoglou M, Battaglia D, Caldarelli M, Tamburrini G (2004). Neurocutaneous melanosis. Childs Nerv Syst 20: 23-28.

466. Di C, Liao S, Adamson DC, Parrett TJ, Broderick DK, Shi Q, Lengauer C, Cummins JM, Velculescu VE, Fults DW, McLendon RE, Bigner DD, Yan H (2005). Identification of OTX2 as a medulloblastoma oncogene whose product can be targeted by all-trans retinoic acid. Cancer Res 65: 919-924.

467. Diaz-Flores L, Alvarez-Arguelles H, Madrid JF, Varela H, Gonzalez MP, Gutierrez R (1997). Perineurial cell tumor (perineurioma) with granular cells. J Cutan Pathol 24: 575-579.

468. Diaz-Insa S, Pineda M, Bestue M, Espada F, Alvarez-Fernandez E (1998). [Neurocutaneous melanosis]. Rev Neurol 26: 769-771.

469. DiCarlo EF, Woodruff JM, Bansal M, Erlandson RA (1986). The purely epithelioid malignant peripheral nerve sheath tumor. Am J Surg Pathol 10: 478-490.

470. Dickey T, Raghaven R, Rushing E (1999). MIB-1 (Ki-67) immunoreactivity as predictor of the risk of recurrence of craniopharyngiomas. J Neuropath Exp Neurol 58: 567-567.

471. Dickson DW, Hart MN, Menezes A, Cancilla PA (1983). Medulloblastoma with glial and rhabdomyoblastic differentiation. A myoglobin and glial fibrillary acidic protein immunohistochemical and ultrastructural study. J Neuropathol Exp Neurol 42: 639-647.

472. Dickson DW, Suzuki KI, Kanner R, Weitz S, Horoupian DS (1986). Cerebral granular cell tumor: immunohistochemical and electron microscopic study. J Neuropathol Exp Neurol 45: 304-314.

473. Dim DC, Lingamfelter DC, Taboada EM, Fiorella RM (2006). Papillary glioneuronal tumor: a case report and review of the literature. Hum Pathol 37: 914-918.

474. Dimopoulos VG, Fountas KN, Robinson JS (2006). Familial intracranial ependymomas. Report of three cases in a family and review of the literature. Neurosurg Focus 20: E8.

475. Dinda AK, Sarkar C, Roy S (1990). Rosenthal fibres: an immunohistochemical, ultrastructural and immunoelectron microscopic study. Acta Neuropathol 79: 456-460.

476. Dirks PB, Jay V, Becker LE, Drake JM, Humphreys RP, Hoffman HJ, Rutka JT (1994). Development of anaplastic changes in low-grade astrocytomas of childhood. Neurosurgery 34: 68-78.

477. Dohrmann GJ, Farwell JR, Flannery JT (1976). Ependymomas and ependymoblastomas in children. J Neurosurg 273-283.

478. Dohrmann GJ, Farwell JR, Flannery JT (1976). Glioblastoma multiforme in children. J Neurosurg 44: 442-448.

479. Dolman CL (1988). Melanotic medulloblastoma. A case report with immunohistochemical and ultrastructural examination. Acta Neuropathol 76: 528-531.

480. Dong S, Pang JC, Hu J, Zhou LF, Ng HK (2002). Transcriptional inactivation of TP73 expression in oligodendroglial tumors. Int J Cancer 98: 370-375.

481. Donner LR, Teshima I (2003). Peripheral medulloepithelioma: an immunohistochemical, ultrastructural, and cytogenetic study of a rare, chemotherapy-sensitive, pediatric tumor. Am J Surg Pathol 27: 1008-1012.

482. Donovan DJ, Prauner RD (2005). Shunt-related abdominal metastases in a child with choroid plexus carcinoma: case report. Neurosurgery 56: E412.

483. Donovan MJ, Yunis EJ, DeGirolami U, Fletcher JA, Schofield DE (1994). Chromosome aberrations in choroid plexus papillomas. Genes Chromosomes Cancer 11: 267-270.

484. Dorsay TA, Rovira MJ, Ho VB, Kelley J (1995). Ependymoblastoma: MR presentation. A case report and review of the literature. Pediatr Radiol 25: 433-435.

485. Drlicek M, Bodenteich A, Urbanits S, Grisold W (2004). Immunohistochemical panel of antibodies in the diagnosis of brain metastases of the unknown primary. Pathol Res Pract 200: 727-734.

486. Dropcho EJ, Soong SJ (1996). The prognostic impact of prior low grade histology in patients with anaplastic gliomas: a case-control study. Neurology 47: 684-690.

487. Ducatman BS, Scheithauer BW (1983). Postirradiation neurofibrosarcoma. Cancer 51: 1028-1033.

488. Ducatman BS, Scheithauer BW (1984). Malignant peripheral nerve sheath tumors with divergent differentiation. Cancer 54: 1049-1057.

489. Ducatman BS, Scheithauer BW, Piepgras DG, Reiman HM (1984). Malignant peripheral nerve sheath tumors in childhood. J Neurooncol 2: 241-248.

490. Ducatman BS, Scheithauer BW, Piepgras DG, Reiman HM, Ilstrup DM (1986). Malignant peripheral nerve sheath tumors. A clinicopathologic study of 120 cases. Cancer 57: 2006-2021.

491. Duerr EM, Rollbrocker B, Hayashi Y, Peters N, Meyer-Puttlitz B, Louis DN, Schramm J, Wiestler OD, Parsons R, Eng C, von Deimling A (1998). PTEN mutations in gliomas and glioneuronal tumors. Oncogene 16: 2259-2264.

492. Dufour H, Bouillot P, Figarella-Branger D, Ndoye N, Regis J, Bugha TN, Grisoli F (1998). [Meningeal hemangiopericytomas. A retrospective review of 20 cases]. Neurochirurgie 44: 5-18.

493. Duinkerke SJ, Slooff JL, Gabreels FJ, Renier WO, Thijssen HO, Biesta JH (1981). Melanotic rhabdomyomedulloblastoma or teratoid tumour of the cerebellar vermis. Clin Neurol Neurosurg 83: 29-33.

494. Dumanski JP, Rouleau GA, Nordenskjold M, Collins VP (1990). Molecular genetic analysis of chromosome 22 in 81 cases of meningioma. Cancer Res 50: 5863-5867.

495. Duncan JA, Hoffman HJ (1995). Intracranial ependymomas. In: Brain Tumors. Kaye AH, Lows ER, Jr., eds. Churchill Livingstone: Edinburgh, pp. 493-504.

496. Duo D, Gasverde S, Benech F, Zenga F, Giordana MT (2003). MIB-1 immunoreactivity in craniopharyngiomas: a clinico-pathological analysis. Clin Neuropathol 22: 229-234.

497. Eberhart CG, Brat DJ, cohen KJ, Burger PC (2000). Pediatric neuroblastic brain tumors containing abundant neuropil and true rosettes. Pediatr Dev Pathol 3: 346-352.

498. Eberhart CG, Burger PC (2003). Anaplasia and grading in medulloblastomas. Brain Pathol 13: 376-385.

499. Eberhart CG, Kaufman WE, Tihan T, Burger PC (2001). Apoptosis, neuronal maturation, and neurotrophin expression within medulloblastoma nodules. J Neuropathol Exp Neurol 60: 462-469.

500. Eberhart CG, Kepner JL, Goldthwaite PT, Kun LE, Duffner PK, Friedman HS, Strother DR, Burger PC (2002). Histopathologic grading of medulloblastomas: a Pediatric Oncology Group study. Cancer 94: 552-560.

501. Eberhart CG, Kratz J, Wang Y, Summers K, Stearns D, Cohen K, Dang CV, Burger PC (2004). Histopathological and molecular prognostic markers in medulloblastoma: c-myc, N-myc, TrkC, and anaplasia. J Neuropathol Exp Neurol 63: 441-449.

502. Eberhart CG, Kratz JE, Schuster A, Goldthwaite P, cohen KJ, Perlman EJ, Burger PC (2002). Comparative genomic hybridization detects an increased number of chromosomal alterations in large cell/anaplastic medulloblastomas. Brain Pathol 12: 36-44.

503. Eberhart CG, Tihan T, Burger PC (2000). Nuclear localization and mutation of beta-catenin in medulloblastomas. J Neuropathol Exp Neurol 59: 333-337.

504. Ebert C, von Haken M, Meyer-Puttlitz B, Wiestler OD, Reifenberger G, Pietsch T, von Deimling A (1999). Molecular genetic analysis of ependymal tumors: NF2 mutations and chromosome 22q loss occur preferentially in intramedullary spinal ependymomas. Am J Pathol 155: 627-632

505. Ebinger M, Senf L, Wachowski O, Scheurlen W (2005). No aberrant methylation of neurofibromatosis 1 gene (NF1) promoter in pilocytic astrocytoma in childhood. Pediatr Hematol Oncol 22: 83-87.

506. Ecker RD, Marsh WR, Pollock BE, Kurtkaya-Yapicier O, McClelland R, Scheithauer BW, Buckner JC (2003). Hemangiopericytoma in the central nervous system: treatment, pathological features, and long-term follow up in 38 patients. J Neurosurg 98: 1182-1187.

507. Eckhardt BP, Brandner S, Zollikofer CL, Wentz KU (2004). Primary cerebral leiomyosarcoma in a child. Pediatr Radiol 34: 495-498.

508. Edwards A, Bermudez C, Piwonka G, Berr ML, Zamorano J, Larrain E, Franck R, Gonzalez M, Alvarez E, Maiers E (2002). Carney's syndrome: complex myxomas. Report of four cases and review of the literature. Cardiovasc Surg 10: 264-275.

509. Ehret M, Jacobi G, Hey A, Segerer S (1987). Embryonal brain neoplasms in the neonatal period and early infancy. Clin Neuropathol 6: 218-223.

510. Eibl RH, Kleihues P, Jat PS, Wiestler OD (1994). A model for primitive neuroectodermal tumors in transgenic neural transplants harboring the SV40 large T antigen. Am J Pathol 144: 556-564.

511. Ekstein D, Ben Yehuda D, Slyusarevsky E, Lossos A, Linetsky E, Siegal T (2006). CSF analysis of IgH gene rearrangement in CNS lymphoma: relationship to the disease course. J Neurol Sci 247: 39-46.

512. Ekstrand AJ, James CD, Cavenee WK, Seliger B, Pettersson RF, Collins VP (1991). Genes for epidermal growth factor receptor, transforming growth factor alpha, and epidermal growth factor and their expression in human gliomas in vivo. Cancer Res 51: 2164-2172.

513. Ekstrand AJ, Sugawa N, James CD, Collins VP (1992). Amplified and rearranged epidermal growth factor receptor genes in human glioblastomas reveal deletions of sequences encoding portions of the N- and/or C-terminal tails. Proc Natl Acad Sci USA 89: 4309-4313.

514. Ellison D (2002). Classifying the medulloblastoma: insights from morphology and molecular genetics. Neuropathol Appl Neurobiol 28: 257-282.

515. Ellison DW, Clifford SC, Gajjar A, Gilbertson RJ (2003). What's new in neuro-oncology? Recent advances in medulloblastoma. Eur J Paediatr Neurol 7: 53-66.

516. Ellison DW, Onilude OE, Lindsey JC, Lusher ME, Weston CL, Taylor RE, Pearson AD, Clifford SC (2005). beta-Catenin status predicts a favorable outcome in childhood medulloblastoma: the United Kingdom Children's Cancer Study Group Brain Tumour Committee. J Clin Oncol 23: 7951-7957.

517. Ellison DW, Zygmunt SC, Weller RO (1993). Neurocytoma/lipoma (neurolipocytoma) of the cerebellum. Neuropathol Appl Neurobiol 19: 95-98.

518. Elmlinger MW, Deininger MH, Schuett BS, Meyermann R, Duffner F, Grote EH, Ranke MB (2001). In vivo expression of insulin-like growth factor-binding protein-2 in human gliomas increases with the tumor grade. Endocrinology 142: 1652-1658.

519. Emory TS, Scheithauer BW, Hirose T, Wood M, Onofrio BM, Jenkins RB (1995). Intraneural perineurioma. A clonal neoplasm associated with abnormalities of chromosome 22. Am J Clin Pathol 103: 696-704.

520. Enam SA, Rosenblum ML, Ho KL (1997). Neurocytoma in the cerebellum. Case report. J Neurosurg 87: 100-102.

521. Eng C (2000). Will the real Cowden syndrome please stand up: revised diagnostic criteria. J Med Genet 37: 828-830.

522. Eng C (2003). PTEN: one gene, many syndromes. Hum Mutat 22: 183-198.

523. Eng C, Murday V, Seal S, Mohammed S, Hodgson SV, Chaudary MA, Fentiman IS, Ponder BA, Eeles RA (1994). Cowden syndrome and Lhermitte-Duclos disease in a family: a single genetic syndrome with pleiotropy? J Med Genet 31: 458-461.

524. Eng DY, DeMonte F, Ginsberg L, Fuller GN, Jaeckle K (1997). Craniospinal dissemination of central neurocytoma - report of two cases. J Neurosurg 86: 547-552.

525. Englund C, Alvord EC, Jr., Folkerth RD, Silbergeld D, Born DE, Small R, Hevner RF (2005). NeuN expression correlates with reduced mitotic index of neoplastic cells in central neurocytomas. Neuropathol Appl Neurobiol 31: 429-438.

526. Enzinger FM, Weiss SW (1995). Paraganglioma. In: Soft Tissue Tumors. Enzinger FM, Weiss SW, eds. Mosby: St. Louis, pp. 965-990.

527. Enzinger FM, Weiss SW (2001). Soft tissue tumors. Mosby: St Louis.

528. Eoli M, Bissola L, Bruzzone MG, Pollo B, Maccagnano C, De Simone T, Valletta L, Silvani A, Bianchessi D, Broggi G, Boiardi A, Finocchiaro G (2006). Reclassification of oligoastrocytomas by loss of heterozygosity studies. Int J Cancer 119: 84-90.

529. Erickson ML, Johnson R, Bannykh SI, de Lotbiniere A, Kim JH (2005). Malignant rhabdoid tumor in a pregnant adult female: literature review of central nervous system rhabdoid tumors. J Neurooncol 74: 311-319.

530. Erlandson RA (1994). Diagnostic Transmission Electron Microscopy of Tumors. Raven Press: New York.

531. Erlandson RA (1994). Paragangliomas. In: Diagnostic Transmission Electron Microscopy of Tumors. Diagnostic Transmission Electron Microscopy of Tumors. Raven Press: New York, pp. 615-622.

532. Erlandson RA, Woodruff JM (1982). Peripheral nerve sheath tumors: an electron microscopic study of 43 cases. Cancer 49: 273-

287.
533. Erman T, Gocer AI, Erdogan S, Tuna M, Ildan F, Zorludemir S (2003). Choroid plexus papilloma of bilateral lateral ventricle. Acta Neurochir 145: 139-143.
534. Ernestus RI, Schroder R, Stutzer H, Klug N (1996). Prognostic relevance of localization and grading in intracranial ependymomas of childhood. Childs Nerv Syst 12: 522-526.
535. Ernestus RI, Schroder R, Stutzer H, Klug N (1997). The clinical and prognostic relevance of grading in intracranial ependymomas. Br J Neurosurg 11: 421-428.
536. Ess KC, Kamp CA, Tu BP, Gutmann DH (2005). Developmental origin of subependymal giant cell astrocytoma in tuberous sclerosis complex. Neurology 64: 1446-1449.
537. Esteller M, Hamilton SR, Burger PC, Baylin SB, Herman JG (1999). Inactivation of the DNA repair gene O6-methylguanine-DNA methyltransferase by promoter hypermethylation is a common event in primary human neoplasia. Cancer Res 59: 793-797.
538. Evans DG, Birch JM, Ramsden RT (1999). Paediatric presentation of type 2 neurofibromatosis. Arch Dis Child 81: 496-499.
539. Evans DG, Farndon PA, Burnell LD, Gattamaneni HR, Birch JM (1991). The incidence of Gorlin syndrome in 173 consecutive cases of medulloblastoma. Br J Cancer 64: 959-961.
540. Evans DG, Huson SM, Donnai D, Neary W, Blair V, Newton V, Harris R (1992). A clinical study of type 2 neurofibromatosis. Q J Med 84: 603-618.
541. Evans DG, Ladusans EJ, Rimmer S, Burnell LD, Thakker N, Farndon PA (1993). Complications of the naevoid basal cell carcinoma syndrome: results of a population based study. J Med Genet 30: 460-464.
542. Evans DG, Mason S, Huson SM, Ponder M, Harding AE, Strachan T (1997). Spinal and cutaneous schwannomatosis is a variant form of type 2 neurofibromatosis: a clinical and molecular study. J Neurol Neurosurg Psychiatry 62: 361-366.
543. Evans DG, Moran A, King A, Saeed S, Gurusinghe N, Ramsden R (2005). Incidence of vestibular schwannoma and neurofibromatosis 2 in the North West of England over a 10-year period: higher incidence than previously thought. Otol Neurotol 26: 93-97.
544. Evans DG, Wallace AJ, Wu CL, Trueman L, Ramsden RT, Strachan T (1998). Somatic mosaicism: a common cause of classic disease in tumor-prone syndromes? Lessons from type 2 neurofibromatosis. Am J Hum Genet 63: 727-736.
545. Fairburn B, Urich H (1971). Malignant gliomas occurring in identical twins. J Neurol Neurosurg Psychiatry 34: 718-722.
546. Fallon KB, Palmer CA, Roth KA, Nabors LB, Wang W, Carpenter M, Banerjee R, Forsyth P, Rich K, Perry A (2004). Prognostic value of 1p, 19q, 9p, 10q, and EGFR-FISH analyses in recurrent oligodendrogliomas. J Neuropathol Exp Neurol 63: 314-322.
547. Fan X, Matsui W, Khaki L, Stearns D, Chun J, Li YM, Eberhart CG (2006). Notch pathway inhibition depletes stem-like cells and blocks engraftment in embryonal brain tumors. Cancer Res 66: 7445-7452.
548. Fan X, Mikolaenko I, Elhassan I, Ni X, Wang Y, Ball D, Brat DJ, Perry A, Eberhart CG (2004). Notch1 and notch2 have opposite effects on embryonal brain tumor growth. Cancer Res 64: 7787-7793.
549. Fan X, Wang Y, Kratz J, Brat DJ, Robitaille Y, Moghrabi A, Perlman EJ, Dang CV, Burger PC, Eberhart CG (2003). hTERT gene amplification and increased mRNA expression in central nervous system embryonal tumors. Am J Pathol 162: 1763-1769.
550. Faro SH, Turtz AR, Koenigsberg RA, Mohamed FB, Chen CY, Stein H (1997). Paraganglioma of the cauda equina with associated intramedullary cyst: MR findings. AJNR Am J Neuroradiol 18: 1588-1590.
551. Farwell J, Flannery JT (1984). Cancer in relatives of children with central-nervous-system neoplasms. N Engl J Med 311: 749-753.
552. Farwell JR, Dohrmann GJ, Flannery JT (1984). Medulloblastoma in childhood: an epidemiological study. J Neurosurg 61: 657-664.
553. Fassett DR, Pingree J, Kestle JR (2005). The high incidence of tumor dissemination in myxopapillary ependymoma in pediatric patients. Report of five cases and review of the literature. J Neurosurg 102: 59-64.
554. Fauchon F, Jouvet A, Paquis P, Saint-Pierre G, Mottolese C, Ben Hassel M, Chauveinc L, Sichez JP, Philippon J, Schlienger M, Bouffet E (2000). Parenchymal pineal tumors: a clinicopathological study of 76 cases. Int J Radiat Oncol Biol Phys 46: 959-968.
555. Favara BE, Feller AC, Pauli M, Jaffe ES, Weiss LM, Arico M, Bucsky P, Egeler RM, Elinder G, Gadner H, Gresik M, Henter JI, Imashuku S, Janka-Schaub G, Jaffe R, Ladisch S, Nezelof C, Pritchard J (1997). Contemporary classification of histiocytic disorders. The WHO Committee On Histiocytic/Reticulum Cell Proliferations. Reclassification Working Group of the Histiocyte Society. Med Pediatr Oncol 29: 157-166.
556. Fecci PE, Mitchell DA, Whitesides JF, Xie W, Friedman AH, Archer GE, Herndon JE, Bigner DD, Dranoff G, Sampson JH (2006). Increased regulatory T-cell fraction amidst a diminished CD4 compartment explains cellular immune defects in patients with malignant glioma. Cancer Res 66: 3294-3302.
557. Fecci PE, Sweeney AE, Grossi PM, Nair SK, Learn CA, Mitchell DA, Cui X, Cummings TJ, Bigner DD, Gilboa E, Sampson JH (2006). Systemic anti-CD25 monoclonal antibody administration safely enhances immunity in murine glioma without eliminating regulatory T cells. Clin Cancer Res 12: 4294-4305.
558. Fecteau AH, Penn I, Hanto DW (1998). Peritoneal metastasis of intracranial glioblastoma via a ventriculoperitoneal shunt preventing organ retrieval: case report and review of the literature. Clin Transplant 12: 348-350.
559. Feigin I, Ransohoff J, Lieberman A (1976). Sarcoma arising in oligodendroglioma of the brain. J Neuropathol Exp Neurol 35: 679-684.
560. Feigin IM, Allen LB, Lipkin L, Gross SW (1958). The endothelial hyperplasia of the cerebral blood vessels, and its sarcomatous transformation. Cancer 11: 264-277.
561. Feigin IM, Gross SW (1955). Sarcoma arising in glioblastoma of the brain. Am J Pathol 31: 633-653.
562. Felix I, Becker LE (1990). Intracranial germ cell tumors in children: an immunohistochemical and electron microscopic study. Pediatr Neurosurg 16: 156-162.
563. Felsberg J, Erkwoh A, Sabel MC, Kirsch L, Fimmers R, Blaschke B, Schlegel U, Schramm J, Wiestler OD, Reifenberger G (2004). Oligodendroglial tumors: refinement of candidate regions on chromosome arm 1p and correlation of 1p/19q status with survival. Brain Pathol 14: 121-130.
564. Fernandez C, Bouvier C, Sevenet N, Liprandi A, Coze C, Lena G, Figarella-Branger D (2002). Congenital disseminated malignant rhabdoid tumor and cerebellar tumor mimicking medulloblastoma in monozygotic twins: pathologic and molecular diagnosis. Am J Surg Pathol 26: 266-270.
565. Fernandez C, Figarella-Branger D, Girard N, Bouvier-Labit C, Gouvernet J, Paz PA, Lena G (2003). Pilocytic astrocytomas in children: prognostic factors—a retrospective study of 80 cases. Neurosurgery 53: 544-553.
566. Fernandez C, Girard N, Paz PA, Bouvier-Labit C, Lena G, Figarella-Branger D (2003). The usefulness of MR imaging in the diagnosis of dysembryoplastic neuroepithelial tumor in children: a study of 14 cases. AJNR Am J Neuroradiol 24: 829-834.
567. Ferraresi S, Servello D, De Lorenzi L, Allegranza A (1989). Familial frontal lobe oligodendroglioma. Case report. J Neurosurg Sci 33: 317-318.
568. Ferrer I, Fabregues I, Coll J, Ribalta T, Rives A (1984). Tuberous sclerosis: a Golgi study of cortical tuber. Clin Neuropathol 3: 47-51.
569. Ferreri AJ, Dell'Oro S, Capello D, Ponzoni M, Iuzzolino P, Rossi D, Pasini F, Ambrosetti A, Orvieto E, Ferrarese F, Arrigoni G, Foppoli M, Reni M, Gaidano G (2004). Aberrant methylation in the promoter region of the reduced folate carrier gene is a potential mechanism of resistance to methotrexate in primary central nervous system lymphomas. Br J Haematol 126: 657-664.
570. Ferretti E, Di Marcotullio L, Gessi M, Mattei T, Greco A, Po A, De Smaele E, Giangaspero F, Riccardi R, Di Rocco C, Pazzaglia S, Maroder M, Alimandi M, Screpanti I, Gulino A (2006). Alternative splicing of the ErbB-4 cytoplasmic domain and its regulation by hedgehog signaling identify distinct medulloblastoma subsets. Oncogene 25: 7267-7273.
571. Fetsch JF, Miettinen M (1997). Sclerosing perineurioma: a clinicopathologic study of 19 cases of a distinctive soft tissue lesion with a predilection for the fingers and palms of young adults. Am J Surg Pathol 21: 1433-1442.
572. Fevre-Montange M, Champier J, Szathmari A, Wierinckx A, Mottolese C, Guyotat J, Figarella-Branger D, Jouvet A, Lachuer J (2006). Microarray analysis reveals differential gene expression patterns in tumors of the pineal region. J Neuropathol Exp Neurol 65: 675-684.
573. Fevre-Montange M, Hasselblatt M, Figarella-Branger D, Chauveinc L, Champier J, Saint-Pierre G, Taillandier L, Coulon A, Paulus W, Fauchon F, Jouvet A (2006). Prognosis and Histopathologic Features in Papillary Tumors of the Pineal Region: A Retrospective Multicenter Study of 31 Cases. J Neuropathol Exp Neurol 65: 1004-1011.
574. Fevre-Montange M, Jouvet A, Privat K, Korf HW, Champier J, Reboul A, Aguera M, Mottolese C (1998). Immunohistochemical, ultrastructural, biochemical and in vitro studies of a pineocytoma. Acta Neuropathol 95: 532-539.
575. Fewings PE, Bhattacharyya D, Crooks D, Morris K (2002). B cell non-Hodgkin cerebral lymphoma associated with an anaplastic oligodendroglioma. Clin Neuropathol 21: 243-247.
576. Figarella-Branger D, Dufour H, Fernandez C, Bouvier-Labit C, Grisoli F, Pellissier JF (2002). Pituicytomas, a mis-diagnosed benign tumor of the neurohypophysis: report of three cases. Acta Neuropathol 104: 313-319.
577. Figarella-Branger D, Gambarelli D, Dollo C, Devictor B, Perez-Castillo AM, Genitori L, Lena G, Choux M, Pellissier JF (1991). Infratentorial ependymomas of childhood. Correlation between histological features, immunohistological phenotype, silver nucleolar organizer region staining values and post-operative survival in 16 cases. Acta Neuropathol 82: 208-216.
578. Figarella-Branger D, Gambarelli D, Perez-Castillo M, Gentet JC, Grisoli F, Pellissier JF (1992). Ectopic intrapelvic medulloepithelioma: case report. Neuropathol Appl Neurobiol 18: 408-414.
579. Figarella B, Durbec PL, Rougon GN (1990). Differential spectrum of expression of neural cell adhesion molecule isoforms and L1 adhesion molecules on human neuroectodermal tumors. Cancer Res 50: 6364-6370.
580. Figarella B, Pellissier JF, Daumas D, Delisle MB, Pasquier B, Parent M, Gambarelli D, Rougon G, Hassoun J (1992). Central neurocytomas. Critical evaluation of a small-cell neuronal tumor. Am J Surg Pathol 16: 97-109.
581. Fine HA, Mayer RJ (1993). Primary central nervous system lymphoma. Ann Intern Med 119: 1093-1104.
582. Fine SW, McClain SA, Li M (2004). Immunohistochemical staining for calretinin is useful for differentiating schwannomas from neurofibromas. Am J Clin Pathol 122: 552-559.
583. Finn WG, Peterson LC, James C, Goolsby CL (1998). Enhanced detection of malignant lymphoma in cerebrospinal fluid by multiparameter flow cytometry. Am J Clin Pathol 110: 341-346.
583A. Fischer I, Gagner JP, Law M, Newcomb EW, Zagzag D (2005). Angiogenesis in gliomas: biology and molecular pathophysiology. Brain Pathol. 15:297-310.
584. Fix SE, Nelson J, Schochet SS, Jr. (1989). Focal leptomeningeal rhabdomyomatosis of the posterior fossa. Arch Pathol Lab Med 113: 872-873.
585. Flament-Durand J, Brion JP (1985). Tanycytes: morphology and functions: a review. Int Rev Cytol 96:121-155.
586. Fletcher CD (2006). The evolving classification of soft tissue tumours: an update based on the new WHO classification. Histopathology 48: 3-12.
587. Fletcher CDM, Unni KK, Mertens F eds. (2002). WHO Classification of Tumours: Pathology and Genetics of Tumours of Soft Tissue and Bone. IARC Press: Lyon.
588. Fogarty MP, Kessler JD, Wechsler-Reya RJ (2005). Morphing into cancer: the role of developmental signaling pathways in brain tumor formation. J Neurobiol 64: 458-475.
589. Foley KM, Woodruff JM, Ellis FT, Posner JB (1980). Radiation-induced malignant and atypical peripheral nerve sheath tumors. Ann Neurol 7: 311-318.
590. Folpe AL, Billings SD, McKenney JK, Walsh SV, Nusrat A, Weiss SW (2002). Expression of claudin-1, a recently described tight junction-associated protein, distinguishes soft tissue perineurioma from potential mimics. Am J Surg Pathol 26: 1620-1626.
591. Font RL, Truong LD (1984). Melanotic schwannoma of soft tissues. Electron-microscopic observations and review of literature. Am J Surg Pathol 8: 129-138.
592. Forsyth PA, Shaw EG, Scheithauer BW, O'Fallon JR, Layton DD, Jr., Katzmann JA (1993). Supratentorial pilocytic astrocytomas. A clinicopathologic, prognostic, and flow cytometric study of 51 patients. Cancer 72: 1335-1342.
593. Fort DW, Tonk VS, Tomlinson GE, Timmons CF, Schneider NR (1994). Rhabdoid tumor of the kidney with primitive neuroectodermal tumor of the central nervous system: associated tumors with different histologic, cytogenetic, and molecular findings. Genes Chromosomes Cancer 11: 146-152.
594. Fortuna A, Celli P, Palma L (1980). Oligodendrogliomas of the spinal cord. Acta Neurochir 52: 305-329.
595. Foster RD, Williams ML, Barkovich AJ, Hoffman WY, Mathes SJ, Frieden IJ (2001). Giant congenital melanocytic nevi: the significance of neurocutaneous melanosis in neurologically asymptomatic children. Plast Reconstr Surg 107: 933-941.
596. Fouladi M, Helton K, Dalton J, Gilger E,

Gajjar A, Merchant T, Kun L, Newsham I, Burger P, Fuller C (2003). Clear cell ependymoma: a clinicopathologic and radiographic analysis of 10 patients. Cancer 98: 2232-2244.
597. Fouladi M, Jenkins J, Burger P, Langston J, Merchant T, Heideman R, Thompson S, Sanford A, Kun L, Gajjar A (2001). Pleomorphic xanthoastrocytoma: favorable outcome after complete surgical resection. Neuro-oncol 3: 184-192.
598. Fountas KN, Kapsalaki E, Kassam M, Feltes CH, Dimopoulos VG, Robinson JS, Smith JR (2006). Management of intracranial meningeal hemangiopericytomas: outcome and experience. Neurosurg Rev 29: 145-153.
599. Fountas KN, Karampelas I, Nikolakakos LG, Troup EC, Robinson JS (2005). Primary spinal cord oligodendroglioma: case report and review of the literature. Childs Nerv Syst 21: 171-175.
600. Fourney DR, Siadati A, Bruner JM, Gokaslan ZL, Rhines LD (2004). Giant cell ependymoma of the spinal cord. Case report and review of the literature. J Neurosurg 100: 75-79.
601. Fowler M, Simpson DA (1962). Malignant melanin-forming tumour of the cerebellum. J Pathol Bacteriol 84: 307-311.
602. Frank AJ, Hernan R, Hollander A, Lindsey JC, Lusher ME, Fuller CE, Clifford SC, Gilbertson RJ (2004). The TP53-ARF tumor suppressor pathway is frequently disrupted in large/cell anaplastic medulloblastoma. Brain Res Mol Brain Res 121: 137-140.
603. Franks AJ (1985). Epithelioid neurilemmoma of the trigeminal nerve: an immunohistochemical and ultrastructural study. Histopathology 9: 1339-1350.
604. Franz DN, Leonard J, Tudor C, Chuck G, Care M, Sethuraman G, Dinopoulos A, Thomas G, Crone KR (2006). Rapamycin causes regression of astrocytomas in tuberous sclerosis complex. Ann Neurol 59: 490-498.
605. Frappaz D, Ricci AC, Kohler R, Bret P, Mottolese C (1999). Diffuse brain stem tumor in an adolescent with multiple enchondromatosis (Ollier's disease). Childs Nerv Syst 15: 222-225.
606. Frebourg T, Barbier N, Yan YX, Garber JE, Dreyfus M, Fraumeni J, Jr., Li FP, Friend SH (1995). Germ-line p53 mutations in 15 families with Li-Fraumeni syndrome. Am J Hum Genet 56: 608-615.
607. Frederick L, Eley G, Wang XY, James CD (2000). Analysis of genomic rearrangements associated with EGFRvIII expression suggests involvement of Alu repeat elements. Neuro-oncol 2: 159-163.
608. Freije WA, Castro-Vargas FE, Fang Z, Horvath S, Cloughesy T, Liau LM, Mischel PS, Nelson SF (2004). Gene expression profiling of gliomas strongly predicts survival. Cancer Res 64: 6503-6510.
609. Freilich RJ, Thompson SJ, Walker RW, Rosenblum MK (1995). Adenocarcinomatous transformation of intracranial germ cell tumors. Am J Surg Pathol 19: 537-544.
610. Frenk E, Marazzi A (1984). Neurofibromatosis of von Recklinghausen: a quantitative study of the epidermal keratinocyte and melanocyte populations. J Invest Dermatol 83: 23-25.
611. Freudenstein D, Wagner A, Bornemann A, Ernemann U, Bauer T, Duffner F (2004). Primary melanocytic lesions of the CNS: report of five cases. Zentralbl Neurochir 65: 146-153.
612. Friede RL (1978). Gliofibroma: a peculiar neoplasia of collagen forming glia-like cells. J Neuropath Exp Neurol 37: 300-313.
613. Friedman HS, Kokkinakis DM, Pluda J, Friedman AH, Cokgor I, Haglund MM, Ashley DM, Rich J, Dolan ME, Pegg AE, Moschel RC, McLendon RE, Kerby T, Herndon JE, Bigner DD, Schold SC, Jr. (1998). Phase I trial of O6-benzylguanine for patients undergoing surgery for malignant glioma. J Clin Oncol 16: 3570-3575.
614. Friedman JA, Lynch JJ, Buckner JC, Scheithauer BW, Raffel C (2001). Management of malignant pineal germ cell tumors with residual mature teratoma. Neurosurgery 48: 518-522.
614A Fritz A, Percy C, Jack A, Shanmugaratham K, Sobin L, Parkin MD, Whelan S (eds.) (2000). International Classification of Diseases fon Oncology, Third Edition, World Health Organisation, Geneva.
615. Frost G, Patel K, Bourne S, Coakham HB, Kemshead JT (1991). Expression of alternative isoforms of the neural cell adhesion molecule (NCAM) on normal brain and a variety of brain tumours. Neuropathol Appl Neurobiol 17: 207-217.
616. Fruhwald MC, Hasselblatt M, Wirth S, Kohler G, Schneppenheim R, Subero JI, Siebert R, Kordes U, Jurgens H, Vormoor J (2006). Non-linkage of familial rhabdoid tumors to SMARCB1 implies a second locus for the rhabdoid tumor predisposition syndrome. Pediatr Blood Cancer 47: 273-278.
617. Fu YS, Chen AT, Kay S, Young H (1974). Is subependymoma (subependymal glomerate astrocytoma) an astrocytoma or ependymoma? A comparative ultrastructural and tissue culture study. Cancer 34: 1992-2008.
618. Fujimaki T, Matsutani M, Funada N, Kirino T, Takakura K, Nakamura O, Tamura A, Sano K (1994). CT and MRI features of intracranial germ cell tumors. J Neurooncol 19: 217-226.
619. Fujimoto K, Ohnishi H, Tsujimoto M, Hoshida T, Nakazato Y (2000). Dysembryoplastic neuroepithelial tumor of the cerebellum and brainstem. Case report. J Neurosurg 93: 487-489.
620. Fujisawa H, Kurrer M, Reis RM, Yonekawa Y, Kleihues P, Ohgaki H (1999). Acqusition of the glioblastoma phenotype during astrocytoma progression is associated with LOH on 10q25-qter. Am J Pathol 155: 387-394.
621. Fujisawa H, Marukawa K, Hasegawa M, Tohma Y, Hayashi Y, Uchiyama N, Tachibana O, Yamashita J (2002). Genetic differences between neurocytoma and dysembryoplastic neuroepithelial tumor and oligodendroglial tumors. J Neurosurg 97: 1350-1355.
622. Fujisawa H, Reis RM, Nakamura M, Colella S, Yonekawa Y, Kleihues P, Ohgaki H (2000). Loss of heterozygosity on chromosome 10 is more extensive in primary (de novo) than in secondary glioblastomas. Lab Invest 80: 65-72.
622A. Fujisawa H, Takabatake Y, Fukusato T, Tachibana O, Tsuchiya Y, Yamashita J (2003). Molecular analysis of the rhabdoid predisposition syndrome in a child: a novel germline hSNF5/INI1 mutation and absence of c-myc amplification. J Neurooncol 63:257-262.
623. Fukunaga M (2001). Unusual malignant perineurioma of soft tissue. Virchows Arch 439: 212-214.
624. Fukushima T, Favereaux A, Huang H, Shimizu T, Yonekawa Y, Nakazato Y, Ohgaki H (2006). Genetic alterations in primary glioblastomas in Japan. J Neuropathol Exp Neurol 65: 12-18.
625. Fulda S, Debatin KM (2006). 5-Aza-2'-deoxycytidine and IFN-gamma cooperate to sensitize for TRAIL-induced apoptosis by upregulating caspase-8. Oncogene 25: 5125-5133.
626. Fulham MJ, Melisi JW, Nishimiya J, Dwyer AJ, Di Chiro G (1993). Neuroimaging of juvenile pilocytic astrocytomas: an enigma. Radiology 189: 221-225.
627. Fuller C, Fouladi M, Gajjar A, Dalton J, Sanford RA, Helton KJ (2006). Chromosome 17 abnormalities in pediatric neuroblastic tumor with abundant neuropil and true rosettes. Am J Clin Pathol 126: 277-283.
628. Fuller CE, Schmidt RE, Roth KA, Burger PC, Scheithauer BW, Banerjee R, Trinkaus K, Lytle R, Perry A (2003). Clinical utility of fluorescence in situ hybridization (FISH) in morphologically ambiguous gliomas with hybrid oligodendroglial/astrocytic features. J Neuropathol Exp Neurol 62: 1118-1128.
629. Fuller GN, Bigner SH (1992). Amplified cellular oncogenes in neoplasms of the human central nervous system. Mutat Res 276: 299-306.
630. Fuller GN, Hess KR, Rhee CH, Yung WK, Sawaya RA, Bruner JM, Zhang W (2002). Molecular classification of human diffuse gliomas by multidimensional scaling analysis of gene expression profiles parallels morphology-based classification, correlates with survival, and reveals clinically-relevant novel glioma subsets. Brain Pathol 12: 108-116.
631. Fuller GN, Su X, Price RE, Cohen ZR, Lang FF, Sawaya R, Majumder S (2005). Many human medulloblastoma tumors overexpress repressor element-1 silencing transcription (REST)/neuron-restrictive silencer factor, which can be functionally countered by REST-VP16. Mol Cancer Ther 4: 343-349.
632. Fults D, Pedone C (1993). Deletion mapping of the long arm of chromosome 10 in glioblastoma multiforme. Genes Chromosomes Cancer 7: 173-177.
633. Fults D, Pedone CA, Thomas GA, White R (1990). Allelotype of human malignant astrocytoma. Cancer Res 50: 5784-5789.
634. Fults D, Pedone CA, Thompson GE, Uchiyama CM, Gumpper KL, Iliev D, Vinson VL, Tavtigian SV, Perry WL, III (1998). Microsatellite deletion mapping on chromosome 10q and mutation analysis of MMAC1, FAS, and MXI1 in human glioblastoma multiforme. Int J Oncol 12: 905-910.
635. Fung KM, Trojanowski JQ (1995). Animal models of medulloblastomas and related primitive neuroectodermal tumors. A review. J Neuropath Exp Neurol 54: 285-296.
636. Furie DM, Provenzale JM (1995). Supratentorial ependymomas and subependymomas: CT and MR appearance. J Comput Assist Tomogr 19: 518-526.
637. Gadish T, Tulchinsky H, Deutsch AA, Rabau M (2005). Pinealoblastoma in a patient with familial adenomatous polyposis: variant of Turcot syndrome type 2? Report of a case and review of the literature. Dis Colon Rectum 48: 2343-2346.
638. Gaffney EF, Doorly T, Dinn JJ (1986). Aggressive oncocytic neuroendocrine tumour ('oncocytic paraganglioma') of the cauda equina. Histopathology 10: 311-319.
639. Gailani MR, Stahle B, Leffell DJ, Glynn M, Zaphiropoulos PG, Pressman C, Unden AB, Dean M, Brash DE, Bale AE, Toftgard R (1996). The role of the human homologue of Drosophila patched in sporadic basal cell carcinomas. Nat Genet 14: 78-81.
640. Gajjar A, Bhargava R, Jenkins JJ, Heideman R, Sanford RA, Langston JW, Walter AW, Kuttesch JF, Muhlbauer M, Kun LE (1995). Low-grade astrocytoma with neuraxis dissemination at diagnosis. J Neurosurg 83: 67-71.
641. Galanis E, Buckner JC, Dinapoli RP, Scheithauer BW, Jenkins RB, Wang CH, O'Fallon JR, Farr G, Jr. (1998). Clinical outcome of gliosarcoma compared with glioblastoma multiforme: North Central Cancer Treatment Group results. J Neurosurg 89: 425-430.
642. Galatioto S, Marafioti T, Cavallari V, Batolo D (1993). Gliomatosis cerebri. Clinical, neuropathological, immunohistochemical and morphometric studies. Zentralbl Pathol 139: 261-267.
643. Galli R, Binda E, Orfanelli U, Cipelletti B, Gritti A, De Vitis S, Fiocco R, Foroni C, Dimeco F, Vescovi A (2004). Isolation and characterization of tumorigenic, stem-like neural precursors from human glioblastoma. Cancer Res 64: 7011-7021.
644. Gander M, Leyvraz S, Decosterd L, Bonfanti M, Marzolini C, Shen F, Lienard D, Perey L, Colella G, Biollaz J, Lejeune F, Yarosh D, Belanich M, D'Incalci M (1999). Sequential administration of temozolomide and fotemustine: depletion of O6-alkyl guanine-DNA transferase in blood lymphocytes and in tumours. Ann Oncol 10: 831-838.
645. Ganesan K, Desai S, Udwadia-Hegde A (2006). Non-infantile variant of desmoplastic ganglioglioma: a report of 2 cases. Pediatr Radiol 36: 541-545.
646. Gao X, Zhang Y, Arrazola P, Hino O, Kobayashi T, Yeung RS, Ru B, Pan D (2002). Tsc tumour suppressor proteins antagonize amino-acid-TOR signalling. Nat Cell Biol 4: 699-704.
647. Garcia B, Cabello A, Guarch R, Ruiz dA, Ezpeleta I (1990). [Melanotic medulloblastoma. Ultrastructural and histochemical study of a case]. Arch Neurobiol Madr 53: 8-12.
648. Garcia DM, Fulling KH (1985). Juvenile pilocytic astrocytoma of the cerebrum in adults. A distinctive neoplasm with favorable prognosis. J Neurosurg 63: 382-386.
649. Garner A, Klinworth GK (1982). Tumors of the orbit, optic nerve and lacrimal sace. In: Pathobiology of ocular disease. Pathobiology of ocular disease. Marcel Dekker: New York, pp. 741.
650. Garty BZ, Laor A, Danon YL (1994). Neurofibromatosis type 1 in Israel: survey of young adults. J Med Genet 31: 853-857.
651. Gaspar L, Scott C, Rotman M, Asbell S, Phillips T, Wasserman T, McKenna WG, Byhardt R (1997). Recursive partitioning analysis (RPA) of prognostic factors in three Radiation Therapy Oncology Group (RTOG) brain metastases trials. Int J Radiat Oncol Biol Phys 37: 745-751.
652. Gaspar LE, Mackenzie IR, Gilbert JJ, Kaufmann JC, Fisher BF, Macdonald DR, Cairncross JG (1993). Primary cerebral fibrosarcomas. Clinicopathologic study and review of the literature. Cancer 72: 3277-3281.
653. Gaspar N, Grill J, Geoerger B, Lellouch-Tubiana A, Michalowski MB, Vassal G (2006). p53 Pathway dysfunction in primary childhood ependymomas. Pediatr Blood Cancer 46: 604-613.
654. Gavrilovic IT, Posner JB (2005). Brain metastases: epidemiology and pathophysiology. J Neurooncol 75: 5-14.
655. Geddes JF, Thom M, Robinson SFD, Revesz T (1996). Granular cell change in astrocytic tumors. Am J Surg Pathol 20: 55-63.
656. Gelabert-Gonzalez M (2005). Paragangliomas of the lumbar region. Report of two cases and review of the literature. J Neurosurg Spine 2: 354-365.
657. Gengler C, Guillou L (2006). Solitary fibrous tumour and haemangiopericytoma: evolution of a concept. Histopathology 48: 63-74.
658. George DH, Scheithauer BW (2001). Central liponeurocytoma. Am J Surg Pathol 25: 1551-1555.
659. George DH, Scheithauer BW, Aker FV, Kurtin PJ, Burger PC, Cameselle-Teijeiro J, McLendon RE, Parisi JE, Paulus W, Roggendorf W, Sotelo C (2003). Primary anaplastic large cell lymphoma of the central nervous system: prognostic effect of ALK-1 expression. Am J Surg Pathol 27: 487-493.
660. Gessi M, Giangaspero F, Pietsch T

(2003). Atypical teratoid/rhabdoid tumors and choroid plexus tumors: when genetics "surprise" pathology. Brain Pathol 13: 409-414.
661. Gessi M, Marani C, Geddes J, Arcella A, Cenacchi G, Giangaspero F (2005). Ependymoma with neuropil-like islands: a case report with diagnostic and histogenetic implications. Acta Neuropathol 109: 231-234.
662. Geyer JR, Sposto R, Jennings M, Boyett JM, Axtell RA, Breiger D, Broxson E, Donahue B, Finlay JL, Goldwein JW, Heier LA, Johnson D, Mazewski C, Miller DC, Packer R, Puccetti D, Radcliffe J, Tao ML, Shiminski-Maher T (2005). Multiagent chemotherapy and deferred radiotherapy in infants with malignant brain tumors: a report from the Children's Cancer Group. J Clin Oncol 23: 7621-7631.
663. Geyer JR, Zeltzer PM, Boyett JM, Rorke LB, Stanley P, Albright AL, Wisoff JH, Milstein JM, Allen JC, Finlay JL, Ayers GD, Shurin SB, Stevens KR, Bleyer WA (1994). Survival of infants with primitive neuroectodermal tumors or malignant ependymomas of the CNS treated with eight drugs in 1 day: a report from the Childrens Cancer Group. J Clin Oncol 12: 1607-1615.
664. Gherardi R, Baudrimont M, Nguyen JP, Gaston A, Cesaro P, Degos JD, Caron JP, Poirier J (1986). Monstrocellular heavily lipidized malignant glioma. Acta Neuropathol 69: 28-32.
665. Gi H, Nagao S, Yoshizumi H, Nishioka T, Uno J, Shingu T, Fujita Y (1990). Meningioma with hypergammaglobulinemia. Case report. J Neurosurg 73: 628-629.
666. Giangaspero F, Cenacchi G, Losi L, Cerasoli S, Bisceglia M, Burger PC (1997). Extraventricular neoplasms with neurocytoma features: A clinicopathological study of11 cases. Am J Surg Pathol 21: 206-212.
667. Giangaspero F, Cenacchi G, Roncaroli F, Rigobello L, Manetto V, Gambacorta M, Allegranza A (1996). Medullocytoma (lipidized medulloblastoma): a cerebellar neoplasm of adults with favorable prognosis. Am J Surg Pathol 20: 656-664.
668. Giangaspero F, Chieco P, Ceccarelli C, Lisignoli G, Pozuolli R, Gambacorta M, Rossi G, Burger PC (1991). "Desmoplastic" versus "classic" medulloblastoma: comparison of DNA content, histopathology and differentiation. Virchows Arch A Pathol Anat Histopathol 418: 207-214.
669. Giangaspero F, Perilongo G, Fondelli MP, Brisigotti M, Carollo C, Burnelli R, Burger PC, Garre ML (1999). Medulloblastoma with extensive nodularity: a variant with favorable prognosis. J Neurosurg 91: 971-977.
670. Giangaspero F, Rigobello L, Badiali M, Loda M, Andreini L, Basso G, Zorzi F, Montaldi A (1992). Large-cell medulloblastomas. A distinct variant with highly aggressive behavior. Am J Surg Pathol 16: 687-693.
671. Giangaspero F, Wellek S, Masuoka J, Gessi M, Kleihues P, Ohgaki H (2006). Stratification of medulloblastoma on the basis of histopathological grading. Acta Neuropathol 112: 5-12.
672. Giani C, Finocchiaro G (1994). Mutation rate of the CDKN2 gene in malignant gliomas. Cancer Res 54: 6338-6339.
673. Giannini C, Hebrink D, Scheithauer BW, Dei Tos AP, James CD (2001). Analysis of p53 mutation and expression in pleomorphic xanthoastrocytoma. Neurogenetics 3: 159-162.
673A. Giannini C, Scheithauer BW, Lopes MBS, Hirose T, Kros M, VandenBerg SR, (2002). Immunophenotype of pleomorphic xanthoastrocytoma. Am J Surg Pathol 26:479-485.
674. Giannini C, Scheithauer BW (1997). Classification and grading of low-grade astrocytic tumors in children. Brain Pathol 7: 785-798.
675. Giannini C, Scheithauer BW, Burger PC, Brat DJ, Wollan PC, Lach B, O'Neill BP (1999). Pleomorphic xanthoastrocytoma: what do we really know about it? Cancer 85: 2033-2045.
676. Giannini C, Scheithauer BW, Burger PC, Christensen MR, Wollan PC, Sebo TJ, Forsyth PA, Hayostek CJ (1999). Cellular proliferation in pilocytic and diffuse astrocytomas. J Neuropathol Exp Neurol 58: 46-53.
677. Giannini C, Scheithauer BW, Jenkins RB, Erlandson RA, Perry A, Borell TJ, Hoda RS, Woodruff JM (1997). Soft-tissue perineurioma. Evidence for an abnormality of chromosome 22, criteria for diagnosis, and review of the literature. Am J Surg Pathol 21: 164-173.
678. Giannini C, Scheithauer BW, Lopes MB, Hirose T, Kros JM, VandenBerg SR (2002). Immunophenotype of pleomorphic xanthoastrocytoma. Am J Surg Pathol 26: 479-485.
679. Giannini C, Scheithauer BW, Steinberg J, Cosgrove TJ (1998). Intraventricular perineurioma: case report. Neurosurgery 43: 1478-1481.
680. Giannini C, Scheithauer BW, Weaver AL, Burger PC, Kros JM, Mork S, Graeber MB, Bauserman S, Buckner JC, Burton J, Riepe R, Tazelaar HD, Nascimento AG, Crotty T, Keeney GL, Pernicone P, Altermatt H (2001). Oligodendrogliomas: reproducibility and prognostic value of histologic diagnosis and grading. J Neuropathol Exp Neurol 60: 248-262.
681. Giese A, Loo MA, Tran N, Haskett D, Coons SW, Berens ME (1996). Dichotomy of astrocytoma migration and proliferation. Int J Cancer 67: 275-282.
682. Gijtenbeek JM, Jacobs B, Sprenger SH, Eleveld MJ, van Kessel AG, Kros JM, Sciot R, Van Calenbergh F, Wesseling P, Jeuken JW (2002). Analysis of von hippel-lindau mutations with comparative genomic hybridization in sporadic and hereditary hemangioblastomas: possible genetic heterogeneity. J Neurosurg 97: 977-982.
683. Gil-Gouveia R, Cristino N, Farias JP, Trindade A, Ruivo NS, Pimentel J (2004). Pleomorphic xanthoastrocytoma of the cerebellum: illustrated review. Acta Neurochir 146: 1241-1244.
684. Gilbertson RJ, Clifford SC (2003). PDGFRB is overexpressed in metastatic medulloblastoma. Nat Genet 35: 197-198.
685. Gilbertson RJ, Jaros E, Perry RH, Kelly PJ, Lunec J, Pearson AD (1997). Mitotic percentage index: a new prognostic factor for childhood medulloblastoma. Eur J Cancer 33: 609-615.
686. Gilbertson RJ, Perry RH, Kelly PJ, Pearson AD, Lunec J (1997). Prognostic significance of HER2 and HER4 coexpression in childhood medulloblastoma. Cancer Res 57: 3272-3280.
687. Giordana MT, Bradac GB, Pagni CA, Marino S, Attanasio A (1995). Primary diffuse leptomeningeal gliomatosis with anaplastic features. Acta Neurochir 132: 154-159.
688. Giordana MT, Cavalla P, Chio A, Marino S, Soffietti R, Vigliani MC, Schiffer D (1995). Prognostic factors in adult medulloblastoma. A clinico- pathologic study. Tumori 81: 338-346.
689. Giordana MT, Schiffer P, Boghi A, Buoncristiani P, Benech F (2000). Medulloblastoma with lipidized cells versus lipomatous medulloblastoma. Clin Neuropathol 19: 273-277.
690. Giordana MT, Schiffer P, Lanotte M, Girardi P, Chio A (1999). Epidemiology of adult medulloblastoma. Int J Cancer 80: 689-692.
691. Giulioni M, Galassi E, Zucchelli M, Volpi L (2005). Seizure outcome of lesionectomy in glioneuronal tumors associated with epilepsy in children. J Neurosurg 102: 288-293.
692. Gjerris F, Klinken L (1978). Long-term prognosis in children with benign cerebellar astrocytoma. J Neurosurg 49: 179-184.
693. Glasker S, Bender BU, Apel TW, Natt E, van Velthoven V, Scheremet R, Zentner J, Neumann HPH (1999). The impact of molecular genetic analysis of the VHL gene in patients with hemangioblastomas of the central nervous system. J Neurol Neurosurg Psychiatry 67: 758-762.
694. Glasker S, Bender BU, Apel TW, van Velthoven V, Mulligan LM, Zentner J, Neumann HP (2001). Reconsideration of biallelic inactivation of the VHL tumour suppressor gene in hemangioblastomas of the central nervous system. J Neurol Neurosurg Psychiatry 70: 644-648.
695. Glasker S, Berlis A, Pagenstecher A, Vougioukas VI, van V, V (2005). Characterization of hemangioblastomas of spinal nerves. Neurosurgery 56: 503-509.
695A. Glasker S, Tran MG, Shively SB, Ikejiri B, Lonser RR, Maxwell PH, Zhuang Z, Oldfield EH, Vortmeyer AO (2006). Epididymal cystadenomas and epithelial tumourlets: effects of VHL deficiency on the human epididymis. J Pathol 210: 32-41.
696. Glasker S, Li J, Xia JB, Okamoto H, Zeng W, Lonser RR, Zhuang Z, Oldfield EH, Vortmeyer AO (2006). Hemangioblastomas share protein expression with embryonal hemangioblast progenitor cell. Cancer Res 66: 4167-4172.
697. Glass J, Hochberg FH, Gruber ML, Louis DN, Smith D, Rattner B (1992). The treatment of oligodendrogliomas and mixed oligodendroglioma- astrocytomas with PCV chemotherapy. J Neurosurg 76: 741-745.
698. Glavac D, Neumann HP, Wittke C, Jaenig H, Masek O, Streicher T, Pausch F, Engelhardt D, Plate KH, Hofler H, Chen F, Zbar B, Brauch H (1996). Mutations in the VHL tumor suppressor gene and associated lesions in families with von Hippel-Lindau disease from central Europe. Hum Genet 98: 271-280.
699. Gleissner B, Chamberlain MC (2006). Neoplastic meningitis. Lancet Neurol 5: 443-452.
700. Gleissner B, Siehl J, Korfel A, Reinhardt R, Thiel E (2002). CSF evaluation in primary CNS lymphoma patients by PCR of the CDR III IgH genes. Neurology 58: 390-396.
701. Glick R, Baker C, Husain S, Hays A, Hibshoosh H (1997). Primary melanocytomas of the spinal cord: a report of seven cases. Clin Neuropathol 16: 127-132.
702. Godard S, Getz G, Delorenzi M, Farmer P, Kobayashi H, Desbaillets I, Nozaki M, Diserens AC, Hamou MF, Dietrich PY, Regli L, Janzer RC, Bucher P, Stupp R, de Tribolet N, Domany E, Hegi ME (2003). Classification of human astrocytic gliomas on the basis of gene expression: a correlated group of genes with angiogenic activity emerges as a strong predictor of subtypes. Cancer Res 63: 6613-6625.
703. Goebel HH, Cravioto H (1972). Ultrastructure of human and experimental ependymomas. A comparative study. J Neuropathol Exp Neurol 31: 54-71.
704. Goldman JE, Corbin E (1991). Rosenthal fibers contain ubiquitinated alpha B-crystallin. Am J Pathol 139: 933-938.
705. Gomez DR, Missett BT, Wara WM, Lamborn KR, Prados MD, Chang S, Berger MS, Haas-Kogan DA (2005). High failure rate in spinal ependymomas with long-term follow-up. Neuro-oncol 7: 254-259.
706. Gomez MR (1991). Phenotypes of the tuberous sclerosis complex with a revision of diagnostic criteria. Ann N Y Acad Sci 615: 1-7.
707. Gonzalez-Campora R, Weller RO (1998). Lipidized mature neuroectodermal tumour of the cerebellum with myoid differentiation. Neuropathol Appl Neurobiol 24: 397-402.
708. Gonzalez-Gomez P, Bello MJ, Arjona D, Alonso ME, Lomas J, Aminoso C, de Campos JM, Sarasa JL, Gutierrez M, Rey JA (2003). CpG island methylation of tumor-related genes in three primary central nervous system lymphomas in immunocompetent patients. Cancer Genet Cytogenet 142: 21-24.
709. Goodrich LV, Scott MP (1998). Hedgehog and patched in neural development and disease. Neuron 21: 1243-1257.
710. Gorlin RJ (1987). Nevoid basal cell carcinoma syndrome. Medicine 66: 98-113.
711. Gorski GK, McMorrow LE, Donaldson MH, Freed M (1992). Multiple chromosomal abnormalities in a case of craniopharyngioma. Cancer Genet Cytogenet 60: 212-213.
712. Gospodarowicz MK, O'Sullivan B, Sobin LH (2006). Prognostic factors in cancer. John Wiley & Sons Ltd: Canada.
713. Goth R, Rajewsky MF (1974). Persistence of O6-ethylguanine in rat-brain DNA: correlation with nervous system-specific carcinogenesis by ethylnitrosourea. Proc Natl Acad Sci U S A 71: 639-643.
714. Goto M, Miller RW, Ishikawa Y, Sugano H (1996). Excess of rare cancers in Werner syndrome (adult progeria). Cancer Epidemiol Biomarkers Prev 5: 239-246.
715. Gottschalk J, Jautzke G, Paulus W, Goebel S, Cervos N (1993). The use of immunomorphology to differentiate choroid plexus tumors from metastatic carcinomas. Cancer 72: 1343-1349.
716. Gould VE, Rorke LB, Jansson DS, Molenaar WM, Trojanowski JQ, Lee VM, Packer RJ, Franke WW (1990). Primitive neuroectodermal tumors of the central nervous system express neuroendocrine markers and may express all classes of intermediate filaments. Hum Pathol 21: 245-252.
717. Graadt van Roggen JF, McMenamin ME, Belchis DA, Nielsen GP, Rosenberg AE, Fletcher CD (2001). Reticular perineurioma: a distinctive variant of soft tissue perineurioma. Am J Surg Pathol 25: 485-493.
717A Graham JF, Stanley L, Matoba A (1999) Primary brain myxoma, an unusual tumor of meningeal origin. Neurosurg 45:166
718. Grant JW (1983). Histiocytic origin of the sarcomatous elements in gliosarcomas. Neuropathol Appl Neurobiol 9: 335.
719. Grant JW, Steart PV, Aguzzi A, Jones DB, Gallagher PJ (1989). Gliosarcoma: an immunohistochemical study. Acta Neuropathol 79: 305-309.
720. Green AJ, Smith M, Yates JR (1994). Loss of heterozygosity on chromosome 16p13.3 in hamartomas from tuberous sclerosis patients. Nat Genet 6: 193-196.
720A. Green WR, Iliff WJ, Trotter RR (1974). Malignant teratoid medulloepithelioma of the optic nerve. 91:451-4.
721. Griffin CA, Burger P, Morsberger L, Yonescu R, Swierczynski S, Weingart JD, Murphy KM (2006). Identification of der(1;19)(q10;p10) in five oligodendrogliomas suggests mechanism of concurrent 1p and 19q loss. J Neuropathol Exp Neurol 65: 988-994.
722. Griffin CA, Hawkins AL, Packer RJ, Rorke LB, Emanuel BS (1988). Chromosome abnormalities in pediatric brain tumors. Cancer Res 48: 175-180.
723. Grill J, Avet-Loiseau H, Lellouch-Tubiana A, Sevenet N, Terrier-Lacombe MJ, Venuat AM, Doz F, Sainte-Rose C, Kalifa C, Vassal G (2002). Comparative genomic hybridization detects specific cytogenetic abnormalities in pediatric ependymomas and choroid plexus papillomas. Cancer Genet Cytogenet 136: 121-125.
724. Grois N, Broadbent V, Favara BE,

D'Angio G (1997). Report of the Histiocyte Society workshop on "Central nervous system (CNS) disease in Langerhans cell histiocytosis (LCH)". Med Pediatr Oncol 29: 73-78.

725. Grois N, Prayer D, Prosch H, Lassmann H (2005). Neuropathology of CNS disease in Langerhans cell histiocytosis. Brain 128: 829-838.

726. Grosse G, Lindner G, Matthies HJ (1976). [Effect of orotic acid on the in vitro cultured nerve tissue]. Z Mikrosk Anat Forsch 90: 499-506.

727. Grossman RI, Yousem DM (1994). Neuroradiology. The Requisites. Mosby-Yearbook: St Louis.

728. Grotzer MA, Hogarty MD, Janss AJ, Liu X, Zhao H, Eggert A, Sutton LN, Rorke LB, Brodeur GM, Phillips PC (2001). MYC messenger RNA expression predicts survival outcome in childhood primitive neuroectodermal tumor/medulloblastoma. Clin Cancer Res 7: 2425-2433.

729. Grove A, Vyberg M (1993). Primary leptomeningeal T-cell lymphoma: a case and a review of primary T-cell lymphoma of the central nervous system. Clin Neuropathol 12: 7-12.

730. Grover WD, Rorke LB (1968). Invasive craniopharyngioma. J Neurol Neurosurg Psychiatry 31: 580-582.

731. Guermazi A, De Kerviler E, Zagdanski AM, Frija J (2000). Diagnostic imaging of choroid plexus disease. Clin Radiol 55: 503-516.

732. Guerrieri C, Jarlsfelt I (1993). Ependymoma of the ovary. A case report with immunohistochemical, ultrastructural, and DNA cytometric findings, as well as histogenetic considerations. Am J Surg Pathol 17: 623-632.

733. Guesmi H, Houtteville JP, Courtheoux P, Derlon JM, Chapon F (1999). [Dysembryoplastic neuroepithelial tumors. Report of 8 cases including two with unusual localization]. Neurochirurgie 45: 190-200.

734. Gultekin SH, Dalmau J, Graus Y, Posner JB, Rosenblum MK (1998). Anti-Hu immunolabeling as an index of neuronal differentiation in human brain tumors: a study of 112 central neuroepithelial neoplasms. Am J Surg Pathol 22: 195-200.

735. Gunny RS, Hayward RD, Phipps KP, Harding BN, Saunders DE (2005). Spontaneous regression of residual low-grade cerebellar pilocytic astrocytomas in children. Pediatr Radiol 35: 1086-1091.

736. Gusella JF, Ramesh V, MacCollin M, Jacoby LB (1996). Neurofibromatosis 2: loss of merlin's protective spell. Curr Opin Genet Dev 6: 87-92.

737. Gusella JF, Ramesh V, MacCollin M, Jacoby LB (1999). Merlin: the neurofibromatosis 2 tumor suppressor. Biochim Biophys Acta 1423: M29-M36.

738. Guthrie BL, Ebersold MJ, Scheithauer BW, Shaw EG (1989). Meningeal hemangiopericytoma: histopathological features, treatment, and long-term follow-up of 44 cases. Neurosurgery 25: 514-522.

739. Gutmann DH, Aylsworth A, Carey JC, Korf B, Marks J, Pyeritz RE, Rubenstein A, Viskochil D (1997). The diagnostic evaluation and multidisciplinary management of neurofibromatosis 1 and neurofibromatosis 2. JAMA 278: 51-57.

740. Gutmann DH, Donahoe J, Brown T, James CD, Perry A (2000). Loss of neurofibromatosis 1 (NF1) gene expression in NF1-associated pilocytic astrocytomas. Neuropathol Appl Neurobiol 26: 361-367.

741. Gutmann DH, Donahoe J, Perry A, Lemke N, Gorse K, Kittiniyom K, Rempel SA, Gutierrez JA, Newsham IF (2000). Loss of DAL-1, a protein 4.1-related tumor suppressor, is an important early event in the pathogenesis

of meningiomas. Hum Mol Genet 9: 1495-1500.

742. Gutmann DH, Hedrick NM, Li J, Nagarajan R, Perry A, Watson MA (2002). Comparative gene expression profile analysis of neurofibromatosis 1-associated and sporadic pilocytic astrocytomas. Cancer Res 62: 2085-2091.

743. Gyure KA, Morrison AL (2000). Cytokeratin 7 and 20 expression in choroid plexus tumors: utility in differentiating these neoplasms from metastatic carcinomas. Mod Pathol 13: 638-643.

744. Gyure KA, Prayson RA (1997). Subependymal giant cell astrocytoma: a clinicopathologic study with HMB-45 and MIB1 immunohistochemistry. Mod Pathol 10: 313-317.

745. Haas JE, Palmer NF, Weinberg AG, Beckwith JB (1981). Ultrastructure of malignant rhabdoid tumor of the kidney. A distinctive renal tumor of children. Hum Pathol 12: 646-657.

746. Haberler C, Jarius C, Lang S, Rossler K, Gruber A, Hainfellner JA, Budka H (2002). Fibrous meningeal tumours with extensive non-calcifying collagenous whorls and glial fibrillary acidic protein expression: the whorling-sclerosing variant of meningioma. Neuropathol Appl Neurobiol 28: 42-47.

747. Haberler C, Laggner U, Slavc I, Czech T, Ambros IM, Ambros PF, Budka H, Hainfellner JA (2006). Immunohistochemical Analysis of INI1 Protein in Malignant Pediatric CNS Tumors: Lack of INI1 in Atypical Teratoid/Rhabdoid Tumors and in a Fraction of Primitive Neuroectodermal Tumors without Rhabdoid Phenotype. Am J Surg Pathol 30: 1462-1468.

748. Haddad E, Sulis ML, Jabado N, Blanche S, Fischer A, Tardieu M (1997). Frequency and severity of central nervous system lesions in hemophagocytic lymphohistiocytosis. Blood 89: 794-800.

749. Haddad SF, Hitchon PW, Godersky JC (1991). Idiopathic and glucocorticoid-induced spinal epidural lipomatosis. J Neurosurg 74: 38-42.

750. Haddad SF, Moore SA, Schelper RL, Goeken JA (1992). Smooth muscle can comprise the sarcomatous component of gliosarcomas. J Neuropathol Exp Neurol 51: 493-498.

751. Haddad SF, Moore SA, Schelper RL, Goeken JA (1992). Vascular smooth muscle hyperplasia underlies the formation of glomeruloid vascular structures of glioblastoma multiforme. J Neuropathol Exp Neurol 51: 488-492.

752. Hage C, Willman CL, Favara BE, Isaacson PG (1993). Langerhans' cell histiocytosis (histiocytosis X): immunophenotype and growth fraction. Hum Pathol 24: 840-845.

753. Hahn H, Wicking C, Zaphiropoulos PG, Gailani MR, Shanley S, Chidambaram A, Vorechovsky I, Holmberg E, Unden AB, Gillies S, Negus K, Smyth I, Pressman C, Leffell DJ, Gerrard B, Goldstein AM, Dean M, Toftgard R, Chenevix T, Wainwright B, Bale AE (1996). Mutations of the human homolog of Drosophila patched in the nevoid basal cell carcinoma syndrome. Cell 85: 841-851.

754. Hahn HP, Bundock EA, Hornick JL (2006). Immunohistochemical staining for claudin-1 can help distinguish meningiomas from histologic mimics. Am J Clin Pathol 125: 203-208.

755. Hahn JF, Sperber EE, Netsky MG (1976). Melanotic neuroectodermal tumors of the brain and skull. J Neuropathol Exp Neurol 35: 508-519.

756. Hair LS, Symmans F, Powers JM, Carmel P (1992). Immunohistochemistry and proliferative activity in Lhermitte- Duclos disease. Acta Neuropathol 84: 570-573.

757. Hallahan AR, Pritchard JI, Hansen S, Benson M, Stoeck J, Hatton BA, Russell TL, Ellenbogen RG, Bernstein ID, Beachy PA,

Olson JM (2004). The SmoA1 mouse model reveals that notch signaling is critical for the growth and survival of sonic hedgehog-induced medulloblastomas. Cancer Res 64: 7794-7800.

758. Halling KC, Scheithauer BW, Halling AC, Nascimento AG, Ziesmer SC, Roche PC, Wollan PC (1996). p53 expression in neurofibroma and malignant peripheral nerve sheath tumor. An immunohistochemical study of sporadic and NF1- associated tumors. Am J Clin Pathol 106: 282-288.

759. Hamazaki S, Nakashima H, Matsumoto K, Taguchi K, Okada S (2001). Metastasis of renal cell carcinoma to central nervous system hemangioblastoma in two patients with von Hippel-Lindau disease. Pathol Int 51: 948-953.

760. Hamilton DW, Lusher ME, Lindsey JC, Ellison DW, Clifford SC (2005). Epigenetic inactivation of the RASSF1A tumour suppressor gene in ependymoma. Cancer Lett 227: 75-81.

761. Hamilton RL, Pollack IF (1997). The molecular biology of ependymomas. Brain Pathol 7: 807-822.

762. Hamilton SR, Liu B, Parsons RE, Papadopoulos N, Jen J, Powell SM, Krush AJ, Berk T, Cohen Z, Tetu B, Burger PC, Wood PA, Tagi F, Booker SV, Peterson GM, Offerhaus GJA, Tersmette AC, Giardiello FM, Vogelstein B, Kinzler RW (1995). The molecular basis of Turcot's syndrome. N Engl J Med 332: 839-847.

763. Hammel PR, Vilgrain V, Terris B, Penfornis A, Sauvanet A, Correas JM, Chauveau D, Balian A, Beigelman C, O'Toole D, Bernades P, Ruszniewski P, Richard S (2000). Pancreatic involvement in von Hippel-Lindau disease. The Groupe Francophone d'Etude de la Maladie de von Hippel-Lindau. Gastroenterology 119: 1087-1095.

764. Hammoud MA, Sawaya R, Shi W, Thall PF, Leeds NE (1996). Prognostic significance of preoperative MRI scans in glioblastoma multiforme. J Neurooncol 27: 65-73.

765. Han DH, Kim DG, Chi JG, Park SH, Jung HW, Kim YG (1992). Malignant triton tumor of the acoustic nerve. Case report. J Neurosurg 76: 874-877.

766. Hanssen AM, Werquin H, Suys E, Fryns JP (1993). Cowden syndrome: report of a large family with macrocephaly and increased severity of signs in subsequent generations. Clin Genet 44: 281-286.

767. Hao C, Beguinot F, Condorelli G, Trencia A, Van Meir EG, Yong VW, Parney IF, Roa WH, Petruk KC (2001). Induction and intracellular regulation of tumor necrosis factor-related apoptosis-inducing ligand (TRAIL) mediated apotosis in human malignant glioma cells. Cancer Res 61: 1162-1170.

768. Harada K, Nishizaki T, Kubota H, Harada K, Suzuki M, Sasaki K (2001). Distinct primary central nervous system lymphoma defined by comparative genomic hybridization and laser scanning cytometry. Cancer Genet Cytogenet 125: 147-150.

769. Hariharan S, Donahue JE, Garre C, Origone P, Grewal RP (2006). Clinicopathologic and genetic analysis of siblings with NF1 and adult-onset gliomas. J Neurol Sci 247: 105-108.

770. Harris BT, Horoupian DS (2000). Spinal cord glioneuronal tumor with "rosetted" neuropil islands and meningeal dissemination: a case report. Acta Neuropathol 100: 575-579.

771. Harris CP, Townsend JJ, Brockmeyer DL, Heilbrun MP (1991). Cerebral granular cell tumor occurring with glioblastoma multiforme: case report. Surg Neurol 36: 202-206.

772. Harrison MJ, Wolfe DE, Lau TS, Mitnick RJ, Sachdev VP (1991). Radiation-induced meningiomas: experience at the Mount Sinai Hospital and review of the literature. J

Neurosurg 75: 564-574.

773. Hart MN, Petito CK, Earle KM (1974). Mixed gliomas. Cancer 33: 134-140.

774. Harter DH, Omeis I, Forman S, Braun A (2006). Endoscopic resection of an intraventricular dysembryoplastic neuroepithelial tumor of the septum pellucidum. Pediatr Neurosurg 42: 105-107.

775. Hartmann C, Bartels G, Gehlhaar C, Holtkamp N, von Deimling A (2005). PIK3CA mutations in glioblastoma multiforme. Acta Neuropathol 109: 639-642.

776. Hartmann C, Numann A, Mueller W, Holtkamp N, Simon M, von Deimling A (2004). Fine mapping of chromosome 22q tumor suppressor gene candidate regions in astrocytoma. Int J Cancer 108: 839-844.

777. Hartmann C, Sieberns J, Gehlhaar C, Simon M, Paulus W, von Deimling A (2006). NF2 mutations in secretory and other rare variants of meningiomas. Brain Pathol 16: 15-19.

778. Hartmann W, Digon-Sontgerath B, Koch A, Waha A, Endl E, Dani I, Denkhaus D, Goodyer CG, Sorensen N, Wiestler OD, Pietsch T (2006). Phosphatidylinositol 3'-kinase/AKT signaling is activated in medulloblastoma cell proliferation and is associated with reduced expression of PTEN. Clin Cancer Res 12: 3019-3027.

779. Hashimoto T, Sasagawa I, Ishigooka M, Kubota Y, Nakada T, Fujita T, Nakai O (1995). Down's syndrome associated with intracranial germinoma and testicular embryonal carcinoma. Urol Int 55: 120-122.

780. Haslam RH, Lamborn KR, Becker LE, Israel MA (1998). Tumor cell apoptosis present at diagnosis may predict treatment outcome for patients with medulloblastoma. J Pediatr Hematol Oncol 20: 520-527.

781. Hasselblatt M, Blumcke I, Jeibmann A, Rickert CH, Jouvet A, van de Nes JA, Kuchelmeister K, Brunn A, Fevre-Montange M, Paulus W (2006). Immunohistochemical profile and chromosomal imbalances in papillary tumours of the pineal region. Neuropathol Appl Neurobiol 32: 278-283.

782. Hasselblatt M, Bohm C, Tatenhorst L, Dinh V, Newrzella D, Keyvani K, Jeibmann A, Buerger H, Rickert CH, Paulus W (2006). Identification of novel diagnostic markers for choroid plexus tumors: a microarray-based approach. Am J Surg Pathol 30: 66-74.

783. Hasselblatt M, Nolte KW, Paulus W (2004). Angiomatous meningioma: a clinicopathologic study of 38 cases. Am J Surg Pathol 28: 390-393.

784. Hasselblatt M, Sepehrnia A, von Falkenhausen M, Paulus W (2003). Intracranial follicular dendritic cell sarcoma. Case report. J Neurosurg 99: 1089-1090.

785. Hassoun J, Devictor B, Gambarelli D, Peragut JC, Toga M (1984). Paired twisted filaments: a new ultrastructural marker of human pinealomas? Acta Neuropathol 65: 163-165.

786. Hassoun J, Gambarelli D, Grisoli F, Pellet W, Salamon G, Pellisier JF, Toga M (1982). Central neurocytoma. An electron-microscopic study of two cases. Acta Neuropathol 56: 151-156.

787. Hassoun J, Gambarelli D, Peragut JC, Toga M (1983). Specific ultrastructural markers of human pinealomas. A study of four cases. Acta Neuropathol 62: 31-40.

788. Hassoun J, Soylemezoglu F, Gambarelli D, Figarella B, von Ammon K, Kleihues P (1993). Central neurocytoma: a synopsis of clinical and histological features. Brain Pathol 3: 297-306.

789. Hattab EM, Tu PH, Wilson JD, Cheng L (2005). OCT4 immunohistochemistry is superior to placental alkaline phosphatase (PLAP) in the diagnosis of central nervous system germinoma. Am J Surg Pathol 29: 368-371.

790. Hattingen E, Pilatus U, Good C, Franz K, Lanfermann H, Zanella FE (2003). An unusual intraventricular haemangiopericytoma: MRI and spectroscopy. Neuroradiology 45: 386-389.

791. Hatva E, Bohling T, Jaaskelainen J, Persico MG, Haltia M, Alitalo K (1996). Vascular growth factors and receptors in capillary hemangioblastomas and hemangiopericytomas. Am J Pathol 148: 763-775.

792. Haupt Y, Maya R, Kazaz A, Oren M (1997). Mdm2 promotes the rapid degradation of p53. Nature 387: 296-299.

793. Hayakawa I, Fujiwara K, Tsuchida T, Aoki M (1979). [Choroid plexus carcinoma with metastasis to bone (author's transl)]. No Shinkei Geka 7: 815-818.

794. Hayashi K, Ohara N, Jeon HJ, Akagi S, Takahashi K, Akagi T, Namba S (1993). Gliosarcoma with features of chondroblastic osteosarcoma. Cancer 72: 850-855.

795. Hayashi S, Kameyama S, Fukuda M, Takahashi H (2000). Ganglioglioma with a tanycytic ependymoma as the glial component. Acta Neuropathol 99: 310-316.

796. Hayashi Y, Iwato M, Hasegawa M, Tachibana O, von Deimling A, Yamashita J (2001). Malignant transformation of a gangliocytoma/ganglioglioma into a glioblastoma multiforme: a molecular genetic analysis. Case report. J Neurosurg 95: 138-142.

797. Hayashi Y, Ueki K, Waha A, Wiestler OD, Louis DN, von Deimling A (1997). Association of EGFR gene amplification and CDKN2 (p16/MTS1) gene deletion in glioblastoma multiforme. Brain Pathol 7: 871-875.

798. Hayostek CJ, Shaw EG, Scheithauer B, O'Fallon JR, Weiland TL, Schomberg PJ, Kelly PJ, Hu TC (1993). Astrocytomas of the cerebellum. A comparative clinicopathologic study of pilocytic and diffuse astrocytomas. Cancer 72: 856-869.

799. He J, Mokhtari K, Sanson M, Marie Y, Kujas M, Huguet S, Leuraud P, Capelle L, Delattre JY, Poirier J, Hoang-Xuan K (2001). Glioblastomas with an oligodendroglial component: a pathological and molecular study. J Neuropathol Exp Neurol 60: 863-871.

800. Heegaard S, Sommer HM, Broholm H, Broendstrup O (1995). Proliferating cell nuclear antigen and Ki-67 immunohistochemistry of oligodendrogliomas with special reference to prognosis. Cancer 76: 1809-1813.

801. Hegi ME, Diserens AC, Gorlia T, Hamou MF, de Tribolet N, Weller M, Kros JM, Hainfellner JA, Mason W, Mariani L, Bromberg JE, Hau P, Mirimanoff RO, Cairncross JG, Janzer RC, Stupp R (2005). MGMT gene silencing and benefit from temozolomide in glioblastoma. N Engl J Med 352: 997-1003.

802. Hegi ME, zur HA, Ruedi D, Malin G, Kleihues P (1997). Hemizygous or homozygous deletion of the chromosomal region containing the p16INK4a gene is associated with amplification of the EGF receptor gene in glioblastomas. Int J Cancer 73: 57-63.

803. Heimdal K, Evensen SA, Fossa SD, Hirscberg H, Langholm R, Brogger A, Moller P (1991). Karyotyping of a hematologic neoplasia developing shortly after treatment for cerebral extragonadal germ cell tumor. Cancer Genet Cytogenet 57: 41-46.

804. Helseth A, Helseth E, Unsgaard G (1989). Primary meningeal melanoma. Acta Oncol 28: 103-104.

805. Helseth A, Mork SJ (1989). Neoplasms of the central nervous system in Norway. III. Epidemiological characteristics of intracranial gliomas according to histology. APMIS 97: 547-555.

806. Helton KJ, Fouladi M, Boop FA, Perry A, Dalton J, Kun L, Fuller C (2004). Medullomyoblastoma: a radiographic and clinicopathologic analysis of six cases and review of the literature. Cancer 101: 1445-1454.

807. Hemminki K, Kyyronen P, Vaittinen P (1999). Parental age as a risk factor of childhood leukemia and brain cancer in offspring. Epidemiology 10: 271-275.

808. Hemminki K, Li X, Vaittinen P, Dong C (2000). Cancers in the first-degree relatives of children with brain tumours. Br J Cancer 83: 407-411.

809. Henn W, Wullich B, Thonnes M, Steudel WI, Feiden W, Zang KD (1993). Recurrent t(12;19)(q13;q13.3) in intracranial and extracranial hemangiopericytoma. Cancer Genet Cytogenet 71: 151-154.

810. Hennessy MJ, Elwes RD, Rabe-Hesketh S, Binnie CD, Polkey CE (2001). Prognostic factors in the surgical treatment of medically intractable epilepsy associated with mesial temporal sclerosis. Acta Neurol Scand 103: 344-350.

811. Henske EP, Scheithauer BW, Short MP, Wollmann R, Nahmias J, Hornigold N, van Slegtenhorst M, Welsh CT, Kwiatkowski DJ (1996). Allelic loss is frequent in tuberous sclerosis kidney lesions but rare in brain lesions. Am J Hum Genet 59: 400-406.

812. Henter JI, Nennesmo I (1997). Neuropathologic findings and neurologic symptoms in twenty-three children with hemophagocytic lymphohistiocytosis. J Pediatr 130: 358-365.

813. Herath SE, Stalboerger PG, Dahl RJ, Parisi JE, Jenkins RB (1994). Cytogenetic studies of four hemangiopericytomas. Cancer Genet Cytogenet 72: 137-140.

814. Hermanson M, Funa K, Hartman M, Claesson W, Heldin CH, Westermark B, Nister M (1992). Platelet-derived growth factor and its receptors in human glioma tissue: expression of messenger RNA and protein suggests the presence of autocrine and paracrine loops. Cancer Res 52: 3213-3219.

815. Herpers MJ, Ramaekers FC, Aldeweireldt J, Moesker O, Slooff J (1986). Co-expression of glial fibrillary acidic protein- and vimentin- type intermediate filaments in human astrocytomas. Acta Neuropathol 70: 333-339.

816. Herpers MJHM, Budka H (1984). Glial fibrillary acidic protein (GFAP) in oligodendroglial tumors: gliofibrillary oligodendroglioma and transitional oligoastrocytoma as subtypes of oligodendroglioma. Acta Neuropathol 64: 265-272.

817. Herregodts P, Vloeberghs M, Schmedding E, Goossens A, Stadnik T, D'Haens J (1991). Solitary dorsal intramedullary schwannoma. Case report. J Neurosurg 74: 816-820.

818. Herrick MK, Rubinstein LJ (1979). The cytological differentiating potential of pineal parenchymal neoplasms (true pinealomas). A clinicopathological study of 28 tumours. Brain 102: 289-320.

819. Herrlinger U, Klingel K, Meyermann R, Kandolf R, Kaiserling E, Kortmann RD, Melms A, Skalej M, Dichgans J, Weller M (2000). Central nervous system Hodgkin's lymphoma without systemic manifestation: case report and review of the literature. Acta Neuropathol 99: 709-714.

820. Herva R, Serlo W, Laitinen J, Becker LE (1996). Intraventricular rhabdomyosarcoma after resection of hyperplastic choroid plexus. Acta Neuropathol 92: 213-216.

821. Hessler RB, Lopes MB, Frankfurter A, Reidy J, VandenBerg SR (1992). Cytoskeletal immunohistochemistry of central neurocytomas. Am J Surg Pathol 16: 1031-1038.

822. Higashino T, Inamura T, Kawashima M, Ikezaki K, Miyazono M, Yoshiura T, Iwaki T, Fukui M (2001). A lateral ventricular gliosarcoma arising in an ependymoma. Clin Neuropathol 20: 219-223.

823. Hilden JM, Meerbaum S, Burger P, Finlay J, Janss A, Scheithauer BW, Walter AW, Rorke LB, Biegel JA (2004). Central nervous system atypical teratoid/rhabdoid tumor: results of therapy in children enrolled in a registry. J Clin Oncol 22: 2877-2884.

824. Hill C, Hunter SB, Brat DJ (2003). Genetic markers in glioblastoma: prognostic significance and future therapeutic implications. Adv Anat Pathol 10: 212-217.

825. Hill DA, Linet MS, Black PM, Fine HA, Selker RG, Shapiro WR, Inskip PD (2004). Meningioma and schwannoma risk in adults in relation to family history of cancer. Neuro-oncol 6: 274-280.

826. Hirato J, Nakazato Y, Iijima M, Yokoo H, Sasaki A, Yokota M, Ono N, Hirato M, Inoue H (1997). An unusual variant of ependymoma with extensive tumor cell vacuolization. Acta Neuropathol 93: 310-316.

827. Hirose T, Giannini C, Scheithauer BW (2001). Ultrastructural features of pleomorphic xanthoastrocytoma: a comparative study with glioblastoma multiforme. Ultrastruct Pathol 25: 469-478.

828. Hirose T, Scheithauer BW (1998). Mixed dysembryoplastic neuroepithelial tumor and ganglioglioma. Acta Neuropathol 95: 649-654.

829. Hirose T, Scheithauer BW (1999). Sclerosing perineurioma: a distinct entity? Int J Surg Pathol. In Press.

830. Hirose T, Scheithauer BW, Lopes MB, Gerber HA, Altermatt HJ, Hukee MJ, VandenBerg SR, Charlesworth JC (1995). Tuber and subependymal giant cell astrocytoma associated with tuberous sclerosis: an immunohistochemical, ultrastructural, and immunoelectron and microscopic study. Acta Neuropathol 90: 387-399.

831. Hirose T, Scheithauer BW, Lopes MB, VandenBerg SR (1994). Dysembryoplastic neuroeptihelial tumor (DNT): an immunohistochemical and ultrastructural study. J Neuropathol Exp Neurol 53: 184-195.

832. Hirose T, Scheithauer BW, Lopes MBS, Gerber HA, Altermatt HJ, VandenBerg SR (1997). Ganglioglioma: An ultrastructural and immunohistochemical study. Cancer 79: 989-1003.

833. Hirose T, Scheithauer BW, Sano T (1998). Perineurial malignant peripheral nerve sheath tumor (MPNST): a clinicopathologic, immunohistochemical, and ultrastructural study of seven cases. Am J Surg Pathol 22: 1368-1378.

834. Hirose T, Tani T, Shimada T, Ishizawa K, Shimada S, Sano T (2003). Immunohistochemical demonstration of EMA/Glut1-positive perineurial cells and CD34-positive fibroblastic cells in peripheral nerve sheath tumors. Mod Pathol 16: 293-298.

835. Hirose Y, Aldape K, Bollen A, James CD, Brat D, Lamborn K, Berger M, Feuerstein BG (2001). Chromosomal abnormalities subdivide ependymal tumors into clinically relevant groups. Am J Pathol 158: 1137-1143.

836. Hirose Y, Aldape KD, Chang S, Lamborn K, Berger MS, Feuerstein BG (2003). Grade II astrocytomas are subgrouped by chromosome aberrations. Cancer Genet Cytogenet 142: 1-7.

837. Hirsch JF, Pierre K (1988). Lumbosacral lipomas with spina bifida. Childs Nerv Syst 4: 354-360.

838. Hitotsumatsu T, Iwaki T, Kitamati T, Mizoguchi M, Suzuki SO, Hamada Y, Fukui M, Tateishi J (1997). Expression of neurofibromatosis 2 protein in human brain tumors: an immunohistochemical study. Acta Neuropathol 93: 225-232.

839. Hjalmars U, Kulldorff M, Wahlqvist Y, Lannering B (1999). Increased incidence rates but no space-time clustering of childhood astrocytoma in Sweden, 1973-1992: a population-based study of pediatric brain tumors. Cancer 85: 2077-2090.

840. Ho DM, Hsu CY, Wong TT, Chiang H (2001). A clinicopathologic study of 81 patients with ependymomas and proposal of diagnostic criteria for anaplastic ependymoma. . J Neurooncol 54: 77-85.

841. Ho DM, Hsu CY, Wong TT, Ting LT, Chiang H (2000). Atypical teratoid/rhabdoid tumor of the central nervous system: a comparative study with primitive neuroectodermal tumor/medulloblastoma. Acta Neuropathol 99: 482-488.

842. Ho DM, Liu HC (1992). Primary intracranial germ cell tumor. Pathologic study of 51 patients. Cancer 70: 1577-1584.

843. Ho KL (1984). Ultrastructure of cerebellar capillary hemangioblastoma. I. Weibel-Palade bodies and stromal cell histogenesis. J Neuropathol Exp Neurol 43: 592-608.

844. Ho KL (1990). Microtubular aggregates within rough endoplasmic reticulum in myxopapillary ependymoma of the filum terminale. Arch Pathol Lab Med 114: 956-960.

845. Ho YS, Wei CH, Tsai MD, Wai YY (1992). Intracerebral malignant fibrous histiocytoma: case report and review of the literature. Neurosurgery 31: 567-571.

846. Hoang-Xuan K, Capelle L, Kujas M, Taillibert S, Duffau H, Lejeune J, Polivka M, Criniere E, Marie Y, Mokhtari K, Carpentier AF, Laigle F, Simon JM, Cornu P, Broet P, Sanson M, Delattre JY (2004). Temozolomide as initial treatment for adults with low-grade oligodendrogliomas or oligoastrocytomas and correlation with chromosome 1p deletions. J Clin Oncol 22: 3133-3138.

847. Hoang MP, Amirkhan RH (2003). Inhibin alpha distinguishes hemangioblastoma from clear cell renal cell carcinoma. Am J Surg Pathol 27: 1152-1156.

848. Hochstrasser H, Boltshauser E, Valavanis A (1988). Brain tumors in children with von Recklinghausen neurofibromatosis. Skeletal Radiol 1: 25-28.

849. Hodaie M, Becker L, Teshima I, Rutka JT (2001). Total resection of an intracerebral hemangioendothelioma in an infant. Case report and review of the literature. Pediatr Neurosurg 34: 104-112.

850. Hoffman HJ, Otsubo H, Hendrick EB, Humphreys RP, Drake JM, Becker LE, Greenberg M, Jenkin D (1991). Intracranial germ-cell tumors in children. J Neurosurg 74: 545-551.

851. Hoffman HJ, Yoshida M, Becker LE, Hendrick EB, Humphreys RP (1983). Pineal region tumors in childhood. Experience at the Hospital for Sick Children. Pediatr Neurosurg 21: 91-103.

852. Hoffman JM, Waskin HA, Schifter T, Hanson MW, Gray L, Rosenfeld S, Coleman RE (1993). FDG-PET in differentiating lymphoma from nonmalignant central nervous system lesions in patients with AIDS. J Nucl Med 34: 567-575.

853. Hoffmann C, Tabrizian S, Wolf E, Eggers C, Stoehr A, Plettenberg A, Buhk T, Stellbrink HJ, Horst HA, Jager H, Rosenkranz T (2001). Survival of AIDS patients with primary central nervous system lymphoma is dramatically improved by HAART-induced immune recovery. AIDS 15: 2119-2127.

854. Hofman S, Heeg M, Klein JP, Krikke AP (1998). Simultaneous occurrence of a supra- and an infratentorial glioma in a patient with

Ollier's disease: more evidence for non-mesodermal tumor predisposition in multiple enchondromatosis. Skeletal Radiol 27: 688-691.

855. Holl T, Kleihues P, Yasargil MG, Wiestler OD (1991). Cerebellar medullomyoblastoma with advanced neuronal differentiation and hamartomatous component. Acta Neuropathol 82: 408-413.

856. Holt SC, Bruner JM, Ordonez NG (1986). Capillary hemangioblastoma. An immunohistochemical study. Am J Clin Pathol 86: 423-429.

857. Homma T, Fukushima T, Vaccarella S, Yonekawa Y, Di Patre PL, Franceschi S, Ohgaki H (2006). Correlation among pathology, genotype, and patient outcomes in glioblastoma. J Neuropathol Exp Neurol 65: 846-854.

858. Honavar M, Janota I (1994). 73 cases of dysembryoplastic neuroepithelial tumour: the range of histological appearances. Brain Pathol 4: 428

859. Honavar M, Janota I, Polkey CE (1999). Histological heterogeneity of dysembryoplastic neuroepithelial tumour: identification and differential diagnosis in a series of 74 cases. Histopathology 34: 342-356.

860. Hong C, Bollen AW, Costello JF (2003). The contribution of genetic and epigenetic mechanisms to gene silencing in oligodendrogliomas. Cancer Res 63: 7600-7605.

861. Hope JK, Armstrong DA, Babyn PS, Humphreys RR, Harwood-Nash DC, Chuang SH, Marks PV (1992). Primary meningeal tumors in children: correlation of clinical and CT findings with histologic type and prognosis. AJNR Am J Neuroradiol 13: 1353-1364.

862. Hopewell JW (1975). The subependymal plate and genesis of gliomas. J Pathol 117: 101-103.

863. Horiguchi H, Hirose T, Sano T, Nagahiro S, Seki K, Fujimoto N, Kaneko F, Kusaka K (2000). Meningioma with granulofilamentous inclusions. Ultrastruct Pathol 24: 267-271.

864. Hormigo A, Gu B, Karimi S, Riedel E, Panageas KS, Edgar MA, Tanwar MK, Rao JS, Fleisher M, DeAngelis LM, Holland EC (2006). YKL-40 and matrix metalloproteinase-9 as potential serum biomarkers for patients with high-grade gliomas. Clin Cancer Res 12: 5698-5704.

865. Horn B, Heideman R, Geyer R, Pollack I, Packer R, Goldwein J, Tomita T, Schomberg P, Ater J, Luchtman-Jones L, Rivlin K, Lamborn K, Prados M, Bollen A, Berger M, Dahl G, McNeil E, Patterson K, Shaw D, Kubalik M, Russo C (1999). A multi-institutional retrospective study of intracranial ependymoma in children: identification of risk factors. J Pediatr Hematol Oncol 21: 203-211.

866. Hornick JL, Fletcher CD (2005). Soft tissue perineurioma: clinicopathologic analysis of 81 cases including those with atypical histologic features. Am J Surg Pathol 29: 845-858.

866A. Hornick JL, Fletcher CD (2005). Intestinal perineuriomas: clinicopathologic definition of a new anatomic subset in a series of 10 cases. Am J Surg Pathol 29:859-65.

867. Horstmann S, Perry A, Reifenberger G, Giangaspero F, Huang H, Hara A, Masuoka J, Rainov NG, Bergmann M, Heppner FL, Brandner S, Chimelli L, Montagna N, Jackson T, Davis DG, Markesbery WR, Ellison DW, Weller RO, Taddei GL, Conti R, Del Bigio MR, Gonzalez-Campora R, Radhakrishnan VV, Soylemezoglu F, Uro-Coste E, Qian J, Kleihues P, Ohgaki H (2004). Genetic and expression profiles of cerebellar liponeurocytomas. Brain Pathol 14: 281-289.

868. Horten BC, Rubinstein LJ (1976). Primary cerebral neuroblastoma. A clinicopathological study of 35 cases. Brain 99: 735-756.

869. Horten BC, Urich H, Rubinstein LJ, Montague SR (1977). The angioblastic meningioma: a reappraisal of a nosological problem. Light-, electron-microscopic, tissue, and organ culture observations. J Neurol Sci 31: 387-410.

870. Hoshino T, Ahn D, Prados MD, Lamborn K, Wilson CB (1993). Prognostic significance of the proliferative potential of intracranial gliomas measured by bromodeoxyuridine labeling. Int J Cancer 53: 550-555.

871. Hoshino T, Wilson BC, Ellis WG (1975). Gemistocytic astrocytes in gliomas. An autoradiographic study. J Neuropathol Exp Neurol 34: 263-281.

872. Hosokawa Y, Tsuchihashi Y, Okabe H, Toyama M, Namura K, Kuga M, Yonezawa T, Fujita S, Ashihara T (1991). Pleomorphic xanthoastrocytoma. Ultrastructural, immunohistochemical and DNA cytofluorometric study of a case. Cancer 68: 853-859.

873. Hoyt WF, Baghdassarian SA (1969). Optic glioma of childhood. Natural history and rationale for conservative management. Br J Ophthalmol 53: 793-798.

874. Hruban RH, Shiu MH, Senie RT, Woodruff JM (1990). Malignant peripheral nerve sheath tumors of the buttock and lower extremity. A study of 43 cases. Cancer 66: 1253-1265.

875. Hsu DW, Efird JT, Hedley Whyte ET (1997). Progesterone and estrogen receptors in meningiomas: prognostic considerations. J Neurosurg 86: 113-120.

876. Hsu DW, Louis DN, Efird JT, Hedley-Whyte ET (1997). Use of MIB-1 (Ki-67) immunoreactivity in differentiating grade II and grade III gliomas. J Neuropathol Exp Neurol 56: 857-865.

877. Huang B, Starostik P, Schraut H, Krauss J, Sorensen N, Roggendorf W (2003). Human ependymomas reveal frequent deletions on chromosomes 6 and 9. Acta Neuropathol 106: 357-362.

878. Huang CI, Chiou WH, Ho DM (1987). Oligodendroglioma occurring after radiation therapy for pituitary adenoma. J Neurol Neurosurg Psychiatry 50: 1619-1624.

879. Huang H, Colella S, Kurrer M, Yonekawa Y, Kleihues P, Ohgaki H (2000). Gene expression profiling of low-grade diffuse astrocytomas by cDNA arrays. Cancer Res 60: 6868-6874.

880. Huang H, Hara A, Homma T, Yonekawa Y, Ohgaki H (2005). Altered expression of immune defense genes in pilocytic astrocytomas. J Neuropathol Exp Neurol 64: 891-901.

881. Huang H, Mahler-Araujo BM, Sankila A, Chimelli L, Yonekawa Y, Kleihues P, Ohgaki H (2000). APC mutations in sporadic medulloblastomas. Am J Pathol 156: 433-437.

882. Huang H, Okamoto Y, Yokoo H, Heppner FL, Vital A, Fevre-Montange M, Jouvet A, Yonekawa Y, Lazaridis EN, Kleihues P, Ohgaki H (2004). Gene expression profiling and subgroup identification of oligodendrogliomas. Oncogene 23: 6012-6022.

883. Huang H, Reis R, Yonekawa Y, Lopes JM, Kleihues P, Ohgaki H (1999). Identification in human brain tumors of DNA sequences specific for SV40 large T antigen. Brain Pathol 9: 33-42.

884. Huang MC, Kubo O, Tajika Y, Takakura K (1996). A clinico-immunohistochemical study of giant cell glioblastoma. Noshuyo Byori 13: 11-16.

885. Hubbard JL, Scheithauer BW, Kispert DB, Carpenter SM, Wick MR, Laws ER, Jr. (1989). Adult cerebellar medulloblastomas: the pathological, radiographic, and clinical disease spectrum. J Neurosurg 70: 536-544.

886. Hufnagel TJ, Kim JH, True LD,

Manuelidis EE (1989). Immunohistochemistry of capillary hemangioblastoma. Immunoperoxidase-labeled antibody staining resolves the differential diagnosis with metastatic renal cell carcinoma, but does not explain the histogenesis of the capillary hemangioblastoma. Am J Surg Pathol 13: 207-216.

887. Hui AB, Lo KW, Yin XL, Poon WS, Ng HK (2001). Detection of multiple gene amplifications in glioblastoma multiforme using array-based comparative genomic hybridization. Lab Invest 81: 717-723.

888. Hui AB, Takano H, Lo KW, Kuo WL, Lam CN, Tong CY, Chang Q, Gray JW, Ng HK (2005). Identification of a novel homozygous deletion region at 6q23.1 in medulloblastomas using high-resolution array comparative genomic hybridization analysis. Clin Cancer Res 11: 4707-4716.

889. Hulette CM (1996). Microglioma, a histiocytic neoplasm of the central nervous system. Mod Pathol 9: 316-319.

890. Hung KL, Wu CM, Huang JS, How SW (1990). Familial medulloblastoma in siblings: report in one family and review of the literature. Surg Neurol 33: 341-346.

891. Hunter S, Young A, Olson J, Brat DJ, Bowers G, Wilcox JN, Jaye D, Mendrinos S, Neish A (2002). Differential expression between pilocytic and anaplastic astrocytomas: identification of apolipoprotein D as a marker for low-grade, non-infiltrating primary CNS neoplasms. J Neuropathol Exp Neurol 61: 275-281.

892. Hunter SB, Varma V, Shehata B, Nolen JD, Cohen C, Olson JJ, Ou CY (2005). Apolipoprotein D expression in primary brain tumors: analysis by quantitative RT-PCR in formalin-fixed, paraffin-embedded tissue. J Histochem Cytochem 53: 963-969.

893. Hurley TR, D'Angelo CM, Clasen RA, Wilkinson SB, Passavoy RD (1994). Magnetic resonance imaging and pathological analysis of a pituicytoma: case report. Neurosurgery 35: 314-317.

894. Hurtt MR, Moossy J, Donovan-Peluso M, Locker J (1992). Amplification of epidermal growth factor receptor gene in gliomas: histopathology and prognosis. J Neuropathol Exp Neurol 51: 84-90.

895. Husain AN, Leestma JE (1986). Cerebral astroblastoma: immunohistochemical and ultrastructural features. Case report. J Neurosurg 64: 657-661.

896. Husemann K, Wolter M, Buschges R, Bostrom J, Sabel M, Reifenberger G (1999). Identification of two distinct deleted regions on the short arm of chromosome 1 and rare mutation of the CDKN2C gene from 1p32 in oligodendroglial tumors. J Neuropathol Exp Neurol 58: 1041-1050.

897. Huson SM (1994). Neurofibromatosis 1: a clinical and genetic overview. In: The Neurofibromatoses. A Pathogenetic and Clinical Overview. Huson SM, Hughes RAC, eds. Chapman & Hall Medical: London, pp. 160-179.

898. Huson SM, Harper PS, Compston DA (1988). Von Recklinghausen neurofibromatosis. A clinical and population study in southeast Wales. Brain 111: 1355-1381.

899. Hussain N, Curran A, Pilling D, Malluci CL, Ladusans EJ, Alfirevic Z, Pizer B (2006). Congenital subependymal giant cell astrocytoma diagnosed on fetal MRI. Arch Dis Child 91: 520.

900. Huttenlocher PR, Heydemann PT (1984). Fine structure of cortical tubers in tuberous sclerosis: a Golgi study. Ann Neurol 16: 595-602.

901. Huynh DP, Maunter V, Baser ME, Stavrou D, Pulst S (1997). Immunohistochemical detection of schwannomin and neu-

rofibromin in vestibular schwannomas, ependymomas and meningiomas. J Neuropath Exp Neurol 56: 382-390.

902. Hyman MH, Whittemore VH (2000). National Institutes of Health consensus conference: tuberous sclerosis complex. Arch Neurol 57: 662-665.

903. Ichimura K, Mungall AJ, Fiegler H, Pearson DM, Dunham I, Carter NP, Collins VP (2006). Small regions of overlapping deletions on 6q26 in human astrocytic tumours identified using chromosome 6 tile path array-CGH. Oncogene 25: 1261-1271.

904. Ichimura K, Schmidt EE, Miyakawa A, Goike HM, Collins VP (1998). Distinct patterns of deletion on 10p and 10q suggest involvement of multiple tumor suppressor genes in the development of astrocytic gliomas of different malignancy grades. Genes Chromosomes Cancer 22: 9-15.

905. Ignatova TN, Kukekov VG, Laywell ED, Suslov ON, Vrionis FD, Steindler DA (2002). Human cortical glial tumors contain neural stem-like cells expressing astroglial and neuronal markers in vitro. Glia 39: 193-206.

906. Ikeda H, Yoshimoto T (2002). Clinicopathological study of Rathke's cleft cysts. Clin Neuropathol 21: 82-91.

907. Ikeda J, Sawamura Y, Van Meir EG (1998). Pineoblastoma presenting in familial adenomatous polyposis (FAP): random association, FAP variant or Turcot syndrome? Br J Neurosurg 12: 576-578.

908. Ilgren EB, Kinnier-Wilson LM, Stiller CA (1985). Gliomas in neurofibromatosis: a series of 89 cases with evidence for enhanced malignancy in associated cerebellar astrocytomas. Pathol Annu 20: 331-358.

909. Ilhan I, Berberoglu S, Kutluay L, Maden HA (1998). Subcutaneous sacrococcygeal myxopapillary ependymoma. Med Pediatr Oncol 30: 81-84.

910. Illerhaus G, Marks R, Ihorst G, Guttenberger R, Ostertag C, Derigs G, Frickhofen N, Feuerhake F, Volk B, Finke J (2006). High-dose chemotherapy with autologous stem-cell transplantation and hyperfractionated radiotherapy as first-line treatment of primary CNS lymphoma. J Clin Oncol. 24: 3865-3870.

911. Im SH, Chung CK, Kim SK, Cho BK, Kim MK, Chi JG (2004). Pleomorphic xanthoastrocytoma: a developmental glioneuronal tumor with prominent glioproliferative changes. J Neurooncol 66: 17-27.

912. Imai H, Kajimoto K, Taniwaki M, Miura I, Hatta Y, Hashizume Y, Watanabe M, Shiraishi T, Nakamura S (2004). Intravascular large B-cell lymphoma presenting with mass lesions in the central nervous system: a report of five cases. Pathol Int 54: 231-236.

913. Imashuku S, Hyakuna N, Funabiki T, Ikuta K, Sako M, Iwai A, Fukushima T, Kataoka S, Yabe M, Muramatsu K, Kohdera U, Nakadate H, Kitazawa K, Toyoda Y, Ishii E (2002). Low natural killer activity and central nervous system disease as a high-risk prognostic indicator in young patients with hemophagocytic lymphohistiocytosis. Cancer 94: 3023-3031.

914. Imbalzano AN, Jones SN (2005). Snf5 tumor suppressor couples chromatin remodeling, checkpoint control, and chromosomal stability. Cancer Cell 7: 294-295.

915. Inda MM, Mercapide J, Munoz J, Coullin P, Danglot G, Tunon T, Martinez-Penuela JM, Rivera JM, Burgos JJ, Bernheim A, Castresana JS (2004). PTEN and DMBT1 homozygous deletion and expression in medulloblastomas and supratentorial primitive neuroectodermal tumors. Oncol Rep 12: 1341-1347.

916. Ingham PW (1998). The patched gene in development and cancer. Curr Opin Genet Dev 8: 88-94.
917. Ironside JW, Jefferson AA, Royds JA, Taylor CB, Timperley WR (1984). Carcinoid tumour arising in a recurrent intradural spinal teratoma. Neuropathol Appl Neurobiol 10: 479-489.
918. Ironside JW, Stephenson TJ, Royds JA, Mills PM, Taylor CB, Rider CC, Timperley WR (1988). Stromal cells in cerebellar haemangioblastomas: an immunocytochemical study. Histopathology 12: 29-40.
919. Isakoff MS, Sansam CG, Tamayo P, Subramanian A, Evans JA, Fillmore CM, Wang X, Biegel JA, Pomeroy SL, Mesirov JP, Roberts CW (2005). Inactivation of the Snf5 tumor suppressor stimulates cell cycle progression and cooperates with p53 loss in oncogenic transformation. Proc Natl Acad Sci U S A 102: 17745-17750.
920. Ishida T, Kuroda M, Motoi T, Oka T, Imamura T, Machinami R (1998). Phenotypic diversity of neurofibromatosis 2: association with plexiform schwannoma. Histopathology 32: 264-270.
921. Ishii E, Ohga S, Imashuku S, Kimura N, Ueda I, Morimoto A, Yamamoto K, Yasukawa M (2005). Review of hemophagocytic lymphohistiocytosis (HLH) in children with focus on Japanese experiences. Crit Rev Oncol Hematol 53: 209-223.
922. Ishiuchi S, Nakazato Y, Iino M, Ozawa S, Tamura M, Ohye C (1998). In vitro neuronal and glial production and differentiation of human central neurocytoma cells. J Neurosci Res 51: 526-535.
923. Ishizawa K, Komori T, Hirose T (2005). Stromal cells in hemangioblastoma: neuroectodermal differentiation and morphological similarities to ependymoma. Pathol Int 55: 377-385.
924. Ishizawa T, Komori T, Shibahara J, Ishizawa K, Adachi J, Nishikawa R, Matsutani M, Hirose T (2006). Papillary glioneuronal tumor with minigemistocytic components and increased proliferative activity. Hum Pathol 37: 627-630.
925. Ismail A, Lamont JM, Tweddle AD, Pearson AD, Clifford SC, Ellison DW (2005). A 7-year-old boy with midline cerebellar mass. Brain Pathol 15: 261-2, 267.
926. Issidorides MR, Havaki S, Chrysanthou-Piterou M, Arvanitis DL (2000). Ultrastructural identification of protein bodies, cellular markers of human catecholamine neurons, in a temporal lobe ganglioglioma. Ultrastruct Pathol 24: 399-405.
927. Ito M, Jamshidi J, Yamanaka K (2001). Does craniopharyngioma metastasize? Case report and review of the literature. Neurosurgery 48: 933-935.
928. Ito S, Chandler KL, Prados MD, Lamborn K, Wynne J, Malec MK, Wilson CB, Davis RL, Hoshino T (1994). Proliferative potential and prognostic evaluation of low-grade astrocytomas. J Neurooncol 19: 1-9.
929. Ito S, Hoshino T, Prados MD, Edwards MS (1992). Cell kinetics of medulloblastomas. Cancer 70: 671-678.
930. Ito S, Hoshino T, Shibuya M, Prados MD, Edwards MS, Davis RL (1992). Proliferative characteristics of juvenile pilocytic astrocytomas determined by bromodeoxyuridine labeling. Neurosurgery 31: 413-418.
931. Itoyama T, Sadamori N, Tsutsumi K, Tokunaga Y, Soda H, Tomonaga M, Yamamori S, Masuda Y, Oshima K, Kikuchi M (1994). Primary central nervous system lymphomas. Immunophenotypic, virologic, and cytogenetic findings of three patients without immune defects. Cancer 73: 455-463.
932. Ivanov SV, Kuzmin I, Wei MH, Pack S, Geil L, Johnson BE, Stanbridge EJ, Lerman MI (1998). Down-regulation of transmembrane carbonic anhydrases in renal cell carcinoma cell lines by wild-type von Hippel-Lindau transgenes. Proc Natl Acad Sci U S A 95: 12596-12601.
933. Ivers LC, Kim AY, Sax PE (2004). Predictive value of polymerase chain reaction of cerebrospinal fluid for detection of Epstein-Barr virus to establish the diagnosis of HIV-related primary central nervous system lymphoma. Clin Infect Dis 38: 1629-1632.
934. Iwabuchi S, Bishara S, Herbison P, Erasmus A, Samejima H (1999). Prognostic factors for supratentorial low grade astrocytomas in adults. Neurol Med Chir (Tokyo) 39: 273-279.
935. Iwai K, Yamanaka K, Kamura T, Minato N, Conaway RC, Conaway JW, Klausner RD, Pause A (1999). Identification of the von Hippel-lindau tumor-suppressor protein as part of an active E3 ubiquitin ligase complex. Proc Natl Acad Sci U S A 96: 12436-12441.
936. Iwaki T, Fukui M, Kondo A, Matsushima T, Takeshita I (1987). Epithelial properties of pleomorphic xanthoastrocytomas determined in ultrastructural and immunohistochemical studies. Acta Neuropathol 74: 142-150.
937. Iwashita T, Enjoji M (1987). Plexiform neurilemmoma: a clinicopathological and immunohistochemical analysis of 23 tumours from 20 patients. Virchows Arch A Pathol Anat Histopathol 411: 305-309.
938. Iwata H, Mori Y, Takagi H, Shirahashi K, Shinoda J, Shimokawa K, Hirose H (2004). Mediastinal growing teratoma syndrome after cisplatin-based chemotherapy and radiotherapy for intracranial germinoma. J Thorac Cardiovasc Surg 127: 291-293.
939. Izuora GI, Ikerionwu S, Saddeqi N, Iloeje SO (1989). Childhood intracranial neoplasms Enugu, Nigeria. West Afr J Med 8: 171-174.
940. Jaaskelainen J (1986). Seemingly complete removal of histologically benign intracranial meningioma: late recurrence rate and factors predicting recurrence in 657 patients. A multivariate analysis. Surg Neurol 26: 461-469.
941. Jaaskelainen J, Haltia M, Servo A (1986). Atypical and anaplastic meningiomas: radiology, surgery, radiotherapy, and outcome. Surg Neurol 25: 233-242.
942. Jaaskelainen J, Paetau A, Pyykko I, Blomstedt G, Palva T, Troupp H (1994). Interface between the facial nerve and large acoustic neurinomas. Immunohistochemical study of the cleavage plane in NF2 and non-NF2 cases. J Neurosurg 80: 541-547.
943. Jaaskelainen J, Servo A, Haltia M, Kallio M, Troupp H (1991). Meningeal hemangiopericytoma. In: Meningiomas and Their Surgical Treatment. Schmidek H, ed. Saunders Company: Orlando, pp. 73-82.
944. Jaaskelainen J, Servo A, Haltia M, Wahlstrom T, Valtonen S (1985). Intracranial hemangiopericytoma: radiology, surgery, radiotherapy, and outcome in 21 patients. Surg Neurol 23: 227-236.
945. Jacks T, Shih TS, Schmitt EM, Bronson RT, Bernards A, Weinberg RA (1994). Tumour predisposition in mice heterozygous for a targeted mutation in Nf1. Nat Genet 7: 353-361.
946. Jackson CG (2001). Glomus tympanicum and glomus jugulare tumors. Otolaryngol Clin North Am 34: 941-970.
947. Jackson TR, Regine WF, Wilson D, Davis DG (2001). Cerebellar liponeurocytoma. Case report and review of the literature. J Neurosurg 95: 700-703.
948. Jacoby LB, Jones D, Davis K, Kronn D, Short MP, Gusella J, MacCollin M (1997). Molecular analysis of the NF2 tumor-suppressor gene in schwannomatosis. Am J Hum Genet 61: 1293-1302.
949. Jacoby LB, MacCollin M, Barone R, Ramesh V, Gusella JF (1996). Frequency and distribution of NF2 mutations in schwannomas. Genes Chromosomes Cancer 17: 45-55.
950. Jacoby LB, MacCollin M, Louis DN, Mohney T, Rubio MP, Pulaski K, Trofatter JA, Kley N, Seizinger B, Ramesh V, et al (1994). Exon scanning for mutation of the NF2 gene in schwannomas. Hum Mol Genet 3: 413-419.
951. Jacoby LB, Pulaski K, Rouleau GA, Martuza RL (1990). Clonal analysis of human meningiomas and schwannomas. Cancer Res 50: 6783-6786.
952. Jacques TS, Eldridge C, Patel A, Saleem NM, Powell M, Kitchen ND, Thom M, Revesz T (2006). Mixed glioneuronal tumour of the fourth ventricle with prominent rosette formation. Neuropathol Appl Neurobiol 32: 217-220.
953. Jacques TS, Valentine A, Bradford R, McLaughlin JE (2004). December 2003: a 70-year-old woman with a recurrent meningeal mass. Recurrent meningioma with rhabdomyosarcomatous differentiation. Brain Pathol 14: 229-230.
954. Jaenisch W, Schreiber D, Guthert H (1988). Primare melanome der ZNS. In: Neuropathologie. Tumoren des Nervensystems. Neuropathologie. Tumoren des Nervensystems. Gustav Fischer: Stuttgart, pp. 347-353.
955. Jaffe ES, Harris NL, Stein H, Vardiman JW eds. (2001). WHO Classification of Tumours: Pathology and Genetics of Tumours of the Haematopoietic and Lymphoid Tissues. IARC Press: Lyon.
956. Jaffey PB, To GT, Xu HJ, Hu SX, Benedict WF, Donoso LA, Campbell GA (1995). Retinoblastoma-like phenotype expressed in medulloblastomas. J Neuropathol Exp Neurol 54: 664-672.
957. Jagadha V, Halliday WC, Becker LE (1986). Glial fibrillary acidic protein (GFAP) in oligodendrogliomas: a reflection of transient GFAP expression by immature oligodendroglia. Can J Neurol Sci 13: 307-311.
958. Jahnke K, Coupland SE, Na IK, Loddenkemper C, Keilholz U, Korfel A, Stein H, Thiel E, Scheibenbogen C (2005). Expression of the chemokine receptors CXCR4, CXCR5, and CCR7 in primary central nervous system lymphoma. Blood 106: 384-385.
959. Jahnke K, Korfel A, O'Neill BP, Blay JY, Abrey LE, Martus P, Poortmans PM, Shenkier TN, Batchelor TT, Neuwelt EA, Raizer JJ, Schiff D, Pels H, Herrlinger U, Stein H, Thiel E (2006). International study on low-grade primary central nervous system lymphoma. Ann Neurol 59: 755-762.
960. Jaing TH, Wang HS, Tsay PK, Tseng CK, Jung SM, Lin KL, Lui TN (2004). Multivariate analysis of clinical prognostic factors in children with intracranial ependymomas. J Neurooncol 68: 255-261.
961. Jaiswal AK, Jaiswal S, Mahapatra AK, Sharma MC (2005). Unusually long survival in a case of medullomyoblastoma. J Clin Neurosci 12: 961-963.
962. Jakacki RI (2005). Treatment strategies for high-risk medulloblastoma and supratentorial primitive neuroectodermal tumors. Review of the literature. J Neurosurg 102: 44-52.
963. Jakobiec FA, Font RL, Johnson FB (1976). Angiomatosis retinae. An ultrastructural study and lipid analysis. Cancer 38: 2042-2056.
964. Jallo GI, Roonprapunt C, Kothbauer K, Freed D, Allen J, Epstein F (2005). Spinal solitary fibrous tumors: a series of four patients: case report. Neurosurgery 57: E195.
965. Jallo GI, Zagzag D, Epstein F (1996). Intramedullary subependymoma of the spinal cord. Neurosurgery 38: 251-257.
966. James CD, Carlbom E, Dumanski JP, Hausen M, Nordenskjold MD, Collins VP, Cavenee WK (1988). Clonal genomic alterations in glioma malignancy stages. Cancer Res 48: 5546-5551.
967. Janisch W, Janda J, Link I (1994). [Primary diffuse leptomeningeal leiomyomatosis]. Zentralbl Pathol 140: 195-200.
968. Janisch W, Schreiber D, Martin H, Gerlach H (1985). [Diencephalic pilocytic astrocytoma with clinical onset in infancy. Biological behavior and pathomorphological findings in 11 children]. Zentralbl Allg Pathol 130: 31-43.
969. Janisch W, Staneczek W (1989). [Primary tumors of the choroid plexus. Frequency, localization and age]. Zentralbl Allg Pathol 135: 235-240.
970. Janka G, Zur SU (2005). Familial and acquired hemophagocytic lymphohistiocytosis. Hematology (Am Soc Hematol Educ Program) :82-8.: 82-88.
971. Janson K, Nedzi LA, David O, Schorin M, Walsh JW, Bhattacharjee M, Pridjian G, Tan L, Judkins AR, Biegel JA (2006). Predisposition to atypical teratoid/rhabdoid tumor due to an inherited INI1 mutation. Pediatr Blood Cancer 47: 279-284.
972. Jaque CM, Kujas M, Poreau A, Raoul M, Collier P, Racadot J, Baumann NA (1979). GFA and S 100 protein levels as an index for malignancy in human gliomas and neurinomas. J Natl Cancer Inst 62: 479-483.
973. Jaros E, Lunec J, Perry RH, Kelly PJ, Pearson AD (1993). p53 protein overexpression identifies a group of central primitive neuroectodermal tumours with poor prognosis. Br J Cancer 68: 801-807.
974. Jaros E, Perry RH, Adam L, Kelly PJ, Crawford PJ, Kalbag RM, Mendelow AD, Sengupta RP, Pearson ADJ (1992). Prognostic implications of p53 protein, epidermal growth factor receptor, and Ki-67 labelling in brain tumours. Br J Cancer 66: 373-385.
975. Jarvella S, Helin H, Haapasalo J, Jarvella T, Junttila TT, Elenius K, Tanner M, Haapasalo H, Isola J (2006). Amplification of the epidermal growth factor receptor in astrocytic tumours by chromogenic in situ hybridization: association with clinicopathological features and patient survival. Neuropathol Appl Neurobiol 32: 441-450.
976. Jaskolsky D, Zawirski M, Papierz W, Kotwica Z (1987). Mixed gliomas. Their clinical course and results of surgery. Zentralbl Neurochir 48: 120-123.
977. Jay V, Edwards V, Squire J, Rutka J (1993). Astroblastoma: report of a case with ultrastructural, cell kinetic, and cytogenetic analysis. Pediatr Pathol 13: 323-332.
978. Jay V, Squire J, Becker LE, Humphreys R (1994). Malignant transformation in a ganglioglioma with anaplastic neuronal and astrocytic components. Report of a case with flow cytometric and cytogenetic analysis. Cancer 73: 2862-2868.
979. Jay V, Edwards V, Hoving E, Rutka J, Becker L, Zielenska M, Teshima I (1999). Central neurocytoma: morphological, flow cytometric, polymerase chain reaction, fluorescence in situ hybridization, and karyotypic analyses. Case report. J Neurosurg 90: 348-354.
980. Jay V, Squire J, Blaser S, Hoffman HJ, Hwang P (1997). Intracranial and spinal metastases from a ganglioglioma with unusual cytogenetic abnormalities in a patient with complex partial seizures. Childs Nerv Syst 13: 550-555.
981. Jayawickreme DP, Hayward RD, Harkness WF (1995). Intracranial ependymomas in childhood: a report of 24 cases followed for 5 years. Childs Nerv Syst 11: 409-413.
982. Jeffs GJ, Lee GY, Wong GT (2003). Functioning paraganglioma of the thoracic spine: case report. Neurosurgery 53: 992-994.

983. Jeibmann A, Hasselblatt M, Gerss J, Wrede B, Egensperger R, Beschorner R, Hans VH, Rickert CH, Wolff JE, Paulus W (2006). Prognostic Implications of Atypical Histologic Features in Choroid Plexus Papilloma. J Neuropathol Exp Neurol 65: 1069-1073.
984. Jellinger K (1986). Vascular malformations of the central nervous system: a morphological overview. Neurosurg Rev 9: 177-216.
985. Jellinger K, Denk H (1974). Blood group isoantigens in angioblastic meningiomas and hemangioblastomas of the central nervous system. Virchows Arch A Pathol Anat Histol 364: 137-144.
986. Jellinger K, Paulus W, Slowik F (1991). The enigma of meningeal hemangiopericytoma. Brain Tumor Pathol 8: 33-43.
987. Jellinger K, Slowik F (1975). Histological subtypes and prognostic problems in meningiomas. J Neurol 208: 279-298.
988. Jenevein EP (1964). A neurohypophyseal tumor originating from pituicytes. Am J Clin Pathol 41:522-6.: 522-526.
989. Jenkins RB, Blair H, Ballman KV, Giannini C, Arusell RM, Law M, Flynn H, Passe S, Felten S, Brown PD, Shaw EG, Buckner JC (2006). A t(1;19)(q10;p10) mediates the combined deletions of 1p and 19q and predicts a better prognosis of patients with oligodendroglioma. Cancer Res 66: 9852-9861.
990. Jenkinson MD, Bosma JJ, Du PD, Ohgaki H, Kleihues P, Warnke P, Rainov NG (2003). Cerebellar liponeurocytoma with an unusually aggressive clinical course: case report. Neurosurgery 53: 1425-1427.
991. Jenkinson MD, du Plessis DG, Smith TS, Joyce KA, Warnke PC, Walker C (2006). Histological growth patterns and genotype in oligodendroglial tumours: correlation with MRI features. Brain 129: 1884-1891.
992. Jennings MT, Frenchman M, Shehab T, Johnson MD, Creasy J, LaPorte K, Dettbarn WD (1995). Gliomatosis cerebri presenting as intractable epilepsy during early childhood. J Child Neurol 10: 37-45.
993. Jensen RL, Caamano E, Jensen EM, Couldwell WT (2006). Development of contrast enhancement after long-term observation of a dysembryoplastic neuroepithelial tumor. J Neurooncol 78: 59-62.
994. Jensen RL, Gillespie D, House P, Layfield L, Shelton C (2004). Endolymphatic sac tumors in patients with and without von Hippel-Lindau disease: the role of genetic mutation, von Hippel-Lindau protein, and hypoxia inducible factor-1alpha expression. J Neurosurg 100: 488-497.
995. Jeuken JW, Sprenger SH, Boerman RH, von Deimling A, Teepen HL, van Overbeeke JJ, Wesseling P (2001). Subtyping of oligo-astrocytic tumours by comparative genomic hybridization. J Pathol 194: 81-87.
996. Jeuken JW, Sprenger SH, Gilhuis J, Teepen HL, Grotenhuis AJ, Wesseling P (2002). Correlation between localization, age, and chromosomal imbalances in ependymal tumours as detected by CGH. J Pathol 197: 238-244.
997. Jeuken JW, von Deimling A, Wesseling P (2004). Molecular pathogenesis of oligodendroglial tumors. J Neurooncol 70: 161-181.
998. Jhanwar SC, Chen Q, Li FP, Brennan MF, Woodruff JM (1994). Cytogenetic analysis of soft tissue sarcomas. Recurrent chromosome abnormalities in malignant peripheral nerve sheath tumors (MPNST). Cancer Genet Cytogenet 78: 138-144.
999. Jiang R, Mircean C, Shmulevich I, Cogdell D, Jia Y, Tabus I, Aldape K, Sawaya R, Bruner JM, Fuller GN, Zhang W (2006). Pathway alterations during glioma progression revealed by reverse phase protein lysate arrays. Proteomics 6: 2964-2971.
1000. Jimenez CL, Carpenter BF, Robb IA (1987). Melanotic cerebellar tumor. Ultrastruct Pathol 11: 751-759.
1001. Johannsson O, Ostermeyer EA, Hakansson S, Friedman LS, Johansson U, Sellberg G, Brondum N, Sele V, Olsson H, King MC, Borg A (1996). Founding BRCA1 mutations in hereditary breast and ovarian cancer in southern Sweden. Am J Hum Genet 58: 441-450.
1002. Johnson JHJ, Hariharan S, Berman J, Sutton LN, Rorke LB, Molloy P, Phillips PC (1997). Clinical outcome of pediatric gangliogliomas: ninety-nine cases over 20 years. Pediatr Neurosurg 27: 203-207.
1003. Johnson M, Pace J, Burroughs JF (2006). Fourth ventricle rosette-forming glioneuronal tumor. Case report. J Neurosurg 105: 129-131.
1004. Johnson MD, Vnencak-Jones CL, Toms SA, Moots PM, Weil R (2003). Allelic losses in oligodendroglial and oligodendroglioma-like neoplasms: analysis using microsatellite repeats and polymerase chain reaction. Arch Pathol Lab Med 127: 1573-1579.
1005. Johnson RL, Rothman AL, Xie J, Goodrich LV, Bare JW, Bonifas JM, Quinn AG, Myers RM, Cox DR, Epstein EH, Jr., Scott MP (1996). Human homolog of patched, a candidate gene for the basal cell nevus syndrome. Science 272: 1668-1671.
1006. Jones AC, Shyamsundar MM, Thomas MW, Maynard J, Idziaszczyk S, Tomkins S, Sampson JR, Cheadle JP (1999). Comprehensive mutation analysis of TSC1 and TSC2-and phenotypic correlations in 150 families with tuberous sclerosis. Am J Hum Genet 64: 1305-1315.
1007. Jones DT, Ichimura K, Liu L, Pearson DM, Plant K, Collins VP (2006). Genomic analysis of pilocytic astrocytomas at 0.97 mb resolution shows an increasing tendency toward chromosomal copy number change with age. J Neuropathol Exp Neurol 65: 1049-1058.
1008. Jones H, Steart PV, Weller RO (1991). Spindle-cell glioblastoma or gliosarcoma? Neuropathol Appl Neurobiol 17: 177-187.
1008A. Jordan CT, Guzman ML, Noble M (2006). Cancer stem cells. N Engl J Med. 355:1253-61.
1009. Joseph JT, Lisle DK, Jacoby LB, Paulus W, Barone R, Cohen ML, Roggendorf WH, Bruner JM, Gusella JF, Louis DN (1995). NF2 gene analysis distinguishes hemangiopericytoma from meningioma. Am J Pathol 147: 1450-1455.
1010. Jouvet A, Fauchon F, Bouffet E, Saint-Pierre G, Champier J, Fevre-Montange M (2006). Tumors of pineal parenchymal and glial cells. In: Russel & Rubinstein's, Pathology of tumors of the nervous system. McLendon RE, Rosenblum MK, Bigner DD, eds. Hodder Arnold: London, pp. 413-424.
1011. Jouvet A, Fauchon F, Liberski P, Saint-Pierre G, Didier-Bazes M, Heitzmann A, Delisle MB, Biassette HA, Vincent S, Mikol J, Streichenberger N, Ahboucha S, Brisson C, Belin MF, Fevre-Montange M (2003). Papillary tumor of the pineal region. Am J Surg Pathol 27: 505-512.
1012. Jouvet A, Fevre-Montange M, Besancon R, Derrington E, Saint-Pierre G, Belin MF, Pialat J, Lapras C (1994). Structural and ultrastructural characteristics of human pineal gland, and pineal parenchymal tumors. Acta Neuropathol 88: 334-348.
1013. Jouvet A, Lellouch-Tubiana A, Boddaert N, Zerah M, Champier J, Fevre-Montange M (2005). Fourth ventricle neurocytoma with lipomatous and ependymal differentiation. Acta Neuropathol 109: 346-351.
1014. Jouvet A, Saint-Pierre G, Fauchon F, Privat K, Bouffet E, Ruchoux MM, Chauveinc L, Fevre-Montange M (2000). Pineal parenchymal tumors: a correlation of histological features with prognosis in 66 cases. Brain Pathol 10: 49-60.
1015. Jozwiak J, Jozwiak S, Skopinski P (2005). Immunohistochemical and microscopic studies on giant cells in tuberous sclerosis. Histol Histopathol 20: 1321-1326.
1016. Judkins AR, Burger PC, Hamilton RL, Kleinschmidt-DeMasters B, Perry A, Pomeroy SL, Rosenblum MK, Yachnis AT, Zhou H, Rorke LB, Biegel JA (2005). INI1 protein expression distinguishes atypical teratoid/rhabdoid tumor from choroid plexus carcinoma. J Neuropathol Exp Neurol 64: 391-397.
1017. Judkins AR, Mauger J, Ht A, Rorke LB, Biegel JA (2004). Immunohistochemical analysis of hSNF5/INI1 in pediatric CNS neoplasms. Am J Surg Pathol 28: 644-650.
1018. Jung SM, Kuo TT (2005). Immunoreactivity of CD10 and inhibin alpha in differentiating hemangioblastoma of central nervous system from metastatic clear cell renal cell carcinoma. Mod Pathol 18: 788-794.
1019. Jungbluth AA, Stockert E, Huang HJ, Collins VP, Coplan K, Iversen K, Kolb D, Johns TJ, Scott AM, Gullick WJ, Ritter G, Cohen L, Scanlan MJ, Cavenee WK, Old LJ (2003). A monoclonal antibody recognizing human cancers with amplification/overexpression of the human epidermal growth factor receptor. Proc Natl Acad Sci U S A 100: 639-644.
1020. Jurco S, III, Nadji M, Harvey DG, Parker JC, Jr., Font RL, Morales AR (1982). Hemangioblastomas: histogenesis of the stromal cell studied by immunocytochemistry. Hum Pathol 13: 13-18.
1021. Kachhara R, Bhattacharya RN, Nair S, Radhakrishnan VV (2003). Liponeurocytoma of the cerebellum—a case report. Neurol India 51: 274-276.
1022. Kadonaga JN, Frieden IJ (1991). Neurocutaneous melanosis: definition and review of the literature. J Am Acad Dermatol 24: 747-755.
1023. Kaido T, Sasaoka Y, Hashimoto H, Taira K (2003). De novo germinoma in the brain in association with Klinefelter's syndrome: case report and review of the literature. Surg Neurol 60: 553-558.
1024. Kakkar N, Vasishta RK, Banerjee AK, Marwaha RK, Thapa BR (2003). Familial hemophagocytic lymphohistiocytosis: an autopsy study. Pediatr Pathol Mol Med 22: 229-242.
1025. Kalifa C, Grill J (2005). The therapy of infantile malignant brain tumors: current status? J Neurooncol 75: 279-285.
1026. Kalimo H, Paljarvi L, Ekfors T, Pelliniemi LJ (1987). Pigmented primitive neuroectodermal tumor with multipotential differentiation in cerebellum (pigmented medullomyoblastoma). A case with light- and electron-microscopic, and immunohistochemical analysis. Pediatr Neurosci 13: 188-195.
1027. Kallio M, Sankila R, Hakulinen T, Jaaskelainen J (1992). Factors affecting operative and excess long-term mortality in 935 patients with intracranial meningioma. Neurosurgery 31: 2-12.
1028. Kalpana GV, Marmon S, Wang W, Crabtree GR, Goff SP (1994). Binding and stimulation of HIV-1 integrase by a human homolog of yeast transcription factor SNF5. Science 266: 2002-2006.
1029. Kaluza V, Rao DS, Said JW, de Vos S (2006). Primary extranodal nasal-type natural killer/T-cell lymphoma of the brain: a case report. Hum Pathol 37: 769-772.
1030. Kalyan R, Olivero WC (1987). Ganglioglioma: a correlative clinicopathological and radiological study of ten surgically treated cases with follow-up. Neurosurgery 20: 428-433.
1031. Kam R, Chen J, Blumcke I, Normann S, Fassunke J, Elger CE, Schramm J, Wiestler OD, Becker AJ (2004). The reelin pathway components disabled-1 and p35 in gangliogliomas—a mutation and expression analysis. Neuropathol Appl Neurobiol 30: 225-232.
1032. Kamakura Y, Hasegawa M, Minamoto T, Yamashita J, Fujisawa H (2006). C-kit gene mutation: common and widely distributed in intracranial germinomas. J Neurosurg 104: 173-180.
1033. Kamijo T, Weber JD, Zambetti G, Zindy F, Roussel MF, Sherr CJ (1998). Functional and physical interactions of the ARF tumor suppressor with p53 and Mdm2. Proc Natl Acad Sci U S A 95: 8292-8297.
1034. Kamiryo T, Tada K, Shiraishi S, Shinojima N, Kochi M, Ushio Y (2004). Correlation between promoter hypermethylation of the O6-methylguanine-deoxyribonucleic acid methyltransferase gene and prognosis in patients with high-grade astrocytic tumors treated with surgery, radiotherapy, and 1-(4-amino-2-methyl-5-pyrimidinyl)methyl-3-(2-chloroethyl)-3-nitrosourea-b ased chemotherapy. Neurosurgery 54: 349-357.
1035. Kamitani H, Masuzawa H, Sato J, Kanazawa I (1987). Capillary hemangioblastoma: histogenesis of stromal cells. Acta Neuropathol 73: 370-378.
1036. Kamura T, Koepp DM, Conrad MN, Skowyra D, Moreland RJ, Iliopoulos O, Lane WS, Kaelin WG, Jr., Elledge SJ, Conaway RC, Harper JW, Conaway JW (1999). Rbx1, a component of the VHL tumor suppressor complex and SCF ubiquitin ligase. Science 284: 657-661.
1037. Kanamori M, Kon H, Nobukuni T, Nomura S, Sugano K, Mashiyama S, Kumabe T, Yoshimoto T, Meuth M, Sekiya T, Murakami Y (2000). Microsatellite instability and the PTEN1 gene mutation in a subset of early onset gliomas carrying germline mutation or promoter methylation of the hMLH1 gene. Oncogene 19: 1564-1571.
1038. Kandt RS, Haines JL, Smith M, Northrup H, Gardner RJ, Short MP, Dumars K, Roach ES, Steingold S, Wall S (1992). Linkage of an important gene locus for tuberous sclerosis to a chromosome 16 marker for polycystic kidney disease. Nat Genet 2: 37-41.
1039. Kanner AA, Staugaitis SM, Castilla EA, Chernova O, Prayson RA, Vogelbaum MA, Stevens G, Peereboom D, Suh J, Lee SY, Tubbs RR, Barnett GH (2006). The impact of genotype on outcome in oligodendroglioma: validation of the loss of chromosome arm 1p as an important factor in clinical decision making. J Neurosurg 104: 542-550.
1040. Kanno H, Kondo K, Ito S, Yamamoto I, Fujii S, Torigoe S, Sakai N, Hosaka M, Shuin T, Yao M (1994). Somatic mutations of the von Hippel-Lindau tumor suppressor gene in sporadic central nervous system hemangioblastomas. Cancer Res 54: 4845-4847.
1041. Kannuki S, Bando K, Soga T, Matsumoto K, Hirose T (1996). [A case report of dysembryoplastic neuroepithelial tumor associated with neurofibromatosis type 1]. No Shinkei Geka 24: 183-188.
1042. Kapadia SB, Frisman DM, Hitchcock CL, Ellis GL, Popek EJ (1993). Melanotic neuroectodermal tumor of infancy. Clinicopathological, immunohistochemical, and flow cytometric study. Am J Surg Pathol 17: 566-573.
1043. Karaki S, Mochida J, Lee YH, Nishimura K, Tsutsumi Y (1999). Low-grade malignant perineurioma of the paravertebral column, transforming into a high-grade malignancy. Pathol Int 49: 820-825.
1044. Karamitopoulou E, Perentes E, Diamantis I, Maraziotis T (1994). Ki-67

immunoreactivity in human central nervous system tumors: a study with MIB 1 monoclonal antibody on archival material. Acta Neuropathol 87: 47-54.

1045. Karch SB, Urich H (1972). Medulloepithelioma: definition of an entity. J Neuropathol Exp Neurol 31: 27-53.

1046. Karim AB, Maat B, Hatlevoll R, Menten J, Rutten EH, Thomas DG, Mascarenhas F, Horiot JC, Parvinen LM, van Reijn M, Jager JJ, Fabrini MG, van Alphen AM, Hamers HP, Gaspar L, Noordman E, Pierart M, van Glabbeke M (1996). A randomized trial on dose-response in radiation therapy of low-grade cerebral glioma: European Organization for Research and Treatment of Cancer (EORTC) Study 22844. Int J Radiat Oncol Biol Phys 36: 549-556.

1047. Karkuzhali P, Deiveegan K, Pari (2005). Melanotic medulloblastoma of cerebellum: a case report. Indian J Pathol Microbiol 48: 243-244.

1048. Karlbom AE, James CD, Boethius J, Cavenee WK, Collins VP, Nordenskjöld M, Larsson C (1993). Loss of heterozygosity in malignant gliomas involves at least three distinct regions on chromosome 10. Hum Genet 92: 169-174.

1049. Karnes PS, Tran TN, Cui MY, Raffel C, Gilles FH, Barranger JA, Ying KL (1992). Cytogenetic analysis of 39 pediatric central nervous system tumors. Cancer Genet Cytogenet 59: 12-19.

1050. Karpinski NC, Yaghmai R, Barba D, Hansen LA (1999). Case of the month: March 1999—A 26 year old HIV positive male with dura based masses. Brain Pathol 9: 609-610.

1051. Karsdorp N, Elderson A, Wittebol P, Hene RJ, Vos J, Feldberg MA, van Gils AP, Jansen Sv, V, Vroom TM, Hoppener JW (1994). Von Hippel-Lindau disease: new strategies in early detection and treatment. Am J Med 97: 158-168.

1052. Kasashima S, Oda Y, Nozaki J, Shirasaki M, Nakanishi I (2000). A case of atypical granular cell tumor of the neurohypophysis. Pathol Int 50: 568-573.

1053. Kato K, Nakatani Y, Kanno H, Inayama Y, Ijiri R, Nagahara N, Miyake T, Tanaka M, Ito Y, Aida N, Tachibana K, Sekido K, Tanaka Y (2004). Possible linkage between specific histological structures and aberrant reactivation of the Wnt pathway in adamantinomatous craniopharyngioma. J Pathol 203: 814-821.

1054. Kato S, Han SY, Liu W, Otsuka K, Shibata H, Kanamaru R, Ishioka C (2003). Understanding the function-structure and function-mutation relationships of p53 tumor suppressor protein by high-resolution missense mutation analysis. Proc Natl Acad Sci U S A 100: 8424-8429.

1055. Kato S, Hirano A, Kato M, Herz F, Ohama E (1993). Comparative study on the expression of stress-response protein (srp) 72, srp 27, alpha B-crystallin and ubiquitin in brain tumours. An immunohistochemical investigation. Neuropathol Appl Neurobiol 19: 436-442.

1056. Kato T, Fujita M, Sawamura Y, Tada M, Abe H, Nagashima K, Nakamura N (1996). Clinicopathological study of choroid plexus tumors: immunohistochemical features and evaluation of proliferative potential by PCNA and Ki-67 immunostaining. Noshuyo Byori 13: 99-105.

1057. Katoh M, Aida T, Sugimoto S, Suwamura Y, Abe H, Isu T, Kaneko S, Mitsumori K, Kojima H, Nakamura N, . (1995). Immunohistochemical analysis of giant cell glioblastoma. Pathol Int 45: 275-282.

1058. Katsetos CD, Del Valle L, Legido A, de Chadarevian JP, Perentes E, Mork SJ (2003). On the neuronal/neuroblastic nature of medul-

loblastomas: a tribute to Pio del Rio Hortega and Moises Polak. Acta Neuropathol 105: 1-13.

1059. Katsetos CD, Herman MM, Frankfurter A, Gass P, Collins VP, Walker CC, Rosemberg S, Barnard RO, Rubinstein LJ (1989). Cerebellar desmoplastic medulloblastomas. A further immunohistochemical characterization of the reticulin-free pale islands. Arch Pathol Lab Med 113: 1019-1029.

1060. Katsetos CD, Herman MM, Krishna L, Vender JR, Vinores SA, Agamanolis DP, Schiffer D, Burger PC, Urich H (1995). Calbindin-D28k in subsets of medulloblastomas and in the human medulloblastoma cell line D283 Med. Arch Pathol Lab Med 119: 734-743.

1061. Katsetos CD, Krishna L (1994). Lobar pilocytic astrocytomas of the cerebral hemispheres: I. Diagnosis and nosology. Clin Neuropathol 13: 295-305.

1062. Katsetos CD, Krishna L, Friedberg E, Reidy J, Karkavelas G, Savory J (1994). Lobar pilocytic astrocytomas of the cerebral hemispheres: II. Pathobiology- Morphogenesis of the eosinophilic granular bodies. Clin Neuropathol 13: 306-314.

1063. Katsetos CD, Legido A, Perentes E, Mork SJ (2003). Class III beta-tubulin isotype: a key cytoskeletal protein at the crossroads of developmental neurobiology and tumor neuropathology. J Child Neurol 18: 851-866.

1064. Katsetos CD, Liu HM, Zacks SI (1988). Immunohistochemical and ultrastructural observations on Homer Wright (neuroblastic) rosettes and the "pale islands" of human cerebellar medulloblastomas. Hum Pathol 19: 1219-1227.

1065. Katsuta T, Inoue T, Nakagaki H, Takeshita M, Morimoto K, Iwaki T (2003). Distinctions between pituicytoma and ordinary pilocytic astrocytoma. Case report. J Neurosurg 98: 404-406.

1066. Kaufman DL, Heinrich BS, Willett C, Perry A, Finseth F, Sobel RA, MacCollin M (2003). Somatic instability of the NF2 gene in schwannomatosis. Arch Neurol 60: 1317-1320.

1067. Kaulich K, Blaschke B, Numann A, von Deimling A, Wiestler OD, Weber RG, Reifenberger G (2002). Genetic alterations commonly found in diffusely infiltrating cerebral gliomas are rare or absent in pleomorphic xanthoastrocytomas. J Neuropathol Exp Neurol 61: 1092-1099.

1068. Kaur B, Khwaja FW, Severson EA, Matheny SL, Brat DJ, Van Meir EG (2005). Hypoxia and the hypoxia-inducible-factor pathway in glioma growth and angiogenesis. Neurooncol 7: 134-153.

1069. Kawamura J, Garcia JH, Kamijyo Y (1973). Cerebellar hemangioblastoma: histogenesis of stroma cells. Cancer 31: 1528-1540.

1070. Kawano N, Yasui Y, Utsuki S, Oka H, Fujii K, Yamashina S (2004). Light microscopic demonstration of the microlumen of ependymoma: a study of the usefulness of antigen retrieval for epithelial membrane antigen (EMA) immunostaining. Brain Tumor Pathol 21: 17-21.

1071. Keith J, Lownie S, Ang LC (2006). Coexistence of paraganglioma and myxopapillary ependymoma of the cauda equina. Acta Neuropathol 111: 617-618

1072. Kelleher T, Aquilina K, Keohane C. O'Sullivan MG (2005). Intramedullary capillary haemangioma. Br J Neurosurg 19: 345-348.

1073. Kelley TW, Prayson RA, Barnett GH, Stevens GH, Cook JR, Hsi ED (2005). Extranodal marginal zone B-cell lymphoma of mucosa-associated lymphoid tissue arising in the lateral ventricle. Leuk Lymphoma 46. 1423-1427.

1074. Kelsey KT, Wrensch M, Zuo ZF, Miike R, Wiencke JK (1997). A population-based case-control study of the CYP2D6 and GSTT1

polymorphisms and malignant brain tumors. Pharmacogenetics 7: 463-468.

1075. Kennedy PG, Watkins BA, Thomas DG, Noble MD (1987). Antigenic expression by cells derived from human gliomas does not correlate with morphological classification. Neuropathol Appl Neurobiol 13: 327-347.

1076. Kepes JJ (1975). The fine structure of hyaline inclusions (pseudopsammoma bodies) in meningiomas. J Neuropathol Exp Neurol 34: 282-294.

1077. Kepes JJ (1978). Transitional cell tumor of the pituitary gland developing from a Rathke's cleft cyst. Cancer 41: 337-343.

1078. Kepes JJ (1979). 'Xanthomatous' lesions of the central nervous system: definition, classification and some recent observations. Prog Neuropathol 4: 179-213.

1079. Kepes JJ (1982). Meningiomas. Biology, Pathology, and Differential Diagnosis. Masson Publishing: New York.

1080. Kepes JJ (1987). Astrocytomas: old and newly recognized variants, their spectrum of morphology and antigen expression. Can J Neurol Sci 14: 109-121.

1081. Kepes JJ (1993). Pleomorphic xanthoastrocytoma: the birth of a diagnosis and a concept. Brain Pathol 3: 269-274.

1082. Kepes JJ, Chen WY, Connors MH, Vogel FS (1988). "Chordoid" meningeal tumors in young individuals with peritumoral lymphoplasmacellular infiltrates causing systemic manifestations of the Castleman syndrome. A report of seven cases. Cancer 62: 391-406.

1083. Kepes JJ, Collins J (1999). Choroid plexus epithelium (normal and neoplastic) expresses synaptophysin. A potentially useful aid in differentiating carcinoma of the choroid plexus from metastatic papillary carcinomas. J Neuropathol Exp Neurol 58: 398-401.

1084. Kepes JJ, Fulling KH, Garcia JH (1982). The clinical significance of "adenoid" formations of neoplastic astrocytes, imitating metastatic carcinoma, in gliosarcomas. A review of five cases. Clin Neuropathol 1: 139-150.

1085. Kepes JJ, Moral LA, Wilkinson SB, Abdullah A, Llena JF (1998). Rhabdoid transformation of tumor cells in meningiomas: a histologic indication of increased proliferative activity: report of four cases. Am J Surg Pathol 22: 231-238.

1086. Kepes JJ, Rengachary SS, Lee SH (1979). Astrocytes in hemangioblastomas of the central nervous system and their relationship to stromal cells. Acta Neuropathol 47: 99-104.

1087. Kepes JJ, Rubinstein LJ (1981). Malignant gliomas with heavily lipidized (foamy) tumor cells: a report of three cases with immunoperoxidase study. Cancer 47: 2451-2459.

1088. Kepes JJ, Rubinstein LJ, Ansbacher L, Schreiber DJ (1989). Histopathological features of recurrent pleomorphic xanthoastrocytomas: further corroboration of the glial nature of this neoplasm. A study of three cases. Acta Neuropathol 78: 585-593.

1089. Kepes JJ, Rubinstein LJ, Chiang H (1984). The role of astrocytes in the formation of cartilage in gliomas. An immunohistochemical study of four cases. Am J Pathol 117: 471-483.

1090. Kepes JJ, Rubinstein LJ, Eng LF (1979). Pleomorphic xanthoastrocytoma: a distinctive meningocerebral glioma of young subjects with relatively favorable prognosis; a study of 12 cases. Cancer 44: 1839-1852.

1091. Kern M, Robbins P, Lee G, Watson P (2006). Papillary tumor of the pineal region - a new pathological entity. Clin Neuropathol 25: 185-192.

1092. Kernohan JW (1931). Primary tumors of the spinal cord and intradural filum terminale. In: Cytology and Cellular Pathology of the

Nervous System. Penfield W, ed. Hoeber: New York, pp. 993.

1093. Kernohan JW, Mabon RF, Svien HJ, Adson AW (1949). A simplified classification of gliomas. Proc Staff Meet Mayo Clin 24: 71-75.

1094. Keyvani K, Rickert CH, von Wild K, Paulus W (2001). Rosetted glioneuronal tumor: a case with proliferating neuronal nodules. Acta Neuropathol 101: 525-528.

1095. Khalili K, Krynska B, Del Valle L, Katsetos CD, Croul S (1999). Medulloblastomas and the human neurotropic polyomavirus JC virus. Lancet 353: 1152-1153.

1096. Khan RB, DeAngelis LM (2003). Brain metastases. In: Cancer Neurology in Clinical Practice. Schiff D, Wen PY, eds. Humana Press: Totowa, NJ, USA.

1097. Khanani MF, Hawkins C, Shroff M, Dirks P, Capra M, Burger PC, Bouffet E (2006). Pilomyxoid astrocytoma in a patient with neurofibromatosis. Pediatr Blood Cancer 46: 377-380.

1098. Kho AT, Zhao Q, Cai Z, Butte AJ, Kim JY, Pomeroy SL, Rowitch DH, Kohane IS (2004). Conserved mechanisms across development and tumorigenesis revealed by a mouse development perspective of human cancers. Genes Dev 18: 629-640.

1099. Khoddami M, Becker LE (1997). Immunohistochemistry of medulloepithelioma and neural tube. Pediatr Pathol Lab Med 17: 913-925.

1100. Khuntia D, Brown P, Li J, Mehta MP (2006). Whole-brain radiotherapy in the management of brain metastasis. J Clin Oncol 24: 1295-1304.

1101. Kida S, Ellison DW, Steart PV, Weller RO (1995). Characterisation of perivascular cells in astrocytic tumours and peritumoral oedematous brain. Neuropathol Appl Neurobiol 21: 121-129.

1102. Kidd EA, Mansur DB, Leonard JR, Michalski JM, Simpson JR, Perry A (2006). The efficacy of radiation therapy in the management of grade I astrocytomas. J Neurooncol 76: 55-58.

1103. Kim DG, Kim JS, Chi JG, Park SH, Jung HW, Choi KS, Han DH (1996). Central neurocytoma: proliferative potential and biological behavior. J Neurosurg 84: 742-747.

1104. Kim DG, Yang HJ, Park IA, Chi JG, Jung HW, Han DH, Choi KS, Cho BK (1998). Gliomatosis cerebri: clinical features, treatment, and prognosis. Acta Neurochir 140: 755-762.

1105. Kim DH, Suh YL (1997). Pseudopapillary neurocytoma of temporal lobe with glial differentiation. Acta Neuropathol 94: 187-191.

1106. Kim HA, Ling B, Ratner N (1997). Nf1-deficient mouse Schwann cells are angiogenic and invasive and can be induced to hyperproliferate: reversion of some phenotypes by an inhibitor of farnesyl protein transferase. Mol Cell Biol 17: 862-872.

1107. Kim JY, Nelson AL, Algon SA, Graves O, Sturla LM, Goumnerova LC, Rowitch DH, Segal RA, Pomeroy SL (2003). Medulloblastoma tumorigenesis diverges from cerebellar granule cell differentiation in patched heterozygous mice. Dev Biol 263: 50-66.

1108. Kim L, Hochberg FH, Thornton AF, Harsh GR, Patel H, Finkelstein D, Louis DN (1996). Procarbazine, lomustine, and vincristine (PCV) chemotherapy for grade III and grade IV oligoastrocytomas. J Neurosurg 85: 602-607.

1109. Kim NR, Im SH, Chung CK, Suh YL, Choe G, Chi JG (2004). Sclerosing meningioma: immunohistochemical analysis of five cases. Neuropathol Appl Neurobiol 30: 126-135.

1110. Kim SD, Nakagawa H, Mizuno J, Inoue T (2005). Thoracic subpial intramedullary schwannoma involving a ventral nerve root: a case report and review of the literature. Surg

Neurol 63: 389-393.
1111. Kim SK, Wang KC, Cho BK, Jung HW, Lee YJ, Chung YS, Lee JY, Park SH, Kim YM, Choe G, Chi JG (2001). Biological behavior and tumorigenesis of subependymal giant cell astrocytomas. J Neurooncol 52: 217-225.
1112. Kimonis VE, Goldstein AM, Pastakia B, Yang ML, Kase R, DiGiovanna JJ, Bale A, Bale SJ (1997). Clinical manifestations in 105 persons with nevoid basal cell carcinoma syndrome. Am J Med Genet 69: 299-308.
1113. Kimura M, Takayasu M, Suzuki Y, Negoro M, Nagasaka T, Nakashima N, Sugita K (1992). Primary choroid plexus papilloma located in the suprasellar region: case report. Neurosurgery 31: 563-566.
1114. Kimura T, Budka H, Soler F (1986). An immunocytochemical comparison of the glia-associated proteins glial fibrillary acidic protein (GFAP) and S-100 protein (S100P) in human brain tumors. Clin Neuropathol 5: 21-27.
1115. Kindblom LG, Ahlden M, Meis K, Stenman G (1995). Immunohistochemical and molecular analysis of p53, MDM2, proliferating cell nuclear antigen and Ki67 in benign and malignant peripheral nerve sheath tumours. Virchows Arch 427: 19-26.
1116. Kirkpatrick PJ, Honavar M, Janota I, Polkey CE (1993). Control of temporal lobe epilepsy following en bloc resection of low-grade tumors. J Neurosurg 78: 19-25.
1117. Kissil JL, Wilker EW, Johnson KC, Eckman MS, Yaffe MB, Jacks T (2003). Merlin, the product of the Nf2 tumor suppressor gene, is an inhibitor of the p21-activated kinase, Pak1. Mol Cell 12: 841-849.
1117A. Kita D, Yonekawa Y, Weller M, Ohgaki H (2007). PIK3CA alterations in primary (de novo) and secondary glioblastomas. Acta Neuropathol 113:295-302.
1118. Kivela T (1999). Trilateral retinoblastoma: a meta-analysis of hereditary retinoblastoma associated with primary ectopic intracranial retinoblastoma. J Clin Oncol 17: 1829-1837.
1119. Klaeboe L, Lonn S, Scheie D, Auvinen A, Christensen HC, Feychting M, Johansen C, Salminen T, Tynes T (2005). Incidence of intracranial meningiomas in Denmark, Finland, Norway and Sweden, 1968-1997. Int J Cancer 117: 996-1001.
1120. Kleihues P, Burger PC, Scheithauer BW eds. (1993). Histological Typing of Tumours of the Central Nervous System. World Health Organization International Histological Classification of Tumours. Springer Verlag: Berlin Heidelberg.
1121. Kleihues P, Burger PC, Scheithauer BW (1993). The new WHO classification of brain tumours. Brain Pathol 3: 255-268.
1122. Kleihues P, Cavenee WK (*eds.*) (2000). WHO Classification of Tumours: Pathology and Genetics of Tumours of the Nervous System. IARC Press: Lyon.
1123. Kleihues P, Kiessling M, Janzer RC (1987). Morphological markers in neuro-oncology. Curr Top Pathol 77: 307-338.
1124. Kleihues P, zur Hausen A, Schauble B, Ohgaki H (1997). Tumours associated with p53 germline mutations. A synopsis of 91 families. Am J Pathol 150: 1-13.
1125. Klein R, Mullges W, Bendszus M, Woydt M, Kreipe H, Roggendorf W (1999). Primary intracerebral Hodgkin's disease: report of a case with Epstein- Barr virus association and review of the literature. Am J Surg Pathol 23: 477-481.
1126. Klein R, Roggendorf W (2001). Increased microglia proliferation separates pilocytic astrocytomas from diffuse astrocytomas: a double labeling study. Acta Neuropathol 101: 245-248.
1127. Kleinman GM, Young RH, Scully RE (1984). Ependymoma of the ovary: report of three cases. Hum Pathol 15: 632-638.
1128. Kleinschmidt-DeMasters BK (2001). Dural metastases. A retrospective surgical and autopsy series. Arch Pathol Lab Med 125: 880-887.
1129. Kleinschmidt-DeMasters BK, Lillehei KO, Breeze RE (2003). Neoplasms involving the central nervous system in the older old. Hum Pathol 34: 1137-1147.
1130. Kleinschmidt D, Lillehei KO (1995). Radiation-induced meningioma with a 63-year latency period. Case report. J Neurosurg 82: 487-488.
1131. Klesse LJ, Parada LF (1998). p21 ras and phosphatidylinositol-3 kinase are required for survival of wild-type and NF1 mutant sensory neurons. J Neurosci 18: 10420-10428.
1132. Kliewer KE, Cochran AJ (1989). A review of the histology, ultrastructure, immunohistology, and molecular biology of extra-adrenal paragangliomas. Arch Pathol Lab Med 113: 1209-1218.
1133. Kliewer KE, Wen DR, Cancilla PA, Cochran AJ (1989). Paragangliomas: assessment of prognosis by histologic, immunohistochemical, and ultrastructural techniques. Hum Pathol 20: 29-39.
1134. Kloub O, Perry A, Tu PH, Lipper M, Lopes MB (2005). Spindle cell oncocytoma of the adenohypophysis: report of two recurrent cases. Am J Surg Pathol 29: 247-253.
1135. Kluwe L, Friedrich R, Mautner V (1999). Loss of NF1 allele in schwann cells but not in fibroblasts derived from a NF1-associated neurofibroma. Genes Chromosomes Cancer 24: 283-285.
1136. Kluwe L, Hagel C, Tatagiba M, Thomas S, Stavrou D, Ostertag H, von Deimling A, Mautner VF (2001). Loss of NF1 alleles distinguish sporadic from NF1-associated pilocytic astrocytomas. J Neuropathol Exp Neurol 60: 917-920.
1137. Kluwe L, MacCollin M, Tatagiba M, Thomas S, Hazim W, Haase W, Mautner VF (1998). Phenotypic variability associated with 14 splice-site mutations in the NF2 gene. Am J Med Genet 77: 228-233.
1138. Kluwe L, Mautner VF (1998). Mosaicism in sporadic neurofibromatosis 2 patients. Hum Mol Genet 7: 2051-2055.
1139. Knobbe CB, Merlo A, Reifenberger G (2002). Pten signaling in gliomas. Neuro-oncol 4: 196-211.
1140. Knobbe CB, Reifenberger G (2003). Genetic alterations and aberrant expression of genes related to the phosphatidyl-inositol-3'-kinase/protein kinase B (Akt) signal transduction pathway in glioblastomas. Brain Pathol 13: 507-518.
1141. Knobbe CB, Trampe-Kieslich A, Reifenberger G (2005). Genetic alteration and expression of the phosphoinositol-3-kinase/Akt pathway genes PIK3CA and PIKE in human glioblastomas. Neuropathol Appl Neurobiol 31: 486-490.
1142. Knott JC, Mahesparan R, Garcia-Cabrera I, Bolge TB, Edvardsen K, Ness GO, Mork S, Lund-Johansen M, Bjerkvig R (1998). Stimulation of extracellular matrix components in the normal brain by invading glioma cells. Int J Cancer 75: 864-872.
1143. Ko LJ, Prives C (1996). p53: puzzle and paradigm. Genes Dev 10: 1054-1072.
1144. Kobayashi C, Oda Y, Takahira T, Izumi T, Kawaguchi K, Yamamoto H, Tamiya S, Yamada T, Oda S, Tanaka K, Matsuda S, Iwamoto Y, Tsuneyoshi M (2006). Chromosomal aberrations and microsatellite instability of malignant peripheral nerve sheath tumors: a study of 10 tumors from nine patients. Cancer Genet Cytogenet 165: 98-105.
1145. Koch A, Tonn J, Kraus JA, Sorensen N, Albrecht NS, Wiestler OD, Pietsch T (1996). Molecular analysis of the lissencephaly gene 1 (LIS-1) in medulloblastomas. Neuropathol Appl Neurobiol 22: 233-242.
1146. Koch A, Waha A, Tonn JC, Sorensen N, Berthold F, Wolter M, Reifenberger J, Hartmann W, Friedl W, Reifenberger G, Wiestler OD, Pietsch T (2001). Somatic mutations of WNT/wingless signaling pathway components in primitive neuroectodermal tumors. Int J Cancer 93: 445-449.
1147. Kochi N, Budka H (1987). Contribution of histiocytic cells to sarcomatous development of the gliosarcoma. An immunohistochemical study. Acta Neuropathol 73: 124-130.
1148. Koen JL, McLendon RE, George TM (1998). Intradural spinal teratoma: evidence for a dysembryogenic origin. Report of four cases. J Neurosurg 89: 844-851.
1149. Koga T, Iwasaki H, Ishiguro M, Matsuzaki A, Kikuchi M (2002). Losses in chromosomes 17, 19, and 22q in neurofibromatosis type 1 and sporadic neurofibromas: a comparative genomic hybridization analysis. Cancer Genet Cytogenet 136: 113-120.
1150. Kolen ER, Horvai A, Perry V, Gupta N (2003). Congenital craniopharyngioma: a role for imaging in the prenatal diagnosis and treatment of an uncommon tumor. Fetal Diagn Ther 18: 270-274.
1151. Kolles H, Niedermayer I, Schmitt C, Henn W, Feld R, Steudel WI, Zang KD, Feiden W (1995). Triple approach for diagnosis and grading of meningiomas: histology, morphometry of Ki-67/Feulgen stainings, and cytogenetics. Acta Neurochir 137: 174-181.
1152. Kollias SS, Ball WSJ, Tzika AA, Harris RE (1994). Familial erythrophagocytic lymphohistiocytosis: neuroradiologic evaluation with pathologic correlation. Radiology 192: 743-754.
1153. Komori T, Scheithauer BW, Anthony DC, Rosenblum MK, McLendon RE, Scott RM, Okazaki H, Kobayashi M (1998). Papillary glioneuronal tumor: a new variant of mixed neuronal-glial neoplasm. Am J Surg Pathol 22: 1171-1183.
1154. Komori T, Scheithauer BW, Anthony DC, Scott RM, Okazaki H, Kobayashi M (1996). Pseudopapillary ganglioneurocytoma. J Neuropathol Exp Neurol 55: 654-654.
1155. Komori T, Scheithauer BW, Hirose T (2002). A rosette-forming glioneuronal tumor of the fourth ventricle: infratentorial form of dysembryoplastic neuroepithelial tumor? Am J Surg Pathol 26: 582-591.
1156. Komori T, Scheithauer BW, Parisi JE, Watterson J, Priest JR (2001). Mixed conventional and desmoplastic infantile ganglioglioma: an autopsied case with 6-year follow-up. Mod Pathol 14: 720-726.
1157. Komotar RJ, Burger PC, Carson BS, Brem H, Olivi A, Goldthwaite PT, Tihan T (2004). Pilocytic and pilomyxoid hypothalamic/chiasmatic astrocytomas. Neurosurgery 54: 72-79.
1158. Komotar RJ, Carson BS, Rao C, Chaffee S, Goldthwaite PT, Tihan T (2005). Pilomyxoid astrocytoma of the spinal cord: report of three cases. Neurosurgery 56: 191.
1159. Komotar RJ, Mocco J, Carson BS, Sughrue ME, Zacharia BE, Sisti AC, Canoll PD, Khandji AG, Tihan T, Burger PC, Bruce JN (2004). Pilomyxoid astrocytoma: a review. MedGenMed 6: 42-
1160. Komuro Y, Mikami M, Sakaiya N, Kurahashi T, Komiyama S, Tei C, Mukai M, Hirose T (2001). Tumor imprint cytology of ovarian ependymoma. A case report. Cancer 92: 3165-3169.
1161. Kondo T (2006). Brain cancer stem-like cells. Eur J Cancer 42: 1237-1242.
1162. Konno S, Oka H, Utsuki S, Kondou K, Tanaka S, Fujii K, Yagishita S (2002). Germinoma with a granulomatous reaction. Problems of differential diagnosis. Clin Neuropathol 21: 248-251.
1163. Konovalov AN, Pitskhelauri DI (2003). Principles of treatment of the pineal region tumors. Surg Neurol 59: 250-268.
1164. Koochekpour S, Jeffers M, Wang PH, Gong C, Taylor GA, Roessler LM, Stearman R, Vasselli JR, Stetler-Stevenson WG, Kaelin WG, Jr., Linehan WM, Klausner RD, Gnarra JR, Vande Woude GF (1999). The von Hippel-Lindau tumor suppressor gene inhibits hepatocyte growth factor/scatter factor-induced invasion and branching morphogenesis in renal carcinoma cells. Mol Cell Biol 19: 5902-5912.
1165. Koperek O, Gelpi E, Birner P, Haberler C, Budka H, Hainfellner JA (2004). Value and limits of immunohistochemistry in differential diagnosis of clear cell primary brain tumors. Acta Neuropathol 108: 24-30.
1166. Koral K, Weprin B, Rollins NK (2006). Sphenoid sinus craniopharyngioma simulating mucocele. Acta Radiol 47: 494-496.
1167. Korf BR, Prasad C, Schneider G, Anthony D (1996). A family with multiple neurofibromas and non-linkage to NF1 and NF2. FASEB Summer Research Conference On Neurofibromatosis, Snowmass, Co, USA
1168. Korhonen K, Salminen T, Raitanen J, Auvinen A, Isola J, Haapasalo H (2006). Female predominance in meningiomas can not be explained by differences in progesterone, estrogen, or androgen receptor expression. J Neurooncol 80: 1-7.
1169. Korogi Y, Takahashi M, Ushio Y (2001). MRI of pineal region tumors. J Neurooncol 54: 251-261.
1170. Korshunov A, Golanov A (2001). The prognostic significance of DNA topoisomerase II-alpha (Ki-S1), p21/Cip-1, and p27/Kip-1 protein immunoexpression in oligodendrogliomas. Arch Pathol Lab Med 125: 892-898.
1171. Korshunov A, Golanov A, Sycheva R, Timirgaz V (2004). The histologic grade is a main prognostic factor for patients with intracranial ependymomas treated in the microneurosurgical era: an analysis of 258 patients. Cancer 100: 1230-1237.
1172. Korshunov A, Golanov A, Timirgaz V (2000). Immunohistochemical markers for intracranial ependymoma recurrence. An analysis of 88 cases. J Neurol Sci 177: 72-82.
1173. Korshunov A, Neben K, Wrobel G, Tews B, Benner A, Hahn M, Golanov A, Lichter P (2003). Gene expression patterns in ependymomas correlate with tumor location, grade, and patient age. Am J Pathol 163: 1721-1727.
1174. Korshunov A, Savostikova M, Ozerov S (2002). Immunohistochemical markers for prognosis of average-risk pediatric medulloblastomas. The effect of apoptotic index, TrkC, and c-myc expression. J Neurooncol 58: 271-279.
1175. Korshunov A, Shishkina L, Golanov A (2003). Immunohistochemical analysis of p16INK4a, p14ARF, p18INK4c, p21CIP1, p27KIP1 and p73 expression in 271 meningiomas correlation with tumor grade and clinical outcome. Int J Cancer 104: 728-734.
1176. Korten AG, ter Berg HJ, Spincemaille GH, van der Laan RT, Van de Wel AM (1998). Intracranial chondrosarcoma: review of the literature and report of 15 cases. J Neurol Neurosurg Psychiatry 65: 88-92.
1177. Koul D, Shen R, Bergh S, Lu Y, de Groot JF, Liu TJ, Mills GB, Yung WK (2005). Targeting integrin-linked kinase inhibits Akt signaling pathways and decreases tumor progression of human glioblastoma. Mol Cancer Ther 4: 1681-1688.

1178. Kourea HP, Bilsky MH, Leung DH, Lewis JJ, Woodruff JM (1998). Subdiaphragmatic and intrathoracic paraspinal malignant peripheral nerve sheath tumors: a clinicopathologic study of 25 patients and 26 tumors. Cancer 82: 2191-2203.

1179. Kourea HP, Cordon-Cardo C, Dudas M, Leung D, Woodruff JM (1999). Expression of p27 (kip) and other cell-cycle regulators in malignant peripheral nerve sheath tumors and neurofibromas: the emerging role of p27KIP in malignant transformation of neurofibromas. Am J Pathol 155: 1885-1891.

1180. Kourea HP, Orlow I, Scheithauer BW, Cordon-Cardo C, Woodruff JM (1999). Deletions of the INK4A gene occur in malignant peripheral nerve sheath tumors but not in neurofibromas. Am J Pathol 155: 1855-1860.

1181. Kowalski RJ, Prayson RA, Mayberg MR (2004). Pituicytoma. Ann Diagn Pathol 8: 290-294.

1182. Kozmik Z, Sure U, Ruedi D, Busslinger M, Aguzzi A (1995). Deregulated expression of PAX5 in medulloblastoma. Proc Natl Acad Sci USA 92: 5709-5713.

1183. Kraus JA, de Millas W, Sorensen N, Herbold C, Schichor C, Tonn JC, Wiestler OD, von Deimling A, Pietsch T (2001). Indications for a tumor suppressor gene at 22q11 involved in the pathogenesis of ependymal tumors and distinct from hSNF5/INI1. Acta Neuropathol 102: 69-74.

1184. Kraus JA, Koopmann J, Kaskel P, Maintz D, Brandner S, Schramm J, Louis DN, Wiestler OD, von Deimling A (1995). Shared allelic losses on chromosomes 1p and 19q suggest a common origin of oligodendroglioma and oligoastrocytoma. J Neuropathol Exp Neurol 54: 91-95.

1185. Kraus JA, Lamszus K, Glesmann N, Beck M, Wolter M, Sabel M, Krex D, Klockgether T, Reifenberger G, Schlegel U (2001). Molecular genetic alterations in glioblastomas with oligodendroglial component. Acta Neuropathol 101: 311-320.

1186. Kraus MD, Haley JC, Ruiz R, Essary L, Moran CA, Fletcher CD (2001). "Juvenile" xanthogranuloma: an immunophenotypic study with a reappraisal of histogenesis. Am J Dermatopathol 23: 104-111.

1187. Krieg M, Marti HH, Plate KH (1998). Coexpression of erythropoietin and vascular endothelial growth factor in nervous system tumors associated with von Hippel-Lindau tumor suppressor gene loss of function. Blood 92: 3388-3393.

1188. Kriho VK, Zang H, Moskal JR, Skalli O (1997). Keratin expression in astrocytomas: an immunofluorescent and biochemical reassessment. Virchows Arch 431:139-147.

1189. Krishnan S, Brown PD, Scheithauer BW, Ebersold MJ, Hammack JE, Buckner JC (2004). Choroid plexus papillomas: a single institutional experience. J Neurooncol 68: 49-55.

1190. Kristof RA, Van Roost D, Wolf HK, Schramm J (1997). Intravascular papillary endothelial hyperplasia of the sellar region. Report of three cases and review of the literature. J Neurosurg 86: 558-563.

1191. Kristopaitis T, Thomas C, Petruzzelli GJ, Lee JM (2000). Malignant craniopharyngioma. Arch Pathol Lab Med 124: 1356-1360.

1192. Kroppenstedt SN, Golfinos J, Sonntag VK, Spetzler RF (2003). Pineal region lesion masquerading choroid plexus papilloma: case report. Surg Neurol 59: 124-127.

1193. Kros J, de Greve K, van Tilborg A, Hop W, Pieterman H, Avezaat C, Lekanne Dit DR, Zwarthoff E (2001). NF2 status of meningiomas is associated with tumour localization and histology. J Pathol 194: 367-372.

1194. Kros JM (2007). Panel review of a set of anaplastic oligodendroglioma of EORTC trial 26951: interobserver variation, correlation with 1p/19q loss and clinical outcome. J Neuropathol Exp Neurol. In Press

1195. Kros JM, Cella F, Bakker SL, Paz YG, Egeler RM (2000). Papillary meningioma with pleural metastasis: case report and literature review. Acta Neurol Scand 102: 200-202.

1196. Kros JM, Delwel EJ, de Jong TH, Tanghe HL, van Run PR, Vissers K, Alers JC (2002). Desmoplastic infantile astrocytoma and ganglioglioma: a search for genomic characteristics. Acta Neuropathol 104: 144-148.

1197. Kros JM, Hop WC, Godschalk JJ, Krishnadath KK (1996). Prognostic value of the proliferation-related antigen Ki-67 in oligodendrogliomas. Cancer 78: 1107-1113.

1198. Kros JM, Lie ST, Stefanko SZ (1994). Familial occurrence of polymorphous oligodendroglioma. Neurosurgery 34: 732-736.

1199. Kros JM, Pieterman H, Van Eden CG, Avezaat CJ (1994). Oligodendroglioma: the Rotterdam-Dijkzigt experience. Neurosurgery 34: 959-966.

1200. Kros JM, Schouten WC, Janssen PJ, van der Kwast TH (1996). Proliferation of gemistocytic cells and glial fibrillary acidic protein (GFAP)-positive oligodendroglial cells in gliomas: a MIB-1/GFAP double labeling study. Acta Neuropathol 91: 99-103.

1201. Kros JM, Stefanko SZ, de Jong AA, van Vroonhoven CC, van der Heul RO, van der Kwast TH (1991). Ultrastructural and immunohistochemical segregation of gemistocytic subsets. Hum Pathol 22: 33-40.

1202. Kros JM, Troost D, Van Eden CG, van der Werf AJ, Uylings HB (1988). Oligodendroglioma. A comparison of two grading systems. Cancer 61: 2251-2259.

1203. Kros JM, van den Brink WA, van Loon-van Luyt JJM, Stefanko SZ (1997). Signet-ring cell oligodendroglioma - report of two cases and discussion of the differential diagnosis. Acta Neuropathol 93: 638-643.

1204. Kros JM, Van Eden CG, Stefanko SZ, Waayer-Van Batenburg M, van der Kwast TH (1990). Prognostic implications of glial fibrillary acidic protein containing cell types in oligodendrogliomas. Cancer 66: 1204-1212.

1205. Kros JM, Vecht CJ, Stefanko SZ (1991). The pleomorphic xanthoastrocytoma and its differential diagnosis: a study of five cases. Hum Pathol 22: 1128-1135.

1206. Kros JM, Zheng P, Dinjens WN, Alers JC (2002). Genetic aberrations in gliomatosis cerebri support monoclonal tumorigenesis. J Neuropathol Exp Neurol 61: 806-814.

1207. Krossnes BK, Wester K, Moen G, Mork SJ (2005). Multifocal dysembryoplastic neuroepithelial tumour in a male with the XYY syndrome. Neuropathol Appl Neurobiol 31: 556-560.

1208. Krouwer HG, Davis RL, Silver P, Prados M (1991). Gemistocytic astrocytomas: a reappraisal. J Neurosurg 74: 399-406.

1209. Krumbholz M, Theil D, Derfuss T, Rosenwald A, Schrader F, Monoranu CM, Kalled SL, Hess DM, Serafini B, Aloisi F, Wekerle H, Hohlfeld R, Meinl E (2005). BAFF is produced by astrocytes and up-regulated in multiple sclerosis lesions and primary central nervous system lymphoma. J Exp Med 201: 195-200.

1210. Krutilkova V, Trkova M, Fleitz J, Gregor V, Novotna K, Krepelova A, Sumerauer D, Kodet R, Siruckova S, Plevova P, Bendova S, Hedvicakova P, Foreman NK, Sedlacek Z (2005). Identification of five new families strengthens the link between childhood choroid plexus carcinoma and germline TP53 mutations. Eur J Cancer 41: 1597-1603.

1211. Krynska B, Del Valle L, Croul S, Gordon J, Katsetos CD, Carbone M, Giordano A, Khalili K (1999). Detection of human neurotropic JC virus DNA sequence and expression of the viral oncogenic protein in pediatric medulloblastomas. Proc Natl Acad Sci U S A 96: 11519-11524.

1212. Kubbutat MHG, Jones SN, Vousden KH (1997). Regulation of p53 stability by Mdm2. Nature 387: 289-303.

1213. Kubo O, Sasahara A, Tajika Y, Kawamura H, Kawabatake H, Takakura K (1996). Pleomorphic xanthoastrocytoma with neurofibromatosis type 1: case report. Noshuyo Byori 13: 79-83.

1214. Kubota T, Hayashi M, Kawano H, Kabuto M, Sato K, Ishise J, Kawamoto K, Shirataki K, Iizuka H, Tsunoda S (1991). Central neurocytoma: immunohistochemical and ultrastructural study. Acta Neuropathol 81: 418-427.

1215. Kubota T, Sato K, Arishima H, Takeuchi H, Kitai R, Nakagawa T (2006). Astroblastoma: immunohistochemical and ultrastructural study of distinctive epithelial and probable tanycytic differentiation. Neuropathology 26: 72-81.

1216. Kuchelmeister K, Demirel T, Schlorer E, Bergmann M, Gullotta F (1995). Dysembryoplastic neuroepithelial tumour of the cerebellum. Acta Neuropathol 89: 385-390.

1217. Kuchelmeister K, Hugens-Penzel M, Jodicke A, Schachenmayr W (2006). Papillary tumour of the pineal region: histodiagnostic considerations. Neuropathol Appl Neurobiol 32: 203-208.

1218. Kuchelmeister K, Nestler U, Siekmann R, Schachenmayr W (2006). Liponeurocytoma of the left lateral ventricle—case report and review of the literature. Clin Neuropathol 25: 86-94.

1219. Kuchelmeister K, Schonmeyr R, Albani M, Schachenmayr W (1998). Anaplastic desmoplastic infantile ganglioglioma. Clin Neuropathol 17: 269-269.

1220. Kuchelmeister K, Steinhauser A, Korf B, Wagner D, Prey N, Schachenmayr W (1996). Anaplastic desmoplastic infantile ganglioglioma: a case report. Clin Neuropathol 15: 280-280.

1221. Kuchelmeister K, von Borcke IM, Klein H, Bergmann M, Gullotta F (1994). Pleomorphic pineocytoma with extensive neuronal differentiation: report of two cases. Acta Neuropathol 88: 448-453.

1222. Kudo H, Oi S, Tamaki N, Nishida Y, Matsumoto S (1990). Ependymoma diagnosed in the first year of life in Japan in collaboration with the International Society for Pediatric Neurosurgery. Childs Nerv Syst 6: 375-378.

1223. Kudo M, Matsumoto M, Terao H (1983). Malignant nerve sheath tumor of acoustic nerve. Arch Pathol Lab Med 107: 293-297.

1224. Kuijten RR, Strom SS, Rorke LB, Boesel CP, Buckley JD, Meadows AT, Bunin GR (1993). Family history of cancer and seizures in young children with brain tumors: a report from the Childrens Cancer Group (United States and Canada). Cancer Causes Control 4: 455-464.

1225. Kujas M, Faillot T, Lalam T, Roncier B, Catala M, Poirier J (2000). Astroblastomas revisited. Report of two cases with immunocytochemical and electron microscopic study. Histogenetic considerations. Neuropathol Appl Neurobiol 26: 295-298.

1226. Kujas M, Lejeune J, Benouaich-Amiel A, Criniere E, Laigle-Donadey F, Marie Y, Mokhtari K, Polivka M, Bernier M, Chretien F, Couvelard A, Capelle L, Duffau H, Cornu P, Broet P, Thillet J, Carpentier AF, Sanson M, Hoang-Xuan K, Delattre JY (2005). Chromosome 1p loss: a favorable prognostic factor in low-grade gliomas. Ann Neurol 58: 322-326.

1227. Kuker W, Nagele T, Korfel A, Heckl S, Thiel E, Bamberg M, Weller M, Herrlinger U (2005). Primary central nervous system lymphomas (PCNSL): MRI features at presentation in 100 patients. J Neurooncol 72: 169-177.

1228. Kulkarni AV, Pierre-Kahn A, Zerah M (2004). Spontaneous regression of congenital spinal lipomas of the conus medullaris. Report of two cases. J Neurosurg 101: 226-227.

1229. Kuppner MC, Hamou MF, de Tribolet N (1990). Activation and adhesion molecule expression on lymphoid infiltrates in human glioblastomas. J Neuroimmunol 29: 229-238.

1230. Kuratsu J, Matsukado Y, Sonoda H (1983). Pseudopsammoma bodies in meningotheliomatous meningioma. A histochemical and ultrastructural study. Acta Neurochir 68: 55-62.

1231. Kuratsu J, Ushio Y (1996). Epidemiological study of primary intracranial tumors in childhood. A population-based survey in Kumamoto Prefecture, Japan. Pediatr Neurosurg 25: 240-246.

1232. Kuratsu J, Ushio Y (1996). Epidemiological study of primary intracranial tumors: a regional survey in Kumamoto Prefecture in the southern part of Japan. J Neurosurg 84: 946-950.

1233. Kurian KM, Summers DM, Statham PF, Smith C, Bell JE, Ironside JW (2005). Third ventricular chordoid glioma: clinicopathological study of two cases with evidence for a poor clinical outcome despite low grade histological features. Neuropathol Appl Neurobiol 31: 354-361.

1234. Kuroiwa T, Bergey GK, Rothman MI, Zoarski GH, Wolf A, Zagardo MT, Kristt DA, Hudson LP, Krumholz A, Barry E (1995). Radiologic appearance of the dysembryoplastic neuroepithelial tumor. Radiology 197: 233-238.

1235. Kurt E, Beute GN, Sluzewski M, van Rooij WJ, Teepen JL (1996). Giant chondroma of the falx. Case report and review of the literature. J Neurosurg 85: 1161-1164.

1236. Kurt E, Zheng PP, Hop WC, van der WM, Bol M, van den Bent MJ, Avezaat CJ, Kros JM (2006). Identification of relevant prognostic histopathologic features in 69 intracranial ependymomas, excluding myxopapillary ependymomas and subependymomas. Cancer 106: 388-395.

1237. Kurtkaya-Yapicier O, Elmaci I, Boran B, Kilic T, Sav A, Pamir MN (2002). Dysembryoplastic neuroepithelial tumor of the midbrain tectum: a case report. Brain Tumor Pathol 19: 97-100.

1238. Kurtkaya-Yapicier O, Scheithauer BW, Van Peteghem KP, Sawicki JE (2002). Unusual case of extradural choroid plexus papilloma of the sacral canal. Case report. J Neurosurg 97: 102-105.

1239. Kurtkaya-Yapicier O, Scheithauer BW, Woodruff JM, Wenger DD, Cooley AM, Dominique D (2003). Schwannoma with rhabdomyoblastic differentiation: a unique variant of malignant triton tumor. Am J Surg Pathol 27: 848-853.

1239A. Kusafuka T, Miao J, Yoneda A, Kuroda S, Fukuzawa M (2004). Novel germline deletion of SNF5/INI1/SMARCB1 gene in neonate presenting with congenital malignant rhabdoid tumor of kidney and brain primitive neuroectodermal tumor. Genes chromosomes Cancer 40:133-139.

1240. Kwiatkowski DJ, Short MP (1994). Tuberous sclerosis. Arch Dermatol 130: 348-354.

1241. Kwon CH, Zhu X, Zhang J, Knoop LL, Tharp R, Smeyne RJ, Eberhart CG, Burger PC, Baker SJ (2001). Pten regulates neuronal soma size: a mouse model of Lhermitte-Duclos disease. Nat Genet 29: 404-411.

1242. Kyritsis AP, Bondy ML, Xiao M, Berman EL, Cunningham JE, Lee PS, Levin VA, Saya H

(1994). Germline p53 gene mutations in subsets of glioma patients. J Natl Cancer Inst 86: 344-349.
1243. Lach B, Duggal N, DaSilva VF, Benoit BG (1996). Association of pleomorphic xanthoastrocytoma with cortical dysplasia and neuronal tumors. A report of three cases. Cancer 78: 2551-2563.
1244. Lach B, Duncan E, Rippstein P, Benoit BG (1994). Primary intracranial pleomorphic angioleiomyoma—a new morphologic variant. An immunohistochemical and electron microscopic study. Cancer 74: 1915-1920.
1245. Lach B, Gregor A, Rippstein P, Omulecka A (1999). Angiogenic histogenesis of stromal cells in hemangioblastoma: ultrastructural and immunohistochemical study. Ultrastruct Pathol 23: 299-310.
1246. Lach B, Sikorska M, Rippstein P, Gregor A, Staines W, Davie TR (1991). Immunoelectron microscopy of Rosenthal fibers. Acta Neuropathol 81: 503-509.
1247. Lack EE (1994). Paragangliomas. In: Diagnostic Surgical Pathology. Sternberg SS, ed. Raven Press: New York, pp. 559-621.
1248. Lack EE, Cubilla AL, Woodruff JM (1979). Paragangliomas of the head and neck region. A pathologic study of tumors from 71 patients. Hum Pathol 10: 191-218.
1249. Lacombe D, Chateil JF, Fontan D, Battin J (1990). Medulloblastoma in the nevoid basal-cell carcinoma syndrome: case reports and review of the literature. Genet Couns 1: 273-277.
1250. Laigle-Donadey F, Taillibert S, Mokhtari K, Hildebrand J, Delattre JY (2005). Dural metastases. J Neurooncol 75: 57-61.
1251. Lakkis MM, Epstein JA (1998). Neurofibromin modulation of ras activity is required for normal endocardial-mesenchymal transformation in the developing heart. Development 125: 4359-4367.
1252. Lam CW, Xie J, To KF, Ng HK, Lee KC, Yuen NW, Lim PL, Chan LY, Tong SF, McCormick F (1999). A frequent activated smoothened mutation in sporadic basal cell carcinomas. Oncogene 18: 833-836.
1253. Laman JD, Leenen PJ, Annels NE, Hogendoorn PC, Egeler RM (2003). Langerhans-cell histiocytosis 'insight into DC biology'. Trends Immunol 24: 190-196.
1254. Lamiell JM, Salazar FG, Hsia YE (1989). von Hippel-Lindau disease affecting 43 members of a single kindred. Medicine (Baltimore) 68: 1-29.
1255. Lamont JM, McManamy CS, Pearson AD, Clifford SC, Ellison DW (2004). Combined histopathological and molecular cytogenetic stratification of medulloblastoma patients. Clin Cancer Res 10: 5482-5493.
1256. Lang FF, Epstein FJ, Ransohoff J, Allen JC, Wisoff J, Abbott IR, Miller DC (1993). Central nervous system gangliogliomas. Part 2: Clinical outcome. J Neurosurg 79: 867-873.
1257. Lang FF, Miller DC, Koslow M, Newcomb EW (1994). Pathways leading to glioblastoma multiforme: a molecular analysis of genetic alterations in 65 astrocytic tumors. J Neurosurg 81: 427-436.
1258. Langford LA (1986). The ultrastructure of the ependymoblastoma. Acta Neuropathol 71: 136-141.
1259. Langford LA, Camel MH (1987). Palisading pattern in cerebral neuroblastoma mimicking the primitive polar spongioblastoma. An ultrastructural study. Acta Neuropathol 73: 153-159.
1260. Lantos PL, Louis DN, Rosenblum MK, Kleihues P (2002). Tumours of the Nervous System. Oxford University Press: London.
1261. Lantos PL, VandenBerg SR, Kleihues P (1996). Tumours of the Nervous System. In: Greenfield's Neuropathology. Graham DI, Lantos PL, eds. Arnold: London, pp. 583-879.
1262. Larson JJ, Tew JM, Jr., Simon M, Menon AG (1995). Evidence for clonal spread in the development of multiple meningiomas. J Neurosurg 83: 705-709.
1263. Laskin WB, Weiss SW, Bratthauer GL (1991). Epithelioid variant of malignant peripheral nerve sheath tumor (malignant epithelioid schwannoma). Am J Surg Pathol 15: 1136-1145.
1264. Lasky JL, Wu H (2005). Notch signaling, brain development, and human disease. Pediatr Res 57: 104R-109R.
1265. Lasser DM, DeVivo DC, Garvin J, Wilhelmsen KC (1994). Turcot's syndrome: evidence for linkage to the adenomatous polyposis coli (APC) locus. Neurology 44: 1083-1086.
1266. Latif F, Tory K, Gnarra J, Yao M, Duh FM, Orcutt ML, Stackhouse T, Kuzmin I, Modi W, Geil L (1993). Identification of the von Hippel-Lindau disease tumor suppressor gene. Science 260: 1317-1320.
1267. Lauer DH, Enzinger FM (1980). Cranial fasciitis of childhood. Cancer 45: 401-406.
1268. Laws ER, Jr., Goldberg WJ, Bernstein JJ (1993). Migration of human malignant astrocytoma cells in the mammalian brain: Scherer revisited. Int J Dev Neurosci 11: 691-697.
1269. Lebrun C, Fontaine D, Ramaioli A, Vandenbos F, Chanalet S, Lonjon M, Michiels JF, Bourg V, Paquis P, Chatel M, Frenay M (2004). Long-term outcome of oligodendrogliomas. Neurology 62: 1783-1787.
1270. Lednicky JA, Garcea RL, Bergsagel DJ, Butel JS (1995). Natural simian virus 40 strains are present in human choroid plexus and ependymoma tumors. Virology 212: 710-717.
1271. Lee A, Kessler JD, Read TA, Kaiser C, Corbeil D, Huttner WB, Johnson JE, Wechsler-Reya RJ (2005). Isolation of neural stem cells from the postnatal cerebellum. Nat Neurosci 8: 723-729.
1272. Lee CJ, Appleby VJ, Orme AT, Chan WI, Scotting PJ (2002). Differential expression of SOX4 and SOX11 in medulloblastoma. J Neurooncol 57: 201-214.
1273. Lee DK, Jung HW, Kim DG, Paek SH, Gwak HS, Choe G (2001). Postoperative spinal seeding of craniopharyngioma. Case report. J Neurosurg 94: 617-620.
1274. Lee DY, Chung CK, Hwang YS, Choe G, Chi JG, Kim HJ, Cho BK (2000). Dysembryoplastic neuroepithelial tumor: radiological findings (including PET, SPECT, and MRS) and surgical strategy. J Neurooncol 47: 167-174.
1275. Lee HY, Yoon CS, Sevenet N, Rajalingam V, Delattre O, Walford NQ (2002). Rhabdoid tumor of the kidney is a component of the rhabdoid predisposition syndrome. Pediatr Dev Pathol 5: 395-399.
1276. Lee JH, Sundaram V, Stein J, Kinney SE, Stacey DW, Golubic M (1997). Reduced expression of schwannomin/merlin in human sporadic meningiomas. Neurosurgery 40: 578-587.
1277. Lee JY, Dong SM, Park WS, Yoo NJ, Kim CS, Jang JJ, Chi JG, Zbar B, Lubensky IA, Linehan WM, Vortmeyer AO, Zhuang Z (1998). Loss of heterozygosity and somatic mutations of the VHL tumor suppressor gene in sporadic cerebellar hemangioblastomas. Cancer Res 58: 504-508.
1278. Lee JY, Wakabayashi T, Yoshida J (2005). Management and survival of pineoblastoma: an analysis of 34 adults from the brain tumor registry of Japan. Neurol Med Chir (Tokyo) 45: 132-141.
1279. Lee R, Kertesz N, Joseph SB, Jegalian A, Wu H (2001). Erythropoietin (Epo) and EpoR expression and 2 waves of erythropoiesis. Blood 98: 1408-1415.
1280. Lee SB, Kim SH, Bell DW, Wahrer DC, Schiripo TA, Jorczak MM, Sgroi DC, Garber JE, Li FP, Nichols KE, Varley JM, Godwin AK, Shannon KM, Harlow E, Haber DA (2001). Destabilization of CHK2 by a missense mutation associated with Li-Fraumeni Syndrome. Cancer Res 61: 8062-8067.
1281. Lee TT, Manzano GR (1997). Third ventricular glioblastoma multiforme: case report. Neurosurg Rev 20: 291-294.
1282. Lee YY, Van Tassel P (1989). Intracranial oligodendrogliomas: imaging findings in 35 untreated cases. AJR Am J Roentgenol 152: 361-369.
1283. Lee YY, Van Tassel P, Bruner JM, Moser RP, Share JC (1989). Juvenile pilocytic astrocytomas: CT and MR characteristics. AJR Am J Roentgenol 152: 1263-1270.
1284. Leeds NE, Lang FF, Ribalta T, Sawaya R, Fuller GN (2006). Origin of chordoid glioma of the third ventricle. Arch Pathol Lab Med 130: 460-464.
1285. Legius E, Dierick H, Wu R, Hall BK, Marynen P, Cassiman JJ, Glover TW (1994). TP53 mutations are frequent in malignant NF1 tumors. Genes Chromosomes Cancer 10: 250-255.
1286. Legius E, Marchuk DA, Collins FS, Glover TW (1993). Somatic deletion of the neurofibromatosis type 1 gene in a neurofibrosarcoma supports a tumour suppressor gene hypothesis. Nat Genet 3: 122-126.
1287. Leisti EL, Pyhtinen J, Poyhonen M (1996). Spontaneous decrease of a pilocytic astrocytoma in neurofibromatosis type I. AJNR Am J Neuroradiol 17: 1691-1694.
1288. Lekanne D, Bianchi AB, Groen NA, Seizinger BR, Hagemeijer A, van Drunen E, Bootsma D, Koper JW, Avezaat CJ, Kley N (1994). Frequent NF2 gene transcript mutations in sporadic meningiomas and vestibular schwannomas. Am J Hum Genet 54: 1022-1029.
1289. Lellouch-Tubiana A, Boddaert N, Bourgeois M, Fohlen M, Jouvet A, Delalande O, Seidenwurm D, Brunelle F, Sainte-Rose C (2005). Angiocentric neuroepithelial tumor (ANET): a new epilepsy-related clinicopathological entity with distinctive MRI. Brain Pathol 15: 281-286.
1290. Lellouch-Tubiana A, Bourgeois M, Vekemans M, Robain O (1995). Dysembryoplastic neuroepithelial tumors in two children with neurofibromatosis type 1. Acta Neuropathol 90: 319-322.
1291. Lemeta S, Pylkkanen L, Sainio M, Niemela M, Saarikoski S, Husgafvel-Pursiainen K, Bohling T (2004). Loss of heterozygosity at 6q is frequent and concurrent with 3p loss in sporadic and familial capillary hemangioblastomas. J Neuropathol Exp Neurol 63: 1072-1079.
1292. Leonard JR, Cai DX, Rivet DJ, Kaufman BA, Park TS, Levy BK, Perry A (2001). Large cell/anaplastic medulloblastomas and medullomyoblastomas: clinicopathological and genetic features. J Neurosurg 95: 82-88.
1292A. Leonard JR, Perry A, Rubin JB, King AA, Chicoine MR, Gutmann DH (2006). The role of surgical biopsy in the diagnosis of glioma in individuals with neurofibromatosis-1. Neurology. 67:1509-12.
1293. Leone PE, Bello MJ, Mendiola M, Kusak ME, de Campos JM, Vaquero J, Sarasa JL, Pestana A, Rey JA (1998). Allelic status of 1p, 14q, and 22q and NF2 gene mutations in sporadic schwannomas. Int J Mol Med 1: 889-892.
1294. Lesniak MS, Viglione MP, Weingart J (2002). Multicentric parenchymal xanthogranuloma in a child: case report and review of the literature. Neurosurgery 51: 1493-1498.
1295. Leung SY, Chan TL, Chung LP, Chan AS, Fan YW, Hung KN, Kwong WK, Ho JW, Yuen ST (1998). Microsatellite instability and mutation of DNA mismatch repair genes in gliomas. Am J Pathol 153: 1181-1188.
1296. Leung SY, Gwi E, Ng HK, Fung CF, Yam KY (1994). Dysembryoplastic neuroepithelial tumor. A tumor with small neuronal cells resembling oligodendroglioma. Am J Surg Pathol 18: 604-614.
1297. Leung SY, Yuen ST, Chan TL, Chan AS, Ho JW, Kwan K, Fan YW, Hung KN, Chung LP, Wyllie AH (2000). Chromosomal instability and p53 inactivation are required for genesis of glioblastoma but not for colorectal cancer in patients with germline mismatch repair gene mutation. Oncogene 19: 4079-4083.
1298. Leverkus M, Kluwe L, Roll EM, Becker G, Brocker EB, Mautner VF, Hamm H (2003). Multiple unilateral schwannomas: segmental neurofibromatosis type 2 or schwannomatosis? Br J Dermatol 148: 804-809.
1299. Levin N, Gomori JM, Siegal T (2004). Chemotherapy as initial treatment in gliomatosis cerebri: results with temozolomide. Neurology 63: 354-356.
1300. Levin N, Lavon I, Zelikovitsh B, Fuchs D, Bokstein F, Fellig Y, Siegal T (2006). Progressive low-grade oligodendrogliomas: response to temozolomide and correlation between genetic profile and O6-methylguanine DNA methyltransferase protein expression. Cancer 106: 1759-1765.
1301. Levine A (1997). p53: the cellular gatekeeper for growth and division. Cell 89: 323-331.
1302. Levy ML, Goldfarb A, Hyder DJ, Gonzales-Gomez I, Nelson M, Gilles FH, McComb JG (2001). Choroid plexus tumors in children: significance of stromal invasion. Neurosurgery 48: 303-309.
1303. Levy RA (1993). Paraganglioma of the filum terminale: MR findings. AJR Am J Roentgenol 160: 851-852.
1304. Lewis JH, Ginsberg AL, Toomey KE (1983). Turcot's syndrome. Evidence for autosomal dominant inheritance. Cancer 51: 524-528.
1305. Lewis JJ, Brennan MF (1996). Soft tissue sarcomas. Curr Probl Surg 33: 817-872.
1306. Lewis RA, Gerson LP, Axelson KA, Riccardi VM, Whitford RP (1984). von Recklinghausen neurofibromatosis. II. Incidence of optic gliomata. Ophthalmology 91: 929-935.
1307. Lhermitte J, Duclos P (1920). Sur un ganglioneurome diffus du coertex du cervelet. Bull Assoc Fran Etude Cancer 9: 99-107.
1308. Li D, Schauble B, Moll C, Fisch U (1996). Intratemporal facial nerve perineurioma. Laryngoscope 106: 328-333.
1309. Li DM, Sun H (1997). TEP1, encoded by a candidate tumor suppressor locus, is a novel protein tyrosine phosphatase regulated by transforming growth factor beta. Cancer Res 57: 2124-2129.
1310. Li FP, Fraumeni JF, Jr., Mulvihill JJ, Blattner WA, Dreyfus MG, Tucker MA, Miller RW (1988). A cancer family syndrome in twenty-four kindreds. Cancer Res 48: 5358-5362.
1311. Li J, Perry A, James CD, Gutmann DH (2001). Cancer-related gene expression profiles in NF1-associated pilocytic astrocytomas. Neurology 56: 885-890.
1312. Li J, Yen C, Liaw D, Podsypanina K, Bose S, Wang SI, Puc J, Miliaresis C, Rodgers L, McCombie R, Bigner SH, Giovanella BC, Ittmann M, Tycko B, Hibshoosh H, Wigler MH, Parsons R (1997). PTEN, a putative protein tyrosine phosphatase gene mutated in human brain, breast, and prostate cancer. Science 275: 1943-1947.
1313. Li MH, Bouffet E, Hawkins CE, Squire JA, Huang A (2005). Molecular genetics of

supratentorial primitive neuroectodermal tumors and pineoblastoma. Neurosurg Focus 19: E3.

1314. Li YS, Ramsay DA, Fan YS, Armstrong RF, Del Maestro RF (1995). Cytogenetic evidence that a tumor suppressor gene in the long arm of chromosome 1 contributes to glioma growth. Cancer Genet Cytogenet 84: 46-50.

1315. Liang L, Korogi Y, Sugahara T, Ikushima I, Shigematsu Y, Okuda T, Takahashi M, Kochi M, Ushio Y (2002). MRI of intracranial germ-cell tumours. Neuroradiology 44: 382-388.

1316. Liang X, Shen D, Huang Y, Yin C, Bojanowski CM, Zhuang Z, Chan CC (2007). Molecular pathology and CXCR4 expression in surgically excised retinal hemangioblastomas associated with von Hippel-Lindau disease. Ophthalmology 114: 147-156.

1317. Liang Y, Diehn M, Watson N, Bollen AW, Aldape KD, Nicholas MK, Lamborn KR, Berger MS, Botstein D, Brown PO, Israel MA (2005). Gene expression profiling reveals molecularly and clinically distinct subtypes of glioblastoma multiforme. Proc Natl Acad Sci USA 102: 5814-5819.

1318. Liaw D, Marsh DJ, Li J, Dahia PLM, Wang SI, Zheng Z, Bose S, Call KM, Tsou HC, Peacocke M, Eng C, Parsons R (1997). Germline mutations of the PTEN gene in Cowden disease, an inherited breast and thyroid cancer syndrome. Nat Genet 16: 64-67.

1319. Lichtenstein L (1953). Histiocytosis X. Integration of eosinophilic granuloma of bone, Letterer-Siwe disease and Schüller-Christian disease as related manifestations of a single nosological entity. Arch Pathol 56: 89-103.

1320. Lieberman KA, Fuller CE, Caruso RD, Schelper RL (2001). Postradiation gliosarcoma with osteosarcomatous components. Neuroradiology 43: 555-558.

1321. Ligon KL, Alberta JA, Kho AT, Weiss J, Kwaan MR, Nutt CL, Louis DN, Stiles CD, Rowitch DH (2004). The oligodendroglial lineage marker OLIG2 is universally expressed in diffuse gliomas. J Neuropathol Exp Neurol 63: 499-509.

1322. Lim SC, Jang SJ (2006). Myxopapillary ependymoma of the fourth ventricle. Clin Neurol Neurosurg 108: 211-214.

1323. Lin SL, Wang JS, Huang CS, Tseng HH (1996). Primary intracerebral leiomyoma: a case with eosinophilic inclusions of actin filaments. Histopathology 28: 365-369.

1324. Lindau A (1926). Studien uber Kleinhirncysten. Bau, Pathogenese und Beziehungen zur Angiomatosis Retinae. Acta Pathol Microbiol Scand Suppl 1.

1325. Lindau A (1931). Discussion on vascular tumors of the brain and spinal cord. Proceedings of the Royal Society of Medicine 24: 363-370.

1326. Lindblom A, Ruttledge M, Collins VP, Nordenskjold M, Dumanski JP (1994). Chromosomal deletions in anaplastic meningiomas suggest multiple regions outside chromosome 22 as important in tumor progression. Int J Cancer 56: 354-357.

1327. Lindstrom E, Shimokawa T, Toftgard R, Zaphiropoulos PG (2006). PTCH mutations: distribution and analyses. Hum Mutat 27: 215-219.

1328. Linehan WM, Zbar B (2004). Focus on kidney cancer. Cancer Cell 6: 223-228.

1329. Linnebank M, Pels H, Kleczar N, Farmand S, Fliessbach K, Urbach H, Orlopp K, Klockgether T, Schmidt-Wolf IG, Schlegel U (2005). MTX-induced white matter changes are associated with polymorphisms of methionine metabolism. Neurology 64: 912-913.

1330. Linnebank M, Schmidt S, Kolsch H, Linnebank A, Heun R, Schmidt-Wolf IG,

Glasmacher A, Fliessbach K, Klockgether T, Schlegel U, Pels H (2004). The methionine synthase polymorphism D919G alters susceptibility to primary central nervous system lymphoma. Br J Cancer 90: 1969-1971.

1331. Lipper S, Decker RE (1984). Paraganglioma of the cauda equina. A histologic, immunohistochemical, and ultrastructural study and review of the literature. Surg Neurol 22: 415-420.

1332. Liss L (1956). The cellular elements of the human neurohypophysis; a study with silvercarbonate. J Comp Neurol 106: 507-525.

1333. Listernick R, Charrow J, Greenwald M, Mets M (1994). Natural history of optic pathway tumors in children with neurofibromatosis type 1: a longitudinal study. J Pediatr 125: 63-66.

1334. Listernick R, Mancini AJ, Charrow J (2003). Segmental neurofibromatosis in childhood. Am J Med Genet A 121: 132-135.

1335. Liszka U, Drlicek M, Hitzenberger P, Machacek E, Mayer H, Stockhammer G, Grisold W (1994). Intravascular lymphomatosis: a clinicopathological study of three cases. J Cancer Res Clin Oncol 120: 164-168.

1336. Liu D, Schelper RL, Carter DA, Poiesz BJ, Shrimpton AE, Frankel BM, Hutchison RE (2003). Primary central nervous system cytotoxic/suppressor T-cell lymphoma: report of a unique case and review of the literature. Am J Surg Pathol 27: 682-688.

1337. Liu HM, Boogs J, Kidd J (1976). Ependymomas of childhood. I. Histological survey and clinicopathological correlation. Childs Brain 2: 92-110.

1338. Liu JM, Garonzik IM, Eberhart CG, Sampath P, Brem H (2002). Ectopic recurrence of craniopharyngioma after an interhemispheric transcallosal approach: case report. Neurosurgery 50: 639-644.

1339. Lloyd KM, Dennis M (1963). Cowden's disease: a possible new symptom complex with multiple system involvement. Ann Intern Med 58: 136-142.

1340. Lodding P, Kindblom LG, Angervall L (1986). Epithelioid malignant schwannoma. A study of 14 cases. Virchows Arch A Pathol Anat Histopathol 409: 433-451.

1341. Lodding P, Kindblom LG, Angervall L, Stenman G (1990). Cellular schwannoma. A clinicopathologic study of 29 cases. Virchows Arch A Pathol Anat Histopathol 416: 237-248.

1342. Lombardi D, Scheithauer BW, Meyer FB, Forbes GS, Shaw EG, Gibney DJ, Katzmann JA (1991). Symptomatic subependymoma: a clinicopathological and flow cytometric study. J Neurosurg 75: 583-588.

1343. Lonergan KM, Iliopoulos O, Ohh M, Kamura T, Conaway RC, Conaway JW, Kaelin WG, Jr. (1998). Regulation of hypoxia-inducible mRNAs by the von Hippel-Lindau tumor suppressor protein requires binding to complexes containing elongins B/C and Cul2. Mol Cell Biol 18: 732-741.

1344. Longatti P, Basaldella L, Orvieto E, Tos AP, Martinuzzi A (2006). Aquaporin 1 expression in cystic hemangioblastomas. Neurosci Lett 392: 178-180.

1345. Longy M, Lacombe D (1996). Cowden disease. Report of a family and review. Ann Genet 39: 35-42.

1346. Lonser RR, Glenn GM, Walther M, Chew EY, Libutti SK, Linehan WM, Oldfield EH (2003). von Hippel-Lindau disease. Lancet 361: 2059-2067.

1347. Lopes MBS, Altermatt HJ, Scheithauer BW, VandenBerg SR (1996). Immunohistochemical characterization of subependymal giant cell astrocytomas. Acta Neuropathol 91: 368-375.

1348. Losa M, Saeger W, Mortini P, Pandolfi C, Terreni MR, Taccagni G, Giovanelli M

(2000). Acromegaly associated with a granular cell tumor of the neurohypophysis: a clinical and histological study. Case report. J Neurosurg 93: 121-126.

1349. Lothe RA, Slettan A, Saeter G, Brogger A, Borresen AL, Nesland JM (1995). Alterations at chromosome 17 loci in peripheral nerve sheath tumors. J Neuropathol Exp Neurol 54: 65-73.

1350. Louis DN, Hamilton AJ, Sobel RA, Ojemann RG (1991). Pseudopsammomatous meningioma with elevated serum carcinoembryonic antigen: a true secretory meningioma. Case report. J Neurosurg 74: 129-132.

1351. Louis DN, Hedley-Whyte ET, Martuza RL (1989). Sarcomatous proliferation of the vasculature in a subependymoma. Acta Neuropathol 78: 332-335.

1352. Louis DN, Ramesh V, Gusella JF (1995). Neuropathology and molecular genetics of neurofibromatosis 2 and related tumors. Brain Pathol 5: 163-172.

1353. Louis DN, von Deimling A (1995). Hereditary tumor syndromes of the nervous system: overview and rare syndromes. Brain Pathol 5: 145-151.

1354. Louis DN, von Deimling A, Dickersin GR, Dooling EC, Seizinger BR (1992). Desmoplastic cerebral astrocytomas of infancy: a histopathologic, immunohistochemical, ultrastructural, and molecular genetic study. Hum Pathol 23: 1402-1409.

1355. Ludemann W, Stan AC, Tatagiba M, Samii M (2000). Sporadic unilateral vestibular schwannoma with islets of meningioma: case report. Neurosurgery 47: 451-452.

1356. Ludwin SK, Rubinstein LJ, Russell DS (1975). Papillary meningioma: a malignant variant of meningioma. Cancer 36: 1363-1373.

1357. Luider TM, Kros JM, Sillevis Smitt PA, van den Bent MJ, Vecht CJ (1999). Glial fibrillary acidic protein and its fragments discriminate astrocytoma from oligodendroglioma. Electrophoresis 20: 1087-1091.

1358. Luse SA, Kernohan JW (1955). Granular-cell tumors of the stalk and posterior lobe of the pituitary gland. Cancer 8: 616-622.

1359. Lusis EA, Watson MA, Chicoine MR, Lyman M, Roerig P, Reifenberger G, Gutmann DH, Perry A (2005). Integrative genomic analysis identifies NDRG2 as a candidate tumor suppressor gene frequently inactivated in clinically aggressive meningioma. Cancer Res 65: 7121-7126.

1360. Luther N, Greenfield JP, Chadburn A, Schwartz TH (2005). Intracranial nasal natural killer/T-cell lymphoma: immunopathologically-confirmed case and review of literature. J Neurooncol 75: 185-188.

1361. Lutterbach J, Liegibel J, Koch D, Madlinger A, Frommhold H, Pagenstecher A (2001). Atypical teratoid/rhabdoid tumors in adult patients: case report and review of the literature. J Neurooncol 52: 49-56.

1362. Luyken C, Blumcke I, Fimmers R, Urbach H, Elger CE, Wiestler OD, Schramm J (2003). The spectrum of long-term epilepsy-associated tumors: long-term seizure and tumor outcome and neurosurgical aspects. Epilepsia 44: 822-830.

1363. Luyken C, Blumcke I, Fimmers R, Urbach H, Wiestler OD, Schramm J (2004). Supratentorial gangliogliomas: histopathologic grading and tumor recurrence in 184 patients with a median follow-up of 8 years. Cancer 101: 146-155.

1364. Lynch HT, Shurin SB, Dahms BB, Izant RJ, Jr., Lynch J, Danes BS (1983). Paravertebral malignant rhabdoid tumor in infancy. In vitro studies of a familial tumor. Cancer 52: 290-296.

1365. Macaulay R, Jay V, Hoffman H, Becker

L (1993). Increase mitotic activity as a negative prognostic indicator in pleomorphic xanthoastrocytoma. J Neurosurg 79: 761-768.

1366. MacCollin M, Chiocca EA, Evans DG, Friedman JM, Horvitz R, Jaramillo D, Lev M, Mautner VF, Niimura M, Plotkin SR, Sang CN, Stemmer-Rachamimov A, Roach ES (2005). Diagnostic criteria for schwannomatosis. Neurology 64: 1838-1845.

1367. MacCollin M, Ramesh V, Jacoby LB, Louis DN, Rubio MP, Pulaski K, Trofatter JA, Short MP, Bove C, Eldridge R, Parry D, Gusella JF (1994). Mutational analysis of patients with neurofibromatosis 2. Am J Hum Genet 55: 314-320.

1368. MacCollin M, Willett C, Heinrich B, Jacoby LB, Acierno JS, Jr., Perry A, Louis DN (2003). Familial schwannomatosis: exclusion of the NF2 locus as the germline event. Neurology 60: 1968-1974.

1369. MacCollin M, Woodfin W, Kronn D, Short MP (1996). Schwannomatosis: a clinical and pathologic study. Neurology 46: 1072-1079.

1370. Macdonald DR, O'Brien RA, Gilbert JJ, Cairncross JG (1989). Metastatic anaplastic oligodendroglioma. Neurology 39: 1593-1596.

1371. MacDonald TJ, Brown KM, LaFleur B, Peterson K, Lawlor C, Chen Y, Packer RJ, Cogen P, Stephan DA (2001). Expression profiling of medulloblastoma: PDGFRA and the RAS/MAPK pathway as therapeutic targets for metastatic disease. Nat Genet 29: 143-152.

1371A. Machein MR, Plate KH (2004). Role of VEGF in developmental angiogenesis and in tumor angiogenesis in the brain. Cancer Treat Res. 117:191-218.

1372. Mack EE, Wilson CB (1993). Meningiomas induced by high-dose cranial irradiation. J Neurosurg 79: 28-31.

1373. Mackenzie IR (1999). Central neurocytoma: histologic atypia, proliferation potential, and clinical outcome. Cancer 85: 1606-1610.

1374. MacKenzie JM (1987). Pleomorphic xanthoastrocytoma in a 62-year-old male. Neuropathol Appl Neurobiol 13: 481-487.

1375. Maddock JR, Moran A, Maher EA, Teare MD, Norman A, Payne SJ, Whitehouse R, Dodd C, Lavin M, Hartely N, Super M, Evans DGR (1996). A genetic register for von Hippel-Lindau disease. J Med Genet 33: 120-127.

1376. Mader I, Stock KW, Radue EW, Steinbrich W (1996). Langerhans cell histiocytosis in monocygote twins: case reports. Neuroradiology 38: 163-165.

1377. Maehama T, Dixon JE (1998). The tumor suppressor, PTEN/MMAC1, dephosphorylates the lipid second messenger, phosphatidylinositol 3,4,5-trisphosphate. J Biol Chem 273: 13375-13378.

1378. Maesawa C, Tamura G, Iwaya T, Ogasawara S, Ishida K, Sato N, Nishizuka S, Suzuki Y, Ikeda K, Aoki K, Saito K, Satodate R (1998). Mutations in the human homologue of the Drosophila patched gene in esophageal squamous cell carcinoma. Genes Chromosomes Cancer 21: 276-279.

1379. Magnani I, Guerneri S, Pollo B, Cirenei N, Colombo BM, Broggi G, Galli C, Bugiani O, DiDonato S, Finocchiaro G (1994). Increasing complexity of the karyotype in 50 human gliomas. Progressive evolution and de novo occurrence of cytogenetic alterations. Cancer Genet Cytogenet 75: 77-89.

1380. Maher ER, Iselius L, Yates JR, Littler M, Benjamin C, Harris R, Sampson J, Williams A, Ferguson Smith MA, Morton N (1991). Von Hippel-Lindau disease: a genetic study. J Med Genet 28: 443-447.

1381. Maher ER, Kaelin WG, Jr. (1997). von Hippel-Lindau disease. Medicine (Baltimore) 76: 381-391.

1382. Maher ER, Yates JR, Ferguson S (1990). Statistical analysis of the two stage mutation model in von Hippel-Lindau disease, and in sporadic cerebellar haemangioblastoma and renal cell carcinoma. J Med Genet 27: 311-314.
1383. Maier D, Comparone D, Taylor E, Zhang Z, Gratzl O, Van Meir EG, Scott RJ, Merlo A (1997). New deletion in low-grade oligodendroglioma at the glioblastoma suppressor locus on chromosome 10q25-26. Oncogene 15: 997-1000.
1384. Maier H, Ofner D, Hittmair A, Kitz K, Budka H (1992). Classic, atypical, and anaplastic meningioma: three histopathological subtypes of clinical relevance. J Neurosurg 77: 616-623.
1385. Maier H, Wanschitz J, Sedivy R, Rossler K, Ofner D, Budka H (1997). Proliferation and DNA fragmentation in meningioma subtypes. Neuropathol Appl Neurobiol 23: 496-506.
1386. Maintz D, Fiedler K, Koopmann J, Rollbrocker B, Nechev S, Lenartz D, Stangl AP, Louis DN, Schramm J, Wiestler OD, von Deimling A (1997). Molecular genetic evidence for subtypes of oligoastrocytomas. J Neuropathol Exp Neurol 56: 1098-1104.
1387. Maiuri F, Stella L, Benvenuti D, Giamundo A, Pettinato G (1990). Cerebral gliosarcomas: correlation of computed tomographic findings, surgical aspect, pathological features, and prognosis. Neurosurgery 26: 261-267.
1388. Majores M, Schick V, Engels G, Fassunke J, Elger CE, Schramm J, Blumcke I, Becker AJ (2005). Mutational and immunohistochemical analysis of ezrin-, radixin-, moesin (ERM) molecules in epilepsy-associated glioneuronal lesions. Acta Neuropathol 110: 537-546.
1389. Makkar HS, Frieden IJ (2002). Congenital melanocytic nevi: an update for the pediatrician. Curr Opin Pediatr 14: 397-403.
1390. Malkin D, Li FP, Strong LC, Fraumeni JF, Nelson CE, Kim DH, Kassel J, Gryka MA, Bishoff FZ, Tainsky MA (1990). Germ line p53 mutations in a familial syndrome of breast cancer, sarcomas, and other neoplasms. Science 250: 1233-1238.
1391. Mallory SB (1995). Cowden syndrome (multiple hamartoma syndrome). Dermatol Clin 13: 27-31.
1392. Mandahl N, Orndal C, Heim S, Willen H, Rydholm A, Bauer HC, Mitelman F (1993). Aberrations of chromosome segment 12q13-15 characterize a subgroup of hemangiopericytomas. Cancer 71: 3009-3013.
1393. Mannoji H, Becker LE (1988). Ependymal and choroid plexus tumors. Cytokeratin and GFAP expression. Cancer 61: 1377-1385.
1394. Mao L, Merlo A, Bedi G, Shapiro GI, Edwards CD, Rollins BJ, Sidransky D (1995). A novel p16INK4A transcript. Cancer Res 55: 2995-2997.
1395. Marano SR, Johnson PC, Spetzler RF (1988). Recurrent Lhermitte-Duclos disease in a child. Case report. J Neurosurg 69: 599-603.
1396. Maraziotis T, Perentes E, Karamitopoulou E, Nakagawa Y, Gessaga EC, Probst A, Frankfurter A (1992). Neuron-associated class III beta-tubulin isotype, retinal S- antigen, synaptophysin, and glial fibrillary acidic protein in human medulloblastomas: a clinicopathological analysis of 36 cases. Acta Neuropathol 84: 355-363.
1397. Marcus DM, Brooks SE, Leff G, McCormick R, Thompson T, Anfinson S, Lasudry J, Albert DM (1998). Trilateral retinoblastoma: insights into histogenesis and management. Surv Ophthalmol 43: 59-70.
1398. Margetts JC, Kalyan R (1989). Giant-celled glioblastoma of brain. A clinico-pathological and radiological study of ten cases (including immunohistochemistry and ultrastructure). Cancer 63: 524-531.
1399. Margison GP, Kleihues P (1975). Chemical carcinogenesis in the nervous system. Preferential accumulation of O6-methylguanine in rat brain deoxyribonucleic acid during repetitive administration of N-methyl-N-nitrosourea. Biochem J 148: 521-525.
1400. Marigo V, Davey RA, Zuo Y, Cunningham JM, Tabin CJ (1996). Biochemical evidence that patched is the Hedgehog receptor. Nature 384: 176-179.
1401. Marino S (2005). Medulloblastoma: developmental mechanisms out of control. Trends Mol Med 11: 17-22.
1402. Markesbery WR, Duffy PE, Cowen D (1973). Granular cell tumors of the central nervous system. J Neuropathol Exp Neurol 32: 92-109.
1403. Markesbery WR, Haugh RM, Young AB (1981). Ultrastructure of pineal parenchymal neoplasms. Acta Neuropathol 55: 143-149.
1404. Marsh A, Wicking C, Wainwright B, Chenevix-Trench G (2005). DHPLC analysis of patients with Nevoid Basal Cell Carcinoma Syndrome reveals novel PTCH missense mutations in the sterol-sensing domain. Hum Mutat 26: 283.
1405. Marsh DJ, Coulon V, Lunetta KL, Rocca-Serra P, Dahia PL, Zheng Z, Liaw D, Caron S, Duboue B, Lin AY, Richardson AL, Bonnetblanc JM, Bressieux JM, Cabarrot-Moreau A, Chompret A, Demange L, Eeles RA, Yahanda AM, Fearon ER, Fricker JP, Gorlin RJ, Hodgson SV, Huson S, Lacombe D, Eng C, . (1998). Mutation spectrum and genotype-phenotype analyses in Cowden disease and Bannayan-Zonana syndrome, two hamartoma syndromes with germline PTEN mutation. Hum Mol Genet 7: 507-515.
1406. Marshman LA, Pollock JR, King A, Chawda SJ (2005). Primary extradural epithelioid leiomyosarcoma of the cervical spine: case report and literature review. Neurosurgery 57: E372
1407. Martin AJ, Summersgill BM, Fisher C, Shipley JM, Dean AF (2002). Chromosomal imbalances in meningeal solitary fibrous tumors. Cancer Genet Cytogenet 135: 160-164.
1408. Martinez-Diaz H, Kleinschmidt-DeMasters BK, Powell SZ, Yachnis AT (2003). Giant cell glioblastoma and pleomorphic xanthoastrocytoma show different immunohistochemical profiles for neuronal antigens and p53 but share reactivity for class III beta-tubulin. Arch Pathol Lab Med 127: 1187-1191.
1409. Martinez-Salazar A, Supler M, Rojiani AM (1997). Primary intracerebral malignant fibrous histiocytoma: immunohistochemical findings and etiopathogenetic considerations. Mod Pathol 10: 149-154.
1410. Martuza RL, Eldridge R (1988). Neurofibromatosis 2 (bilateral acoustic neurofibromatosis). N Engl J Med 318: 684-688.
1411. Masuoka J, Brandner S, Paulus W, Soffer D, Vital A, Chimelli L, Jouvet A, Yonekawa Y, Kleihues P, Ohgaki H (2001). Germline SDHD mutation in paraganglioma of the spinal cord. Oncogene 20: 5084-5086.
1412. Mathews T, Moossy J (1974). Gliomas containing bone and cartilage. J Neuropathol Exp Neurol 33: 456-471.
1413. Matsuda M, Yasui K, Nagashima K, Mori W (1987). Origin of the medulloblastoma experimentally induced by human polyomavirus JC. J Natl Cancer Inst 79: 585-591.
1414. Matsuno A, Fujimaki T, Sasaki T, Nagashima T, Ide T, Asai A, Matsuura R, Utsunomiya H, Kirino T (1996). Clinical and histopathological analysis of proliferative potentials of recurrent and non-recurrent meningiomas. Acta Neuropathol 91: 504-510.
1415. Matsutani M (2001). Combined chemotherapy and radiation therapy for CNS germ cell tumors—the Japanese experience. J Neurooncol 54: 311-316.
1416. Matsutani M, Sano K, Takakura K, Fujimaki T, Nakamura O, Funata N, Seto T (1997). Primary intracranial germ cell tumors: a clinical analysis of 153 histologically verified cases. J Neurosurg 86: 446-455.
1417. Matthies C, Samii M (1997). Management of 1000 vestibular schwannomas (acoustic neuromas): clinical presentation. Neurosurgery 40: 1-9.
1418. Mautner VF, Kluwe L, Thakker SD, Leark RA (2002). Treatment of ADHD in neurofibromatosis type 1. Dev Med Child Neurol 44: 164-170.
1419. Mawrin C (2005). Molecular genetic alterations in gliomatosis cerebri: what can we learn about the origin and course of the disease? Acta Neuropathol 110: 527-536.
1420. Mawrin C, Lins H, Kirches E, Schildhaus HU, Scherlach C, Kanakis D, Dietzmann K (2003). Distribution of p53 alterations in a case of gliomatosis cerebri. Hum Pathol 34: 102-106.
1420A. Maxwell PH (2005). A common pathway for genetic events leading to pheochromocytoma. Cancer Cell 8:91-93
1421. Maxwell PH, Wiesener MS, Chang G-W, Clifford SC, Vaux EC, Cockman ME, Wykoff CC, Pugh CW, Maher ER, Ratcliffe PJ (1999). The tumor suppressor gene VHL targets hypoxia-inducible factors for oxygen-dependent proteolysis. Nature 399: 271-275.
1422. Mayer-Proschel M, Kalyani AJ, Mujtaba T, Rao MS (1997). Isolation of lineage-restricted neuronal precursors from multipotent neuroepithelial stem cells. Neuron 19: 773-785.
1423. Mazal PR, Hainfellner JA, Preiser J, Czech T, Simonitsch I, Radaszkiewicz T, Budka H (1996). Langerhans cell histiocytosis of the hypothalamus: diagnostic value of immunohistochemistry. Clin Neuropathol 15: 87-91.
1424. Mazur MA, Gururangan S, Bridge JA, Cummings TJ, Mukundan S, Fuchs H, Larrier N, Halperin EC (2005). Intracranial Ewing sarcoma. Pediatr Blood Cancer 45: 850-856.
1425. McCabe MG, Ichimura K, Liu L, Plant K, Backlund LM, Pearson DM, Collins VP (2006). High-resolution array-based comparative genomic hybridization of medulloblastomas and supratentorial primitive neuroectodermal tumors. J Neuropathol Exp Neurol 65: 549-561.
1426. McCall T, Binning M, Blumenthal DT, Jensen RL (2006). Variations of disseminated choroid plexus papilloma: 2 case reports and a review of the literature. Surg Neurol 66: 62-67.
1427. McClatchey AI, Giovannini M (2005). Membrane organization and tumorigenesis—the NF2 tumor suppressor, Merlin. Genes Dev 19: 2265-2277.
1428. McDonald JD, Daneshvar L, Willert JR, Matsumura K, Waldman F, Cogen PH (1994). Physical mapping of chromosome 17p13.3 in the region of a putative tumor suppressor gene important in medulloblastoma. Genomics 23: 229-232.
1429. McDonald JM, Dunlap S, Cogdell D, Dunmire V, Wei Q, Starzinski-Powitz A, Sawaya R, Bruner J, Fuller GN, Aldape K, Zhang W (2006). The SHREW1 gene, frequently deleted in oligodendrogliomas, functions to inhibit cell adhesion and migration. Cancer Biol Ther 5: 300-304.
1430. McDonald JM, Dunmire V, Taylor E, Sawaya R, Bruner J, Fuller GN, Aldape K, Zhang W (2005). Attenuated expression of DFFB is a hallmark of oligodendrogliomas with 1p-allelic loss. Mol Cancer 4:35.: 35
1431. McGarvey TW, Maruta Y, Tomaszewski JE, Linnenbach AJ, Malkowicz SB (1998). PTCH gene mutations in invasive transitional cell carcinoma of the bladder. Oncogene 17: 1167-1172.
1432. McGirr SJ, Kelly PJ, Scheithauer BW (1987). Stereotactic resection of juvenile pilocytic astrocytomas of the thalamus and basal ganglia. Neurosurgery 20: 447-452.
1433. McKusick VA (1994). Mendelian Inheritance in Man: a Catalogue of Human Genes and Genetic Disorders. The John Hopkins University Press: Baltimore & London.
1434. McLean CA, Laidlaw JD, Brownbill DS, Gonzales MF (1990). Recurrence of acoustic neurilemoma as a malignant spindle-cell neoplasm. Case report. J Neurosurg 73: 946-950.
1435. McManamy CS, Lamont JM, Taylor RE, Cole M, Pearson AD, Clifford SC, Ellison DW (2003). Morphophenotypic variation predicts clinical behavior in childhood non-desmoplastic medulloblastomas. J Neuropathol Exp Neurol 62: 627-632.
1436. McMenamin ME, Fletcher CD (2001). Expanding the spectrum of malignant change in schwannomas: epithelioid malignant change, epithelioid malignant peripheral nerve sheath tumor, and epithelioid angiosarcoma: a study of 17 cases. Am J Surg Pathol 25: 13-25.
1437. McNatt SA, Gonzalez-Gomez I, Nelson MD, McComb JG (2005). Synchronous multicentric pleomorphic xanthoastrocytoma: case report. Neurosurgery 57: E191.
1438. McNeil DE, Cote TR, Clegg L, Rorke LB (2002). Incidence and trends in pediatric malignancies medulloblastoma/primitive neuroectodermal tumor: a SEER update. Surveillance Epidemiology and End Results. Med Pediatr Oncol 39: 190-194.
1439. McPherson CM, Brown J, Kim AW, DeMonte F (2006). Regression of intracranial rosai-dorfman disease following corticosteroid therapy. Case report. J Neurosurg 104: 840-844.
1440. Medhkour A, Traul D, Husain M (2002). Neonatal subependymal giant cell astrocytoma. Pediatr Neurosurg 36: 271-274.
1441. Megdiche BH, Nagi S, Zouauoi W, Belghith L, Sebai R, Touibi S (2005). [Cerebellar liponeurocytoma. Case report]. Tunis Med 83: 120-122.
1442. Megyesi JF, Kachur E, Lee DH, Zlatescu MC, Betensky RA, Forsyth PA, Okada Y, Sasaki H, Mizoguchi M, Louis DN, Cairncross JG (2004). Imaging correlates of molecular signatures in oligodendrogliomas. Clin Cancer Res 10: 4303-4306.
1443. Meis JM, Ho KL, Nelson JS (1990). Gliosarcoma: a histologic and immunohistochemical reaffirmation. Mod Pathol 3: 19-24.
1444. Meis JM, Martz KL, Nelson JS (1991). Mixed glioblastoma multiforme and sarcoma. A clinicopathologic study of 26 radiation therapy oncology group cases. Cancer 67: 2342-2349.
1445. Mellemkjaer L, Hasle H, Gridley G, Johansen C, Kjaer SK, Frederiksen K, Olsen JH (2006). Risk of cancer in children with the diagnosis immaturity at birth. Paediatr Perinat Epidemiol 20: 231-237.
1446. Mellinghoff IK, Wang MY, Vivanco I, Haas-Kogan DA, Zhu S, Dia EQ, Lu KV, Yoshimoto K, Huang JH, Chute DJ, Riggs BL, Horvath S, Liau LM, Cavenee WK, Rao PN, Beroukhim R, Peck TC, Lee JC, Sellers WR, Stokoe D, Prados M, Cloughesy TF, Sawyers CL, Mischel PS (2005). Molecular determinants of the response of glioblastomas to EGFR kinase inhibitors. N Engl J Med 353: 2012-2024.
1447. Mellon CD, Carter JE, Owen DB (1988). Ollier's disease and Maffucci's syndrome: distinct entities or a continuum. Case report: enchondromatosis complicated by an

intracranial glioma. J Neurol 235: 376-378.
1448. Memoli VA, Brown EF, Gould VE (1984). Glial fibrillary acidic protein (GFAP) immunoreactivity in peripheral nerve sheath tumors. Ultrastruct Pathol 7: 269-275.
1449. Mena H, Morrison AL, Jones RV, Gyure KA (2001). Central neurocytomas express photoreceptor differentiation. Cancer 91: 136-143.
1450. Mena H, Ribas JL, Enzinger FM, Parisi JE (1991). Primary angiosarcoma of the central nervous system. Study of eight cases and review of the literature. J Neurosurg 75: 73-76.
1451. Mena H, Ribas JL, Pezeshkpour GH, Cowan DN, Parisi JE (1991). Hemangiopericytoma of the central nervous system: a review of 94 cases. Hum Pathol 22: 84-91.
1452. Mena H, Rushing EJ, Ribas JL, Delahunt B, McCarthy WF (1995). Tumors of pineal parenchymal cells: a correlation of histological features, including nucleolar organizer regions, with survival in 35 cases. Hum Pathol 26: 20-30.
1453. Mendrzyk F, Korshunov A, Benner A, Toedt G, Pfister S, Radlwimmer B, Lichter P (2006). Identification of gains on 1q and epidermal growth factor receptor overexpression as independent prognostic markers in intracranial ependymoma. Clin Cancer Res 12: 2070-2079.
1454. Mendrzyk F, Radlwimmer B, Joos S, Kokocinski F, Benner A, Stange DE, Neben K, Fiegler H, Carter NP, Reifenberger G, Korshunov A, Lichter P (2005). Genomic and protein expression profiling identifies CDK6 as novel independent prognostic marker in medulloblastoma. J Clin Oncol 23: 8853-8862.
1455. Menko FH, Kaspers GL, Meijer GA, Claes K, van Hagen JM, Gille JJ (2004). A homozygous MSH6 mutation in a child with cafe-au-lait spots, oligodendroglioma and rectal cancer. Fam Cancer 3: 123-127.
1456. Menon AG, Anderson KM, Riccardi VM, Chung RY, Whaley JM, Yandell DW, Farmer GE, Freiman RN, Lee JK, Li FP, Barker DF, Ledbetter DH, Kleider A, Martuza RL, Gusella JF, Seizinger BR (1990). Chromosome 17p deletions and p53 gene mutations associated with the formation of malignant neurofibrosarcomas in von Recklinghausen neurofibromatosis. Proc Natl Acad Sci USA 87: 5435-5439.
1457. Menon AG, Rutter JL, von Sattel JP, Synder H, Murdoch C, Blumenfeld A, Martuza RL, von Deimling A, Gusella JF, Houseal TW (1997). Frequent loss of chromosome 14 in atypical and malignant meningioma: Identification a putative'tumor progression' locus. Oncogene 14: 611-616.
1458. Merchant TE, Jenkins JJ, Burger PC, Sanford RA, Sherwood SH, Jones-Wallace D, Heideman RL, Thompson SJ, Helton KJ, Kun LE (2002). Influence of tumor grade on time to progression after irradiation for localized ependymoma in children. Int J Radiat Oncol Biol Phys 53: 52-57.
1459. Mercuri S, Gazzeri R, Galarza M, Esposito S, Giordano M (2005). Primary meningeal pheochromocytoma: case report. J Neurooncol 73: 169-172.
1460. Merel P, Khe HX, Sanson M, Bijlsma E, Rouleau G, Laurent P, Pulst S, Baser M, Lenoir G, Sterkers JM (1995). Screening for germ-line mutations in the NF2 gene. Genes Chromosomes Cancer 12: 117-127.
1461. Merrell R, Nabors LB, Perry A, Palmer CA (2006). 1p/19q chromosome deletions in metastatic oligodendroglioma. J Neurooncol 80: 203-207.
1462. Mertens F, Rydholm A, Bauer HF, Limon J, Nedoszytko B, Szadowska A, Willen H, Heim S, Mitelman F, Mandahl N (1995). Cytogenetic findings in malignant peripheral nerve sheath tumors. Int J Cancer 61: 793-798.
1463. Messiaen LM, Callens T, Mortier G, Beysen D, Vandenbroucke I, van Roy N, Speleman F, Paepe AD (2000). Exhaustive mutation analysis of the NF1 gene allows identification of 95% of mutations and reveals a high frequency of unusual splicing defects. Hum Mutat 15: 541-555.
1464. Meyer-Puttlitz B, Hayashi Y, Waha A, Rollbrocker B, Bostrom J, Wiestler OD, Louis DN, Reifenberger G, von Deimling A (1997). Molecular genetic analysis of giant cell glioblastomas. Am J Pathol 151: 853-857.
1465. Meyer P, Eberle MM, Probst A, Tolnay M (2000). [Ganglioglioma of optic nerve in neurofibromatosis type 1. Case report and review of the literature]. Klin Monatsbl Augenheilkd 217: 55-58.
1466. Meyers SP, Khademian ZP, Biegel JA, Chuang SH, Korones DN, Zimmerman RA (2006). Primary intracranial atypical teratoid/rhabdoid tumors of infancy and childhood: MRI features and patient outcomes. AJNR Am J Neuroradiol 27: 962-971.
1467. Meyers SP, Khademian ZP, Chuang SH, Pollack IF, Korones DN, Zimmerman RA (2004). Choroid plexus carcinomas in children: MRI features and patient outcomes. Neuroradiology 46: 770-780.
1467A. Mezey E, Key S, Vogelsang G, Szalayova I, Lange GD, Crain B (2003). Transplanted bone marrow generates new neurons in human brains. Proc Natl Acad Sci USA 100:1364-9.
1468. Michalowski MB, de Fraipont F, Michelland S, Entz-Werle N, Grill J, Pasquier B, Favrot MC, Plantaz D (2006). Methylation of RASSF1A and TRAIL pathway-related genes is frequent in childhood intracranial ependymomas and benign choroid plexus papilloma. Cancer Genet Cytogenet 166: 74-81.
1469. Miettinen M, Shekitka KM, Sobin LH (2001). Schwannomas in the colon and rectum: a clinicopathologic and immunohistochemical study of 20 cases. Am J Surg Pathol 25: 846-855.
1470. Miettinen MM, el Rifai W, Sarlomo-Rikala M, Andersson LC, Knuutila S (1997). Tumor size-related DNA copy number changes occur in solitary fibrous tumors but not in hemangiopericytomas. Mod Pathol 10: 1194-1200.
1471. Migheli A, Cavalla P, Marino S, Schiffer D (1994). A study of apoptosis in normal and pathologic nervous tissue after in situ endlabeling of DNA strand breaks. J Neuropathol Exp Neurol 53: 606-616.
1472. Milbouw G, Born JD, Martin D, Collignon J, Hans P, Reznik M, Bonnal J (1988). Clinical and radiological aspects of dysplastic gangliocytoma (Lhermitte-Duclos disease): a report of two cases with review of the literature. Neurosurgery 22: 124-128.
1473. Miller CA, Torack RM (1970). Secretory ependymoma of the filum terminale. Acta Neuropathol 15: 240-250.
1474. Miller CR, Dunham CP, Scheithauer BW, Perry A (2006). Significance of necrosis in grading of oligodendroglial neoplasms: A clinicopathological and genetic study of newly-diagnosed high-grade gliomas. J Clin Oncol 24: 5419-5426.
1475. Miller CR, Dunham CP, Scheithauer BW, Perry A. (2006). Significance of necrosis in grading of oligodendroglial neoplasms: A clinicopathological and genetic study of 1093 newly-diagnosed high-grade gliomas. J Clin Oncol 24 :5419-26.
1476. Miller DC, Hochberg FH, Harris NL, Gruber ML, Louis DN, Cohen H (1994). Pathology with clinical correlations of primary central nervous system non-Hodgkin's lymphoma. The Massachusetts General Hospital experience 1958-1989. Cancer 74: 1383-1397.
1477. Miller DC, Lang FF, Epstein FJ (1993). Central nervous system gangliogliomas. Part 1: Pathology. J Neurosurg 79: 859-866.
1478. Min KW, Scheithauer BW (1990). Pineal germinomas and testicular seminoma: a comparative ultrastructural study with special references to early carcinomatous transformation. Ultrastruct Pathol 14: 483-496.
1479. Min KW, Scheithauer BW (1997). Clear cell ependymoma: a mimic of oligodendroglioma: clinicopathologic and ultrastructural considerations. Am J Surg Pathol 21: 820-826.
1480. Min KW, Scheithauer BW, Bauserman SC (1994). Pineal parenchymal tumors: an ultrastructural study with prognostic implications. Ultrastruct Pathol 18: 69-85.
1481. Min KW, Seo IS, Song J (1987). Postnatal evolution of the human pineal gland. An immunohistochemical study. Lab Invest 57: 724-728.
1482. Minehan KJ, Shaw EG, Scheithauer BW, Davis DL, Onofrio BM (1995). Spinal cord astrocytoma: pathological and treatment considerations. J Neurosurg 83: 590-595.
1483. Ming JE, Kaupas ME, Roessler E, Brunner HG, Nance WE, Stratton RF, Sujanski E, Bale SJ, Muenke M (1998). Mutations of PATCHED in holoprosencephaly. Am J Hum Genet 63: A140-A140.
1484. Miralbell R, Tolnay M, Bieri S, Probst A, Sappino AP, Berchtold W, Pepper MS, Pizzolato G (1999). Pediatric medulloblastoma: prognostic value of p53, bcl-2, Mib-1, and microvessel density. J Neurooncol 45: 103-110.
1485. Miranda RN, Glantz LK, Myint MA, Levy N, Jackson CL, Rhodes CH, Glantz MJ, Medeiros LJ (1996). Stage IE non-Hodgkin's lymphoma involving the dura: A clinicopathologic study of five cases. Arch Pathol Lab Med 120: 254-260.
1486. Mirimanoff RO, Gorlia T, Mason W, van den Bent MJ, Kortmann RD, Fisher B, Reni M, Brandes AA, Curschmann J, Villa S, Cairncross G, Allgeier A, Lacombe D, Stupp R (2006). Radiotherapy and temozolomide for newly diagnosed glioblastoma: recursive partitioning analysis of the EORTC 26981/22981-NCIC CE3 phase III randomized trial. J Clin Oncol 24: 2563-2569.
1487. Mischel PS, Shai R, Shi T, Horvath S, Lu KV, Choe G, Seligson D, Kremen TJ, Palotie A, Liau LM, Cloughesy TF, Nelson SF (2003). Identification of molecular subtypes of glioblastoma by gene expression profiling. Oncogene 22: 2361-2373.
1488. Mishima K, Nakamura M, Nakamura H, Nakamura O, Funata N, Shitara N (1992). Leptomeningeal dissemination of cerebellar pilocytic astrocytoma. Case report. J Neurosurg 77: 788-791.
1489. Misra A, Pellarin M, Nigro J, Smirnov I, Moore D, Lamborn KR, Pinkel D, Albertson DG, Feuerstein BG (2005). Array comparative genomic hybridization identifies genetic subgroups in grade 4 human astrocytoma. Clin Cancer Res 11: 2907-2918.
1490. Mitchell A, Scheithauer BW, Ebersold MJ, Forbes GS (1991). Intracranial fibromatosis. Neurosurgery 29: 123-126.
1491. Mitchell A, Scheithauer BW, Unni KK, Forsyth PJ, Wold LE, McGivney DJ (1993). Chordoma and chondroid neoplasms of the spheno-occiput. An immunohistochemical study of 41 cases with prognostic and nosologic implications. Cancer 72: 2943-2949.
1492. Mittheisz E, Seidl R, Prayer D, Waldenmair M, Neophytou B, Potschger U, Minkov M, Steiner M, Prosch H, Wnorowski M, Gadner H, Grois N (2007). Central nervous system-related permanent consequences in patients with Langerhans cell histiocytosis. Pediatr Blood Cancer 48: 50-56.
1493. Miyagami M, Katayama Y, Nakamura S (2000). Clinicopathological study of vascular endothelial growth factor (VEGF), p53, and proliferative potential in familial von Hippel-Lindau disease and sporadic hemangioblastomas. Brain Tumor Pathol 17: 111-120.
1494. Miyagi Y, Suzuki SO, Iwaki T, Shima F, Ishido K, Araki T, Kamikaseda K (2001). Pleomorphic xanthoastrocytoma with predominantly exophytic growth: case report. Surg Neurol 56: 330-332.
1495. Miyakawa A, Ichimura K, Schmidt EE, Varmeh-Ziaie S, Collins VP (2000). Multiple deleted regions on the long arm of chromosome 6 in astrocytic tumours. Br J Cancer 82: 543-549.
1496. Miyaki M, Nishio J, Konishi M, Kikuchi-Yanoshita R, Tanaka K, Muraoka M, Nagato M, Chong JM, Koike M, Terada T, Kawahara Y, Fukutome A, Tomiyama J, Chuganji Y, Momoi M, Utsunomiya J (1997). Drastic genetic instability of tumors and normal tissues in Turcot syndrome. Oncogene 15: 2877-2881.
1497. Miyamori T, Mizukoshi H, Yamano K, Takayanagi N, Sugino M, Hayase H, Ito H (1990). Intracranial chondrosarcoma—case report. Neurol Med Chir Tokyo 30: 263-267.
1498. Miyanohara O, Takeshima H, Kaji M, Hirano H, Sawamura Y, Kochi M, Kuratsu J (2002). Diagnostic significance of soluble c-kit in the cerebrospinal fluid of patients with germ cell tumors. J Neurosurg 97: 177-183.
1499. Miyashita K, Hayashi Y, Fujisawa H, Hasegawa M, Yamashita J (2004). Recurrent intracranial solitary fibrous tumor with cerebrospinal fluid dissemination. Case report. J Neurosurg 101: 1045-1048.
1500. Mizoguchi M, Nutt CL, Mohapatra G, Louis DN (2004). Genetic alterations of phosphoinositide 3-kinase subunit genes in human glioblastomas. Brain Pathol 14: 372-377.
1501. Mizuno J, Iwata K, Takei Y (1993). Immunohistochemical study of hemangioblastoma with special reference to its cytogenesis. Neurol Med Chir (Tokyo) 33: 420-424.
1502. Mobley BC, Roulston D, Shah GV, Bijwaard KE, McKeever PE (2006). Peripheral primitive neuroectodermal tumor/Ewing's sarcoma of the craniospinal vault: case reports and review. Hum Pathol 37: 845-853.
1503. Modena P, Lualdi E, Facchinetti F, Galli L, Teixeira MR, Pilotti S, Sozzi G (2005). SMARCB1/INI1 tumor suppressor gene is frequently inactivated in epithelioid sarcomas. Cancer Res 65: 4012-4019.
1504. Mokhtari K, Paris S, Aguirre-Cruz L, Privat N, Criniere E, Marie Y, Hauw JJ, Kujas M, Rowitch D, Hoang-Xuan K, Delattre JY, Sanson M (2005). Olig2 expression, GFAP, p53 and 1p loss analysis contribute to glioma subclassification. Neuropathol Appl Neurobiol 31: 62-69.
1505. Molenaar WM, de Leij L, Trojanowski JQ (1991). Neuroectodermal tumors of the peripheral and the central nervous system share neuroendocrine N-CAM-related antigens with small cell lung carcinomas. Acta Neuropathol 83: 46-54.
1506. Mollemann M, Wolter M, Felsberg J, Collins VP, Reifenberger G (2005). Frequent promoter hypermethylation and low expression of the MGMT gene in oligodendroglial tumors. Int J Cancer 113: 379-385.
1507. Mollenhauer J, Holmskov U, Wiemann S, Krebs I, Herbertz S, Madsen J, Kioschis P, Coy JF, Poustka A (1999). The genomic structure of the DMBT1 gene: evidence for a region with susceptibility to genomic instability. Oncogene 18: 6233-6240.
1508. Mollenhauer J, Wiemann S, Scheurlen W, Korn B, Hayashi Y, Wilgenbus KK, von Deimling A, Poustka A (1997). DMBT1, a new

member of the SRCR superfamily, on chromosome 10q25.3-26.1 is deleted in malignant brain tumours. Nat Genet 17: 32-39.

1509. Molloy PT, Yachnis AT, Rorke LB, Dattilo JJ, Needle MN, Millar WS, Goldwein JW, Sutton LN, Phillips PC (1996). Central nervous system medulloepithelioma: a series of eight cases including two arising in the pons. J Neurosurg 84: 430-436.

1510. Momand J, Zambetti GP, Olson DC, George D, Levine AJ (1992). The mdm-2 oncogene product forms a complex with the p53 protein and inhibits p53-mediated transactivation. Cell 69: 1237-1245.

1511. Monabati A, Rakei SM, Kumar P, Taghipoor M, Rahimi A (2002). Primary burkitt lymphoma of the brain in an immunocompetent patient. Case report. J Neurosurg 96: 1127-1129.

1512. Monteferrante ML, Shimkin PM, Fichtenbaum C, Kleinman GM, Lipow KI (1991). Tentorial traversal by ependymoblastoma. AJNR Am J Neuroradiol 12: 181.

1513. Montesinos-Rongen M, Akasaka T, Zuhlke-Jenisch R, Schaller C, Van Roost D, Wiestler OD, Siebert R, Deckert M (2003). Molecular characterization of BCL6 breakpoints in primary diffuse large B-cell lymphomas of the central nervous system identifies GAPD as novel translocation partner. Brain Pathol 13: 534-538.

1514. Montesinos-Rongen M, Besleaga R, Heinsohn S, Siebert R, Kabisch H, Wiestler OD, Deckert M (2004). Absence of simian virus 40 DNA sequences in primary central nervous system lymphoma in HIV-negative patients. Virchows Arch 444: 436-438.

1515. Montesinos-Rongen M, Hans VH, Eis-Hubinger AM, Prinz M, Schaller C, Van Roost D, Aguzzi A, Wiestler OD, Deckert M (2001). Human herpes virus-8 is not associated with primary central nervous system lymphoma in HIV-negative patients. Acta Neuropathol 102: 489-495.

1516. Montesinos-Rongen M, Kuppers R, Schluter D, Spieker T, Van Roost D, Schaller C, Reifenberger G, Wiestler OD, Deckert-Schluter M (1999). Primary central nervous system lymphomas are derived from germinal-center B cells and show a preferential usage of the V4-34 gene segment. Am J Pathol 155: 2077-2086.

1517. Montesinos-Rongen M, Schmitz R, Courts C, Stenzel W, Bechtel D, Niedobitek G, Blumcke I, Reifenberger G, von Deimling A, Jungnickel B, Wiestler OD, Kuppers R, Deckert M (2005). Absence of immunoglobulin class switch in primary lymphomas of the central nervous system. Am J Pathol 166: 1773-1779.

1518. Montesinos-Rongen M, Van Roost D, Schaller C, Wiestler OD, Deckert M (2004). Primary diffuse large B-cell lymphomas of the central nervous system are targeted by aberrant somatic hypermutation. Blood 103: 1869-1875.

1519. Montesinos-Rongen M, Zuhlke-Jenisch R, Gesk S, Martin-Subero JI, Schaller C, Van Roost D, Wiestler OD, Deckert M, Siebert R (2002). Interphase cytogenetic analysis of lymphoma-associated chromosomal breakpoints in primary diffuse large B-cell lymphomas of the central nervous system. J Neuropathol Exp Neurol 61: 926-933.

1519A. Montgomery P, Kuhn JP, Berger PE (1985). Rhabdoid tumor of the kidney: a case report. Urol Radiol. 7(1): 42-44.

1520. Moran CA, Rush W, Mena H (1997). Primary spinal paragangliomas: a clinicopathological and immunohistochemical study of 30 cases. Histopathology 31: 167-173.

1521. Morantz RA, Feigin I, Ransohoff J, III (1976). Clinical and pathological study of 24 cases of gliosarcoma. J Neurosurg 45: 398-408.

1522. Morgan DR, Gregg KL (2002). Microvessel density and angiogenic promoters in relation to metastatic urological carcinoma. Is there a difference between lymph node and more distant metastases subgroups? Histopathology 41: 170-171.

1523. Mori T, Nagase H, Horii A, Miyoshi Y, Shimano T, Nakatsuru S, Aoki T, Arakawa H, Yanagisawa A, Ushio Y, Takano S, Ogaura M, Karamura M, Shibuya M, Nishikawa R, Matsutani M, Hayashi Y, Jakahashi H, Ikuta F, Nishihara T, Mori S, Nakamura Y (1994). Germ-line and somatic mutations of the APC gene in patients with Turcot syndrome and analysis of APC mutations in brain tumors. Genes Chromosomes Cancer 9: 168-172.

1524. Morimura T, Maier H, Budka H (1996). Intermediate filament protein expression in gliomas: Correlation with proliferation rate. Virchows Arch

1525. Mork SJ, Rubinstein LJ (1985). Ependymoblastoma. A reappraisal of a rare embryonal tumor. Cancer 55: 1536-1542.

1526. Mork SJ, Rubinstein LJ, Kepes JJ, Perentes E, Uphoff DF (1988). Patterns of epithelial metaplasia in malignant gliomas II. Squamous differentiation of epithelial-like formations in gliosarcomas and glioblastomas. J Neuropath Exp Neurol 47: 101-118.

1527. Moskowitz SI, Jin T, Prayson RA (2006). Role of MIB1 in predicting survival in patients with glioblastomas. J Neurooncol 76: 193-200.

1528. Moss TH (1984). Observations on the nature of subependymoma: an electron microscopic study. Neuropathol Appl Neurobiol 10: 63-75.

1529. Motoi M, Yoshino T, Hayashi K, Nose S, Horie Y, Ogawa K (1985). Immunohistochemical studies on human brain tumors using anti-Leu 7 monoclonal antibody in paraffin-embedded specimens. Acta Neuropathol 66: 75-77.

1530. Mott RT, Goodman BK, Burchette JL, Cummings TJ (2005). Loss of chromosome 13 in a case of soft tissue perineurioma. Clin Neuropathol 24: 69-76.

1531. Mrak RE (2002). The Big Eye in the 21st century: the role of electron microscopy in modern diagnostic neuropathology. J Neuropathol Exp Neurol 61: 1027-1039.

1532. Mrak RE, Flanigan S, Collins CL (1994). Malignant acoustic schwannoma. Arch Pathol Lab Med 118: 557-561.

1533. Mueller W, Eum JH, Lass U, Paulus W, Sarkar C, Bruck W, von Deimling A (2004). No evidence of hSNF5/INI1 point mutations in choroid plexus papilloma. Neuropathol Appl Neurobiol 30: 304-307.

1534. Mueller W, Hartmann C, Hoffmann A, Lanksch W, Kiwit J, Tonn J, Veelken J, Schramm J, Weller M, Wiestler OD, Louis DN, von Deimling A (2002). Genetic signature of oligoastrocytomas correlates with tumor location and denotes distinct molecular subsets. Am J Pathol 161: 313-319.

1535. Muller W, Afra D, Schroder R, Slowik F, Wilcke O, Klug N (1982). Medulloblastoma: survey of factors possibly influencing the prognosis. Acta Neurochir 64: 215-224.

1536. Munoz EL, Eberhard DA, Lopes MBS, Schneider BF, Gonzalez F, VandenBerg SR (1996). Proliferative activity and p53 mutation as prognostic indicators in pleomorphic xanthoastrocytoma. J Neuropathol Exp Neurol 55: 606.

1537. Murphy MN, Dhalla SS, Diocee M, Halliday W, Wiseman NE, deSa DJ (1987). Congenital ependymoblastoma presenting as a sacrococcygeal mass in a newborn: an immunohistochemical, light and electron microscopic study. Clin Neuropathol 6: 169-173.

1538. Murray JM, Morgello S (2004). Polyomaviruses and primary central nervous system lymphomas. Neurology 63: 1299-1301.

1539. Murthy A, Gonzalez-Agosti C, Cordero E, Pinney D, Candia C, Solomon F, Gusella J, Ramesh V (1998). NHE-RF, a regulatory cofactor for Na(+)-H+ exchange, is a common interactor for merlin and ERM (MERM) proteins. J Biol Chem 273: 1273-1276.

1540. Musa BS, Pople IK, Cummins BH (1995). Intracranial meningiomas following irradiation—a growing problem? Br J Neurosurg 9: 629-637.

1541. Mut M, Schiff D, Shaffrey ME (2005). Metastasis to nervous system: spinal epidural and intramedullary metastases. J Neurooncol 75: 43-56.

1542. Muta T, Yamano Y (2004). Fulminant hemophagocytic syndrome with a high interferon gamma level diagnosed as macrophage activation syndrome. Int J Hematol 79: 484-487.

1543. Muttaqin Z, Uozumi T, Kuwabara S, Kiya K, Arita K, Ogasawara H, Takechi A (1991). Intraventricular hemangiopericytoma - case report. Neurol Med Chir (Tokyo) 31: 662-665.

1544. Myers MP, Stolarov JP, Eng C, Li J, Wang SI, Wigler MH, Parsons R, Tonks NK (1997). P-TEN, the tumor suppressor from human chromosome 10q23, is a dual- specificity phosphatase. Proc Natl Acad Sci U S A 94: 9052-9057.

1545. Nagao K, Togawa N, Fujii K, Uchikawa H, Kohno Y, Yamada M, Miyashita T (2005). Detecting tissue-specific alternative splicing and disease-associated aberrant splicing of the PTCH gene with exon junction microarrays. Hum Mol Genet 14: 3379-3388.

1546. Nagao K, Toyoda M, Takeuchi-Inoue K, Fujii K, Yamada M, Miyashita T (2005). Identification and characterization of multiple isoforms of a murine and human tumor suppressor, patched, having distinct first exons. Genomics 85: 462-471.

1547. Nagashima T, Hoshino T, Cho KG (1987). Proliferative potential of vascular components in human glioblastoma multiforme. Acta Neuropathol 73: 301-305.

1548. Nagashima Y, Miyagi Y, Udagawa K, Taki A, Misugi K, Sakai N, Kondo K, Kaneko S, Yao M, Shuin T (1996). Von Hippel-Lindau tumour suppressor gene. Localization of expression by in situ hybridization. J Pathol 180: 271-274.

1549. Naggara O, Varlet P, Page P, Oppenheim C, Meder JF (2005). Suprasellar paraganglioma: a case report and review of the literature. Neuroradiology 47: 753-757.

1550. Naidich MJ, Walker MT, Gottardi-Littell NR, Han G, Chandler JP (2004). Cerebellar pleomorphic xanthoastrocytoma in a patient with neurofibromatosis type 1. Neuroradiology 46: 825-829.

1551. Naitoh Y, Sasajima T, Kinouchi H, Mikawa S, Mizoi K (2002). Medulloblastoma with extensive nodularity: single photon emission CT study with iodine-123 metaiodobenzylguanidine. AJNR Am J Neuroradiol 23: 1564-1567.

1552. Nakagawa H, Lockman JC, Frankel WL, Hampel H, Steenblock K, Burgart LJ, Thibodeau SN, de la CA (2004). Mismatch repair gene PMS2: disease-causing germline mutations are frequent in patients whose tumors stain negative for PMS2 protein, but paralogous genes obscure mutation detection and interpretation. Cancer Res 64: 4721-4727.

1553. Nakagawa Y, Perentes E, Rubinstein LJ (1986). Immunohistochemical characterization of oligodendrogliomas: an analysis of multiple markers. Acta Neuropathol 72: 15-22.

1554. Nakagawa Y, Perentes E, Rubinstein LJ (1987). Non-specificity of anti-carbonic anhydrase C antibody as a marker in human neurooncology. J Neuropathol Exp Neurol 46: 451-460.

1555. Nakama S, Higashi T, Kimura A, Yamamuro K, Kikkawa I, Hoshino Y (2005). Double myxopapillary ependymoma of the cauda equina. J Orthop Sci 10: 543-545.

1556. Nakamura H, Takeshima H, Makino K, Kuratsu J (2005). C-kit expression in germinoma: an immunohistochemistry-based study. J Neurooncol 75: 163-167.

1557. Nakamura M, Chiba K, Matsumoto M, Ikeda E, Toyama Y (2006). Pleomorphic xanthoastrocytoma of the spinal cord. Case report. J Neurosurg Spine 5: 72-75.

1558. Nakamura M, Ishida E, Shimada K, Kishi M, Nakase H, Sakaki T, Konishi N (2005). Frequent LOH on 22q12.3 and TIMP-3 inactivation occur in the progression to secondary glioblastomas. Lab Invest 85: 165-175.

1559. Nakamura M, Ishida E, Shimada K, Nakase H, Sakaki T, Konishi N (2006). Defective expression of HRK is associated with promoter methylation in primary central nervous system lymphomas. Oncology 70: 212-221.

1560. Nakamura M, Kishi M, Sakaki T, Hashimoto H, Nakase H, Shimada K, Ishida E, Konishi N (2003). Novel tumor suppressor loci on 6q22-23 in primary central nervous system lymphomas. Cancer Res 63: 737-741.

1561. Nakamura M, Saeki N, Iwadate Y, Sunami K, Osato K, Yamaura A (2000). Neuroradiological characteristics of pineocytoma and pineoblastoma. Neuroradiology 42: 509-514.

1562. Nakamura M, Watanabe T, Klangby U, Asker C, Wiman K, Yonekawa Y, Kleihues P, Ohgaki H (2001). p14ARF deletion and methylation in genetic pathways to glioblastomas. Brain Pathol 11: 159-168.

1563. Nakamura M, Watanabe T, Yonekawa Y, Kleihues P, Ohgaki H (2001). Promoter methylation of the DNA repair gene MGMT in astrocytomas is frequently associated with G:C —> A:T mutations of the TP53 tumor suppressor gene. Carcinogenesis 22: 1715-1719.

1564. Nakamura M, Yang F, Fujisawa H, Yonekawa Y, Kleihues P, Ohgaki H (2000). Loss of heterozygosity on chromosome 19 in secondary glioblastomas. in preparation. 59: 539-543.

1565. Nakamura M, Yonekawa Y, Kleihues P, Ohgaki H (2001). Promoter hypermethylation of the RB1 gene in glioblastomas. Lab Invest 81: 77-82.

1566. Nakamura Y, Becker LE, Mancer K, Gillespie R (1982). Peripheral medulloepithelioma. Acta Neuropathol 57: 137-142.

1567. Nakano I, Kondo A, Iwasaki K (1997). Choroid plexus papilloma in the posterior third ventricle: case report. Neurosurgery 40: 1279-1282.

1568. Nakasu S, Nakasu Y, Nioka H, Nakajima M, Handa J (1994). bcl-2 protein expression in tumors of the central nervous system. Acta Neuropathol 88: 520-526.

1569. Nakasu Y, Nakasu S, Saito A, Horiguchi S, Kameya T (2006). Pituicytoma. Two case reports. Neurol Med Chir (Tokyo) 46: 152-156.

1570. Narod SA, Parry DM, Parboosingh J, Lenoir GM, Ruttledge M, Fischer G, Eldridge R, Martuza RL, Frontali M, Haines J (1992). Neurofibromatosis type 2 appears to be a genetically homogeneous disease. Am J Hum Genet 51: 486-496.

1571. Nathoo N, Chahlavi A, Barnett GH, Toms SA (2005). Pathobiology of brain metastases. J Clin Pathol 58: 237-242.

1572. Naudin tC, Vermeij K, Smit DA, Cohen O, Gerssen S, Dijkhuizen T (1995). Intracranial teratoma with multiple fetuses: pre- and post-

natal appearance. Hum Pathol 26: 804-807.
1573. Neben K, Korshunov A, Benner A, Wrobel G, Hahn M, Kokocinski F, Golanov A, Joos S, Lichter P (2004). Microarray-based screening for molecular markers in medulloblastoma revealed STK15 as independent predictor for survival. Cancer Res 64: 3103-3111.
1574. Neder L, Colli BO, Machado HR, Carlotti CG, Jr., Santos AC, Chimelli L (2004). MIB-1 labeling index in astrocytic tumors—a clinicopathologic study. Clin Neuropathol 23: 262-270.
1575. Neder L, Marie SK, Carlotti CG, Jr., Gabbai AA, Rosemberg S, Malheiros SM, Siqueira RP, Oba-Shinjo SM, Uno M, Aguiar PH, Miura F, Chammas R, Colli BO, Silva WA, Jr., Zago MA (2004). Galectin-3 as an immunohistochemical tool to distinguish pilocytic astrocytomas from diffuse astrocytomas, and glioblastomas from anaplastic oligodendrogliomas. Brain Pathol 14: 399-405.
1576. Neff BA, Willcox Jr TO, Sataloff RT (2003). Intralabyrinthine schwannomas. Otol Neurotol 24: 299-307.
1577. Nelen MR, Kremer H, Konings IB, Schoute F, van Essen AJ, Koch R, Woods CG, Fryns JP, Hamel B, Hoefsloot LH, Peeters EA, Padberg GW (1999). Novel PTEN mutations in patients with Cowden disease: absence of clear genotype-phenotype correlations. Eur J Hum Genet 7: 267-273.
1578. Nelen MR, Padberg GW, Peeters EAJ, Lin AY, van den Helm B, Frants RR, Coulon V, Goldstein AM, van Reen MMM, Easton DF, Eeles RA, Hodgson S, Mulvihill JJ, Murday VA, Tucker MA, Mariman ECM, Starink TM, Ponder BAJ, Ropers HH, Kremer H, Longy M, Eng C (1996). Localization of the gene for Cowden disease to chromosome 10q22-23. Nat Genet 13: 114-116.
1579. Nemes Z (1992). Fibrohistiocytic differentiation in capillary hemangioblastoma. Hum Pathol 23: 805-810.
1580. Nestor SL, Perry A, Kurtkaya O, Abell-Aleff P, Rosemblat AM, Burger PC, Scheithauer BW (2003). Melanocytic colonization of a meningothelial meningioma: histopathological and ultrastructural findings with immunohistochemical and genetic correlation: case report. Neurosurgery 53: 211-214.
1581. Neumann HP, Bender BU (1998). Genotype-phenotype correlations in von Hippel-Lindau disease. J Intern Med 243: 541-545.
1582. Neumann HP, Wiestler OD (1994). Von Hippel-Lindau disease: a syndrome providing insights into growth control and tumorigenesis. Nephrol Dial Transplant 9: 1832-1833.
1583. Neves S, Mazal PR, Wanschitz J, Rudnay AC, Drlicek M, Czech T, Wustinger C, Budka H (2001). Pseudogliomatous growth pattern of anaplastic small cell carcinomas metastatic to the brain. Clin Neuropathol 20: 38-42.
1584. Nevin S (1938). Glimatosis cerebri. Brain 61: 170-191.
1585. Newcomb EW, Alonso M, Sung T, Miller DC (2000). Incidence of p14ARF gene deletion in high-grade adult and pediatric astrocytomas. Hum Pathol 31: 115-119.
1586. Newcomb EW, Bhalla SK, Parrish CL, Hayes RL, Cohen H, Miller DC (1997). bcl-2 protein expression in astrocytomas in relation to patient survival and p53 gene status. Acta Neuropathol 94: 369-375.
1587. Ng HK, Poon WS (1990). Gliosarcoma of the posterior fossa with features of a malignant fibrous histiocytoma. Cancer 65: 1161-1166.
1588. Ng HK, Poon WS (1999). Diffuse leptomeningeal gliomatosis with oligodendroglioma. Pathology 31: 59-63.
1589. Ng TH, Fung CF, Ma LT (1990). The pathological spectrum of desmoplastic infantile gangliogliomas. Histopathology 16: 235-241.
1590. Nicholson JC, Ross FM, Kohler JA, Ellison DW (1999). Comparative genomic hybridization and histological variation in primitive neuroectodermal tumours. Br J Cancer 80: 1322-1331.
1591. Nielsen GP, Stemmer-Rachmaninov AO, Ino Y, Moller MB, Rosenberg AE, Louis DN (1999). Malignant transformation of neurofibromas in neurofibromatosis 1 is associated with CDKN2A/p16 inactivation. Am J Pathol 155: 1879-1884.
1592. Niemela M, Lemeta S, Sainio M, Rauma S, Pukkala E, Kere J, Bohling T, Laatikainen L, Jaaskelainen J, Summanen P (2000). Hemangioblastomas of the retina: impact of von Hippel-Lindau disease. Invest Ophthalmol Vis Sci 41: 1909-1915.
1593. Nigro JM, Misra A, Zhang L, Smirnov I, Colman H, Griffin C, Ozburn N, Chen M, Pan E, Koul D, Yung WK, Feuerstein BG, Aldape KD (2005). Integrated array-comparative genomic hybridization and expression array profiles identify clinically relevant molecular subtypes of glioblastoma. Cancer Res 65: 1678-1686.
1594. Niida Y, Stemmer-Rachamimov AO, Logrip M, Tapon D, Perez R, Kwiatkowski DJ, Sims K, MacCollin M, Louis DN, Ramesh V (2001). Survey of somatic mutations in tuberous sclerosis complex (TSC) hamartomas suggests different genetic mechanisms for pathogenesis of TSC lesions. Am J Hum Genet 69: 493-503.
1595. Nijssen PC, Deprez RH, Tijssen CC, Hagemeijer A, Arnoldus EP, Teepen JL, Holl R, Niermeyer MF (1994). Familial anaplastic ependymoma: evidence of loss of chromosome 22 in tumour cells. J Neurol Neurosurg Psychiatry 57: 1245-1248.
1596. Nishikawa R, Furnari FB, Lin H, Arap W, Berger MS, Cavenee WK, Su H (1995). Loss of P16INK4 expression is frequent in high grade gliomas. Cancer Res 55: 1941-1945.
1597. Nishio S, Morioka T, Inamura T, Takeshita I, Fukui M, Sasaki M, Nakamura K, Wakisaka S (1998). Radiation-induced brain tumours: potential late complications of radiation therapy for brain tumours. Acta Neurochir 140: 763-770.
1598. Nishio S, Takeshita I, Kaneko Y, Fukui M (1992). Cerebral neurocytoma. A new subset of benign neuronal tumors of the cerebrum. Cancer 70: 529-537.
1599. Nishioka H, Ito H, Miki T (1996). Difficulties in the antemortem diagnosis of gliomatosis cerebri: report of a case with diffuse increase of gemistocyte-like cells, mimicking reactive gliosis. Br J Neurosurg 10: 103-107.
1600. Nishizaki T, Ozaki S, Harada K, Ito H, Arai H, Beppu T, Sasaki K (1998). Investigation of genetic alterations associated with the grade of astrocytic tumor by comparative genomic hybridization. Genes Chromosomes Cancer 21: 340-346.
1601. Nitta H, Hayase H, Moriyama Y, Yamashima T, Yamashita J (1993). Gliosarcoma of the posterior cranial fossa: MRI findings. Neuroradiology 35: 279-280.
1602. Nolan MA, Sakuta R, Chuang N, Otsubo H, Rutka JT, Snead OC, III, Hawkins CE, Weiss SK (2004). Dysembryoplastic neuroepithelial tumors in childhood: long-term outcome and prognostic features. Neurology 62: 2270-2276.
1603. Nomura M, Hasegawa M, Kita D, Yamashita J, Minato H, Nakazato Y (2006). Cerebellar gliofibroma with numerous psammoma bodies. Clin Neurol Neurosurg 108: 421-425.
1604. Nora FE, Scheithauer BW (1996). Primary epithelioid hemangioendothelioma of the brain. Am J Surg Pathol 20: 707-714.
1605. Norman MG, Harrison KJ, Poskitt KJ, Kalousek DK (1995). Duplication of 9P and hyperplasia of the choroid plexus: a pathologic, radiologic, and molecular cytogenetics study. Pediatr Pathol Lab Med 15: 109-120.
1606. Norris LS, Snodgrass S, Miller DC, Wisoff J, Garvin J, Rorke LB, Finlay JL (2005). Recurrent central nervous system medulloepithelioma: response and outcome following marrow-ablative chemotherapy with stem cell rescue. J Pediatr Hematol Oncol 27: 264-266.
1607. Nozaki M, Tada M, Matsumoto R, Sawamura Y, Abe H, Iggo RD (1998). Rare occurrence of inactivating p53 gene mutations in primary non- astrocytic tumors of the central nervous system: reappraisal by yeast functional assay. Acta Neuropathol 95: 291-296.
1608. Numoto RT (1994). Pineal parenchymal tumors: cell differentiation and prognosis. J Cancer Res Clin Oncol 120: 683-690.
1609. Nunes F, Shen Y, Niida Y, Beauchamp R, Stemmer-Rachamimov AO, Ramesh V, Gusella J, MacCollin M (2005). Inactivation patterns of NF2 and DAL-1/4.1B (EPB41L3) in sporadic meningioma. Cancer Genet Cytogenet 162: 135-139.
1610. O'Malley S, Weitman D, Olding M, Sekhar L (1994). Multiple neoplasms following craniospinal irradiation for medulloblastoma in a patient with nevoid basal cell carcinoma syndrome. Case report. J Neurosurg 86: 286-288.
1611. O'Marcaigh AS, Ledger GA, Roche PC, Parisi JE, Zimmerman D (1995). Aromatase expression in human germinomas with possible biological effects. J Clin Endocrinol Metab 80: 3763-3766.
1612. Oberstrass J, Reifenberger G, Reifenberger J, Wechsler W, Collins VP (1996). Mutation of the Von Hippel-Lindau tumour suppressor gene in capillary haemangioblastomas of the central nervous system. J Pathol 179: 151-156.
1613. Oblinger JL, Pearl DK, Boardman CL, Saqr H, Prior TW, Scheithauer BW, Jenkins RB, Burger PC, Yates AJ (2006). Diagnostic and prognostic value of glycosyltransferase mRNA in glioblastoma multiforme patients. Neuropathol Appl Neurobiol 32: 410-418.
1614. Offiah CJ, Laitt RD (2006). Case report: Intracranial meningeal melanocytoma: a cause of high signal on T1- and low signal on T2-weighted MRI. Clin Radiol 61: 294-298.
1615. Ogasawara H, Inagawa T, Yamamoto M, Kamiya K, Yano T, Utsunomiya H (1988). Medulloblastoma in infancy associated with omphalocele, malrotation of the intestine, and extrophy of the bladder. Childs Nerv Syst 4: 108-111.
1616. Ogawa K, Shikama N, Toita T, Nakamura K, Uno T, Onishi H, Itami J, Kakinohana Y, Kinjo T, Yoshii Y, Ito H, Murayama S (2004). Long-term results of radiotherapy for intracranial germinoma: a multi-institutional retrospective review of 126 patients. Int J Radiat Oncol Biol Phys 58: 705-713.
1617. Ogawa K, Toita T, Nakamura K, Uno T, Onishi H, Itami J, Shikama N, Saeki N, Yoshii Y, Murayama S (2003). Treatment and prognosis of patients with intracranial nongerminomatous malignant germ cell tumors: a multiinstitutional retrospective analysis of 41 patients. Cancer 98: 369-376.
1618. Ogihara S, Seichi A, Iwasaki M, Kawaguchi H, Kitagawa T, Tajiri Y, Nakamura K (2003). Concurrent spinal schwannomas and meningiomas. Case illustration. J Neurosurg 98: 300.
1619. Oguzkan S, Terzi YK, Cinbis M, Anlar B, Aysun S, Ayter S (2006). Molecular genetic analyses in neurofibromatosis type 1 patients with tumors. Cancer Genet Cytogenet 165: 167-171.
1620. Ohgaki H, Dessen P, Jourde B, Horstmann S, Nishikawa T, Di Patre PL, Burkhard C, Schuler D, Probst-Hensch NM, Maiorka PC, Baeza N, Pisani P, Yonekawa Y, Yasargil MG, Lutolf UM, Kleihues P (2004). Genetic pathways to glioblastoma: a population-based study. Cancer Res 64: 6892-6899.
1621. Ohgaki H, Eibl RH, Schwab M, Reichel MB, Mariani L, Gehring M, Petersen I, Holl T, Wiestler OD, Kleihues P (1993). Mutations of the p53 tumor suppressor gene in neoplasms of the human nervous system. Mol Carcinog 8: 74-80.
1622. Ohgaki H, Eibl RH, Wiestler OD, Yasargil MG, Newcomb EW, Kleihues P (1991). p53 mutations in nonastrocytic human brain tumors. Cancer Res 51: 6202-6205.
1623. Ohgaki H, Huang H, Haltia M, Vainio H, Kleihues P (2000). More about: cell and molecular biology of simian virus 40: implications for human infections and disease. J Natl Cancer Inst 92: 495-497.
1624. Ohgaki H, Kleihues P (2005). Epidemiology and etiology of gliomas. Acta Neuropathol 109: 93-108.
1625. Ohgaki H, Kleihues P (2005). Population-based studies on incidence, survival rates, and genetic alterations in astrocytic and oligodendroglial gliomas. J Neuropathol Exp Neurol 64: 479-489.
1625A. Ohgaki H, Kleihues P (2007). Genetic pathways to primary and secondary glioblastoma. Am J Pathol 170: 1445-1453.
1626. Ohgaki H, Schauble B, zur H, von Ammon K, Kleihues P (1995). Genetic alterations associated with the evolution and progression of astrocytic brain tumours. Virchows Arch 427: 113-118.
1627. Ohgaki H, Watanabe K, Peraud A, Biernat W, von Deimling A, Yasargil MG, Yonekawa Y, Kleihues P (1999). A case history of glioma progression. Acta Neuropathol 97: 525-532.
1628. Ohh M, Kaelin WG, Jr. (1999). The von Hippel-Lindau tumour suppressor protein: new perspectives. Mol Med Today 5: 257-263.
1629. Ohh M, Yauch RL, Lonergan KM, Whaley JM, Stemmer-Rachamimov AO, Louis DN, Gavin BJ, Kley N, Kaelin WG, Jr., Iliopoulos O (1998). The von Hippel-Lindau tumor suppressor protein is required for proper assembly of an extracellular fibronectin matrix. Mol Cell 1: 959-968.
1630. Ohji H, Sasagawa I, Iciyanagi O, Suzuki Y, Nakada T (2001). Tumour angiogenesis and Ki-67 expression in phaeochromocytoma. BJU Int 87: 381-385.
1631. Ohta T, Watanabe T, Katayama Y, Kurihara J, Yoshino A, Nishimoto H, Kishimoto H (2006). TrkA expression is associated with an elevated level of apoptosis in classic medulloblastomas. Neuropathology 26: 170-177.
1632. Oikonomou E, Barreto DC, Soares B, De Marco L, Buchfelder M, Adams EF (2005). Beta-catenin mutations in craniopharyngiomas and pituitary adenomas. J Neurooncol 73: 205-209.
1633. Okada Y, Nishikawa R, Matsutani M, Louis DN (2002). Hypomethylated X chromosome gain and rare isochromosome 12p in diverse intracranial germ cell tumors. J Neuropathol Exp Neurol 61: 531-538.
1634. Okamoto Y, Di Patre PL, Burkhard C, Horstmann S, Jourde B, Fahey M, Schuler D, Probst-Hensch NM, Yasargil MG, Yonekawa Y, Lutolf UM, Kleihues P, Ohgaki H (2004). Population-based study on incidence, survival rates, and genetic alterations of low-grade diffuse astrocytomas and oligodendrogliomas. Acta Neuropathol 108: 49-56.
1635. Oliner JD, Kinzler KW, Meltzer PS, George DL, Vogelstein B (1992). Amplification

of a gene encoding a p53-associated protein in human sarcomas. Nature 358: 80-83.

1636. Oliveira AM, Scheithauer BW, Salomao DR, Parisi JE, Burger PC, Nascimento AG (2002). Primary sarcomas of the brain and spinal cord: a study of 18 cases. Am J Surg Pathol 26: 1056-1063.

1637. Oliver TG, Read TA, Kessler JD, Mehmeti A, Wells JF, Huynh TT, Lin SM, Wechsler-Reya RJ (2005). Loss of patched and disruption of granule cell development in a preneoplastic stage of medulloblastoma. Development 132: 2425-2439.

1638. Olivier M, Eeles R, Hollstein M, Khan MA, Harris CC, Hainaut P (2002). The IARC TP53 database: new online mutation analysis and recommendations to users. Hum Mutat 19: 607-614.

1639. Olivier M, Goldgar DE, Sodha N, Ohgaki H, Kleihues P, Hainaut P, Eeles RA (2003). Li-Fraumeni and related syndromes: correlation between tumor type, family structure, and TP53 genotype. Cancer Res 63: 6643-6650.

1640. Olivier M, Hussain SP, Caron dF, Hainaut P, Harris CC (2004). TP53 mutation spectra and load: a tool for generating hypotheses on the etiology of cancer. IARC Sci Publ 247-270.

1641. Olschwang S, Richard S, Boisson S, Giraud S, Laurent-Puig P, Resche F, Thomas G (1998). Germline mutation profile of the VHL gene in von Hippel-Lindau disease and in sporadic hemangioblastomas. Hum Mutat 12: 424-430.

1642. Olson JD, Riedel E, DeAngelis LM (2000). Long-term outcome of low-grade oligodendroglioma and mixed glioma. Neurology 54: 1442-1448.

1643. Olson JM, Breslow NE, Barce J (1993). Cancer in twins of Wilms tumor patients. Am J Med Genet 47: 91-94.

1644. Omulecka A, Lach B, Alwasiak J, Gregor A (1995). Immunohistochemical and ultrastructural studies of stromal cells in hemangioblastoma. Folia Neuropathol 33: 41-50.

1645. Onda K, Davis RL, Wilson CB, Hoshino T (1994). Regional differences in bromodeoxyuridine uptake, expression of Ki-67 protein, and nucleolar organizer region counts in glioblastoma multiforme. Acta Neuropathol 87: 586-593.

1646. Onguru O, Deveci S, Sirin S, Timurkaynak E, Gunhan O (2003). Dysembryoplastic neuroepithelial tumor in the left lateral ventricle. Minim Invasive Neurosurg 46: 306-309.

1647. Ono Y, Ueki K, Joseph JT, Louis DN (1996). Homozygous deletions of the CDKN2/p16 gene in dural hemangiopericytomas. Acta Neuropathol 91: 221-225.

1648. Oro AE, Higgins KM, Hu Z, Bonifas JM, Epstein EH, Jr., Scott MP (1997). Basal cell carcinomas in mice overexpressing Sonic hedgehog. Science 276: 817-821.

1649. Ortega-Aznar A, Romero-Vidal FJ, de la TJ, Castellvi J, Nogues P (2001). Neonatal tumors of the CNS: a report of 9 cases and a review. Clin Neuropathol 20: 181-189.

1650. Oruckaptan HH, Berker M, Soylemezoglu F, Ozcan OE (2001). Parafalcine chondrosarcoma: an unusual localization for a classical variant. Case report and review of the literature. Surg Neurol 55: 174-179.

1651. Osborne AG (1994). Diagnostic Neuroradiology. Mosby, St Louis.

1652. Ostergaard JR, Sunde L, Okkels H (2005). Neurofibromatosis von Recklinghausen type I phenotype and early onset of cancers in siblings compound heterozygous for mutations in MSH6. Am J Med Genet A 139: 96-105.

1653. Ostertun B, Wolf HK, Campos MG,

Matus C, Solymosi L, Elger CE, Schramm J, Schild HH (1996). Dysembryoplastic neuroepithelial tumors: MR and CT evaluation. AJNR Am J Neuroradiol 17: 419-430.

1654. Ota S, Crabbe DC, Tran TN, Triche TJ, Shimada H (1993). Malignant rhabdoid tumor. A study with two established cell lines. Cancer 71: 2862-2872.

1655. Oviedo A, Pang D, Zovickian J, Smith M (2005). Clear cell meningioma: case report and review of the literature. Pediatr Dev Pathol 8: 386-390.

1656. Owen G, Webb DK (1995). Evidence of clonality in a child with haemophagocytic lymphohistiocytosis. Br J Haematol 89: 681-682.

1657. Owler BK, Makeham JM, Shingde M, Besser M (2005). Cerebellar liponeurocytoma. J Clin Neurosci 12: 326-329.

1658. Ozek MM, Sav A, Pamir MN, Ozer AF, Ozek E, Erzen C (1993). Pleomorphic xanthoastrocytoma associated with von Recklinghausen neurofibromatosis. Childs Nerv Syst 9: 39-42.

1659. Ozolek JA, Finkelstein SD, Couce ME (2004). Gliosarcoma with epithelial differentiation: immunohistochemical and molecular characterization. A case report and review of the literature. Mod Pathol 17: 739-745.

1660. Ozoren N, El Deiry WS (2003). Cell surface Death Receptor signaling in normal and cancer cells. Semin Cancer Biol 13: 135-147.

1661. Packer RJ (1999). Childhood medulloblastoma: progress and future challenges. Brain Dev 21: 75-81.

1662. Packer RJ, Sutton LN, Elterman R, Lange B, Goldwein J, Nicholson HS, Mulne L, Boyett J, D'Angio G, Wechsler Jentzsch K, et al (1994). Outcome for children with medulloblastoma treated with radiation and cisplatin, CCNU, and vincristine chemotherapy. J Neurosurg 81: 690-698.

1663. Packer RJ, Sutton LN, Rorke LB, Zimmerman RA, Littman P, Bruce DA, Schut L (1985). Oligodendroglioma of the posterior fossa in childhood. Cancer 56: 195-199.

1664. Padberg GW, Schot JD, Vielvoye GJ, Bots GT, de Beer FC (1991). Lhermitte-Duclos disease and Cowden disease: a single phakomatosis. Ann Neurol 29: 517-523.

1665. Paek SH, Kim SH, Chang KH, Park CK, Kim JE, Kim DG, Park SH, Jung HW (2005). Microcystic meningiomas: radiological characteristics of 16 cases. Acta Neurochir 147: 965-972.

1666. Pagni CA, Giordana MT, Canavero S (1991). Benign recurrence of a pilocytic cerebellar astrocytoma 36 years after radical removal: case report. Neurosurgery 28: 606-609.

1667. Pahapill PA, Ramsay DA, Del Maestro RF (1996). Pleomorphic xanthoastrocytoma: case report and analysis of the literature concerning the efficacy of resection and the significance of necrosis. Neurosurgery 38: 822-828.

1668. Pakos EE, Goussia AC, Zina VP, Pitouli EJ, Tsekeris PG (2005). Multi-focal gliosarcoma: a case report and review of the literature. J Neurooncol 74: 301-304.

1669. Palma L, Celli P, Maleci A, Di Lorenzo N, Cantore G (1989). Malignant monstrocellular brain tumours. A study of 42 surgically treated cases. Acta Neurochir 97: 17-25.

1670. Palma L, Di Lorenzo N, Guidetti B (1978). Lymphocytic infiltrates in primary glioblastomas and recidivous gliomas: Incidence, fate, and relevance to prognosis in 228 operated cases. J Neurosurg 49: 854-861.

1671. Palma L, Maleci A, Di Lorenzo N, Lauro GM (1985). Pleomorphic xanthoastrocytoma with 18-year survival. Case report. J Neurosurg 63: 808-810.

1671A. Palma L, Russo A, Mercuri S (1983). Cystic cerebral astrocytomas in infancy and

childhood: long-term results. Childs Brain 10: 79-91.

1672. Palma L, Russo A, Celli P (1984). Prognosis of the so-called "diffuse" cerebellar astrocytoma. Neurosurgery 15: 315-317.

1673. Palmedo H, Urbach H, Bender H, Schlegel U, Schmidt-Wolf IG, Matthies A, Linnebank M, Joe A, Bucerius J, Biersack HJ, Pels H (2006). FDG-PET in immunocompetent patients with primary central nervous system lymphoma: correlation with MRI and clinical follow-up. Eur J Nucl Med Mol Imaging 33: 164-168.

1674. Pang JC, Dong Z, Zhang R, Liu Y, Zhou LF, Chan BW, Poon WS, Ng HK (2003). Mutation analysis of DMBT1 in glioblastoma, medulloblastoma and oligodendroglial tumors. Int J Cancer 105: 76-81.

1675. Pang LM, Roebuck DJ, Ng HK, Chan YL (2001). Sellar and suprasellar medulloepithelioma. Pediatr Radiol 31: 594-596.

1676. Paraf F, Jothy S, Van Meir EG (1997). Brain tumor-polyposis syndrome: two genetic diseases? J Clin Oncol 15: 2744-58.

1677. Parham DM, Weeks DA, Beckwith JB (1994). The clinicopathologic spectrum of putative extrarenal rhabdoid tumors. An analysis of 42 cases studied with immunohistochemistry or electron microscopy. Am J Surg Pathol 18: 1010-1029.

1678. Park DH, Park YK, Oh JI, Kwon TH, Chung HS, Cho HD, Suh YL (2002). Oncocytic paraganglioma of the cauda equina in a child. Case report and review of the literature. Pediatr Neurosurg 36: 260-265.

1679. Park SH, Park HR, Chi JG (1996). Papillary ependymoma: its differential diagnosis from choroid plexus papilloma. J Korean Med Sci 11: 415-421.

1680. Parkash V, Gerald WL, Parma A, Miettinen M, Rosai J (1995). Desmoplastic small round cell tumor of the pleura. Am J Surg Pathol 19: 659-665.

1680A. Parkin DM, Whelan SL, Ferlay J, Raymond L, Young J eds. (1997). Cancer incidence in five continents Volume VII. IARC Scientific Publications No. 143, Lyon.

1681. Parkinson D, Hall CW (1962). Case Reports. Oligodendrogliomas. Simultaneous appearance in frontal lobes of siblings. J Neurosurg 19: 424-426.

1682. Parkkila AK, Herva R, Parkkila S, Rajaniemi H (1995). Immunohistochemical demonstration of human carbonic anhydrase isoenzyme II in brain tumours. Histochem J 27: 974-982.

1682A. Parry DM, Eldridge R, Kaiser-Kuper MI, Bouzas EA, Pikus A, Patronas N (1994). Neurofibromatosis 2 (NF2): clinical characteristics fo 63 affected individuals and clinical evidence for heterogeneity. AM J Med Genet 52:450-61.

1683. Parry L, Maynard JH, Patel A, Hodges AK, von Deimling A, Sampson JR, Cheadle JP (2000). Molecular analysis of the TSC1 and TSC2 tumour suppressor genes in sporadic glial and glioneuronal tumours. Hum Genet 107: 350-356.

1684. Paspala AB, Sundaram C, Purohit AK, Immaneni D (1999). Exclusive CNS involvement by lymphomatoid granulomatosis in a 12-year-old boy: a case report. Surg Neurol 51: 258-260.

1685. Pasquier B, Couderc P, Pasquier D, Panh MH, N'Golet A (1978). Sarcoma arising in oligodendroglioma of the brain: a case with intramedullary and subarachnoid spinal metastases. Cancer 42: 2753-2758.

1686. Pasquier B, Gasnier F, Pasquier D, Keddari E, Morens A, Couderc P (1986). Papillary meningioma. Clinicopathologic study of seven cases and review of the literature.

Cancer 58: 299-305.

1687. Pasquier B, Pasquier D, Golet AN, Panh MH, Couderc P (1980). Extraneural metastases of astrocytomas and glioblastomas: clinicopathological study of two cases and review of the literature. Cancer 45: 112-125.

1688. Pasquier B, Pasquier D, N'Golet A, Panh MH, Couderc P (1979). [The metastatic potential of primary central nervous tumours (author's transl)]. Rev Neurol Paris 135: 263-278.

1689. Pasquier B, Peoc'h M, Fabre-Bocquentin B, Bensaadi L, Pasquier D, Hoffmann D, Kahane P, Tassi L, Le Bas JF, Benabid AL (2002). Surgical pathology of drug-resistant partial epilepsy. A 10-year-experience with a series of 327 consecutive resections. Epileptic Disord 4: 99-119.

1690. Pasquier B, Peoc'h M, Morrison AL, Gay E, Pasquier D, Grand S, Sindou M, Kopp N (2002). Chordoid glioma of the third ventricle: a report of two new cases, with further evidence supporting an ependymal differentiation, and review of the literature. Am J Surg Pathol 26: 1330-1342.

1691. Passone E, Pizzolitto S, D'Agostini S, Skrap M, Gardiman MP, Nocerino A, Scarzello G, Perilongo G (2006). Non-anaplastic pleomorphic xanthoastrocytoma with neuroradiological evidences of leptomeningeal dissemination. Childs Nerv Syst 22: 614-618.

1692. Patil A, Yamanashi W (1992). Stereotactic microsurgical resection of intracranial tumors using the electromagnetic field focusing system. Stereotact Funct Neurosurg 59: 128-134.

1693. Patriarca F, Zaja F, Silvestri F, Sperotto A, Scalise A, Gigli G, Fanin R (2001). Meningeal and cerebral involvement in multiple myeloma patients. Ann Hematol 80: 758-762.

1694. Paulli M, Bergamaschi G, Tonon L, Viglio A, Rosso R, Facchetti F, Geerts ML, Magrini U, Cazzola M (1995). Evidence for a polyclonal nature of the cell infiltrate in sinus histiocytosis with massive lymphadenopathy (Rosai-Dorfman disease). Br J Haematol 91: 415-418.

1695. Paulus W, Bayas A, Ott G, Roggendorf W (1994). Interphase cytogenetics of glioblastoma and gliosarcoma. Acta Neuropathol 88: 420-425.

1696. Paulus W, Brandner S (1999). Synaptophysin in choroid plexus epithelial cells: no useful aid in differential diagnosis. J Neuropathol Exp Neurol 58: 1111-1112.

1697. Paulus W, Honegger J, Keyvani K, Fahlbusch R (1999). Xanthogranuloma of the sellar region: a clinicopathological entity different from adamantinomatous craniopharyngioma. Acta Neuropathol 97: 377-382.

1698. Paulus W, Janisch W (1990). Clinicopathologic correlations in epithelial choroid plexus neoplasms: a study of 52 cases. Acta Neuropathol 80: 635-641.

1699. Paulus W, Jellinger K (1993). Comparison of integrin adhesion molecules expressed by primary brain lymphomas and nodal lymphomas. Acta Neuropathol 86: 360-364.

1700. Paulus W, Jellinger K, Hallas C, Ott G, Muller Hermelink HK (1993). Human herpesvirus-6 and Epstein-Barr virus genome in primary cerebral lymphomas. Neurology 43: 1591-1593.

1701. Paulus W, Kirchner T, Michaela M, Kuhl J, Warmuth-Metz M, Sorensen N, Muller-Hermelink HK, Roggendorf W (1992). Histiocytic tumor of Meckel's cave. An intracranial equivalent of juvenile xanthogranuloma of the skin. Am J Surg Pathol 16: 76-83.

1702. Paulus W, Lisle DK, Tonn JC, Wolf HK, Roggendorf W, Reeves SA, Louis DN (1996). Molecular genetic alterations in pleomorphic xanthoastrocytoma. Acta Neuropathol 91: 293-

297.
1703. Paulus W, Schlote W, Perentes E, Jacobi G, Warmuth Metz M, Roggendorf W (1992). Desmoplastic supratentorial neuroepithelial tumours of infancy. Histopathology 21: 43-49.
1704. Paulus W, Slowik F, Jellinger K (1991). Primary intracranial sarcomas: histopathological features of 19 cases. Histopathology 18: 395-402.
1705. Pause A, Lee S, Lonergan KM, Klausner RD (1998). The von Hippel-Lindau tumor suppressor gene is required for cell cycle exit upon serum withdrawal. Proc Natl Acad Sci U S A 95: 993-998.
1706. Pause A, Lee S, Worrel RA, Chen DYT, Burgess WH, Linehan WM, Klausner RD (1997). The von Hippel-Lindau tumor-suppressor gene product forms a stable complex with human CUL-2, a member of the Cdc53 family of proteins. Proc Natl Acad Sci USA 94: 2156-2161.
1707. Pearl GS, Takei Y, Bakay RA, Davis P (1985). Intraventricular primary cerebral neuroblastoma in adults: report of three cases. Neurosurgery 16: 847-849.
1708. Pedersen PH, Rucklidge GJ, Mork SJ, Terzis AJ, Engebraaten O, Lund J, Backlund EO, Laerum OD, Bjerkvig R (1994). Leptomeningeal tissue: a barrier against brain tumor cell invasion. J Natl Cancer Inst 86: 1593-1599.
1708A. Pelloski CE, Mahajan A, Maor M, Chang EL, Woo S, Gilbert M, Colman h, Yang H, Ledoux A, Blair H, Passe S, Jenkins RB, Aldape KD (2005). YKL-40 expression is associated with poorer response to radiation and shorter overall survival in glioblastoma. Clin Cancer Res. 11:3326-34.
1709. Pels H, Schlegel U (2006). Primary central nervous system lymphoma. Curr Treat Options Neurol 8: 346-357.
1710. Pels H, Schmidt-Wolf IG, Glasmacher A, Schulz H, Engert A, Diehl V, Zellner A, Schackert G, Reichmann H, Kroschinsky F, Vogt-Schaden M, Egerer G, Bode U, Schaller C, Deckert M, Fimmers R, Helmstaedter C, Atasoy A, Klockgether T, Schlegel U (2003). Primary central nervous system lymphoma: results of a pilot and phase II study of systemic and intraventricular chemotherapy with deferred radiotherapy. J Clin Oncol 21: 4489-4495.
1711. Penn I, Porat G (1995). Central nervous system lymphomas in organ allograft recipients. Transplantation 59: 240-244.
1712. Peraud A, Ansari H, Bise K, Reulen HJ (1998). Clinical outcome of supratentorial astrocytoma WHO grade II. Acta Neurochir 140: 1213-1222.
1713. Peraud A, Kreth FW, Wiestler OD, Kleihues P, Reulen HJ (2002). Prognostic impact of TP53 mutations and P53 protein overexpression in supratentorial WHO grade II astrocytomas and oligoastrocytomas. Clin Cancer Res 8: 1117-1124.
1714. Peraud A, Watanabe K, Plate KH, Yonekawa Y, Kleihues P, Ohgaki H (1997). p53 Mutations versus EGF receptor expression in giant cell glioblastomas. J Neuropath Exp Neurol 56: 1235-1241.
1715. Peraud A, Watanabe K, Schwechheimer K, Yonekawa Y, Kleihues P, Ohgaki H (1999). Genetic profile of the giant cell glioblastoma. Lab Invest 79: 123-129.
1716. Perentes E, Rubinstein LJ, Herman MM, Donoso LA (1986). S-antigen immunoreactivity in human pineal glands and pineal parenchymal tumors. A monoclonal antibody study. Acta Neuropathol 71: 224-227.
1717. Perilongo G, Carollo C, Salviati L, Murgia A, Pillon M, Basso G, Gardiman M, Laverda AM (1997). Diencephalic syndromoe and disseminated juvenile pilocytic astrocytomas of the hypothalamic-optic chiasm region. Cancer 80: 142-146.
1718. Perkins GH, Schomer DF, Fuller GN, Allen PK, Maor MH (2003). Gliomatosis cerebri: improved outcome with radiotherapy. Int J Radiat Oncol Biol Phys 56: 1137-1146.
1719. Perrone F, Tabano S, Colombo F, Dagrada G, Birindelli S, Gronchi A, Colecchia M, Pierotti MA, Pilotti S (2003). p15INK4b, p14ARF, and p16INK4a inactivation in sporadic and neurofibromatosis type 1-related malignant peripheral nerve sheath tumors. Clin Cancer Res 9: 4132-4138.
1720. Perry A, Aldape KD, George DH, Burger PC (2004). Small cell astrocytoma: an aggressive variant that is clinicopathologically and genetically distinct from anaplastic oligodendroglioma. Cancer 101: 2318-2326.
1721. Perry A, Banerjee R, Lohse CM, Kleinschmidt-DeMasters BK, Scheithauer BW (2002). A role for chromosome 9p21 deletions in the malignant progression of meningiomas and the prognosis of anaplastic meningiomas. Brain Pathol 12: 183-190.
1722. Perry A, Cai DX, Scheithauer BW, Swanson PE, Lohse CM, Newsham IF, Weaver A, Gutmann DH (2000). Merlin, DAL-1, and progesterone receptor expression in clinicopathologic subsets of meningioma: a correlative immunohistochemical study of 175 cases. J Neuropathol Exp Neurol 59: 872-879.
1723. Perry A, Fuller CE, Judkins AR, Dehner LP, Biegel JA (2005). INI1 expression is retained in composite rhabdoid tumors, including rhabdoid meningiomas. Mod Pathol 18: 951-958.
1724. Perry A, Giannini C, Raghavan R, Scheithauer BW, Banerjee R, Margraf L, Bowers DC, Lytle RA, Newsham IF, Gutmann DH (2001). Aggressive phenotypic and genotypic features in pediatric and NF2-associated meningiomas: a clinicopathologic study of 53 cases. J Neuropathol Exp Neurol 60: 994-1003.
1725. Perry A, Giannini C, Scheithauer BW, Rojiani AM, Yachnis AT, Seo IS, Johnson PC, Kho J, Shapiro S (1997). Composite pleomorphic xanthoastrocytoma and ganglioglioma: report of four cases and review of the literature. Am J Surg Pathol 21: 763-771.
1726. Perry A, Gutmann DH, Reifenberger G (2004). Molecular pathogenesis of meningiomas. J Neurooncol 70: 183-202.
1727. Perry A, Jenkins RB, Dahl RJ, Moertel CA, Scheithauer BW (1996). Cytogenetic analysis of aggressive meningiomas: possible diagnostic and prognostic implications. Cancer 77: 2567-2573.
1728. Perry A, Kunz SN, Fuller CE, Banerjee R, Marley EF, Liapis H, Watson MA, Gutmann DH (2002). Differential NF1, p16, and EGFR patterns by interphase cytogenetics (FISH) in malignant peripheral nerve sheath tumor (MPNST) and morphologically similar spindle cell neoplasms. J Neuropathol Exp Neurol 61: 702-709.
1729. Perry A, Lusis EA, Gutmann DH (2005). Meningothelial hyperplasia: a detailed clinicopathologic, immunohistochemical and genetic study of 11 cases. Brain Pathol 15: 109-115.
1730. Perry A, Roth KA, Banerjee R, Fuller CE, Gutmann DH (2001). NF1 deletions in S-100 protein-positive and negative cells of sporadic and neurofibromatosis 1 (NF1)-associated plexiform neurofibromas and malignant peripheral nerve sheath tumors. Am J Pathol 159: 57-61.
1731. Perry A, Scheithauer BW, Macaulay RJ, Raffel C, Roth KA, Kros JM (2002). Oligodendrogliomas with neurocytic differentiation. A report of 4 cases with diagnostic and histogenetic implications. J Neuropathol Exp Neurol 61: 947-955.
1732. Perry A, Scheithauer BW, Nascimento AG (1997). The immunophenotypic spectrum of meningeal hemangiopericytoma: a comparison with fibrous meningioma and solitary fibrous tumor of meninges. Am J Surg Pathol 21: 1354-1360.
1733. Perry A, Scheithauer BW, Stafford SL, Abell-Aleff PC, Meyer FB (1998). "Rhabdoid" meningioma: an aggressive variant. Am J Surg Pathol 22: 1482-1490.
1734. Perry A, Scheithauer BW, Stafford SL, Lohse CM, Wollan PC (1999). "Malignancy" in meningiomas: a clinicopathologic study of 116 patients, with grading implications. Cancer 85: 2046-2056.
1735. Perry A, Scheithauer BW, Szczesniak DM, Atkinson JL, Wald JT, Hammak JE (2001). Combined oligodendroglioma/pleomorphic xanthoastrocytoma: a probable collision tumor: case report. Neurosurgery 48: 1358-1361.
1736. Perry A, Stafford SL, Scheithauer BW, Suman VJ, Lohse CM (1997). Meningioma grading: an analysis of histologic parameters. Am J Surg Pathol 21: 1455-1465.
1737. Perry A, Stafford SL, Scheithauer BW, Suman VJ, Lohse CM (1998). The prognostic significance of MIB-1, p53, and DNA flow cytometry in completely resected primary meningiomas. Cancer 82: 2262-2269.
1738. Perry JR, Ang LC, Bilbao JM, Muller PJ (1995). Clinicopathologic features of primary and postirradiation cerebral gliosarcoma. Cancer 75: 2910-2918.
1739. Peters O, Gnekow AK, Rating D, Wolff JE (2004). Impact of location on outcome in children with low-grade oligodendroglioma. Pediatr Blood Cancer 43: 250-256.
1740. Petersen I, Hidalgo A, Petersen S, Schluns K, Schewe C, Pacyna-Gengelbach M, Goeze A, Krebber B, Knosel T, Kaufmann O, Szymas J, von Deimling A (2000). Chromosomal imbalances in brain metastases of solid tumors. Brain Pathol 10: 395-401.
1741. Phan RT, Dalla-Favera R (2004). The BCL6 proto-oncogene suppresses p53 expression in germinal-centre B cells. Nature 432: 635-639.
1742. Phillips HS, Kharbanda S, Chen R, Forrest WF, Soriano RH, Wu TD, Misra A, Nigro JM, Colman H, Soroceanu L, Williams PM, Modrusan Z, Feuerstein BG, Aldape K (2006). Molecular subclasses of high-grade glioma predict prognosis, delineate a pattern of disease progression, and resemble stages in neurogenesis. Cancer Cell 9: 157-173.
1743. Picksley SM, Lane DP (1993). The p53-mdm2 autoregulatory feedback loop: a paradigm for the regulation of growth control by p53? Bioessays 15: 689-690.
1744. Pierallini A, Bonamini M, Pantano P, Palmeggiani F, Raguso M, Osti MF, Anaveri G, Bozzao L (1998). Radiological assessment of necrosis in glioblastoma: variability and prognostic value. Neuroradiology 40: 150-153.
1745. Piercecchi-Marti MD, Mohamed H, Liprandi A, Gambarelli D, Grisoli F, Pellissier JF (2002). Intracranial meningeal melanocytoma associated with ipsilateral nevus of Ota. Case report. J Neurosurg 96: 619-623.
1746. Pierre K, Hirsch JF, Roux FX, Renier D, Sainte R (1983). Intracranial ependymomas in childhood. Survival and functional results of 47 cases. Childs Brain 10: 145-156.
1747. Pietsch T, Waha A, Koch A, Kraus J, Albrecht S, Tonn J, Sorensen N, Berthold F, Henk B, Schmandt N, Wolf HK, von Deimling A, Wainwright B, Chenevix-Trench G, Wiestler OD, Wicking C (1997). Medulloblastomas of the desmoplastic variant carry mutations of the human homologue of Drosoophila patched. Cancer Res 57:2085-2088.
1748. Pilarski R, Eng C (2004). Will the real Cowden syndrome please stand up (again)? Expanding mutational and clinical spectra of the PTEN hamartoma tumour syndrome. J Med Genet 41: 323-326.
1749. Pillai A, Rajeev K, Chandi S, Unnikrishnan M (2004). Intrinsic brainstem choroid plexus papilloma. Case report. J Neurosurg 100: 1076-1078.
1750. Pimentel J, Tavora L, Cristina ML, Antunes JA (1988). Intraventricular schwannoma. Childs Nerv Syst 4: 373-375.
1751. Pinto D, Clevers H (2005). Wnt control of stem cells and differentiation in the intestinal epithelium. Exp Cell Res 306: 357-363.
1752. Pirotte B, Krischek B, Levivier M, Bolyn S, Brucher JM, Brotchi J (1998). Diagnostic and microsurgical presentation of intracranial angiolipomas. Case report and review of the literature. J Neurosurg 88: 129-132.
1753. Pirotte B, Levivier M, Goldman S, Brucher JM, Brotchi J, Hildebrand J (1997). Glucocorticoid-induced long-term remission in primary cerebral lymphoma: case report and review of the literature. J Neurooncol 63-69.
1754. Pitkethly DT, Major MC, Hardman JM, Kempe LG, Earle KM (1970). Angioblastic meningiomas. Clinicopathologic study of 81 cases. J Neurosurg 32: 539-544.
1755. Pitt MA, Jones AW, Reeve RS, Cowie RA (1992). Oligodendroglioma of the fourth ventricle with intracranial and spinal oligodendrogliomatosis: a case report. Br J Neurosurg 6: 371-374.
1756. Pizem J, Cor A, Zadravec ZL, Popovic M (2005). Prognostic significance of apoptosis in medulloblastoma. Neurosci Lett 381: 69-73.
1757. Pizer BL, Moss T, Oakhill A, Webb D, Coakham HB (1995). Congenital astroblastoma: an immunohistochemical study. Case report. J Neurosurg 83: 550-555.
1758. Plank TL, Logginidou H, Klein-Szanto A, Henske EP (1999). The expression of hamartin, the product of the TSC1 gene, in normal human tissues and in TSC1- and TSC2-linked angiomyolipomas. Mod Pathol 12: 539-545.
1759. Plank TL, Yeung RS, Henske EP (1998). Hamartin, the product of the tuberous sclerosis 1 (TSC1) gene, interacts with tuberin and appears to be localized to cytoplasmic vesicles. Cancer Res 58: 4766-4770.
1760. Plate KH (1999). Mechanisms of angiogenesis in the brain. J Neuropathol Exp Neurol 58: 313-320.
1761. Platten M, Giordano MJ, Dirven CM, Gutmann DH, Louis DN (1996). Up-regulation of specific NF 1 gene transcripts in sporadic pilocytic astrocytomas. Am J Pathol 149: 621-627.
1762. Plowman PN, Pizer B, Kingston JE (2004). Pineal parenchymal tumours: II. On the aggressive behaviour of pineoblastoma in patients with an inherited mutation of the RB1 gene. Clin Oncol (R Coll Radiol) 16: 244-247.
1763. Plukker JT, Koops HS, Molenaar I, Vermey A, ten Kate LP, Oldhoff J (1988). Malignant hemangiopericytoma in three kindred members of one family. Cancer 61: 841-844.
1764. Poe LB, Dubowy RL, Hochhauser L, Collins GH, Crosley CJ, Kanzer MD, Oliphant M, Hodge CJ, Jr. (1994). Demyelinating and gliotic cerebellar lesions in Langerhans cell histiocytosis. Am J Neuroradiol 15: 1921-1928.
1765. Pohl U, Cairncross JG, Louis DN (1999). Homozygous deletions of the CDKN2C/p18INK4C gene on chromosome 1p in anaplastic oligodendrogliomas. Brain Pathol 9 :639-43.
1766. Pollack IF, Claassen D, al Shboul Q, Janosky JE, Deutsch M (1995). Low-grade gliomas of the cerebral hemispheres in children: an analysis of 71 cases. J Neurosurg 82:

536-547.
1767. Pollack IF, Finkelstein SD, Burnham J, Holmes EJ, Hamilton RL, Yates AJ, Finlay JL, Sposto R (2001). Age and TP53 mutation frequency in childhood malignant gliomas: results in a multi-institutional cohort. Cancer Res 61: 7404-7407.
1768. Pollack IF, Gerszten PC, Martinez AJ, Lo KH, Shultz B, Albright AL, Janosky J, Deutsch M (1995). Intracranial ependymomas of childhood: long-term outcome and prognostic factors. Neurosurgery 37: 655-666.
1769. Pollack IF, Hoffman HJ, Humphreys RP, Becker L (1993). The long-term outcome after surgical treatment of dorsally exophytic brain-stem gliomas. J Neurosurg 78: 859-863.
1770. Pollack IF, Hurtt M, Pang D, Albright AL (1994). Dissemination of low grade intracranial astrocytomas in children. Cancer 73: 2869-2878.
1771. Pollak A, Friede RL (1977). Fine structure of medulloepithelioma. J Neuropathol Exp Neurol 36: 712-725.
1772. Pomerantz J, Schreiber-Agus N, Liegeois NJ, Silverman A, Alland L, Chin L, Potes J, Chen K, Orlow I, Lee HW, Cordon-Cardo C, DePinho RA (1998). The Ink4a tumor suppressor gene product, p19Arf, interacts with MDM2 and neutralizes MDM2's inhibition of p53. Cell 92: 713-723.
1773. Pomeroy SL, Tamayo P, Gaasenbeek M, Sturla LM, Angelo M, McLaughlin ME, Kim JY, Goumnerova LC, Black PM, Lau C, Allen JC, Zagzag D, Olson JM, Curran T, Wetmore C, Biegel JA, Poggio T, Mukherjee S, Rifkin R, Califano A, Stolovitzky G, Louis DN, Mesirov JP, Lander ES, Golub TR (2002). Prediction of central nervous system embryonal tumour outcome based on gene expression. Nature 415: 436-442.
1774. Pommepuy I, Delage-Corre M, Moreau JJ, Labrousse F (2006). A report of a desmoplastic ganglioglioma in a 12-year-old girl with review of the literature. J Neurooncol 76: 271-275.
1775. Pomper MG, Passe TJ, Burger PC, Scheithauer BW, Brat DJ (2001). Chordoid glioma: a neoplasm unique to the hypothalamus and anterior third ventricle. AJNR Am J Neuroradiol 22: 464-469.
1776. Pompili A, Calvosa F, Caroli F, Mastrostefano R, Occhipinti E, Raus L, Sciaretta F (1993). The transdural extension of gliomas. J Neurooncol 15: 67-74.
1777. Ponzoni M, Ferreri AJ (2006). Intravascular lymphoma: a neoplasm of 'homeless' lymphocytes? Hematol Oncol 24: 105-112.
1778. Pope LZ, Tatsui CE, Moro MS, Neto AC, Bleggi-Torres LF (2003). Meningioma with extensive noncalcifying collagenous whorls and glial fibrillary acidic protein expression: new variant of meningioma diagnosed by smear preparation. Diagn Cytopathol 28: 274-277.
1779. Poremba C, Dockhorn-Dworniczak B, Merritt V, Li CY, Heidl G, Tauber PF, Bocker W, Yandell DW (1993). Immature teratomas of different origin carried by a pregnant mother and her fetus. Diagn Mol Pathol 2: 131-136.
1780. Powell SZ, Yachnis AT, Rorke LB, Rojiani AM, Eskin TA (1996). Divergent differentiation in pleomorphic xanthoastrocytoma. Evidence for a neuronal element and possible relationship to ganglion cell tumors. Am J Surg Pathol 20: 80-85.
1781. Prabhu SS, Lynch PG, Keogh AJ, Parekh HC (1993). Intracranial meningeal melanocytoma: a report of two cases and a review of the literature. Surg Neurol 40: 516-521.
1782. Prabhu VC, Brown HG (2005). The pathogenesis of craniopharyngiomas. Childs Nerv Syst 21: 622-627.
1783. Prados MD, Krouwer HG, Edwards MS, Cogen PH, Davis RL, Hoshino T (1992). Proliferative potential and outcome in pediatric astrocytic tumors. J Neurooncol 13: 277-282.
1784. Pramanik P, Sharma MC, Mukhopadhyay P, Singh VP, Sarkar C (2003). A comparative study of classical vs. desmoplastic medulloblastomas. Neurol India 51: 27-34.
1785. Prayer D, Grois N, Prosch H, Gadner H, Barkovich AJ (2004). MR imaging presentation of intracranial disease associated with Langerhans cell histiocytosis. AJNR Am J Neuroradiol 25: 880-891.
1786. Prayson RA (1996). Gliofibroma: a distinct entity or a subtype of desmoplastic astrocytoma? Hum Pathol 27: 610-613.
1787. Prayson RA (1997). Myxopapillary ependymomas: a clinicopathologic study of 14 cases including MIB-1 and p53 immunoreactivity. Mod Pathol 10: 304-310.
1788. Prayson RA (1999). Clinicopathologic study of 61 patients with ependymoma including MIB-1 immunohistochemistry. Ann Diagn Pathol 3: 11-18.
1789. Prayson RA (1999). Composite ganglioglioma and dysembryoplastic neuroepithelial tumor. Arch Pathol Lab Med 123: 247-250.
1790. Prayson RA (2000). Papillary glioneuronal tumor. Arch Pathol Lab Med 124: 1820-1823.
1791. Prayson RA (2004). Cyclooxygenase-2, Bcl-2, and chromosome 1p analysis in protoplasmic astrocytomas. Hum Pathol 35: 317-321.
1792. Prayson RA, Abramovich CM (2000). Glioneuronal tumor with neuropil-like islands. Hum Pathol 31: 1435-1438.
1793. Prayson RA, Castilla EA, Hartke M, Pettay J, Tubbs RR, Barnett GH (2002). Chromosome 1p allelic loss by fluorescence in situ hybridization is not observed in dysembryoplastic neuroepithelial tumors. Am J Clin Pathol 118: 512-517.
1794. Prayson RA, Chahlavi A, Luciano M (2004). Cerebellar paraganglioma. Ann Diagn Pathol 8: 219-223.
1795. Prayson RA, Estes ML (1992). Dysembryoplastic neuroepithelial tumor. Am J Clin Pathol 97: 398-401.
1796. Prayson RA, Estes ML (1995). Protoplasmic astrocytoma. A clinicopathologic study of 16 tumors. Am J Clin Pathol 103: 705-709.
1797. Prayson RA, Estes ML (1996). MIB1 and p53 immunoreactivity in protoplasmic astrocytomas. Pathol Int 46: 862-866.
1798. Prayson RA, Khajavi K, Comair YG (1995). Cortical architectural abnormalities and MIB1 immunoreactivity in gangliogliomas: a study of 60 patients with intracranial tumors. J Neuropathol Exp Neurol 54: 513-520.
1799. Preusser M, Dietrich W, Czech T, Prayer D, Budka H, Hainfellner JA (2003). Rosette-forming glioneuronal tumor of the fourth ventricle. Acta Neuropathol 106: 506-508.
1799A. Preusser M, Hoischen A, Novak K, Czech T, Prayer D, Hainfellner JA, Baumgartner C, Woermann FG, Tuxhorn IE, Pannek HW, Bergmann M, Radlwimmer B, Villagran R, Weber RG, Hans VH (2007). Angiocentric glioma: report of clinico-pathologic and genetic findings in 8 cases. Am J Surg Pathol. In Press.
1800. Preusser M, Laggner U, Haberler C, Heinzl H, Budka H, Hainfellner JA (2006). Comparative analysis of NeuN immunoreactivity in primary brain tumours: conclusions for rational use in diagnostic histopathology. Histopathology 48: 438-444.
1801. Prevot S, Bienvenu L, Vaillant JC, Saint-Maur PP (1999). Benign schwannoma of the digestive tract: a clinicopathologic and immunohistochemical study of five cases, including a case of esophageal tumor. Am J Surg Pathol 23: 431-436.
1802. Probst-Cousin S, Bergmann M, Schroder R, Kuchelmeister K, Schmid KW, Ernestus RJ, Janus J (1996). Ki-67 and biological behaviour in meningeal haemangiopericytomas. Histopathology 29: 57-61.
1803. Proescholdt MA, Mayer C, Kubitza M, Schubert T, Liao SY, Stanbridge EJ, Ivanov S, Oldfield EH, Brawanski A, Merrill MJ (2005). Expression of hypoxia-inducible carbonic anhydrases in brain tumors. Neuro-oncol 7: 465-475.
1804. Proust F, Laquerriere A, Constantin B, Ruchoux MM, Vannier JP, Freger P (1999). Simultaneous presentation of atypical teratoid/rhabdoid tumor in siblings. J Neurooncol 43: 63-70.
1805. Pruchon E, Chauveinc L, Sabatier L, Dutrillaux AM, Ricoul M, Delattre JY, Vega F, Poisson M, Hor F, Dutrillaux B (1994). A cytogenetic study of 19 recurrent gliomas. Cancer Genet Cytogenet 76: 85-92.
1806. Pulst SM, Rouleau GA, Marineau C, Fain P, Sieb JP (1993). Familial meningioma is not allelic to neurofibromatosis 2. Neurology 43: 2096-2098.
1807. Pummi KP, Aho HJ, Laato MK, Peltonen JT, Peltonen SA (2006). Tight junction proteins and perineurial cells in neurofibromas. J Histochem Cytochem 54: 53-61.
1808. Purav P, Ganapathy K, Mallikarjuna VS, Annapurneswari S, Kalyanaraman S, Reginald J, Natarajan P, Bapu KR, Balamurugan M (2005). Rosai-Dorfman disease of the central nervous system. J Clin Neurosci 12: 656-659.
1809. Pyhtinen J, Paakko E (1996). A difficult diagnosis of gliomatosis cerebri. Neuroradiology 38: 444-448.
1810. Pykett MJ, Murphy M, Harnish PR, George DL (1994). Identification of a microsatellite instability phenotype in meningiomas. Cancer Res 54: 6340-6343.
1811. Qian XC, Brent TP (1997). Methylation hot spots in the 5' flanking region denote silencing of the O6-methylguanine-DNA methyltransferase gene. Cancer Res 57: 3672-3677.
1812. Queiroz LS, Faria AV, Zanardi VA, Netto JR (2005). Lipidized giant-cell glioblastoma of cerebellum. Clin Neuropathol 24: 262-6.
1813. Rades D, Fehlauer F, Lamszus K, Schild SE, Hagel C, Westphal M, Alberti W (2005). Well-differentiated neurocytoma: what is the best available treatment? Neuro-oncol 7: 77-83.
1814. Rades D, Fehlauer F, Schild SE (2004). Treatment of atypical neurocytomas. Cancer 100: 814-817.
1815. Rades D, Schild SE, Fehlauer F (2004). Prognostic value of the MIB-1 labeling index for central neurocytomas. Neurology 62: 987-989.
1816. Raffel C, Jenkins RB, Frederick L, Hebrink D, Alderete BE, Fults DW, James CD (1997). Sporadic medulloblastomas contain PTCH mutations. Cancer Res 57: 842-845.
1817. Ragel BT, Jensen RL (2005). Molecular genetics of meningiomas. Neurosurg Focus 19: E9.
1818. Ragel BT, Osborn AG, Whang K, Townsend JJ, Jensen RL, Couldwell WT (2006). Subependymomas: an analysis of clinical and imaging features. Neurosurgery 58: 881-890.
1819. Raghavan R, Balani J, Perry A, Margraf L, Vono MB, Cai DX, Wyatt RE, Rushing EJ, Bowers DC, Hynan LS, White CL, III (2003). Pediatric oligodendrogliomas: a study of molecular alterations on 1p and 19q using fluorescence in situ hybridization. J Neuropathol Exp Neurol 62: 530-537.
1820. Raghavan R, Steart PV, Weller RO (1990). Cell proliferation patterns in the diagnosis of astrocytomas, anaplastic astrocytomas and glioblastoma multiforme: a Ki-67 study. Neuropathol Appl Neurobiol 16: 123-133.
1821. Rainho CA, Rogatto SR, de Moraes LC, Barbieri-Neto J (1992). Cytogenetic study of a pineocytoma. Cancer Genet Cytogenet 64: 127-132.
1822. Rainov NG, Lubbe J, Renshaw J, Pritchard J, Luthy AR, Aguzzi A (1995). Association of Wilms' tumor with primary brain tumor in siblings. J Neuropathol Exp Neurol 54: 214-223.
1823. Raisanen J, Biegel JA, Hatanpaa KJ, Judkins A, White CL, Perry A (2005). Chromosome 22q deletions in atypical teratoid/rhabdoid tumors in adults. Brain Pathol 15: 23-28.
1824. Rajan B, Ashley S, Gorman C, Jose CC, Horwich A, Bloom HJ, Marsh H, Brada M (1993). Craniopharyngioma—a long-term results following limited surgery and radiotherapy. Radiother Oncol 26: 1-10.
1825. Rajaram V, Brat DJ, Perry A (2004). Anaplastic meningioma versus meningeal hemangiopericytoma: immunohistochemical and genetic markers. Hum Pathol 35: 1413-1418.
1826. Rajcan-Separovic E, Maguire J, Loukianova T, Nisha M, Kalousek D (2003). Loss of 1p and 7p in radiation-induced meningiomas identified by comparative genomic hybridization. Cancer Genet Cytogenet 144: 6-11.
1827. Raney RB, Ater JL, Herman L, Leeds NE, Cleary KR, Womer RB, Rorke LM (1994). Primary intraspinal soft-tissue sarcoma in childhood: report of two cases with a review of the literature. Med Pediatr Oncol 23: 359-364.
1828. Rankine AJ, Filion PR, Platten MA, Spagnolo DV (2004). Perineurioma: a clinicopathological study of eight cases. Pathology 36: 309-315.
1829. Ransom DT, Ritland SR, Kimmel DW, Moertel CA, Dahl RJ, Scheithauer BW, Kelly PJ, Jenkins RB (1992). Cytogenetic and loss of heterozygosity studies in ependymomas, pilocytic astrocytomas, and oligodendrogliomas. Genes Chromosomes Cancer 5: 348-356.
1830. Rao C, Friedlander ME, Klein E, Anzil AP, Sher JH (1990). Medullomyoblastoma in an adult. Cancer 65: 157-163.
1831. Rao UN, Surti U, Hoffner L, Yaw K (1996). Cytogenetic and histologic correlation of peripheral nerve sheath tumors of soft tissue. Cancer Genet Cytogenet 88: 17-25.
1832. Rasheed BK, McLendon RE, Friedman HS, Friedman AH, Fuchs HE, Bigner DD, Bigner SH (1995). Chromosome 10 deletion mapping in human gliomas: a common deletion region in 10q25. Oncogene 10: 2243-2246.
1833. Rasheed BK, Wiltshire RN, Bigner SH, Bigner DD (1999). Molecular pathogenesis of malignant gliomas. Curr Opin Oncol 11: 162-167.
1834. Rasmussen A, Nava-Salazar S, Yescas P, Alonso E, Revuelta R, Ortiz I, Canizales-Quinteros S, Tusie-Luna MT, Lopez-Lopez M (2006). Von Hippel-Lindau disease germline mutations in Mexican patients with cerebellar hemangioblastoma. J Neurosurg 104: 389-394.
1835. Rauhut F, Reinhardt V, Budach V, Wiedemayer H, Nau HE (1989). Intramedullary pilocytic astrocytomas—a clinical and morphological study after combined surgical and photon or neutron therapy. Neurosurg Rev 12: 309-313.
1836. Rausing A, Ybo W, Stenflo J (1970). Intracranial meningioma - a population study of ten years. Acta Neurol Scand 46: 102-110.
1837. Rawlings CE, III, Giangaspero F, Burger PC, Bullard DE (1988). Ependymomas: a clinicopathologic study. Surg Neurol 29: 271-281.
1838. Rawlinson DG, Herman MM, Rubinstein LJ (1973). The fine structure of a myxopapillary ependymoma of the filum terminale. Acta Neuropathol 25: 1-13.

1839. Raymond AA, Halpin SF, Alsanjari N, Cook MJ, Kitchen ND, Fish DR, Stevens JM, Harding BN, Scaravilli F, Kendall B (1994). Dysembryoplastic neuroepithelial tumor. Features in 16 patients. Brain 117: 461-475.
1840. Raza SM, Lang FF, Aggarwal BB, Fuller GN, Wildrick DM, Sawaya R (2002). Necrosis and glioblastoma: a friend or a foe? A review and a hypothesis. Neurosurgery 51: 2-12.
1841. Regis J, Bouillot P, Rouby V, Figarella B, Dufour H, Peragut JC (1996). Pineal region tumors and the role of stereotactic biopsy: review of the mortality, morbidity, and diagnostic rates in 370 cases. Neurosurgery 39: 907-912.
1842. Reifenberger G (1991). Immunhistochemie der Tumoren des Zentralnervensystems. Springer-Verlag: Berlin.
1843. Reifenberger G, Kaulich K, Wiestler OD, Blumcke I (2003). Expression of the CD34 antigen in pleomorphic xanthoastrocytomas. Acta Neuropathol 105: 358-364.
1844. Reifenberger G, Liu L, Ichimura K, Schmidt EE, Collins VP (1993). Amplification and overexpression of the MDM2 gene in a subset of human malignant gliomas without p53 mutations. Cancer Res 53: 2736-2739.
1845. Reifenberger G, Louis DN (2003). Oligodendroglioma: toward molecular definitions in diagnostic neuro-oncology. J Neuropathol Exp Neurol 62: 111-126.
1846. Reifenberger G, Reifenberger J, Ichimura K, Meltzer PS, Collins VP (1994). Amplification of multiple genes from chromosomal region 12q13-14 in human malignant gliomas: preliminary mapping of the amplicons shows preferential involvement of CDK4, SAS, and MDM2. Cancer Res 54: 4299-4303.
1847. Reifenberger G, Szymas J, Wechsler W (1987). Differential expression of glial- and neuronal-associated antigens in human tumors of the central and peripheral nervous system. Acta Neuropathol 74: 105-123.
1848. Reifenberger G, Weber T, Weber RG, Wolter M, Brandis A, Kuchelmeister K, Pilz P, Reusche E, Lichter P, Wiestler OD (1999). Chordoid glioma of the third ventricle: immunohistochemical and molecular genetic characterization of a novel tumor entity. Brain Pathol 9: 617-626.
1849. Reifenberger J, Reifenberger G, Ichimura K, Schmidt EE, Wechsler W, Collins VP (1996). Epidermal growth factor receptor expression in oligodendroglial tumors. Am J Pathol 149: 29-35.
1850. Reifenberger J, Reifenberger G, Liu L, James CD, Wechsler W, Collins VP (1994). Molecular genetic analysis of oligodendroglial tumors shows preferential allelic deletions on 19q and 1p. Am J Pathol 145: 1175-1190.
1851. Reifenberger J, Ring GU, Gies U, Cobbers L, Oberstrass J, An HX, Niederacher D, Wechsler W, Reifenberger G (1996). Analysis of p53 mutation and epidermal growth factor receptor amplification in recurrent gliomas with malignant progression. J Neuropathol Exp Neurol 55: 822-831.
1852. Reifenberger J, Wolter M, Weber RG, Megahed M, Ruzicka T, Lichter P, Reifenberger G (1998). Missense mutations in SMOH in sporadic basal cell carcinomas of the skin and primitive neuroectodermal tumors of the central nervous system. Cancer Res 58: 1798-1803.
1853. Reilly KM, Jacks T (2001). Genetically engineered mouse models of astrocytoma: GEMs in the rough? Semin Cancer Biol 11: 177-191.
1854. Reis-Filho JS, Faoro LN, Carrilho C, Bleggi-Torres LF, Schmitt FC (2000). Evaluation of cell proliferation, epidermal growth factor receptor, and bcl-2 immunoexpression as prognostic factors for patients with World Health Organization grade 2 oligodendroglioma. Cancer 88: 862-869.
1855. Reis RM, Hara A, Kleihues P, Ohgaki H (2001). Genetic evidence of the neoplastic nature of gemistocytes in astrocytomas. Acta Neuropathol 102: 422-425.
1856. Reis RM, Konu-Lebleblicioglu D, Lopes JM, Kleihues P, Ohgaki H (2000). Genetic profile of the gliosarcoma. Am J Pathol 156: 425-432.
1857. Reithmeier T, Gumprecht H, Stolzle A, Lumenta CB (2000). Intracerebral paraganglioma. Acta Neurochir 142: 1063-1066.
1858. Rempel SA, Schwechheimer K, Davis RL, Cavenee WK, Rosenblum ML (1993). Loss of heterozygosity for loci on chromosome 10 is associated with morphologically malignant meningioma progression. Cancer Res 53: 2386-2392.
1859. Rencic A, Gordon J, Otte J, Curtis M, Kovatich A, Zoltick P, Khalili K, Andrews D (1996). Detection of JC virus DNA sequence and expression of the viral oncoprotein, tumor antigen, in brain of immunocompetent patient with oligoastrocytoma. Proc Natl Acad Sci USA 93: 7352-7357.
1860. Reni M, Ferreri AJ, Zoldan MC, Villa E (1997). Primary brain lymphomas in patients with a prior or concomitant malignancy. J Neurooncol 32: 135-142.
1861. Renshaw AA, Paulus W, Joseph JT (1995). CD34 and epithelial membrane antigen distinguish dural hemangiopericytoma and meningioma. Appl Immunohistochem 3: 108-114.
1862. Resta N, Lauriola L, Puca A, Susca FC, Albanese A, Sabatino G, Di Giacomo MC, Gessi M, Guanti G (2006). Ganglioglioma arising in a Peutz-Jeghers patient: a case report with molecular implications. Acta Neuropathol 112: 106-111.
1863. Reyes-Mugica M, Chou P, Byrd S, Ray V, Castelli M, Gattuso P, Gonzalez Crussi F (1993). Nevomelanocytic proliferations in the central nervous system of children. Cancer 72: 2277-2285.
1864. Reyes-Mugica M, Chou P, Gonzalez C, Tomita T (1992). Fibroma of the meninges in a child: immunohistological and ultrastructural study. Case report. J Neurosurg 76: 143-147.
1865. Rhodes RH, Cole M, Takaoka Y, Roessmann U, Cotes EE, Simon J (1994). Intraventricular cerebral neuroblastoma. Analysis of subtypes and comparison with hemispheric neuroblastoma. Arch Pathol Lab Med 118: 897-911.
1866. Ribalta T, Fuller GN (2006). Brain metastases; histopathological evaluation and diagnostic pitfalls. In: Sawaya R, ed. Blackwell Futura Publishing: Malden, MA, USA.
1867. Ribeiro RC, Sandrini F, Figueiredo B, Zambetti GP, Michalkiewicz E, Lafferty AR, DeLacerda L, Rabin M, Cadwell C, Sampaio G, Cat I, Stratakis CA, Sandrini R (2001). An inherited p53 mutation that contributes in a tissue-specific manner to pediatric adrenal cortical carcinoma. Proc Natl Acad Sci U S A 98: 9330-9335.
1868. Riccardi VM (1981). Von Recklinghausen neurofibromatosis. N Engl J Med 305: 1617-1627.
1869. Ricci A, Jr., Parham DM, Woodruff JM, Callihan T, Green A, Erlandson RA (1984). Malignant peripheral nerve sheath tumors arising from ganglioneuromas. Am J Surg Pathol 8: 19-29.
1870. Rich JN, Hans C, Jones B, Iversen ES, McLendon RE, Rasheed BK, Dobra A, Dressman HK, Bigner DD, Nevins JR, West M (2005). Gene expression profiling and genetic markers in glioblastoma survival. Cancer Res 65: 4051-4058.
1871. Rich JN, Reardon DA, Peery T, Dowell JM, Quinn JA, Penne KL, Wikstrand CJ, Van Duyn LB, Dancey JE, McLendon RE, Kao JC, Stenzel TT, Rasheed BK, Tourt-Uhlig SE, Herndon JE, Vredenburgh JJ, Sampson JH, Friedman AH, Bigner DD, Friedman HS (2004). Phase II trial of gefitinib in recurrent glioblastoma. J Clin Oncol 22: 133-142.
1872. Richard S, David P, Marsot-Dupuch K, Giraud S, Beroud C, Resche F (2000). Central nervous system hemangioblastomas, endolymphatic sac tumors, and von Hippel-Lindau disease. Neurosurg Rev 23: 1-22.
1873. Rickert CH, Dockhorn-Dworniczak B, Simon R, Paulus W (1999). Chromosomal imbalances in primary lymphomas of the central nervous system. Am J Pathol. 155: 1445-1451.
1874. Rickert CH, Jasper M, Sepehrnia A, Jeibmann A (2006). Rosetted glioneuronal tumour of the spine: clinical, histological and cytogenetic data. Acta Neuropathol 112: 231-233.
1875. Rickert CH, Korshunov A, Paulus W (2006). Chromosomal imbalances in clear cell ependymomas. Mod Pathol 19: 958-962.
1876. Rickert CH, Paulus W (2001). Epidemiology of central nervous system tumors in childhood and adolescence based on the new WHO classification. Childs Nerv Syst 17: 503-511.
1877. Rickert CH, Paulus W (2001). Tumors of the choroid plexus. Microsc Res Tech 52: 104-111.
1878. Rickert CH, Paulus W (2002). Genetic characterisation of granular cell tumours. Acta Neuropathol 103: 309-312.
1879. Rickert CH, Paulus W (2002). No chromosomal imbalances detected by comparative genomic hybridisation in a case of fetal immature teratoma. Childs Nerv Syst 18: 639-643.
1880. Rickert CH, Paulus W (2003). Lack of chromosomal imbalances in adamantinomatous and papillary craniopharyngiomas. J Neurol Neurosurg Psychiatry 74: 260-261.
1881. Rickert CH, Paulus W (2004). Comparative genomic hybridization in central and peripheral nervous system tumors of childhood and adolescence. J Neuropathol Exp Neurol 63: 399-417.
1882. Rickert CH, Simon R, Bergmann M, Dockhorn-Dworniczak B, Paulus W (2000). Comparative genomic hybridization in pineal germ cell tumors. J Neuropathol Exp Neurol 59: 815-821.
1883. Rickert CH, Simon R, Bergmann M, Dockhorn-Dworniczak B, Paulus W (2001). Comparative genomic hybridization in pineal parenchymal tumors. Genes Chromosomes Cancer 30: 99-104.
1884. Rickert CH, Strater R, Kaatsch P, Wassmann H, Jurgens H, Dockhorn-Dworniczak B, Paulus W (2001). Pediatric high-grade astrocytomas show chromosomal imbalances distinct from adult cases. Am J Pathol 158: 1525-1532.
1885. Rickert CH, Wiestler OD, Paulus W (2002). Chromosomal imbalances in choroid plexus tumors. Am J Pathol 160: 1105-1113.
1886. Rickman DS, Bobek MP, Misek DE, Kuick R, Blaivas M, Kurnit DM, Taylor J, Hanash SM (2001). Distinctive molecular profiles of high-grade and low-grade gliomas based on oligonucleotide microarray analysis. Cancer Res 61: 6885-6891.
1887. Riemenschneider MJ, Koy TH, Reifenberger G (2004). Expression of oligodendrocyte lineage genes in oligodendroglial and astrocytic gliomas. Acta Neuropathol 107: 277-282.
1888. Rienstein S, Adams EF, Pilzer D, Goldring AA, Goldman B, Friedman E (2003). Comparative genomic hybridization analysis of craniopharyngiomas. J Neurosurg 98: 162-164.
1889. Rieske P, Zakrzewska M, Piaskowski S, Jaskolski D, Sikorska B, Papierz W, Zakrzewski K, Liberski PP (2003). Molecular heterogeneity of meningioma with INI1 mutation. Mol Pathol 56: 299-301.
1890. Riffaud L, Vinchon M, Ragragui O, Delestret I, Ruchoux MM, Dhellemmes P (2002). Hemispheric cerebral gliomas in children with NF1: arguments for a long-term follow-up. Childs Nerv Syst 18: 43-47.
1891. Ringertz J (1950). Grading of gliomas. Acta Pathol Microbiol Scand 27: 51-64.
1892. Risdall RJ, Dehner LP, Duray P, Kobrinsky N, Robison L, Nesbit ME, Jr. (1983). Histiocytosis X (Langerhans' cell histiocytosis). Prognostic role of histopathology. Arch Pathol Lab Med 107: 59-63.
1893. Ritter JH, Mills SE, Nappi O, Wick MR (1995). Angiosarcoma-like neoplasms of epithelial organs: true endothelial tumors or variants of carcinoma? Semin Diagn Pathol 12: 270-282.
1894. Roach ES, DiMario FJ, Kandt RS, Northrup H (1999). Tuberous Sclerosis Consensus Conference: recommendations for diagnostic evaluation. National Tuberous Sclerosis Association. J Child Neurol 14: 401-407.
1895. Roach ES, Sparagana SP (2004). Diagnosis of tuberous sclerosis complex. J Child Neurol 19: 643-649.
1896. Robbins P, Segal A, Narula S, Stokes B, Lee M, Thomas W, Caterina P, Sinclair I, Spagnolo D (1995). Central neurocytoma. A clinicopathological, immunohistochemical and ultrastructural study of 7 cases. Pathol Res Pract 191: 100-111.
1897. Roberts CW, Orkin SH (2004). The SWI/SNF complex—chromatin and cancer. Nat Rev Cancer 4: 133-142.
1898. Roberts RO, Lynch CF, Jones MP, Hart MN (1991). Medulloblastoma: a population-based study of 532 cases. J Neuropathol Exp Neurol 50: 134-144.
1899. Robertson PL, Zeltzer PM, Boyett JM, Rorke LB, Allen JC, Geyer JR, Stanley P, Li H, Albright AL, McGuire-Cullen P, Finlay JL, Stevens KR, Jr., Milstein JM, Packer RJ, Wisoff J (1998). Survival and prognostic factors following radiation therapy and chemotherapy for ependymomas in children: a report of the Children's Cancer Group. J Neurosurg 88: 695-703.
1899A Robin YM, Guilllou L, Michels JJ, Coindre JM (2004). Human herpesvirus 8 immunostaining: a sensitive and specific method for diagnosing Kaposi sarcoma in paraffin-embedded sections. Am J Clin Pathol 121:330-4.
1900. Robinson JC, Challa VR, Jones DS, Kelly DL, Jr. (1996). Pericytosis and edema generation: a unique clinicopathological variant of meningioma. Neurosurgery 39: 700-706.
1901. Roche PH, Figarella B, Regis J, Peragut JC (1996). Cauda equina paraganglioma with subsequent intracranial and intraspinal metastases. Acta Neurochir 138: 475-479.
1902. Rodriguez-Pereira C, Borras-Moreno JM, Pesudo-Martinez JV, Vera-Roman JM (2005). Cerebral solitary Langerhans cell histiocytosis: report of two cases and review of the literature. Br J Neurosurg 19: 192-197.
1903. Rodriguez FJ, Scheithauer BW, Abell-Aleff PC, Elamin E, Erlandson RA (2006). Low grade malignant peripheral nerve sheath tumor with smooth muscle differentiation. Acta Neuropathol. In Press.
1904. Rodriguez HA, Berthrong M (1966). Multiple primary intracranial tumors in von Recklinghausen's neurofibromatosis. Arch Neurol 14: 467-475.
1905. Rodriguez LA, Edwards MS, Levin VA (1990). Management of hypothalamic gliomas in children: an analysis of 33 cases.

Neurosurgery 26: 242-246.
1906. Roelvink NC, Kamphorst W, Lindhout D, Ponssen H (1986). Concordant cerebral oligodendroglioma in identical twins. J Neurol Neurosurg Psychiatry 49: 706-708.
1907. Roerig P, Nessling M, Radlwimmer B, Joos S, Wrobel G, Schwaenen C, Reifenberger G, Lichter P (2005). Molecular classification of human gliomas using matrix-based comparative genomic hybridization. Int J Cancer 117: 95-103.
1908. Roessler E, Belloni E, Gaudenz K, Jay P, Berta P, Scherer SW, Tsui LC, Muenke M (1996). Mutations in the human Sonic Hedgehog gene cause holoprosencephaly. Nat Genet 14: 357-360.
1909. Roessler K, Bertalanffy A, Jezan H, Ba-Ssalamah A, Slavc I, Czech T, Budka H (2002). Proliferative activity as measured by MIB-1 labeling index and long-term outcome of cerebellar juvenile pilocytic astrocytomas. J Neurooncol 58: 141-146.
1910. Rogers L, Pattisapu J, Smith RR, Parker P (1988). Medulloblastoma in association with the Coffin-Siris syndrome. Childs Nerv Syst 4: 41-44.
1911. Rohringer M, Sutherland GR, Louw DF, Sima AA (1989). Incidence and clinicopathological features of meningioma. J Neurosurg 71: 665-672.
1912. Rollins KE, Kleinschmidt-DeMasters BK, Corboy JR, Damek DM, Filley CM (2005). Lymphomatosis cerebri as a cause of white matter dementia. Hum Pathol 36: 282-290.
1913. Rollison DE, Utaipat U, Ryschkewitsch C, Hou J, Goldthwaite P, Daniel R, Helzlsouer KJ, Burger PC, Shah KV, Major EO (2005). Investigation of human brain tumors for the presence of polyomavirus genome sequences by two independent laboratories. Int J Cancer 113: 769-774.
1914. Roncaroli F, Riccioni L, Cerati M, Capella C, Calbucci F, Trevisan C, Eusebi V (1997). Oncocytic meningioma. Am J Surg Pathol 21: 375-382.
1915. Roncaroli F, Scheithauer BW, Cenacchi G, Horvath E, Kovacs K, Lloyd RV, Abell-Aleff P, Santi M, Yates AJ (2002). 'Spindle cell oncocytoma' of the adenohypophysis: a tumor of folliculostellate cells? Am J Surg Pathol 26: 1048-1055.
1916. Roncaroli F, Scheithauer BW, Papazoglou S (2001). Primary polymorphous hemangioendothelioma of the spinal cord. Case report. J Neurosurg 95: 93-95.
1917. Rong Y, Durden DL, Van Meir EG, Brat DJ (2006). 'Pseudopalisading' necrosis in glioblastoma: a familiar morphologic feature that links vascular pathology, hypoxia, and angiogenesis. J Neuropathol Exp Neurol 65: 529-539.
1918. Rongioletti F, Drago F, Rebora A (1989). Multiple cutaneous plexiform schwannomas with tumors of the central nervous system. Arch Dermatol 125: 431-432.
1919. Rood BR, Zhang H, Weitman DM, Cogen PH (2002). Hypermethylation of HIC-1 and 17p allelic loss in medulloblastoma. Cancer Res 62: 3794-3797.
1920. Roosen N, De La Porte C, Van Vyve M, Solheid C, Selosse P (1984). Familial oligodendroglioma. Case report. J Neurosurg 60: 848-849.
1921. Rorke LB (1983). The cerebellar medulloblastoma and its relationship to primitive neuroectodermal tumors. J Neuropathol Exp Neurol 42: 1-15.
1922. Rorke LB, Biegel JA (2000). Atypical teratoid/rhabdoid tumours. In: Pathology and Genetics - Tumours of the Nervous System. Kleihues P, Cavenee WK, eds. IARC: Lyon, pp.
1923. Rorke LB, Gilles FH, Davis RL, Becker LE (1985). Revision of the World Health Organization classification of brain tumors for childhood brain tumors. Cancer 56: 1869-1886.
1924. Rorke LB, Packer RJ, Biegel JA (1996). Central nervous system atypical teratoid/rhabdoid tumors of infancy and childhood: definition of an entity. J Neurosurg 85: 56-65.
1925. Rosemberg S, Fujiwara D (2005). Epidemiology of pediatric tumors of the nervous system according to the WHO 2000 classification: a report of 1,195 cases from a single institution. Childs Nerv Syst 21: 940-944.
1926. Rosemberg S, Vieira GS (1998). [Dysembryoplastic neuroepithelial tumor. An epidemiological study from a single institution]. Arq Neuropsiquiatr 56: 232-236.
1927. Rosenberg AS, Langee CL, Stevens GL, Morgan MB (2002). Malignant peripheral nerve sheath tumor with perineurial differentiation: "malignant perineurioma". J Cutan Pathol 29: 362-367.
1928. Rosenberg DS, Demarquay G, Jouvet A, Le Bars D, Streichenberger N, Sindou M, Kopp N, Mauguiere F, Ryvlin P (2005). [11C]-Methionine PET: dysembryoplastic neuroepithelial tumours compared with other epileptogenic brain neoplasms. J Neurol Neurosurg Psychiatry 76: 1686-1692.
1929. Rosenberg JE, Lisle DK, Burwick JA, Ueki K, von Deimling A, Mohrenweiser HW, Louis DN (1996). Refined deletion mapping of the chromosome 19q glioma tumor suppressor gene to the D19S412-STD interval. Oncogene 13: 2483-2485.
1930. Rosenblum MK (1998). Ependymal tumors: A review of their diagnostic surgical pathology. Pediatr Neurosurg 28: 160-165.
1931. Rosenblum MK, Erlandson RA, Aleksic SN, Budzilovich GN (1990). Melanotic ependymoma and subependymoma. Am J Surg Pathol 14: 729-736.
1932. Rosenblum MK, Erlandson RA, Budzilovich GN (1991). The lipid-rich epithelioid glioblastoma. Am J Surg Pathol 15: 925-934.
1933. Roser F, Nakamura M, Bellinzona M, Rosahl SK, Ostertag H, Samii M (2004). The prognostic value of progesterone receptor status in meningiomas. J Clin Pathol 57: 1033-1037.
1934. Roser F, Nakamura M, Brandis A, Hans V, Vorkapic P, Samii M (2004). Transition from meningeal melanocytoma to primary cerebral melanoma. Case report. J Neurosurg 101: 528-531.
1935. Rosser T, Packer RJ (2002). Intracranial neoplasms in children with neurofibromatosis 1. J Child Neurol 17: 630-637.
1936. Rossi A, Cama A, Consales A, Gandolfo C, Garre ML, Milanaccio C, Pavanello M, Piatelli G, Ravegnani M, Tortori-Donati P (2006). Neuroimaging of pediatric craniopharyngiomas: a pictorial essay. J Pediatr Endocrinol Metab 19 Suppl 1:299-319.: 299-319.
1937. Rossi ML, Jones NR, Candy E, Nicoll JA, Compton JS, Hughes JT, Esiri MM, Moss TH, Cruz S, Coakham HB (1989). The mononuclear cell infiltrate compared with survival in high- grade astrocytomas. Acta Neuropathol 78: 189-193.
1938. Rossi MR, Conroy J, McQuaid D, Nowak NJ, Rutka JT, Cowell JK (2006). Array CGH analysis of pediatric medulloblastomas. Genes Chromosomes Cancer 45: 290-303.
1939. Rossitch E, Jr., Zeidman SM, Burger PC, Curnes JT, Harsh C, Anscher M, Oakes WJ (1990). Clinical and pathological analysis of spinal cord astrocytomas in children. Neurosurgery 27: 193-196.
1940. Rostomily RC, Bermingham-McDonogh O, Berger MS, Tapscott SJ, Reh TA, Olson JM (1997). Expression of neurogenic basic helix-loop-helix genes in primitive neuroectodermal tumors. Cancer Res 57: 3526-3531.
1941. Rouleau GA, Merel P, Lutchman M, Sanson M, Zucman J, Marineau C, Hoang X, Demczuk S, Desmaze C, Plougastel B (1993). Alteration in a new gene encoding a putative membrane-organizing protein causes neurofibromatosis type 2. Nature 363: 515-521.
1942. Rousseau E, Ruchoux MM, Scaravilli F, Chapon F, Vinchon M, De Smet C, Godfraind C, Vikkula M (2003). CDKN2A, CDKN2B and p14ARF are frequently and differentially methylated in ependymal tumours. Neuropathol Appl Neurobiol 29: 574-583.
1943. Roussy G, Oberling C (1930). Les tumeurs angiomateuses des centres nerveux. Presse Med 38: 179-185.
1944. Rowsell EH, Zekry N, Liwnicz BH, Cao JD, Huang Q, Wang J (2004). Primary anaplastic lymphoma kinase-negative anaplastic large cell lymphoma of the brain in a patient with acquired immunodeficiency syndrome. Arch Pathol Lab Med 128: 324-327.
1945. Roy S, Chu A, Trojanowski JQ, Zhang PJ (2005). D2-40, a novel monoclonal antibody against the M2A antigen as a marker to distinguish hemangioblastomas from renal cell carcinomas. Acta Neuropathol 109: 497-502.
1946. Rubenstein JL, Fridlyand J, Shen A, Aldape K, Ginzinger D, Batchelor T, Treseler P, Berger M, McDermott M, Prados M, Karch J, Okada C, Hyun W, Parikh S, Haqq C, Shuman M (2006). Gene expression and angiotropism in primary CNS lymphoma. Blood 107: 3716-3723.
1947. Rubin JB, Gutmann DH (2005). Neurofibromatosis type 1 - a model for nervous system tumour formation? Nat Rev Cancer 5: 557-564.
1948. Rubinstein LJ (1970). The definition of the ependymoblastoma. Arch Pathol 90: 35-45.
1949. Rubinstein LJ (1986). The malformative central nervous system lesions in the central and peripheral forms of neurofibromatosis. A neuropathological study of 22 cases. Ann N Y Acad Sci 486: 14-29.
1950. Rubinstein LJ, Northfield DWC (1964). The medulloblastoma and the so-called "arachnoidal cerebellar sarcoma". A critical re-examination of a nosological problem. Brain 87: 379-412.
1951. Rubio MP, Correa KM, Ramesh V, MacCollin MM, Jacoby LB, von Deimling A, Gusella JF, Louis DN (1994). Analysis of the neurofibromatosis 2 gene in human ependymomas and astrocytomas. Cancer Res 54: 45-47.
1952. Ruchoux MM, Kepes JJ, Dhellemmes P, Hamon M, Maurage CA, Lecomte M, Gall CM, Chilton J (1998). Lipomatous differentiation in ependymomas: a report of three cases and comparison with similar changes reported in other central nervous system neoplasms of neuroectodermal origin. Am J Surg Pathol 22: 338-346.
1953. Ruckert RI, Fleige B, Rogalla P, Woodruff JM (2000). Schwannoma with angiosarcoma. Report of a case and comparison with other types of nerve tumors with angiosarcoma. Cancer 89: 1577-1585.
1954. Rueda P, Heifetz SA, Sesterhenn IA, Clark GB (1987). Primary intracranial germ cell tumors in the first two decades of life. A clinical, light-microscopic, and immunohistochemical analysis of 54 cases. Perspect Pediatr Pathol 10: 160-207.
1955. Ruggieri M (2001). Mosaic (segmental) neurofibromatosis type 1 (NF1) and type 2 (NF2): no longer neurofibromatosis type 5 (NF5). Am J Med Genet 101: 178-180.
1956. Rushing EJ, Armonda RA, Ansari Q, Mena H (1996). Mesenchymal chondrosarcoma: a clinicopathologic and flow cytometric study of 13 cases presenting in the central nervous system. Cancer 77: 1884-1891.
1957. Rushing EJ, Rorke LB, Sutton L (1993). Problems in the nosology of desmoplastic tumors of childhood. Pediatr Neurosurg 19: 57-62.
1958. Rushing EJ, Thompson LD, Mena H (2003). Malignant transformation of a dysembryoplastic neuroepithelial tumor after radiation and chemotherapy. Ann Diagn Pathol 7: 240-244.
1959. Russell DS, Rubinstein LJ (1989). Pathology of Tumours of the Nervous System. Edward Arnold: London.
1960. Russo C, Pellarin M, Tingby O, Bollen AW, Lamborn KR, Mohapatra G, Collins VP, Feuerstein BG (1999). Comparative genomic hybridization in patients with supratentorial and infratentorial primitive neuroectodermal tumors. Cancer 86: 331-339.
1961. Rutka JT, Giblin JR, Apodaca G, DeArmond SJ, Stern R, Rosenblum ML (1987). Inhibition of growth and induction of differentiation in a malignant human glioma cell line by normal leptomeningeal extracellular matrix proteins. Cancer Res 47: 3515-3522.
1962. Rutka JT, Kuo JS, Carter M, Ray A, Ueda S, Mainprize TG (2004). Advances in the treatment of pediatric brain tumors. Expert Rev Neurother 4: 879-893.
1963. Rutkowski S, Bode U, Deinlein F, Ottensmeier H, Warmuth-Metz M, Soerensen N, Graf N, Emser A, Pietsch T, Wolff JE, Kortmann RD, Kuehl J (2005). Treatment of early childhood medulloblastoma by postoperative chemotherapy alone. N Engl J Med 352: 978-986.
1964. Ruttledge MH, Xie YG, Han FY, Peyrard M, Collins VP, Nordenskjold M, Dumanski JP (1994). Deletions on chromosome 22 in sporadic meningioma. Genes Chromosomes Cancer 10: 122-130.
1965. Ryken TC, Robinson RA, VanGilder JC (1994). Familial occurrence of subependymoma. Report of two cases. J Neurosurg 80: 1108-1111.
1966. Sabel M, Reifenberger J, Weber RG, Reifenberger G, Schmitt HP (2001). Long-term survival of a patient with giant cell glioblastoma. Case report. J Neurosurg 94: 605-611.
1967. Sabin FR (2002). Preliminary note on the differentiation of angioblasts and the method by which they produce blood-vessels, blood-plasma and red blood-cells as seen in the living chick. 1917. J Hematother Stem Cell Res 11: 5-7.
1968. Sacktor N, Lyles RH, Skolasky R, Kleeberger C, Selnes OA, Miller EN, Becker JT, Cohen B, McArthur JC (2001). HIV-associated neurologic disease incidence changes:: Multicenter AIDS Cohort Study, 1990-1998. Neurology 56: 257-260.
1969. Saesue P, Chankaew E, Chawalparit O, Na Ayudhya NS, Muangsomboon S, Sangruchi T (2004). Primary extraskeletal osteosarcoma in the pineal region. Case report. J Neurosurg 101: 1061-1064.
1970. Sainz J, Figueroa K, Baser ME, Mautner VF, Pulst SM (1995). High frequency of nonsense mutations in the NF2 gene caused by C to T transitions in five CGA codons. Hum Mol Genet 4: 137-139.
1971. Sainz J, Huynh DP, Figueroa K, Ragge NK, Baser ME, Pulst SM (1994). Mutations of the neurofibromatosis type 2 gene and lack of the gene product in vestibular schwannomas. Hum Mol Genet 3: 885-891.
1972. Sakaguchi N, Sano K, Ito M, Baba T, Fukuzawa M, Hotchi M (1996). A case of von Recklinghausen's disease with bilateral pheochromocytoma- malignant peripheral nerve sheath tumors of the adrenal and gastrointestinal autonomic nerve tumors. Am J Surg Pathol 20: 889-897.
1973. Sakashita N, Takeya M, Kishida T, Stackhouse TM, Zbar B, Takahashi K (1999).

Expression of von Hippel-Lindau protein in normal and pathological human tissues. Histochem J 31: 133-144.
1974. Sakuta R, Otsubo H, Nolan MA, Weiss SK, Hawkins C, Rutka JT, Chuang NA, Chuang SH, Snead OC, III (2005). Recurrent intractable seizures in children with cortical dysplasia adjacent to dysembryoplastic neuroepithelial tumor. J Child Neurol 20: 377-384.
1975. Salvati M, Caroli E, Raco A, Giangaspero F, Delfini R, Ferrante L (2005). Gliosarcomas: analysis of 11 cases do two subtypes exist? J Neurooncol 74: 59-63.
1976. Salvati M, Ciappetta P, Raco A (1993). Osteosarcomas of the skull. Clinical remarks on 19 cases. Cancer 71: 2210-2216.
1977. Salvati M, Oppido PA, Artizzu S, Fiorenza F, Puzzilli F, Orlando ER (1991). Multicentric gliomas. Report of seven cases. Tumori 77: 518-522.
1978. Samuels Y, Wang Z, Bardelli A, Silliman N, Ptak J, Szabo S, Yan H, Gazdar A, Powell SM, Riggins GJ, Willson JK, Markowitz S, Kinzler KW, Vogelstein B, Velculescu VE (2004). High frequency of mutations of the PIK3CA gene in human cancers. Science 304: 554.
1979. Sanai N, Alvarez-Buylla A, Berger MS (2005). Neural stem cells and the origin of gliomas. N Engl J Med 353: 811-822.
1980. Sancak O, Nellist M, Goedbloed M, Elfferich P, Wouters C, Maat-Kievit A, Zonnenberg B, Verhoef S, Halley D, van den OA (2005). Mutational analysis of the TSC1 and TSC2 genes in a diagnostic setting: genotype—phenotype correlations and comparison of diagnostic DNA techniques in Tuberous Sclerosis Complex. Eur J Hum Genet 13: 731-741.
1981. Sandberg DI, Ragheb J, Dunoyer C, Bhatia S, Olavarria G, Morrison G (2005). Surgical outcomes and seizure control rates after resection of dysembryoplastic neuroepithelial tumors. Neurosurg Focus 18: E5-
1982. Sanford RA (1994). Craniopharyngioma: results of survey of the American Society of Pediatric Neurosurgery. Pediatr Neurosurg 21 Suppl 1: 39-43.
1983. Sankhla S, Khan GM (2004). Cauda equina paraganglioma presenting with intracranial hypertension: case report and review of the literature. Neurol India 52: 243-244.
1984. Sano K (1999). Pathogenesis of intracranial germ cell tumors reconsidered. J Neurosurg 90: 258-264.
1985. Sanoudou D, Tingby O, Ferguson-Smith MA, Collins VP, Coleman N (2000). Analysis of pilocytic astrocytoma by comparative genomic hybridization. Br J Cancer 82: 1218-1222.
1986. Sanson M, Cartalat-Carel S, Taillibert S, Napolitano M, Djafari L, Cougnard J, Gervais H, Laigle F, Carpentier A, Mokhtari K, Taillandier L, Chinot O, Duffau H, Honnorat J, Hoang-Xuan K, Delattre JY (2004). Initial chemotherapy in gliomatosis cerebri. Neurology 63: 270-275.
1987. Santi M, Quezado M, Ronchetti R, Rushing EJ (2005). Analysis of chromosome 7 in adult and pediatric ependymomas using chromogenic in situ hybridization. J Neurooncol 72: 25-28.
1988. Sarkar C, Deb P, Sharma MC (2005). Recent advances in embryonal tumours of the central nervous system. Childs Nerv Syst 21: 272-293.
1989. Sarkar C, Pramanik P, Karak AK, Mukhopadhyay P, Sharma MC, Singh VP, Mehta VS (2002). Are childhood and adult medulloblastomas different? A comparative study of clinicopathological features, proliferation index and apoptotic index. J Neurooncol 59: 49-61.
1990. Sarkar C, Sharma MC, Gaikwad S, Sharma C, Singh VP (1999). Choroid plexus papilloma: a clinicopathological study of 23 cases. Surg Neurol 52: 37-39.
1991. Sarkar C, Sharma MC, Sudha K, Gaikwad S, Varma A (1997). A clinico-pathological study of 29 cases of gliosarcoma with special reference to two unique variants. Indian J Med Res 106:229-35: 229-235.
1992. Sartoretti-Schefer S, Wichmann W, Aguzzi A, Valavanis A (1997). MR differentiation of adamantinous and squamous-papillary craniopharyngiomas. AJNR Am J Neuroradiol 18: 77-87.
1993. Sasaki H, Zlatescu MC, Betensky RA, Ino Y, Cairncross JG, Louis DN (2001). PTEN is a target of chromosome 10q loss in anaplastic oligodendrogliomas and PTEN alterations are associated with poor prognosis. Am J Pathol 159: 359-367.
1994. Sasaki H, Zlatescu MC, Betensky RA, Johnk LB, Cutone AN, Cairncross JG, Louis DN (2002). Histopathological-molecular genetic correlations in referral pathologist-diagnosed low-grade "oligodendroglioma". J Neuropathol Exp Neurol 61: 58-63.
1995. Sato H, Ohmura K, Mizushima M, Ito J, Kuyama H (1983). Myxopapillary ependymoma of the lateral ventricle. A study on the mechanism of its stromal myxoid change. Acta Pathol Jpn 33: 1017-1025.
1996. Sato K, Kubota T (1999). Fine structure of ossification in craniopharyngiomas. Ultrastruct Pathol 23: 395-399.
1997. Sato K, Kubota T, Ishida M, Yoshida K, Takeuchi H, Handa Y (2003). Immunohistochemical and ultrastructural study of chordoid glioma of the third ventricle: its tanycytic differentiation. Acta Neuropathol 106: 176-180.
1997A. Savla J, Chen TT, Schneider NR, Timmons CF, Delattre O, Tomlinson GE (2000). Mutations of the hSNF5/INI1 gene in renal rhabdoid tumors with second primary brain tumors. J Natl Cancer Inst 92:648:650.
1998. Sawada S, Florell S, Purandare SM, Ota M, Stephens K, Viskochil D (1996). Identification of NF1 mutations in both alleles of a dermal neurofibroma. Nat Genet 14: 110-112.
1999. Sawamura Y, Hamou MF, Kuppner MC, de Tribolet N (1989). Immunohistochemical and in vitro functional analysis of pineal-germinoma infiltrating lymphocytes: report of a case. Neurosurgery 25: 454-457.
2000. Sawamura Y, Ikeda J, Shirato H, Tada M, Abe H (1998). Germ cell tumours of the central nervous system: treatment consideration based on 111 cases and their long-term clinical outcomes. Eur J Cancer 34: 104-110.
2001. Sawin PD, Theodore N, Rekate HL (1999). Spinal cord ganglioglioma in a child with neurofibromatosis type 2. Case report and literature review. J Neurosurg 90: 231-233.
2002. Sawyer JR, Roloson GJ, Chadduck WM, Boop FA (1991). Cytogenetic findings in a pleomorphic xanthoastrocytoma. Cancer Genet Cytogenet 55: 225-230.
2003. Sawyer JR, Thomas EL, Roloson GJ, Chadduck WM, Boop FA (1992). Telomeric associations evolving to ring chromosomes in a recurrent pleomorphic xanthoastrocytoma. Cancer Genet Cytogenet 60: 152-157.
2004. Scheil S, Bruderlein S, Eicker M, Herms J, Herold-Mende C, Steiner HH, Barth TF, Moller P (2001). Low frequency of chromosomal imbalances in anaplastic ependymomas as detected by comparative genomic hybridization. Brain Pathol 11: 133-143.
2005. Scheinker IM (1945). Subependymoma (a newly recognized tumor of subependymal derivation). J Neurosurg 2: 232-240.
2006. Scheithauer BW (1978). Symptomatic subependymoma. Report of 21 cases with review of the literature. J Neurosurg 49: 689-696.
2007. Scheithauer BW, Halling KC, Nascimento AG, Hill EM, Sin FH, Katzmann JA (1995). Neurofibroma and malignant preipheral nerve sheath tumor: a proliferation index and DNA ploidy study. Pathol Res Pract 19: 177-177.
2008. Scheithauer BW, Horvath E, Kovacs K (1992). Ultrastructure of the neurohypophysis. Microsc Res Tech 20: 177-186.
2009. Scheithauer BW, Rubinstein LJ (1978). Meningeal mesenchymal chondrosarcoma: report of 8 cases with review of the literature. Cancer 42: 2744-2752.
2010. Scheithauer BW, Rubinstein LJ (1979). Cerebral medulloepithelioma. Report of a case with multiple divergent neuroepithelial differentiation. Childs Brain 5: 62-71.
2011. Scheithauer BW, Woodruff JM, Erlandson RA (1999). Tumors of the Peripheral Nervous System. Armed Forces Institute of Pathology: Washington,D.C.
2012. Scherer HJ (1938). Structural development in gliomas. Am J Cancer 34: 333-351.
2013. Scherer HJ (1940). Cerebral astrocytomas and their derivatives. Am J Cancer 40: 159-198.
2014. Scherer HJ (1940). The forms of growth in gliomas and their practical significance. Brain 63: 1-35.
2015. Scheurlen WG, Schwabe GC, Joos S, Mollenhauer J, Sorensen N, Kuhl J (1998). Molecular analysis of childhood primitive neuroectodermal tumors defines markers associated with poor outcome. J Clin Oncol 16: 2478-2485.
2016. Scheurlen WG, Seranski P, Minchera A, Kuhl J, Sorensen N, Krauss J, Lichter P, Poustka A, Wilgenbus KK (1997). High-resolution deletion mapping of chromosome arm 17p in childhood primitive neuroectodermal tumors reveals a common chromosomal disruption within the Smith-Magenis Region, an unstable region in chromosome band 17p11.2. Genes Chromosomes Cancer 18: 50-58.
2017. Schiff D (2003). Spinal metastases. In: Cancer Neurology in Clinical Practice. Schiff D, Wen PY, eds. Humana Press: Totowa, NJ, USA.
2018. Schiffer D (1997). Brain Tumors. Biology, Pathology, and Clinical References. Springer: Berlin.
2019. Schiffer D, Cavalla P, Chio A, Giordana MT, Marino S, Mauro A, Migheli A (1994). Tumor cell proliferation and apoptosis in medulloblastoma. Acta Neuropathol 87: 362-370.
2020. Schiffer D, Cavalla P, Migheli A, Chio A, Giordana MT, Marino S, Attanasio A (1995). Apoptosis and cell proliferation in human neuroepithelial tumors. Neurosci Lett 195: 81-84.
2021. Schiffer D, Cavalla P, Migheli A, Giordana MT, Chiado-Piat L (1996). Bcl-2 distribution in neuroepithelial tumors: an immunohistochemical study. J Neurooncol 27: 101-109.
2022. Schiffer D, Chio A, Cravioto H, Giordana MT, Migheli A, Soffietti R, Vigliani MC (1991). Ependymoma: internal correlations among pathological signs: the anaplastic variant. Neurosurgery 29: 206-210.
2023. Schiffer D, Chio A, Giordana MT, Leone M, Soffietti R (1988). Prognostic value of histologic factors in adult cerebral astrocytoma. Cancer 61: 1386-1393.
2024. Schiffer D, Chio A, Giordana MT, Migheli A, Palma L, Pollo B, Soffietti R, Tribolo A (1991). Histologic prognostic factors in ependymoma. Childs Nerv Syst 7: 177-182.
2025. Schiffer D, Cravioto H, Giordana MT, Migheli A, Pezzulo T, Vigliani MC (1993). Is polar spongioblastoma a tumor entity? J Neurosurg 78: 587-591.
2026. Schiffer D, Dutto A, Cavalla P, Bosone I, Chio A, Villani R, Bellotti C (1997). Prognostic factors in oligodendroglioma. Can J Neurol Sci 24: 313-319.
2027. Schiffer D, Giordana MT (1998). Prognosis of ependymoma. Childs Nerv Syst 14: 357-361.
2028. Schiffer D, Giordana MT, Mauro A, Migheli A (1984). GFAP, F VIII/RAg, laminin, and fibronectin in gliosarcomas: an immunohistochemical study. Acta Neuropathol 63: 108-116.
2029. Schiffer D, Giordana MT, Pezzotta S, Pezzulo T, Vigliani MC (1992). Medullomyoblastoma: report of two cases. Childs Nerv Syst 8: 268-272.
2030. Schild SE, Scheithauer BW, Haddock MG, Wong WW, Lyons MK, Marks LB, Norman MG, Burger PC (1996). Histologically confirmed pineal tumors and other germ cell tumors of the brain. Cancer 78: 2564-2571.
2031. Schild SE, Scheithauer BW, Schomberg PJ, Hook CC, Kelly PJ, Frick L, Robinow JS, Buskirk SJ (1993). Pineal parenchymal tumors. Clinical, pathologic, and therapeutic aspects. Cancer 72: 870-880.
2032. Schmidt MC, Antweiler S, Urban N, Mueller W, Kuklik A, Meyer-Puttlitz B, Wiestler OD, Louis DN, Fimmers R, von Deimling A (2002). Impact of genotype and morphology on the prognosis of glioblastoma. J Neuropathol Exp Neurol 61: 321-328.
2033. Schmitz U, Mueller W, Weber M, Sevenet N, Delattre O, von Deimling A (2001). INI1 mutations in meningiomas at a potential hotspot in exon 9. Br J Cancer 84: 199-201.
2034. Schneider DT, Zahn S, Sievers S, Alemazkour K, Reifenberger G, Wiestler OD, Calaminus G, Gobel U, Perlman EJ (2006). Molecular genetic analysis of central nervous system germ cell tumors with comparative genomic hybridization. Mod Pathol 19: 864-873.
2035. Schofield D, West DC, Anthony DC, Marshal R, Sklar J (1995). Correlation of loss of heterozygosity at chromosome 9q with histological subtype in medulloblastomas. Am J Pathol 146: 472-480.
2036. Schouten LJ, Rutten J, Huveneers HA, Twijnstra A (2002). Incidence of brain metastases in a cohort of patients with carcinoma of the breast, colon, kidney, and lung and melanoma. Cancer 94: 2698-2705.
2037. Schrock E, Blume C, Meffert MC, du MS, Bersch W, Kiessling M, Lozanowa T, Thiel G, Witkowski R, Ried T, Cremer T (1996). Recurrent gain of chromosome arm 7q in low-grade astrocytic tumors studied by comparative genomic hybridization. Genes Chromosomes Cancer 15: 199-205.
2038. Schroder R, Bien K, Kott R, Meyers I, Vossing R (1991). The relationship between Ki-67 labeling and mitotic index in gliomas and meningiomas: demonstration of the variability of the intermitotic cycle time. Acta Neuropathol 82: 389-394.
2039. Schroder R, Firsching R, Kochanek S (1986). Hemangiopericytoma of meninges. II. General and clinical data. Zentralbl Neurochir 47: 191-199.
2040. Schuller U, Schober F, Kretzschmar HA, Herms J (2004). Bcl-2 expression inversely correlates with tumour cell differentiation in medulloblastoma. Neuropathol Appl Neurobiol 30: 513-521.
2041. Schultz AB, Brat DJ, Oyesiku NM, Hunter SB (2001). Intrasellar pituicytoma in a patient with other endocrine neoplasms. Arch Pathol Lab Med 125: 527-530.
2042. Schwechheimer K, Huang S, Cavenee WK (1995). EGFR gene amplification—rearrangement in human glioblastomas. Int J Cancer 62: 145-148.
2043. Schwindt H, Akasaka T, Zuhlke-Jenisch

R, Hans V, Schaller C, Klapper W, Dyer MJ, Siebert R, Deckert M (2006). Chromosomal translocations fusing the BCL6 gene to different partner loci are recurrent in primary central nervous system lymphoma and may be associated with aberrant somatic hypermutation or defective class switch recombination. J Neuropathol Exp Neurol 65: 776-782.
2044. Sciot R, Cin PD, Hagemeijer A, De Smet L, Van Damme B, Van den BH (1999). Cutaneous sclerosing perineurioma with cryptic NF2 gene deletion. Am J Surg Pathol 23: 849-853.
2045. Seizinger BR, Martuza RL, Gusella JF (1986). Loss of genes on chromosome 22 in tumorigenesis of human acoustic neuroma. Nature 322: 644-647.
2046. Seizinger BR, Rouleau GA, Ozelius LJ, Lane AH, Faryniarz AG, Chao MV, Huson S, Korf BR, Parry DM, Pericak V, Collins FS, Hobbs WJ, Falcone BG, Ianazzi JA, Roy JC, St, Tanzi RE, Bothwell MA, Upadhyaya M, Harper P, Goldstein AE, Hoover DL, Bader JL, Spence MA, Mulvihill JJ, Aylsworth AS, Vance JM, Rossenwasser GOD, Gaskell PC, Roses AD, Martuza RL, Breakefield XO, Gusella JF (1987). Genetic linkage of von Recklinghausen neurofibromatosis to the nerve growth factor receptor gene. Cell 49: 589-594.
2047. Sekine S, Shibata T, Kokubu A, Morishita Y, Noguchi M, Nakanishi Y, Sakamoto M, Hirohashi S (2002). Craniopharyngiomas of adamantinomatous type harbor beta-catenin gene mutations. Am J Pathol 161: 1997-2001.
2048. Sener RN (2002). Astroblastoma: diffusion MRI, and proton MR spectroscopy. Comput Med Imaging Graph 26: 187-191.
2049. Seppala MT, Haltia MJ, Sankila RJ, Jaaskelainen JE, Heiskanen O (1995). Long-term outcome after removal of spinal neurofibroma. J Neurosurg 82: 572-577.
2050. Seppala MT, Sainio MA, Haltia MJ, Kinnunen JJ, Setala KH, Jaaskelainen JE (1998). Multiple schwannomas: schwannomatosis or neurofibromatosis type 2? J Neurosurg 89: 36-41.
2051. Serra E, Ars E, Ravella A, Sanchez A, Puig S, Rosenbaum T, Estivill X, Lazaro C (2001). Somatic NF1 mutational spectrum in benign neurofibromas: mRNA splice defects are common among point mutations. Hum Genet 108: 416-429.
2052. Serra E, Puig S, Otero D, Gaona A, Kruyer H, Ars E, Estivill X, Lazaro C (1997). Confirmation of a double-hit model for the NF1 gene in benign neurofibromas. Am J Hum Genet 61: 512-519.
2053. Serra E, Rosenbaum T, Nadal M, Winner U, Ars E, Estivill X, Lazaro C (2001). Mitotic recombination effects homozygosity for NF1 germline mutations in neurofibromas. Nat Genet 28: 294-296.
2054. Serrano M, Hannon GJ, Beach D (1993). A new regulatory motif in cell-cycle control causing specific inhibition of cyclin D/CDK4. Nature 336: 704-707.
2055. Setzer M, Lang J, Turowski B, Marquardt G (2002). Primary meningeal osteosarcoma: case report and review of the literature. Neurosurgery 51: 488-492.
2056. Sevenet N, Lellouch-Tubiana A, Schofield D, Hoang-Xuan K, Gessler M, Birnbaum D, Jeanpierre C, Jouvet A, Delattre O (1999). Spectrum of hSNF5/INI1 somatic mutations in human cancer and genotype-phenotype correlations. Hum Mol Genet 8: 2359-2368.
2057. Sevenet N, Sheridan E, Amram D, Schneider P, Handgretinger R, Delattre O (1999). Constitutional mutations of the hSNF5/INI1 gene predispose to a variety of cancers. Am J Hum Genet 65: 1342-1348.
2058. Shaffrey ME, Farace E, Schiff D, Larner JM, Mut M, Lopes MB (2005). The Ki-67 labeling index as a prognostic factor in Grade II oligoastrocytomas. J Neurosurg 102: 1033-1039.
2059. Shaffrey ME, Lanzino G, Lopes BS, Hessler RB, Kassel NF, VandenBerg SR (1996). Maturation of intracranial teratomas. Report of two cases. J Neurosurg 85: 672-676.
2060. Shafqat S, Hedley-Whyte ET, Henson JW (1999). Age-dependent rate of anaplastic transformation in low-grade astrocytoma. Neurology 52: 867-869.
2061. Shah B, Lipper MH, Laws ER, Lopes MB, Spellman MJ, Jr. (2005). Posterior pituitary astrocytoma: a rare tumor of the neurohypophysis: a case report. AJNR Am J Neuroradiol 26: 1858-1861.
2062. Shanklin WM (1953). The origin, histology and senescence of tumorettes in the human neurohypophysis. Acta Anat (Basel) 18: 1-20.
2063. Shanley S, Ratcliffe J, Hockey A, Haan E, Oley C, Ravine D, Martin N, Wicking C, Chenevix T (1994). Nevoid basal cell carcinoma syndrome: review of 118 affected individuals. Am J Med Genet 50: 282-290.
2064. Sharma M, Ralte A, Arora R, Santosh V, Shankar SK, Sarkar C (2004). Subependymal giant cell astrocytoma: a clinicopathological study of 23 cases with special emphasis on proliferative markers and expression of p53 and retinoblastoma gene proteins. Pathology 36: 139-144.
2065. Sharma MC, Agarwal M, Suri A, Gaikwad S, Mukhopadhyay P, Sarkar C (2002). A melanotic desmoplastic medulloblastoma: report of a rare case and review of the literature. Brain Tumor Pathol 19: 93-96.
2066. Sharma MC, Agarwal M, Suri A, Gaikwad S, Mukhopadhyay P, Sarkar C (2002). Lipomedulloblastoma in a child: a controversial entity. Hum Pathol 33: 564-569.
2067. Sharma MC, Gaikwad S, Mehta VS, Dhar J, Sarkar C (1998). Gliofibroma: mixed glial and mesenchymal tumour. Report of three cases. Clin Neurol Neurosurg 100: 153-159.
2068. Sharma MC, Mahapatra AK, Gaikwad S, Jain AK, Sarkar C (1998). Pigmented medulloepithelioma: report of a case and review of the literature. Childs Nerv Syst 14: 74-78.
2069. Sharma MC, Ralte AM, Gaekwad S, Santosh V, Shankar SK, Sarkar C (2004). Subependymal giant cell astrocytoma—a clinicopathological study of 23 cases with special emphasis on histogenesis. Pathol Oncol Res 10: 219-224.
2070. Sharma MK, Watson MA, Lyman M, Perry A, Aldape KD, Deak F, Gutmann DH (2006). Matrilin-2 expression distinguishes clinically relevant subsets of pilocytic astrocytoma. Neurology 66: 127-130.
2071. Sharma MK, Zehnbauer BA, Watson MA, Gutmann DH (2005). RAS pathway activation and an oncogenic RAS mutation in sporadic pilocytic astrocytoma. Neurology 65: 1335-1336.
2072. Sharma S, Abbott RI, Zagzag D (1998). Malignant intracerebral nerve sheath tumor: a case report and review of the literature. Cancer 82: 545-552.
2073. Shaw EG, Scheithauer BW, O'Fallon JR, Davis DH (1994). Mixed oligoastrocytomas: a survival and prognostic factor analysis. Neurosurg 34: 577-582.
2074. Shaw EG, Scheithauer BW, O'Fallon JR, Tazelaar HD, Davis DH (1992). Oligodendrogliomas: the Mayo Clinic experience. J Neurosurg 76: 428-434.
2075. Shaw RJ, Paez JG, Curto M, Yaktine A, Pruitt WM, Saotome I, O'Bryan JP, Gupta V, Ratner N, Der CJ, Jacks T, McClatchey AI (2001). The Nf2 tumor suppressor, merlin, functions in Rac-dependent signaling. Dev Cell 1: 63-72.
2076. Shenkier TN, Blay JY, O'Neill BP, Poortmans P, Thiel E, Jahnke K, Abrey LE, Neuwelt E, Tsang R, Batchelor T, Harris N, Ferreri AJ, Ponzoni M, O'Brien P, Rubenstein J, Connors JM (2005). Primary CNS lymphoma of T-cell origin: a descriptive analysis from the international primary CNS lymphoma collaborative group. J Clin Oncol 23: 2233-2239.
2077. Shepherd CW, Houser OW, Gomez MR (1995). MR findings in tuberous sclerosis complex and correlation with seizure development and mental impairment. AJNR Am J Neuroradiol 16: 149-155.
2078. Shepherd CW, Scheithauer BW, Gomez MR, Altermatt HJ, Katzmann JA (1991). Subependymal giant cell astrocytoma: a clinical, pathological, and flow cytometric study. Neurosurgery 28: 864-868.
2079. Sherr CJ, Roberts JM (1999). CDK inhibitors: positive and negative regulators of G1-phase progression. Genes Dev 13: 1501-1512.
2080. Shibahara J, Todo T, Morita A, Mori H, Aoki S, Fukayama M (2004). Papillary neuroepithelial tumor of the pineal region. A case report. Acta Neuropathol 108: 337-340.
2081. Shibamoto Y, Takahashi M, Sasai K (1997). Prognosis of intracranial germinoma with syncytiotrophoblastic giant cells treated by radiation therapy. Int J Radiat Oncol Biol Phys 37: 505-510.
2082. Shih AH, Holland EC (2004). Developmental neurobiology and the origin of brain tumors. J Neurooncol 70: 125-136.
2083. Shimada Y, Kubo O, Tajika Y, Hiyama H, Atuji S, Takakura K (1997). Clinicopathological study of mixed oligoastrocytoma. In: Brain tumor research and therapy. Nagai M, ed. Springer-Verlag: Tokyo, pp. 51-60.
2084. Shimbo Y, Takahashi H, Hayano M, Kumagai T, Kameyama S (1997). Temporal lobe lesion demonstrating features of dysembryoplastic neuroepithelial tumor and ganglioglioma: a transitional form? Clin Neuropathol 16: 65-68.
2085. Shimoji K, Yasuma Y, Mori K, Eguchi M, Maeda M (1999). Unique radiological appearance of a microcystic meningioma. Acta Neurochir 141: 1119-1121.
2086. Shin YM, Chang KH, Han MH, Myung NH, Chi JG, Cha SH, Han MC (1993). Gliomatosis cerebri: comparison of MR and CT features. AJR Am J Roentgenol 161: 859-862.
2087. Shinoda J, Murase S, Takenaka K, Sakai N (2005). Isolated central nervous system hemophagocytic lymphohistiocytosis: case report. Neurosurgery 56: 187
2088. Shinojima N, Kochi M, Hamada J, Nakamura H, Yano S, Makino K, Tsuiki H, Tada K, Kuratsu J, Ishimaru Y, Ushio Y (2004). The influence of sex and the presence of giant cells on postoperative long-term survival in adult patients with supratentorial glioblastoma multiforme. J Neurosurg 101: 219-226.
2089. Shinojima N, Ohta K, Yano S, Nakamura H, Kochi M, Ishimaru Y, Nakazato Y, Ushio Y (2002). Myofibroblastoma in the suprasellar region. Case report. J Neurosurg 97: 1203-1207.
2090. Shishiba T, Niimura M, Ohtsuka F, Tsuru N (1984). Multiple cutaneous neurilemmomas as a skin manifestation of neurilemmomatosis. J Am Acad Dermatol 10: 744-754.
2091. Shiurba RA, Buffinger NS, Spencer EM, Urich H (1991). Basic fibroblast growth factor and somatomedin C in human medulloepithelioma. Cancer 68: 798-808.
2092. Shlomit R, Ayala AG, Michal D, Ninett A, Frida S, Boleslaw G, Gad B, Gideon R, Shlomi C (2000). Gains and losses of DNA sequences in childhood brain tumors analyzed by comparative genomic hybridization. Cancer Genet Cytogenet 121: 67-72.
2093. Short MP, Richardson EP, Jr., Haines JL, Kwiatkowski DJ (1995). Clinical, neuropathological and genetic aspects of the tuberous sclerosis complex. Brain Pathol 5: 173-179.
2094. Shoshan Y, Chernova O, Juen SS, Somerville RP, Israel Z, Barnett GH, Cowell JK (2000). Radiation-induced meningioma: a distinct molecular genetic pattern? J Neuropathol Exp Neurol 59: 614-620.
2095. Shuangshoti S, Kasantikul V, Suwanwela N (1987). Spontaneous penetretion of dura mater and bone by glioblastoma multiforme. J Surg Oncol 36: 36-44.
2096. Shuangshoti S, Rushing EJ, Mena H, Olsen C, Sandberg GD (2005). Supratentorial extraventricular ependymal neoplasms: a clinicopathologic study of 32 patients. Cancer 103: 2598-2605.
2097. Siami-Namini K, Shuey-Drake R, Wilson D, Francel P, Perry A, Fung KM (2005). A 15-year-old female with progressive myelopathy. Brain Pathol 15: 265-267.
2098. Sidransky D, Mikkelsen T, Schwechheimer K, Rosenblum ML, Cavenee WK, Vogelstein B (1992). Clonal expansion of p53 mutant cells is associated with brain tumour progression. Nature 355: 846-847.
2099. Silva AJ, Frankland PW, Marowitz Z, Friedman E, Lazlo G, Cioffi D, Jacks T, Bourtchuladze R (1997). A mouse model for the learning and memory deficits associated with neurofibromatosis type I. Nat Genet 15: 281-284.
2100. Simon M, Kokkino AJ, Warnick RE, Tew JM, Jr., von Deimling A, Menon AG (1996). Role of genomic instability in meningioma progression. Genes Chromosomes Cancer 16: 265-269.
2101. Simon M, von Deimling A, Larson JJ, Wellenreuther R, Kaskel P, Waha A, Warnick RW, Tew JM, Menon AG (1995). Allelic losses on chromosomes 14, 10, and 1 in atypical and malignant meningiomas: a genetic model of meningioma progression. Cancer Res 55: 4696-4701.
2102. Simon SL, Moonis G, Judkins AR, Scobie J, Burnett MG, Riina HA, Judy KD (2005). Intracranial capillary hemangioma: case report and review of the literature. Surg Neurol 64: 154-159.
2103. Simpson L, Parsons R (2001). PTEN: life as a tumor suppressor. Exp Cell Res 264: 29-41.
2104. Singh SK, Clarke ID, Hide T, Dirks PB (2004). Cancer stem cells in nervous system tumors. Oncogene 23: 7267-7273.
2105. Singh SK, Hawkins C, Clarke ID, Squire JA, Bayani J, Hide T, Henkelman RM, Cusimano MD, Dirks PB (2004). Identification of human brain tumour initiating cells. Nature 432: 396-401.
2106. Sinson G, Gennarelli TA, Wells GB (1998). Suprasellar osteolipoma: case report. Surg Neurol 50: 457-460.
2107. Skotheim RI, Kallioniemi A, Bjerkhagen B, Mertens F, Brekke HR, Monni O, Mousses S, Mandahl N, Soeter G, Nesland JM, Smeland S, Kallioniemi OP, Lothe RA (2003). Topoisomerase-II alpha is upregulated in malignant peripheral nerve sheath tumors and associated with clinical outcome. J Clin Oncol 21: 4586-4591.
2108. Skullerud K, Stenwig AE, Brandtzaeg P, Nesland JM, Kerty E, Langmoen I, Saeter G (1995). Intracranial primary leiomyosarcoma arising in a teratoma of the pineal area. Clin Neuropathol 14: 245-248.
2109. Skuse GR, Kosciolek BA, Rowley PT (1989). Molecular genetic analysis of tumors in

von Recklinghausen neurofibromatosis: loss of heterozygosity for chromosome 17. Genes Chromosomes Cancer 1: 36-41.
2110. Skuse GR, Kosciolek BA, Rowley PT (1991). The neurofibroma in von Recklinghausen neurofibromatosis has a unicellular origin. Am J Hum Genet 49: 600-607.
2111. Slowik F, Jellinger K, Gaszo L, Fischer J (1985). Gliosarcomas: histological, immunohistochemical, ultrastructural, and tissue culture studies. Acta Neuropathol 201-210.
2112. Smith JR, Braziel RM, Paoletti S, Lipp M, Uguccioni M, Rosenbaum JT (2003). Expression of B-cell-attracting chemokine 1 (CXCL13) by malignant lymphocytes and vascular endothelium in primary central nervous system lymphoma. Blood 101: 815-821.
2113. Smith JS, Perry A, Borell TJ, Lee HK, O'Fallon J, Hosek SM, Kimmel D, Yates A, Burger PC, Scheithauer BW, Jenkins RB (2000). Alterations of chromosome arms 1p and 19q as predictors of survival in oligodendrogliomas, astrocytomas, and mixed oligoastrocytomas. J Clin Oncol 18: 636-645.
2114. Smith JS, Tachibana I, Passe SM, Huntley BK, Borell TJ, Iturria N, O'Fallon JR, Schaefer PL, Scheithauer BW, James CD, Buckner JC, Jenkins RB (2001). PTEN mutation, EGFR amplification, and outcome in patients with anaplastic astrocytoma and glioblastoma multiforme. J Natl Cancer Inst 93: 1246-1256.
2115. Smith MT, Ludwig CL, Godfrey AD, Armbrustmacher VW (1983). Grading of oligodendrogliomas. Cancer 52: 2107-2114.
2116. Smith T, Davidson R (1984). Medullomyoblastoma. A histologic, immunohistochemical, and ultrastructural study. Cancer 54: 323-332.
2117. Smith WT, Hughes B, Ermocilla R (1966). Chemodectoma of the pineal region, with observations on the pineal body and chemoreceptor tissue. J Pathol Bacteriol 92: 69-76.
2118. Smyth I, Narang MA, Evans T, Heimann C, Nakamura Y, Chenevix-Trench G, Pietsch T, Wicking C, Wainwright BJ (1999). Isolation and characterization of human patched 2 (PTCH2), a putative tumour suppressor gene inbasal cell carcinoma and medulloblastoma on chromosome 1p32. Hum Mol Genet 8: 291-297.
2119. Snipes GJ, Steinberg GK, Lane B, Horoupian DS (1991). Gliofibroma. Case report. J Neurosurg 75: 642-646.
2120. Sobrido MJ, Pereira CR, Barros F, Forteza J, Carracedo A, Lema M (2000). Low frequency of replication errors in primary nervous system tumours. J Neurol Neurosurg Psychiatry 69: 369-375.
2121. Solecki DJ, Liu XL, Tomoda T, Fang Y, Hatten ME (2001). Activated Notch2 signaling inhibits differentiation of cerebellar granule neuron precursors by maintaining proliferation. Neuron 31: 557-568.
2122. Somasundaram K, Reddy SP, Vinnakota K, Britto R, Subbarayan M, Nambiar S, Hebbar A, Samuel C, Shetty M, Sreepathi HK, Santosh V, Hegde AS, Hegde S, Kondaiah P, Rao MR (2005). Upregulation of ASCL1 and inhibition of Notch signaling pathway characterize progressive astrocytoma. Oncogene 24: 7073-7083.
2123. Somerville RP, Shoshan Y, Eng C, Barnett G, Miller D, Cowell JK (1998). Molecular analysis of two putative tumour suppressor genes, PTEN and DMBT, which have been implicated in glioblastoma multiforme disease progression. Oncogene 17: 1755-1757.
2123A. Sonier CB, Feve JR, De Kersaint-Gilly A, Ruchoux MM, Rymer R, Auffray E (1992). Lhermitte-duclos disease. A rare cause of intracranial hypertension in adults. J Neuroradiol 19: 133-138.
2124. Sonneland PR, Scheithauer BW, LeChago J, Crawford BG, Onofrio BM (1986). Paraganglioma of the cauda equina region. Clinicopathologic study of 31 cases with special reference to immunocytology and ultrastructure. Cancer 58: 1720-1735.
2125. Sonneland PR, Scheithauer BW, Onofrio BM (1985). Myxopapillary ependymoma. A clinicopathologic and immunocytochemical study of 77 cases. Cancer 56: 883-893.
2126. Soussain C, Suzan F, Hoang-Xuan K, Cassoux N, Levy V, Azar N, Belanger C, Achour E, Ribrag V, Gerber S, Delattre JY, Leblond V (2001). Results of intensive chemotherapy followed by hematopoietic stem-cell rescue in 22 patients with refractory or recurrent primary CNS lymphoma or intraocular lymphoma. J Clin Oncol 19: 742-749.
2127. Soylemezoglu F, Kleihues P, Esteve J, Scheithauer BW (1997). Atypical central neurocytoma. J Neuropath Exp Neurol 56: 551-556.
2128. Soylemezoglu F, Onder S, Tezel GG, Berker M (2003). Neuronal nuclear antigen (NeuN): a new tool in the diagnosis of central neurocytoma. Pathol Res Pract 199: 463-468.
2129. Soylemezoglu F, Soffer D, Onol B, Schwechheimer K, Kleihues P (1996). Lipomatous medulloblastoma in adults: a distinct clinicopathological entity. Am J Surg Pathol 20: 413-418.
2130. Soylemezoglu F, Tezel GG, Koybasoglu F, Er U, Akalan N (2001). Cranial infantile myofibromatosis: report of three cases. Childs Nerv Syst 17: 524-527.
2131. Specht CS, Smith TW, DeGirolami U, Price JM (1986). Myxopapillary ependymoma of the filum terminale. A light and electron microscopic study. Cancer 58: 310-317.
2132. Spence AM, Rubinstein LJ (1975). Cerebellar capillary hemangioblastoma: its histogenesis studied by organ culture and electron microscopy. Cancer 35: 326-341.
2133. Sperfeld AD, Hein C, Schroder JM, Ludolph AC, Hanemann CO (2002). Occurrence and characterization of peripheral nerve involvement in neurofibromatosis type 2. Brain 125: 996-1004.
2134. Spiegel E (1920). Hyperplasie des Kleinhirns. Beitr Path Anat 67: 539-548.
2135. Squire JA, Arab S, Marrano P, Bayani J, Karaskova J, Taylor M, Becker L, Rutka J, Zielenska M (2001). Molecular cytogenetic analysis of glial tumors using spectral karyotyping and comparative genomic hybridization. Mol Diagn 6: 93-108.
2136. St Croix B, Kerbel RS (1997). Cell adhesion and drug resistance in cancer. Curr Opin Oncol 9: 549-556.
2137. Stahlberger R, Friede RL (1977). Fine structure of myomedulloblastoma. Acta Neuropathol 37: 43-48.
2138. Stambolic V, Ruel L, Woodgett JR (1996). Lithium inhibits glycogen synthase kinase-3 activity and mimics wingless signalling in intact cells. Curr Biol 6: 1664-1668.
2139. Stander M, Peraud A, Leroch B, Kreth FW (2004). Prognostic impact of TP53 mutation status for adult patients with supratentorial World Health Organization Grade II astrocytoma or oligoastrocytoma: a long-term analysis. Cancer 101: 1028-1035.
2140. Stanescu CR, Varlet P, Beuvon F, Daumas DC, Devaux B, Chassoux F, Fredy D, Meder JF (2001). Dysembryoplastic neuroepithelial tumors: CT, MR findings and imaging follow-up: a study of 53 cases. J Neuroradiol 28: 230-240.
2141. Stangl AP, Wellenreuther R, Lenartz D, Kraus JA, Menon AG, Schramm J, Wiestler OD, von Deimling A (1997). Clonality of multiple meningioma. J Neurosurg 86: 853-858.
2142. Starzyk J, Starzyk B, Bartnik-Mikuta A, Urbanowicz W, Dziatkowiak H (2001). Gonadotropin releasing hormone-independent precocious puberty in a 5 year-old girl with suprasellar germ cell tumor secreting beta-hCG and alpha-fetoprotein. J Pediatr Endocrinol Metab 14: 789-796.
2143. Stavrou T, Bromley CM, Nicholson HS, Byrne J, Packer RJ, Goldstein AM, Reaman GH (2001). Prognostic factors and secondary malignancies in childhood medulloblastoma. J Pediatr Hematol Oncol 23: 431-436.
2144. Stebbins CE, Kaelin WG, Jr., Pavletich NP (1999). Structure of the VHL-ElonginC-ElonginB complex: implications for VHL tumor suppressor function. Science 284: 455-461.
2145. Steck PA, Pershouse MA, Jasser SA, Yung WKA, Lin H, Ligon AH, Langford LA, Baumgard ML, Hattier T, Davis T, Frye C, Hu R, Swedlund B, Teng DHF, Tavtigian SV (1997). Identification of a candidate tumour suppressor gene, MMAC1, at chromosome 10q23.3 that is mutated in multiple advanced cancers. Nature Genet 15: 356-362.
2146. Steel TR, Botterill P, Sheehy JP (1994). Paraganglioma of the cauda equina with associated syringomyelia: case report. Surg Neurol 42: 489-493.
2147. Stefanko SZ, Vuzevski VD, Maas AI, van Vroonhoven CC (1986). Intracerebral malignant schwannoma. Acta Neuropathol 71: 321-325.
2148. Stein AA, Schilp AO, Whitfield RD (1960). The histogenesis of hemangioblastoma of the brain. A review of twenty-one cases. J Neurosurg 17:751-761.
2149. Stemmer-Rachamimov AO, Gonzalez-Agosti C, Xu L, Burwick JA, Beauchamp R, Pinney D, Louis DN, Ramesh V (1997). Expression of NF2-encoded merlin and related ERM family proteins in the human central nervous system. J Neuropathol Exp Neurol 56: 735-742.
2150. Stemmer-Rachamimov AO, Horgan MA, Taratuto AL, Munoz DG, Smith TW, Frosch MP, Louis DN (1997). Meningioangiomatosis is associated with Neurofibromatosis 2 but not with somatic alterations of the NF2 gene. J Neuropathol Exp Neurol 56: 485-489.
2151. Stemmer-Rachamimov AO, Ino Y, Lim ZY, Jacoby LB, MacCollin M, Gusella JF, Ramesh V, Louis DN (1998). Loss of the NF2 gene and merlin occur by the tumorlet stage of schwannoma development in neurofibromatosis 2. J Neuropathol Exp Neurol 57: 1164-1167.
2152. Stenzel W, Pels H, Staib P, Impekoven P, Bektas N, Deckert M (2004). Concomitant manifestation of primary CNS lymphoma and Toxoplasma encephalitis in a patient with AIDS. J Neurol 251: 764-766.
2153. Stern J, Jakobiec FA, Housepian EM (1980). The architecture of optic nerve gliomas with and without neurofibromatosis. Arch Ophthalmol 98: 505-511.
2154. Stevens MC, Cameron AH, Muir KR, Parkes SE, Reid H, Whitwell H (1991). Descriptive epidemiology of primary central nervous system tumours in children: a population-based study. Clin Oncol (R Coll Radiol) 3: 323-329.
2155. Stolle C, Glenn G, Zbar B, Humphrey JS, Choyke P, Walther M, Pack S, Hurley K, Andrey C, Klausner R, Linehan WM (1998). Improved detection of germline mutations in the von Hippel-Lindau disease tumor suppressor gene. Hum Mutat 12: 417-423.
2156. Stone DM, Hynes M, Armanini M, Swanson TA, Gu Q, Johnson RL, Scott MP, Pennica D, Goddard A, Phillips H, Noll M, Hooper JE, de Sauvage F, Rosenthal A (1996). The tumour-suppressor gene patched encodes a candidate receptor for Sonic hedgehog. Nature 384: 129-134.
2157. Stone S, Jiang P, Dayananth P, Tavtigian SV, Katcher H, Parry D, Peters G, Kamb A (1995). Complex structure and regulation of the P16 (MTS1) locus. Cancer Res 55: 2988-2994.
2158. Storlazzi CT, Von Steyern FV, Domanski HA, Mandahl N, Mertens F (2005). Biallelic somatic inactivation of the NF1 gene through chromosomal translocations in a sporadic neurofibroma. Int J Cancer 117: 1055-1057.
2159. Stott FJ, Bates S, James MC, McConnell BB, Starborg M, Brookes S, Palmero I, Ryan K, Hara E, Vousden KH, Peters G (1998). The alternative product from the human CDKN2A locus, p14(ARF), participates in a regulatory feedback loop with p53 and MDM2. EMBO J 17: 5001-5014.
2160. Stout AP, Murray MR (1942). Hemangiopericytoma. A vascular tumor featuring Zimmermann's pericytes. Ann Surg 116: 26-33.
2161. Stratakis CA (2002). Mutations of the gene encoding the protein kinase A type I-alpha regulatory subunit (PRKAR1A) in patients with the "complex of spotty skin pigmentation, myxomas, endocrine overactivity, and schwannomas" (Carney complex). Ann N Y Acad Sci 968:3-21.: 3-21.
2162. Stratton MR, Darling J, Lantos PL, Cooper CS, Reeves BR (1989). Cytogenetic abnormalities in human ependymomas. Int J Cancer 44: 579-581.
2163. Strojan P, Popovic M, Surlan K, Jereb B (2004). Choroid plexus tumors: a review of 28-year experience. Neoplasma 51: 306-312.
2164. Strommer KN, Brandner S, Sarioglu AC, Sure U, Yonekawa Y (1995). Symptomatic cerebellar metastasis and late local recurrence of a cauda equina paraganglioma. Case report. J Neurosurg 83: 166-169.
2165. Stumpf DA, Alksne JF, Annegers JF (1988). Neurofibromatosis. NIH consensus development conference statement. Arch Neurol 45: 575-578.
2166. Stupp R, Mason WP, van den Bent MJ, Weller M, Fisher B, Taphoorn MJ, Belanger K, Brandes AA, Marosi C, Bogdahn U, Curschmann J, Janzer RC, Ludwin SK, Gorlia T, Allgeier A, Lacombe D, Cairncross JG, Eisenhauer E, Mirimanoff RO (2005). Radiotherapy plus concomitant and adjuvant temozolomide for glioblastoma. N Engl J Med 352: 987-996.
2167. Su X, Gopalakrishnan V, Stearns D, Aldape K, Lang FF, Fuller G, Snyder E, Eberhart CG, Majumder S (2006). Abnormal expression of REST/NRSF and Myc in neural stem/progenitor cells causes cerebellar tumors by blocking neuronal differentiation. Mol Cell Biol 26: 1666-1678.
2168. Subramanian A, Harris A, Piggott K, Shieff C, Bradford R (2002). Metastasis to and from the central nervous system—the 'relatively protected site'. Lancet Oncol 3: 498-507.
2169. Sugawa N, Ekstrand AJ, James CD, Collins VP (1990). Identical splicing of aberrant epidermal growth factor receptor transcripts from amplified rearranged genes in human glioblastomas. Proc Natl Acad Sci USA 87: 8602-8606.
2170. Sugita Y, Kepes JJ, Shigemori M, Kuramoto S, Reifenberger G, Kiwit JC, Wechsler W (1990). Pleomorphic xanthoastrocytoma with desmoplastic reaction: angiomatous variant. Report of two cases. Clin Neuropathol 9: 271-278.
2171. Sugita Y, Terasaki M, Shigemori M, Morimatsu M, Honda E, Oshima Y (2002). Astroblastoma with unusual signet-ring-like cell components: a case report and literature

review. Neuropathology 22: 200-205.

2172. Sugiyama K, Arita K, Shima T, Nakaoka M, Matsuoka T, Taniguchi E, Okamura T, Yamasaki H, Kajiwara Y, Kurisu K (2002). Good clinical course in infants with desmoplastic cerebral neuroepithelial tumor treated by surgery alone. J Neurooncol 59: 63-69.

2173. Suh YL, Koo H, Kim TS, Chi JG, Park SH, Khang SK, Choe G, Lee MC, Hong EK, Sohn YK, Chae YS, Kim DS, Huh GY, Lee SS, Lee YS (2002). Tumors of the central nervous system in Korea: a multicenter study of 3221 cases. J Neurooncol 56: 251-259.

2174. Suki D (2004). The epidemiology of brain metastases. In: Intracranial metastases; Current management strategies. Sawaya R, ed. Blackwell Futura Publishing: Malden, MA, USA.

2175. Sun W, Nordberg ML, Fowler MR (2003). Histiocytic sarcoma involving the central nervous system: clinical, immunohistochemical, and molecular genetic studies of a case with review of the literature. Am J Surg Pathol 27: 258-265.

2176. Sundaram C, Vydehi BV, Jaganmohan RJ, Reddy AK (2003). Medulloepithelioma: a case report. Neurol India 51: 546-547.

2177. Sundgren P, Annertz M, Englund E, Stromblad LG, Holtas S (1999). Paragangliomas of the spinal canal. Neuroradiology 41: 788-794.

2178. Sung CC, Collins R, Li J, Pearl DK, Coons SW, Scheithauer BW, Johnson PC, Yates AJ (1996). Glycolipids and myelin proteins in human oligodendrogliomas. Glycoconj J 13: 433-443.

2179. Sung JH, Mastri AR, Segal EL (1973). Melanotic medulloblastoma of the cerebellum. J Neuropathol Exp Neurol 32: 437-445.

2180. Sung T, Miller DC, Hayes RL, Alonso M, Yee H, Newcomb EW (2000). Preferential inactivation of the p53 tumor suppressor pathway and lack of EGFR amplification distinguish de novo high grade pediatric astrocytomas from de novo adult astrocytomas. Brain Pathol 10: 249-259.

2181. Surace EI, Lusis E, Murakami Y, Scheithauer BW, Perry A, Gutmann DH (2004). Loss of tumor suppressor in lung cancer-1 (TSLC1) expression in meningioma correlates with increased malignancy grade and reduced patient survival. J Neuropathol Exp Neurol 63: 1015-1027.

2182. Sure U, Berghorn WJ, Bertalanffy H, Wakabayashi T, Yoshida J, Sugita K, Seeger W (1995). Staging, scoring and grading of medulloblastoma. A postoperative prognosis predicting system based on the cases of a single institute. Acta Neurochir 132: 59-65.

2183. Suresh TN, Santosh V, Yasha TC, Anandh B, Mohanty A, Indiradevi B, Sampath S, Shankar SK (2004). Medulloblastoma with extensive nodularity: a variant occurring in the very young-clinicopathological and immunohistochemical study of four cases. Childs Nerv Syst 20: 55-60.

2184. Suster D, Plaza JA, Shen R (2005). Low-grade malignant perineurioma (perineurial sarcoma) of soft tissue: a potential diagnostic pitfall on fine needle aspiration. Ann Diagn Pathol 9: 197-201.

2185. Suzuki S, Oka H, Kawano N, Tanaka S, Utsuki S, Fujii K (2001). Prognostic value of Ki-67 (MIB-1) and p53 in ependymomas. Brain Tumor Pathol 18: 151-154.

2186. Suzuki SO, Iwaki T (2000). Amplification and overexpression of mdm2 gene in ependymomas. Mod Pathol 13: 548-553.

2187. Suzuki T, Izumoto S, Fujimoto Y, Maruno M, Ito Y, Yoshimine T (2005). Clinicopathological study of cellular proliferation and invasion in gliomatosis cerebri: important role of neural cell adhesion molecule L1 in

tumour invasion. J Clin Pathol 58: 166-171.

2188. Swanson PE, Lillemoe TJ, Manivel JC, Wick MR (1990). Mesenchymal chondrosarcoma. An immunohistochemical study. Arch Pathol Lab Med 114: 943-948.

2189. Swensen AR, Bushhouse SA (1998). Childhood cancer incidence and trends in Minnesota, 1988-1994. Minn Med 81: 27-32.

2190. Szeifert GT, Pasztor E (1993). Could craniopharyngiomas produce pituitary hormones? Neurol Res 15: 68-69.

2191. Szudek J, Joe H, Friedman JM (2002). Analysis of intrafamilial phenotypic variation in neurofibromatosis 1 (NF1). Genet Epidemiol 23: 150-164.

2192. Tachibana O, Lampe K, Kleihues P, Ohgaki H (1996). Preferential expression of Fas/APO1 (CD95) and apoptotic cell death in perinecrotic cells of the glioblastoma multiforme. Acta Neuropathol 92: 431-434.

2193. Tachibana O, Yamashima T, Yamashita J, Takabatake Y (1994). Immunohistochemical expression of human chorionic gonadotropin and P-glycoprotein in human pituitary glands and craniopharyngiomas. J Neurosurg 80: 79-84.

2194. Tada K, Kochi M, Saya H, Kuratsu J, Shiraishi S, Kamiryo T, Shinojima N, Ushio Y (2003). Preliminary observations on genetic alterations in pilocytic astrocytomas associated with neurofibromatosis 1. Neuro-oncol 5: 228-234.

2195. Tada T, Katsuyama T, Aoki T (1987). Mixed glioblastoma and sarcoma with osteoid-chondral tissue. Clin Neuropathol 6: 160-163.

2196. Taillibert S, Chodkiewicz C, Laigle-Donadey F, Napolitano M, Cartalat-Carel S, Sanson M (2006). Gliomatosis cerebri: a review of 296 cases from the ANOCEF database and the literature. J Neurooncol 76: 201-205.

2197. Taillibert S, Laigle-Donadey F, Chodkiewicz C, Sanson M, Hoang-Xuan K, Delattre JY (2005). Leptomeningeal metastases from solid malignancy: a review. J Neurooncol 75: 85-99.

2198. Taipale J, Cooper MK, Maiti T, Beachy PA (2002). Patched acts catalytically to suppress the activity of Smoothened. Nature 418: 892-897.

2199. Tajima Y, Molina RPJ, Rorke LB, Kaplan DR, Radeke M, Feinstein SC, Lee VM, Trojanowski JQ (1998). Neurotrophins and neuronal versus glial differentiation in medulloblastomas and other pediatric brain tumors. Acta Neuropathol 95: 325-332.

2200. Takahashi A, Hong SC, Seo DW, Hong SB, Lee M, Suh YL (2005). Frequent association of cortical dysplasia in dysembryoplastic neuroepithelial tumor treated by epilepsy surgery. Surg Neurol 64: 419-427.

2201. Takei H, Goodman JC, Tanaka S, Bhattacharjee MB, Bahrami A, Powell SZ (2005). Pituicytoma incidentally found at autopsy. Pathol Int 55: 745-749.

2202. Takei Y, Mirra SS, Miles ML (1976). Eosinophilic granular cells in oligodendrogliomas. An ultrastructural study. Cancer 38: 1968-1976.

2203. Takei Y, Seyama S, Pearl GS, Tindall GT (1980). Ultrastructural study of the human neurohypophysis. II. Cellular elements of neural parenchyma, the pituicytes. Cell Tissue Res 205: 273-287.

2204. Takeshima H, Kawahara Y, Hirano H, Obara S, Niiro M, Kuratsu J (2003). Postoperative regression of desmoplastic infantile gangliogliomas: report of two cases. Neurosurgery 53: 979-983.

2205. Takeuchi H, Kubota T, Sato K, Arishima H (2004). Ultrastructure of capillary endothelium in pilocytic astrocytomas. Brain Tumor Pathol 21: 23-26.

2206. Taliansky-Aronov A, Bokstein F, Lavon

I, Siegal T (2006). Temozolomide treatment for newly diagnosed anaplastic oligodendrogliomas: a clinical efficacy trial. J Neurooncol 79: 153-157.

2207. Tamura M, Gu J, Matsumoto K, Aota S, Parsons R, Yamada KM (1998). Inhibition of cell migration, spreading, and focal adhesions by tumor suppressor PTEN. Science 280: 1614-1617.

2208. Tanaka K, Waga S, Itho H, Shimizu DM, Namiki H (1989). Superficial location of malignant glioma with heavily lipidized (foamy) tumor cells: a case report. J Neurooncol 7: 293-297.

2209. Tanaka M, Suda M, Ishikawa Y, Fujitake J, Fuji H, Tatsuoka Y (1996). Idiopathic hypertrophic cranial pachymeningitis associated with hydrocephalus and myocarditis: remarkable steroid-induced remission of hypertrophic dura mater. Neurology 46: 554-556.

2210. Tanaka Y, Yokoo H, Komori T, Makita Y, Ishizawa T, Hirose T, Ebato M, Shibahara J, Tsukayama C, Shibuya M, Nakazato Y (2005). A distinct pattern of Olig2-positive cellular distribution in papillary glioneuronal tumors: a manifestation of the oligodendroglial phenotype? Acta Neuropathol 110: 39-47.

2211. Tancredi A, Mangiola A, Guiducci A, Peciarolo A, Ottaviano P (2000). Oligodendrocytic gliomatosis cerebri. Acta Neurochir 142: 469-472.

2212. Tang Y, Eng C (2006). p53 down-regulates phosphatase and tensin homologue deleted on chromosome 10 protein stability partially through caspase-mediated degradation in cells with proteasome dysfunction. Cancer Res 66: 6139-6148.

2213. Tang Y, Eng C (2006). PTEN autoregulates its expression by stabilization of p53 in a phosphatase-independent manner. Cancer Res 66: 736-742.

2214. Tanimura A, Nakamura Y, Hachisuka H, Tanimura Y, Fukumura A (1984). Hemangioblastoma of the central nervous system: nature of the stromal cells as studied by the immunoperoxidase technique. Hum Pathol 15: 866-869.

2215. Taratuto AL, Molina HA, Diez B, Zuccaro G, Monges J (1985). Primary rhabdomyosarcoma of brain and cerebellum. Report of four cases in infants: an immunohistochemical study. Acta Neuropathol 66: 98-104.

2216. Taratuto AL, Monges J, Lylyk P, Leiguarda R (1982). Meningocerebral astrocytoma attached to dura with "desmoplastic" reaction. Proceedings of the IX International Congress of Neuropathology (Viena) 5-10.

2217. Taratuto AL, Monges J, Lylyk P, Leiguarda R (1984). Superficial cerebral astrocytoma attached to dura. Report of six cases in infants. Cancer 54: 2505-2512.

2218. Taratuto AL, Pomata H, Sevlever G, Gallo G, Monges J (1995). Dysembryoplastic neuroepithelial tumor: morphological, immunocytochemical, and deoxyribonucleic acid analyses in a pediatric series. Neurosurgery 36: 474-481.

2219. Taratuto AL, Sevlever G, Schultz M (1987). Monoclonal antibodies in superficial desmoplastic cerebral astrocytoma attached to dura in infants. J Neuropathol Exp Neurol 46: 395-395.

2220. Taratuto AL, Sevlever G, Schultz M, Gutierrez M, Monges J, Sanchez M (1994). Desmoplastic cerebral astrocytoma of infancy (DCAI). Survival data of the original series and report of two additional cases, DNA, kinetic and molecular genetic studies. Brain Pathol 4: 423.

2221. Taruscio D, Danesi R, Montaldi A, Cerasoli S, Cenacchi G, Giangaspero F (1997). Nonrandom gain of chromosome 7 in central neurocytoma: a chromosomal analysis and fluorescence in situ hybridization study. Virchows

Arch 430: 47-51.

2222. Tatke M, Suri VS, Malhotra V, Sharma A, Sinha S, Kumar S (2001). Dysembryoplastic neuroepithelial tumors: report of 10 cases from a center where epilepsy surgery is not done. Pathol Res Pract 197: 769-774.

2223. Tatter SB, Borges LF, Louis DN (1994). Central neurocytomas of the cervical spinal cord. Report of two cases. J Neurosurg 81: 288-293.

2224. Tavangar SM, Larijani B, Mahta A, Hosseini SM, Mehrazine M, Bandarian F (2004). Craniopharyngioma: a clinicopathological study of 141 cases. Endocr Pathol 15: 339-344.

2225. Taylor MD, Gokgoz N, Andrulis IL, Mainprize TG, Drake JM, Rutka JT (2000). Familial posterior fossa brain tumors of infancy secondary to germline mutation of the hSNF5 gene. Am J Hum Genet 66: 1403-1406.

2226. Taylor MD, Liu L, Raffel C, Hui CC, Mainprize TG, Zhang X, Agatep R, Chiappa S, Gao L, Lowrance A, Hao A, Goldstein AM, Stavrou T, Scherer SW, Dura WT, Wainwright B, Squire JA, Rutka JT, Hogg D (2002). Mutations in SUFU predispose to medulloblastoma. Nat Genet 31: 306-310.

2227. Taylor MD, Mainprize TG, Rutka JT, Becker L, Bayani J, Drake JM (2001). Medulloblastoma in a child with Rubenstein-Taybi Syndrome: case report and review of the literature. Pediatr Neurosurg 35: 235-238.

2228. Taylor MD, Perry J, Zlatescu MC, Stemmer-Rachamimov AO, Ang LC, Ino Y, Schwartz M, Becker LE, Louis DN, Cairncross JG (1999). The hPMS2 exon 5 mutation and malignant glioma. Case report. J Neurosurg 90: 946-950.

2229. Taylor MD, Poppleton H, Fuller C, Su X, Liu Y, Jensen P, Magdaleno S, Dalton J, Calabrese C, Board J, Macdonald T, Rutka J, Guha A, Gajjar A, Curran T, Gilbertson RJ (2005). Radial glia cells are candidate stem cells of ependymoma. Cancer Cell 8: 323-335.

2230. Tee AR, Fingar DC, Manning BD, Kwiatkowski DJ, Cantley LC, Blenis J (2002). Tuberous sclerosis complex-1 and -2 gene products function together to inhibit mammalian target of rapamycin (mTOR)-mediated downstream signaling. Proc Natl Acad Sci U S A 99: 13571-13576.

2231. Tekautz TM, Fuller CE, Blaney S, Fouladi M, Broniscer A, Merchant TE, Krasin M, Dalton J, Hale G, Kun LE, Wallace D, Gilbertson RJ, Gajjar A (2005). Atypical teratoid/rhabdoid tumors (ATRT): improved survival in children 3 years of age and older with radiation therapy and high-dose alkylator-based chemotherapy. J Clin Oncol 23: 1491-1499.

2232. Telera S, Carosi M, Cerasoli V, Facciolo F, Occhipinti E, Vidiri A, Pompili A (2006). Hemothorax presenting as a primitive thoracic paraganglioma. Case illustration. J Neurosurg Spine 4: 515.

2233. Telfeian AE, Judkins A, Younkin D, Pollock AN, Crino P (2004). Subependymal giant cell astrocytoma with cranial and spinal metastases in a patient with tuberous sclerosis. Case report. J Neurosurg 100: 498-500.

2234. Teng DH, Hu R, Lin H, Davis T, Iliev D, Frye C, Swedlund B, Hansen KL, Vinson VL, Gumpper KL, Ellis L, El-Naggar A, Frazier M, Jasser S, Langford LA, Lee J, Mills GB, Pershouse MA, Pollack RE, Tornos C, Troncoso P, Yung WK, Fujii G, Berson A, Steck PA (1997). MMAC1/PTEN mutations in primary tumor specimens and tumor cell lines. Cancer Res 57: 5221-5225.

2235. Tenreiro P, Kamath SV, Knorr JR, Ragland RL, Smith TW, Lau KY (1995). Desmoplastic infantile ganglioglioma: CT and MRI features. Pediatr Radiol 25: 540-543.

2235A. Teo JG, Gultekin SH, Bilsky M, Gutin P,

Rosenblum MK (1999). A distinctive glioneuronal tumor of the adult cerebrum with neuropil-like (including "rosetted") islands: report of 4 cases. Am J Surg Pathol 23: 502-510.

2236. Teresi RE, Shaiu CW, Chen CS, Chatterjee VK, Waite KA, Eng C (2006). Increased PTEN expression due to transcriptional activation of PPARgamma by Lovastatin and Rosiglitazone. Int J Cancer 118: 2390-2398.

2237. Thiel G, Losanowa T, Kintzel D, Nisch G, Martin H, Vorpahl K, Witkowski R (1992). Karyotypes in 90 human gliomas. Cancer Genet Cytogenet 58: 109-120.

2238. Thiessen B, Finlay J, Kulkarni R, Rosenblum MK (1998). Astroblastoma: does histology predict biologic behavior? J Neurooncol 40: 59-65.

2239. Thines L, Lejeune JP, Ruchoux MM, Assaker R (2006). Management of delayed intracranial and intraspinal metastases of intradural spinal paragangliomas. Acta Neurochir 148: 63-66.

2240. Thom M, Gomez-Anson B, Revesz T, Harkness W, O'Brien CJ, Kett-White R, Jones EW, Stevens J, Scaravilli F (1999). Spontaneous intralesional haemorrhage in dysembryoplastic neuroepithelial tumours: a series of five cases. J Neurol Neurosurg Psychiatry 67: 97-101.

2241. Thomas C, Kristopaitis T, Petruzelli G, Lee J (1999). Malignant craniopharyngioma. J Neuropath Exp Neurol 58: 567-567.

2242. Thomas PK, King RH, Chiang TR, Scaravilli F, Sharma AK, Downie AW (1990). Neurofibromatous neuropathy. Muscle Nerve 13: 93-101.

2243. Thompsett AR, Ellison DW, Stevenson FK, Zhu D (1999). V(H) gene sequences from primary central nervous system lymphomas indicate derivation from highly mutated germinal center B cells with ongoing mutational activity. Blood 94: 1738-1746.

2244. Thompson MC, Fuller C, Hogg TL, Dalton J, Finkelstein D, Lau CC, Chintagumpala M, Adesina A, Ashley DM, Kellie SJ, Taylor MD, Curran T, Gajjar A, Gilbertson RJ (2006). Genomics identifies medulloblastoma subgroups that are enriched for specific genetic alterations. J Clin Oncol 24: 1924-1931.

2245. Tihan T, Burger PC (1998). A variant of "pilocytic astrocytoma" - a possible distinct clinicopathological entity with a less favorable outcome. J Neuropath Exp Neurol 57: 500-500.

2246. Tihan T, Davis R, Elowitz E, DiCostanzo D, Moll U (2000). Practical value of Ki-67 and p53 labeling indexes in stereotactic biopsies of diffuse and pilocytic astrocytomas. Arch Pathol Lab Med 124: 108-113.

2247. Tihan T, Fisher PG, Kepner JL, Godfraind C, McComb RD, Goldthwaite PT, Burger PC (1999). Pediatric astrocytomas with monomorphous pilomyxoid features and a less favorable outcome. J Neuropathol Exp Neurol 58: 1061-1068.

2248. Tihan T, Viglione M, Rosenblum MK, Olivi A, Burger PC (2003). Solitary fibrous tumors in the central nervous system. A clinicopathologic review of 18 cases and comparison to meningeal hemangiopericytomas. Arch Pathol Lab Med 127: 432-439.

2249. Tihan T, Vohra P, Berger MS, Keles GE (2006). Definition and diagnostic implications of gemistocytic astrocytomas: a pathological perspective. J Neurooncol 76: 175-183.

2250. Timmermann B, Kortmann RD, Kuhl J, Rutkowski S, Meisner C, Pietsch T, Deinlein F, Urban C, Warmuth-Metz M, Bamberg M (2006). Role of radiotherapy in supratentorial primitive neuroectodermal tumor in young children: results of the German HIT-SKK87 and HIT-SKK92 trials. J Clin Oncol 24: 1554-1560.

2251. Tirakotai W, Mennel HD, Celik I, Hellwig D, Bertalanffy H, Riegel T (2006). Secretory meningioma: immunohistochemical findings and evaluation of mast cell infiltration. Neurosurg Rev 29: 41-48.

2252. Tohma Y, Gratas C, Biernat W, Peraud A, Fukuda M, Yonekawa Y, Kleihues P, Ohgaki H (1998). PTEN (MMAC1) mutations are frequent in primary glioblastomas (de novo) but not in secondary glioblastomas. J Neuropathol Exp Neurol 57: 684-689.

2253. Tohma Y, Gratas C, Van Meir EG, Desbaillets I, Tenan M, Tachibana O, Kleihues P, Ohgaki H (1998). Necrogenesis and Fas/APO-1(CD95) expression in primary (de novo) and secondary glioblastomas. J Neuropath Exp Neurol 57: 239-245.

2254. Tohyama T, Lee VM, Rorke LB, Marvin M, McKay RD, Trojanowski JQ (1992). Nestin expression in embryonic human neuroepithelium and in human neuroepithelial tumor cells. Lab Invest 66: 303-313.

2255. Tomita T, Gates E (1999). Pituitary adenomas and granular cell tumors. Incidence, cell type, and location of tumor in 100 pituitary glands at autopsy. Am J Clin Pathol 111: 817-825.

2256. Tomlinson FH, Scheithauer BW, Hayostek CJ, Parisi JE, Meyer FB, Shaw EG, Weiland TL, Katzmann JA, Jack CR, Jr. (1994). The significance of atypia and histologic malignancy in pilocytic astrocytoma of the cerebellum: a clinicopathologic and flow cytometric study. J Child Neurol 9: 301-310.

2257. Tomlinson FH, Scheithauer BW, Kelly PJ, Forbes GS (1991). Subependymoma with rhabdomyosarcomatous differentiation: report of a case and literature review. Neurosurgery 28: 761-768.

2258. Tomura N, Hirano H, Watanabe O, Watarai J, Itoh Y, Mineura K, Kowada M (1997). Central neurocytoma with clinically malignant behavior. AJNR Am J Neuroradiol 18: 1175-1178.

2259. Tong CY, Hui AB, Yin XL, Pang JC, Zhu XL, Poon WS, Ng HK (2004). Detection of oncogene amplifications in medulloblastomas by comparative genomic hybridization and array-based comparative genomic hybridization. J Neurosurg 100: 187-193.

2260. Tong CY, Ng HK, Pang JC, Hu J, Hui AB, Poon WS (2000). Central neurocytomas are genetically distinct from oligodendrogliomas and neuroblastomas. Histopathology 37: 160-165.

2261. Torres CF, Korones DN, Pilcher W (1997). Multiple ependymomas in a patient with Turcot's syndrome. Med Pediatr Oncol 28: 59-61.

2262. Trassard M, Le D, V, Bui BN, Coindre JM (1996). Angiosarcoma arising in a solitary schwannoma (neurilemoma) of the sciatic nerve. Am J Surg Pathol 20: 1412-1417.

2263. Trehan G, Bruge H, Vinchon M, Khalil C, Ruchoux MM, Dhellemmes P, Ares GS (2004). MR imaging in the diagnosis of desmoplastic infantile tumor: retrospective study of six cases. AJNR Am J Neuroradiol 25: 1028-1033.

2264. Tresser N, Parveen T, Roessmann U (1993). Intracranial lipomas with teratomatous elements. Arch Pathol Lab Med 117: 918-920.

2265. Trimbath JD, Petersen GM, Erdman SH, Ferre M, Luce MC, Giardiello FM (2001). Cafe-au-lait spots and early onset colorectal neoplasia: a variant of HNPCC? Fam Cancer 1: 101-105.

2266. Trofatter JA, MacCollin MM, Rutter JL, Murrell JR, Duyao MP, Parry DM, Eldridge R, Kley N, Menon AG, Pulaski K (1993). A novel moesin-, ezrin-, radixin-like gene is a candidate for the neurofibromatosis 2 tumor suppressor. Cell 72: 791-800.

2267. Trojanowski JQ, Tascos NA, Rorke LB (1982). Malignant pineocytoma with prominent papillary features. Cancer 50: 1789-1793.

2268. Troost D, Jansen GH, Dingemans KP (1990). Cerebral medulloepithelioma—electron microscopy and immunohistochemistry. Acta Neuropathol 80: 103-107.

2269. Trouillard O, Aguirre-Cruz L, Hoang-Xuan K, Marie Y, Delattre JY, Sanson M (2004). Parental 19q loss and PEG3 expression in oligodendrogliomas. Cancer Genet Cytogenet 151: 182-183.

2270. Tsirikos AI, Saifuddin A, Noordeen MH (2005). Spinal deformity in neurofibromatosis type-1: diagnosis and treatment. Eur Spine J 14: 427-439.

2271. Tso CL, Freije WA, Day A, Chen Z, Merriman B, Perlina A, Lee Y, Dia EQ, Yoshimoto K, Mischel PS, Liau LM, Cloughesy TF, Nelson SF (2006). Distinct transcription profiles of primary and secondary glioblastoma subgroups. Cancer Res 66: 159-167.

2272. Tsuchida T, Matsumoto M, Shirayama Y, Imahori T, Kasai H, Kawamoto K (1996). Neuronal and glial characteristics of central neurocytoma: electron microscopical analysis of two cases. Acta Neuropathol 91: 573-577.

2273. Tsukayama C, Arakawa Y (2002). A papillary glioneuronal tumor arising in an elderly woman: a case report. Brain Tumor Pathol 19: 35-39.

2274. Tsumanuma I, Sato M, Okazaki H, Tanaka R, Washiyama K, Kawasaki T, Kumanishi T (1995). The analysis of p53 tumor suppressor gene in pineal parenchymal tumors. Noshuyo Byori 12: 39-43.

2275. Tsumanuma I, Tanaka R, Abe S, Kawasaki T, Washiyama K, Kumanishi T (1997). Infrequent mutation of Waf1/p21 gene, a CDK inhibitor gene, in brain tumors. Neurol Med Chir (Tokyo) 37: 150-156.

2276. Tsumanuma I, Tanaka R, Washiyama K (1999). Clinicopathological study of pineal parenchymal tumors: correlation between histopathological features, proliferative potential, and prognosis. Brain Tumor Pathol 16: 61-68.

2277. Tu PH, Giannini C, Judkins AR, Schwalb JM, Burack R, O'Neill BP, Yachnis AT, Burger PC, Scheithauer BW, Perry A (2005). Clinicopathologic and genetic profile of intracranial marginal zone lymphoma: a primary low-grade CNS lymphoma that mimics meningioma. J Clin Oncol 23: 5718-5727.

2278. Tucker T, Wolkenstein P, Revuz J, Zeller J, Friedman JM (2005). Association between benign and malignant peripheral nerve sheath tumors in NF1. Neurology 65: 205-211.

2279. Turcot J, Despres JP, St (1959). Malignant tumors of the central nervous system associated with familial polyposis of the colon. Dis Colon Rectum 2: 465-468.

2280. Turhan T, Oner K, Yurtseven T, Akalin T, Ovul I (2004). Spinal meningeal melanocytoma. Report of two cases and review of the literature. J Neurosurg 100: 287-290.

2281. Uchikawa H, Toyoda M, Nagao K, Miyauchi H, Nishikawa R, Fujii K, Kohno Y, Yamada M, Miyashita T (2006). Brain- and heart-specific Patched-1 containing exon 12b is a dominant negative isoform and is expressed in medulloblastomas. Biochem Biophys Res Commun 349: 277-283.

2282. Ueki K, Ono Y, Henson JW, Efird JT, von Deimling A, Louis DN (1996). CDKN2/p16 or RB alterations occur in the majority of glioblastomas and are inversely correlated. Cancer Res 56: 150-153.

2283. Uesaka T, Miyazono M, Nishio S, Iwaki T (2002). Astrocytoma of the pituitary gland (pituicytoma): case report. Neuroradiology 44: 123-125.

2284. Ullrich A, Coussens L, Hayflick JS, Dull TJ, Gray A, Tam AW, Lee J, Yarden Y, Libermann TA, Schlessinger J (1984). Human epidermal growth factor receptor cDNA sequence and aberrant expression of the amplified gene in A431 epidermoid carcinoma cells. Nature 309: 418-425.

2285. Ulm AJ, Yachnis AT, Brat DJ, Rhoton AL, Jr. (2004). Pituicytoma: report of two cases and clues regarding histogenesis. Neurosurgery 54: 753-757.

2286. Ulrich J, Heitz PU, Fischer T, Obrist E, Gullotta F (1987). Granular cell tumors: evidence for heterogeneous tumor cell differentiation. An immunocytochemical study. Virchows Arch B Cell Pathol Incl Mol Pathol 53: 52-57.

2287. Uluc K, Arsava EM, Ozkan B, Cila A, Zorlu F, Tan E (2004). Primary leptomeningeal sarcomatosis; a pathology proven case with challenging MRI and clinical findings. J Neurooncol 66: 307-312.

2288. Unni KK (2002). Schwannoma. In: WHO Classification of Tumours: Pathology and Genetics of Tumours of Soft Tissue and Bone. Fletcher CDM, Unni KK, Mertens F eds. IARC Press: Lyon, pp. 331.

2289. Uno K, Takita J, Yokomori K, Tanaka Y, Ohta S, Shimada H, Gilles FH, Sugita K, Abe S, Sako M, Hashizume K, Hayashi Y (2002). Aberrations of the hSNF5/INI1 gene are restricted to malignant rhabdoid tumors or atypical teratoid/rhabdoid tumors in pediatric solid tumors. Genes Chromosomes Cancer 34: 33-41.

2290. Upadhyaya M, Han S, Consoli C, Majounie E, Horan M, Thomas NS, Potts C, Griffiths S, Ruggieri M, von Deimling A, Cooper DN (2004). Characterization of the somatic mutational spectrum of the neurofibromatosis type 1 (NF1) gene in neurofibromatosis patients with benign and malignant tumors. Hum Mutat 23: 134-146.

2291. Upadhyaya M, Spurlock G, Majounie E, Griffiths S, Forrester N, Baser M, Huson SM, Gareth ED, Ferner R (2006). The heterogeneous nature of germline mutations in NF1 patients with malignant peripheral serve sheath tumours (MPNSTs). Hum Mutat 27: 716.

2292. Usul H, Kuzeyli K, Cakir E, Caylan R, Sayin OC, Peksoylu B, Karaarslan G (2005). Giant cranial extradural primary fibroxanthoma: a case report. Surg Neurol 63: 281-284.

2293. Uzal D, Ozyar E, Tukul A, Genc M, Soylemezoglu F, Atahan IL, Onol B (1996). Familial glioma in two siblings. Radiat Med 14: 43-47.

2294. Vahteristo P, Tamminen A, Karvinen P, Eerola H, Eklund C, Aaltonen LA, Blomqvist C, Aittomaki K, Nevanlinna H (2001). p53, CHK2, and CHK1 genes in Finnish families with Li-Fraumeni syndrome: further evidence of CHK2 in inherited cancer predisposition. Cancer Res 61: 5718-5722.

2295. Vajaranant TS, Mafee MF, Kapur R, Rapoport M, Edward DP (2005). Medulloepithelioma of the ciliary body and optic nerve: clinicopathologic, CT, and MR imaging features. Neuroimaging Clin N Am 15: 69-83.

2296. Vajtai I, Varga Z, Aguzzi A (1996). MIB-1 immunoreactivity reveals different labelling in low-grade and in malignant epithelial neoplasms of the choroid plexus. Histopathology 29: 147-151.

2297. Vajtai I, Kappeler A, Lukes A, Arnold M, Luthy AR, Leibundgut K (2006). Papillary glioneuronal tumor. Pathol Res Pract 202: 107-112.

2298. Vajtai I, Sahli R, Kappeler A (2006). Spindle cell oncocytoma of the adenohypophysis: Report of a case with a 16-year follow-up. Pathol Res Pract 202: 745-750.

2298A. Val-Bernal JF, Hernando M, Garijo MF, Villa P (1997). Renal perineurinoma in childhood. Gen Diagn Pathol. 143:75-81.

2299. Valenti MP, Froelich S, Armspach JP, Chenard MP, Dietemann JL, Kerhli P, Marescaux C, Hirsch E, Namer IJ (2002).

Contribution of SISCOM imaging in the presurgical evaluation of temporal lobe epilepsy related to dysembryoplastic neuroepithelial tumors. Epilepsia 43: 270-276.

2300. Valery CA, Sakka LJ, Poirier J (2004). Problematic differential diagnosis between cerebellar liponeurocytoma and anaplastic oligodendroglioma. Br J Neurosurg 18: 300-303.

2301. van den Bent MJ, Carpentier AF, Brandes AA, Sanson M, Taphoorn MJ, Bernsen HJ, Frenay M, Tijssen CC, Grisold W, Sipos L, Haaxma-Reiche H, Kros JM, van Kouwenhoven MC, Vecht CJ, Allgeier A, Lacombe D, Gorlia T (2006). Adjuvant procarbazine, lomustine, and vincristine improves progression-free survival but not overall survival in newly diagnosed anaplastic oligodendrogliomas and oligoastrocytomas: a randomized European Organisation for Research and Treatment of Cancer phase III trial. J Clin Oncol 24: 2715-2722.

2302. van den Bent MJ, Stupp R, Mason W, Mirimanoff RO, Lacombe D, Gorlia T (2005). Impact of extent of resection on overall survival in newly diagnosed glioblastoma after chemoirradiation with temozolomide: Further analysis of EORTC study 26981. Eur J Cancer Suppl3: 134.

2303. Van Es S, North KN, McHugh K, De Silva M (1996). MRI findings in children with neurofibromatosis type 1: a prospective study. Pediatr Radiol 26: 478-487.

2304. Van Meir EG (1998). "Turcot's syndrome": phenotype of brain tumors, survival and mode of inheritance. Int J Cancer 75: 162-164.

2305. Van Meir EG, Oosterhuis JW, Looijenga LHJ (1998). Genesis and genetics of intracranial germ cell tumors. In: Intracranial Germ Cell Tumors. Sawamura Y, Shirato H, de Tribolet N, eds. Springer Verlag: Wien New York, pp. 45-76.

2306. van Nielen KM, de Jong BM (1999). A case of Ollier's disease associated with two intracerebral low-grade gliomas. Clin Neurol Neurosurg 101: 106-110.

2307. van Slegtenhorst M, de Hoogt R, Hermans C, Nellist M, Janssen B, Verhoef S, Lindhout D, van den OA, Halley D, Young J, Burley M, Jeremiah S, Woodward K, Nahmias J, Fox M, Ekong R, Osborne J, Wolfe J, Povey S, Snell RG, Cheadle JP, Jones AC, Tachataki M, Ravine D, Kwiatkowski DJ (1997). Identification of the tuberous sclerosis gene TSC1 on chromosome 9q34. Science 277: 805-808.

2308. van Slegtenhorst M, Verhoef S, Tempelaars A, Bakker L, Wang Q, Wessels M, Bakker R, Nellist M, Lindhout D, Halley D, van den OA (1999). Mutational spectrum of the TSC1 gene in a cohort of 225 tuberous sclerosis complex patients: no evidence for genotype-phenotype correlation. J Med Genet 36: 285-289.

2309. van Tilborg AA, Morolli B, Giphart-Gassler M, de Vries A, van Geenen DA, Lurkin I, Kros JM, Zwarthoff EC (2006). Lack of genetic and epigenetic changes in meningiomas without NF2 loss. J Pathol 208: 564-573.

2310. van Veelen ML, Avezaat CJ, Kros JM, van Putten W, Vecht C (1998). Supratentorial low grade astrocytoma: prognostic factors, dedifferentiation, and the issue of early versus late surgery. J Neurol Neurosurg Psychiatry 64: 581-587.

2311. VandenBerg SR (1991). Desmoplastic infantile ganglioglioma: a clinicopathologic review of sixteen cases. Brain Tumor Pathol 8: 25-31.

2312. VandenBerg SR (1993). Desmoplastic infantile ganglioglioma and desmoplastic cerebral astrocytoma of infancy. Brain Pathol 3: 275-281.

2313. VandenBerg SR, Herman MM, Rubinstein LJ (1987). Embryonal central neuroepithelial tumors: current concepts and future challenges. Cancer Metastasis Rev 5: 343-365.

2314. VandenBerg SR, May EE, Rubinstein LJ, Herman MM, Perentes E, Vinores SA, Collins VP, Park TS (1987). Desmoplastic supratentorial neuroepithelial tumors of infancy with divergent differentiation potential ("desmoplastic infantile gangliogliomas"). Report on 11 cases of a distinctive embryonal tumor with favorable prognosis. J Neurosurg 66: 58-71.

2315. Vandewalle G, Brucher JM, Michotte A (1995). Intracranial facial nerve rhabdomyoma. Case report. J Neurosurg 83: 919-922.

2316. Vang R, Heck K, Fuller GN, Medeiros LJ (2000). Granular cell tumor of intracranial meninges. Clin Neuropathol 19: 41-44.

2317. Vaquero J, Coca S, Martinez R, Escandon J (1990). Papillary pineocytoma. Case report. J Neurosurg 73: 135-137.

2318. Varley JM, McGown G, Thorncroft M, Santibanez-Koref MF, Kelsey AM, Tricker KJ, Evans DG, Birch JM (1997). Germ-line mutations of TP53 in Li-Fraumeni families: an extended study of 39 families. Cancer Res 57: 3245-3252.

2319. Vasen HF, Sanders EA, Taal BG, Nagengast FM, Griffioen G, Menko FH, Kleibeuker JH, Houwing-Duistermaat JJ, Meera KP (1996). The risk of brain tumours in hereditary non-polyposis colorectal cancer (HNPCC). Int J Cancer 65: 422-425.

2320. Vates GE, Chang S, Lamborn KR, Prados M, Berger MS (2003). Gliomatosis cerebri: a review of 22 cases. Neurosurgery 53: 261-271.

2321. Vazquez M, Miller DC, Epstein F, Allen JC, Budzilovich GN (1991). Glioneurofibroma: renaming the pediatric "gliofibroma": a neoplasm composed of Schwann cells and astrocytes. Mod Pathol 4: 519-523.

2322. Versteege I, Sevenet N, Lange J, Rousseau-Merck MF, Ambros P, Handgretinger R, Aurias A, Delattre O (1998). Truncating mutations of hSNF5/INI1 in aggressive paediatric cancer. Nature 394: 203-206.

2323. Verstegen MJ, Leenstra DT, Ijlst-Keizers H, Bosch DA (2002). Proliferation- and apoptosis-related proteins in intracranial ependymomas: an immunohistochemical analysis. J Neurooncol 56: 21-28.

2324. Vertosick FT, Jr., Selker RG, Arena VC (1991). Survival of patients with well-differentiated astrocytomas diagnosed in the era of computed tomography. Neurosurgery 28: 496-501.

2325. Vescovi AL, Galli R, Reynolds BA (2006). Brain tumour stem cells. Nat Rev Cancer 6: 425-436.

2326. Vincent S, Dhellemmes P, Maurage CA, Soto-Ares G, Hassoun J, Ruchoux MM (2002). Intracerebral medulloepithelioma with a long survival. Clin Neuropathol 21: 197-205.

2327. Vinchon M, Blond S, Lejeune JP, Krivosik I, Fossati P, Assaker R, Christiaens JL (1994). Association of Lhermitte-Duclos and Cowden disease: report of a new case and review of the literature. J Neurol Neurosurg Psychiatry 57: 699-704.

2328. Vital A, Vital C, Martin N, McGrogan G, Bioulac P, Trojani M, Loiseau H, Rougier A (1994). Lhermitte-Duclos type cerebellum hamartoma and Cowden disease. Clin Neuropathol 13: 229-231.

2329. Vlodavsky E, Konstantinesku M, Soustiel JF (2006). Gliosarcoma with liposarcomatous differentiation: the new member of the lipid-containing brain tumors family. Arch Pathol Lab Med 130: 381-384.

2330. Vogelbaum MA, Suh JH (2006). Resectable brain metastases. J Clin Oncol 24: 1289-1294.

2331. Vogelgesang S, Junge MH, Pahnke J, Gaab MR, Warzok RW (2002). Sellar/suprasellar mass in a 59-year-old woman. Brain Pathol 12: 135-6, 139.

2332. von Deimling A, Bender B, Jahnke R, Waha A, Kraus J, Albrecht S, Wellenreuther R, Fassbender F, Nagel J, Menon AG, Louis DN, Lenartz D, Schramm J, Wiestler OD (1994). Loci associated with malignant progression in astrocytomas: a candidate on chromosome 19q1. Cancer Res 54: 1397-1401.

2333. von Deimling A, Eibl RH, Ohgaki H, Louis DN, von Ammon K, Petersen I, Kleihues P, Chung RY, Wiestler OD, Seizinger BR (1992). p53 mutations are associated with 17p allelic loss in grade II and grade III astrocytoma. Cancer Res 52: 2987-2990.

2334. von Deimling A, Fimmers R, Schmidt MC, Bender B, Fassbender F, Nagel J, Jahnke R, Kaskel P, Duerr EM, Koopmann J, Maintz D, Steinbeck S, Wick W, Platten M, Muller DJ, Przkora R, Waha A, Blumcke B, Wellenreuther R, Meyer-Puttlitz B, Schmidt O, Mollenhauer J, Poustka A, Stangl AP, Lenartz D, von Ammon K (2000). Comprehensive allelotype and genetic anaysis of 466 human nervous system tumors. J Neuropathol Exp Neurol 59: 544-558.

2335. von Deimling A, Janzer R, Kleihues P, Wiestler OD (1990). Patterns of differentiation in central neurocytoma. An immunohistochemical study of eleven biopsies. Acta Neuropathol 79: 473-479.

2336. von Deimling A, Kleihues P, Saremaslani P, Yasargil MG, Spoerri O, Sudhof TC, Wiestler OD (1991). Histogenesis and differentiation potential of central neurocytomas. Lab Invest 64: 585-591.

2337. von Deimling A, Kraus JA, Stangl AP, Wellenreuther R, Lenartz D, Schramm J, Louis DN, Ramesh V, Gusella JF, Wiestler OD (1995). Evidence for subarachnoid spread in the development of multiple meningiomas. Brain Pathol 5: 11-14.

2338. von Deimling A, Larson J, Wellenreuther R, Stangl AP, van V, V, Warnick R, Tew J, Jr., Balko G, Menon AG (1999). Clonal origin of recurrent meningiomas. Brain Pathol 9: 645-650.

2339. von Deimling A, Louis DN, von Ammon K, Petersen I, Wiestler OD, Seizinger BR (1992). Evidence for a tumor suppressor gene on chromosome 19q associated with human astrocytomas, oligodendrogliomas, and mixed gliomas. Cancer Res 52: 4277-4279.

2340. von Deimling A, Nagel J, Bender B, Lenartz D, Schramm J, Louis DN, Wiestler OD (1994). Deletion mapping of chromosome 19 in human gliomas. Int J Cancer 57: 676-680.

2341. von Deimling A, von Ammon K, Schoenfeld D, Wiestler OD, Seizinger BR, Louis DN (1993). Subsets of glioblastoma multiforme defined by molecular genetic analysis. Brain Pathol 3: 19-26.

2342. von Haken MS, White EC, Daneshvar S, Sih S, Choi E, Kalra R, Cogen PH (1996). Molecular genetic analysis of chromosome arm 17p and chromosome arm 22q DNA sequences in sporadic pediatric ependymomas. Genes Chromosomes Cancer 17: 37-44.

2343. von Hippel E (1904). Uber eine sehr seltene Erkrankung der Netzhaut. Graefe's Arch 59: 83-86.

2344. von Koch CS, Gulati M, Aldape K, Berger MS (2002). Familial medulloblastoma: case report of one family and review of the literature. Neurosurgery 51: 227-233.

2345. Vorechovsky I, Tingby O, Hartman M, Stromberg B, Nister M, Collins VP, Toftgard R (1997). Somatic mutations in the human homologue of Drosophila patched in primitive neuroectodermal tumours. Oncogene 15: 361-366.

2346. Vorechovsky I, Unden AB, Sandstedt

B, Toftgard R, Stahle-Backdahl M (1997). Trichoepitheliomas contain somatic mutations in the overexpressed PTCH gene: support for a gatekeeper mechanism in skin tumorigenesis. Cancer Res 57: 4677-4681.

2347. Vortmeyer AO, Frank S, Jeong SY, Yuan K, Ikejiri B, Lee YS, Bhowmick D, Lonser RR, Smith R, Rodgers G, Oldfield EH, Zhuang Z (2003). Developmental arrest of angioblastic lineage initiates tumorigenesis in von Hippel-Lindau disease. Cancer Res 63: 7051-7055.

2348. Vortmeyer AO, Gnarra JR, Emmert-Buck MR, Katz D, Linehan WM, Oldfield EH, Zhuang Z (1997). von Hippel-Lindau gene deletion detected in the stromal cell component of a cerebellar hemangioblastoma associated with von Hippel-Lindau disease. Hum Pathol 28: 540-543.

2349. Vortmeyer AO, Tran MGB, Zeng W, Glasker S, Riley C, Tsokos M, Ikejiri B, Merrill MJ, Raffeld M, Zhuang Z, Lonser RR, Maxwell PH, Oldfield EH (2006). Evolution of VHL tumorigenesis in nerve root tissue. J Pathol 210: 374-382.

2350. Vortmeyer AO, Yuan Q, Lee YS, Zhuang Z, Oldfield EH (2004). Developmental effects of von Hippel-Lindau gene deficiency. Ann Neurol 55: 721-728.

2351. Vredenburgh JJ, Desjardins A, Herndon JE, Dowell JM, Reardon DV, Quinn JA, Rich JN, Sathornsumetee S, Gururangan S, Bigner DD, Friedman AH, Friedmqn HS (2007). Phase II trial of bevacizumab and irinotecan in recurrent malignant glioma. Clin Cancer Res 13: 1253-9.

2352. Vuorinen V, Sallinen P, Haapasalo H, Visakorpi T, Kallio M, Jaaskelainen J (1996). Outcome of 31 intracranial hemangiopericytomas: poor predictive value of cell proliferation indices. Acta Neurochir 138: 1399-1408.

2353. Wacker MR, Cogen PH, Etzell JE, Daneshvar L, Davis RL, Prados MD (1992). Diffuse leptomeningeal involvement by a ganglioglioma in a child. Case report. J Neurosurg 77: 302-306.

2354. Wada C, Kurata A, Hirose R, Tazaki Y, Kan S, Ishihara Y, Kameya T (1986). Primary leptomeningeal ependymoblastoma. Case report. J Neurosurg 64: 968-973.

2355. Waha A, Koch A, Hartmann W, Mack H, Schramm J, Sorensen N, Berthold F, Wiestler OD, Pietsch T, Waha A (2004). Analysis of HIC-1 methylation and transcription in human ependymomas. Int J Cancer 110: 542-549.

2356. Waha A, Waha A, Koch A, Meyer-Puttlitz B, Weggen S, Sorensen N, Tonn JC, Albrecht S, Goodyer CG, Berthold F, Wiestler OD, Pietsch T (2003). Epigenetic silencing of the HIC-1 gene in human medulloblastomas. J Neuropathol Exp Neurol 62: 1192-1201.

2357. Waite KA, Eng C (2002). Protean PTEN: form and function. Am J Hum Genet 70: 829-844.

2358. Waldron JS, Tihan T (2003). Epidemiology and pathology of intraventricular tumors. Neurosurg Clin N Am 14: 469-482.

2359. Walker C, Joyce KA, Thompson-Hehir J, Davies MP, Gibbs FE, Halliwell N, Lloyd BH, Machell Y, Roebuck MM, Salisbury J, Sibson DR, Du PD, Broome J, Rossi ML (2001). Characterisation of molecular alterations in microdissected archival gliomas. Acta Neuropathol 101: 321-333.

2360. Walker L, Thompson D, Easton D, Ponder B, Ponder M, Frayling I, Baralle D (2006). A prospective study of neurofibromatosis type 1 cancer incidence in the UK. Br J Cancer 95: 233-238.

2361. Wang H, Wang H, Shen W, Huang H, Hu L, Ramdas L, Zhou YH, Liao WS, Fuller GN, Zhang W (2003). Insulin-like growth factor binding protein 2 enhances glioblastoma invasion

by activating invasion-enhancing genes. Cancer Res 63: 4315-4321.
2362. Wang H, Wang H, Zhang W, Fuller GN (2006). Overexpression of IGFBP5, but not IGFBP3, correlates with the histologic grade of human diffuse glioma: a tissue microarray and immunohistochemical study. Technol Cancer Res Treat 5: 195-199.
2363. Wang JL, Zhang ZJ, Hartman M, Smits A, Westermark B, Muhr C, Nister M (1995). Detection of TP53 gene mutation in human meningiomas: a study using immunohistochemistry, polymerase chain reaction/single-strand conformation polymorphism and DNA sequencing techniques on paraffin-embedded samples. Int J Cancer 64: 223-228.
2364. Wang M, Tihan T, Rojiani AM, Bodhireddy SR, Prayson RA, Iacuone JJ, Alles AJ, Donahue DJ, Hessler RB, Kim JH, Haas M, Rosenblum MK, Burger PC (2005). Monomorphous angiocentric glioma: a distinctive epileptogenic neoplasm with features of infiltrating astrocytoma and ependymoma. J Neuropathol Exp Neurol 64: 875-881.
2365. Wanschitz J, Schmidbauer M, Maier H, Rossler K, Vorkapic P, Budka H (1995). Suprasellar meningioma with expression of glial fibrillary acidic protein: a peculiar variant. Acta Neuropathol 90: 539-544.
2366. Warnick RE, Raisanen J, Adornato BT, Prados MD, Davis RL, Larson DA, Gutin PH (1993). Intracranial myxopapillary ependymoma: case report. J Neurooncol 15: 251-256.
2367. Warren C, James LA, Ramsden RT, Wallace A, Baser ME, Varley JM, Evans DG (2003). Identification of recurrent regions of chromosome loss and gain in vestibular schwannomas using comparative genomic hybridisation. J Med Genet 40: 802-806.
2368. Wasdahl DA, Scheithauer BW, Andrews BT, Jeffrey RA, Jr. (1994). Cerebellar pleomorphic xanthoastrocytoma: case report. Neurosurgery 35: 947-950.
2369. Watanabe K, Ogata N, von Ammon K, Yonekawa Y, Nagai M, Ohgaki H, Kleihues P (1996). Immunohistochemical assessments of P53 protein accumulation and tumor growth fraction during the progression of astrocytomas. In: Brain Tumour Research and Therapy. Nagai M, ed. Springer-Verlag: Tokyo, pp. 255-262.
2370. Watanabe K, Peraud A, Gratas C, Wakai S, Kleihues P, Ohgaki H (1998). p53 and PTEN gene mutations in gemistocytic astrocytomas. Acta Neuropathol 95: 559-564.
2371. Watanabe K, Sato K, Biernat W, Tachibana O, von Ammon K, Ogata N, Yonekawa Y, Kleihues P, Ohgaki H (1997). Incidence and timing of p53 mutations during astrocytoma progression in patients with multiple biopsies. Clin Cancer Res 3: 523-530.
2372. Watanabe K, Tachibana O, Sato K, Yonekawa Y, Kleihues P, Ohgaki H (1996). Overexpression of the EGF receptor and p53 mutations are mutually exclusive in the evolution of primary and secondary glioblastomas. Brain Pathol 6: 217-224.
2373. Watanabe K, Tachibana O, Yonekawa Y, Kleihues P, Ohgaki H (1997). Role of gemistocytes in astrocytoma progression. Lab Invest 76: 277-284.
2374. Watanabe T, Makiyama Y, Nishimoto H, Matsumoto M, Kikuchi A, Tsubokawa T (1995). Metachronous ovarian dysgerminoma after a suprasellar germ-cell tumor treated by radiation therapy. Case report. J Neurosurg 83: 149-153.
2375. Watanabe T, Oda Y, Tamiya S, Kinukawa N, Masuda K, Tsuneyoshi M (2001). Malignant peripheral nerve sheath tumours: high Ki67 labelling index is the significant prognostic indicator. Histopathology 39: 187-197.
2376. Weary PE, Gorlin RJ, Gentry WC, Jr., Comer JE, Greer KE (1972). Multiple hamartoma syndrome (Cowden's disease). Arch Dermatol 106: 682-690.
2377. Weber M, Stockhammer F, Schmitz U, von Deimling A (2001). Mutational analysis of INI1 in sporadic human brain tumors. Acta Neuropathol 101: 479-482.
2378. Weber RG, Bostrom J, Wolter M, Baudis M, Collins VP, Reifenberger G, Lichter P (1997). Analysis of genomic alterations in benign, atypical, and anaplastic meningiomas: toward a genetic model of meningioma progression. Proc Natl Acad Sci U S A 94: 14719-14724.
2379. Weber RG, Hoischen A, Ehrler M, Zipper P, Kaulich K, Blaschke B, Becker AJ, Weber-Mangal S, Jauch A, Radlwimmer B, Schramm J, Wiestler OD, Lichter P, Reifenberger G (2007). Frequent loss of chromosome 9, homozygous CDKN2A/p14(ARF)/CDKN2B deletion and low TSC1 mRNA expression in pleomorphic xanthoastrocytomas. Oncogene 26:1088-97.
2380. Weber T, Weber RG, Kaulich K, Actor B, Meyer-Puttlitz B, Lampel S, Buschges R, Weigel R, Deckert-Schluter M, Schmiedek P, Reifenberger G, Lichter P (2000). Characteristic chromosomal imbalances in primary central nervous system lymphomas of the diffuse large B-cell type. Brain Pathol 10: 73-84.
2381. Webster AR, Maher ER, Bird AC, Gregor ZJ, Moore AT (1999). A clinical and molecular genetic analysis of solitary ocular angioma. Ophthalmology 106: 623-629.
2382. Wechsler-Reya RJ, Scott MP (1999). Control of neuronal precursor proliferation in the cerebellum by Sonic Hedgehog. Neuron 22: 103-114.
2383. Wechsler J, Lantieri L, Zeller J, Voisin MC, Martin-Garcia N, Wolkenstein P (2003). Aberrant axon neurofilaments in schwannomas associated with phacomatoses. Virchows Arch 443: 768-773.
2384. Weggen S, Bayer TA, von Deimling A, Reifenberger G, Wiestler OD, Pietsch T (2000). Low frequency of SV40, JC and BK polyoma virus sequences in human medulloblastomas, meningiomas and ependymomas. Brain Pathol 10: 85-92.
2385. Wei YQ, Hang ZB, Liu KF (1992). In situ observation of inflammatory cell-tumor cell interaction in human seminomas (germinomas): light, electron microscopic, and immunohistochemical study. Hum Pathol 23: 421-428.
2386. Weidauer S, Stuckrad-Barre S, Dettmann E, Zanella FE, Lanfermann H (2003). Cerebral Erdheim-Chester disease: case report and review of the literature. Neuroradiology 45: 241-245.
2387. Weiner HL, Wisoff JH, Rosenberg ME, Kupersmith MJ, Cohen H, Zagzag D, Shiminski M, Flamm ES, Epstein FJ, Miller DC (1994). Craniopharyngiomas: a clinicopathological analysis of factors predictive of recurrence and functional outcome. Neurosurgery 35: 1001-1010.
2388. Weiner HL, Zagzag D, Babu R, Weinreb HJ, Ransohoff J (1993). Schwannoma of the fourth ventricle presenting with hemifacial spasm. A report of two cases. J Neurooncol 15: 37-43.
2389. Weintraub M, Bhatia KG, Chandra RS, Magrath IT, Ladisch S (1998). p53 expression in Langerhans cell histiocytosis. J Pediatr Hematol Oncol 20: 12-17.
2390. Weiss SW, Langloss JM, Enzinger FM (1983). Value of S-100 protein in the diagnosis of soft tissue tumors with particular reference to benign and malignant Schwann cell tumors. Lab Invest 49: 299-308.
2391. Weiss WA, Israel M, Cobbs C, Holland E, James CD, Louis DN, Marks C, McClatchey AI, Roberts T, Van Dyke T, Wetmore C, Chiu IM, Giovannini M, Guha A, Higgins RJ, Marino S, Radovanovic I, Reilly K, Aldape K (2002). Neuropathology of genetically engineered mice: consensus report and recommendations from an international forum. Oncogene 21: 7453-7463.
2392. Weldon-Linne GM, Victor TA, Groothuis DR, Vick NA (1983). Pleomorphic xanthoastrocytoma: ultrastructural and immunohistochemical study of a case with a rapidly fatal outcome following surgery. Cancer 52: 2055-2063.
2393. Wellenreuther R, Kraus JA, Lenartz D, Menon AG, Schramm J, Louis DN, Ramesh V, Gusella JF, Wiestler OD, von Deimling A (1995). Analysis of the neurofibromatosis 2 gene reveals molecular variants of meningioma. Am J Pathol 146: 827-832.
2394. Wellons JC, III, Reddy AT, Tubbs RS, Abdullatif H, Oakes WJ, Blount JP, Grabb PA (2004). Neuroendoscopic findings in patients with intracranial germinomas correlating with diabetes insipidus. J Neurosurg 100: 430-436.
2395. Werness BA, Guccion JG (1997). Tumor of the broad ligament in von Hippel-Lindau disease of probable mullerian origin. Int J Gynecol Pathol 16: 282-285.
2396. Wesseling P, Schlingemann RO, Rietveld FJ, Link M, Burger PC, Ruiter DJ (1995). Early and extensive contribution of pericytes/vascular smooth muscle cells to microvascular proliferation in glioblastoma multiforme: an immuno-light and immuno-electron microscopic study. J Neuropathol Exp Neurol 54: 304-310.
2397. West CR, Bruce DA, Duffner PK (1985). Ependymomas. Factors in clinical and diagnostic staging. Cancer 56: 1812-1816.
2398. Wester DJ, Falcone S, Green BA, Camp A, Quencer RM (1993). Paraganglioma of the filum: MR appearance. J Comput Assist Tomogr 17: 967-969.
2399. Westphal M, Stavrou D, Nausch H, Valdueza JM, Herrmann HD (1994). Human neurocytoma cells in culture show characteristics of astroglial differentiation. J Neurosci Res 38: 698-704.
2400. Wharton SB, Chan KK, Anderson JR, Stoeber K, Williams GH (2001). Replicative Mcm2 protein as a novel proliferation marker in oligodendrogliomas and its relationship to Ki67 labelling index, histological grade and prognosis. Neuropathol Appl Neurobiol 27: 305-313.
2401. Wharton SB, Chan KK, Hamilton FA, Anderson JR (1998). Expression of neuronal markers in oligodendrogliomas: an immunohistochemical study. Neuropathol Appl Neurobiol 24: 302-308.
2402. White FV, Dehner LP, Belchis DA, Conard K, Davis MM, Stocker JT, Zuppan CW, Biegel JA, Perlman EJ (1999). Congenital disseminated malignant rhabdoid tumor: a distinct clinicopathologic entity demonstrating abnormalities of chromosome 22q11. Am J Surg Pathol 23: 249-256.
2403. White W, Shiu MH, Rosenblum MK, Erlandson RA, Woodruff JM (1990). Cellular schwannoma. A clinicopathologic study of 57 patients and 58 tumors. Cancer 66: 1266-1275.
2404. Whittle IR, Dow GR, Lammie GA, Wardlaw J (1999). Dsyembryoplastic neuroepithelial tumour with discrete bilateral multifocality: further evidence for a germinal origin. Br J Neurosurg 13: 508-511.
2405. Whittle IR, Gordon A, Misra BK, Shaw JF, Steers AJ (1989). Pleomorphic xanthoastrocytoma: report of four cases. J Neurosurg 70: 463-468.
2406. Wick W, Naumann U, Weller M (2006). Transforming growth factor-beta: a molecular target for the future therapy of glioblastoma. Curr Pharm Des 12: 341-349.
2407. Wicking C, Evans T, Henk B, Hayward N, Simms LA, Chenevix-Trench G, Pietsch T, Wainwright B (1998). No evidence for the H133Y mutation in SONIC HEDGEHOG in a collection of common tumour types. Oncogene 16: 1091-1093.
2408. Wicking C, Gillies S, Smyth I, Shanley S, Fowles L, Ratcliffe J, Wainwright B, Chenevix-Trench G (1997). De novo mutations of the patched gene in nevoid basal cell carcinoma syndrome help to define phenotype. Am J Med Genet 73: 304-307.
2409. Wicking C, Shanley S, Smyth I, Gillies S, Negus K, Graham S, Suthers G, Haites N, Edwards M, Wainwright B, Chenevix T (1997). Most germ-line mutations in the nevoid basal cell carcinoma syndrome lead to a premature termination of the PATCHED protein, and no genotype-phenotype correlations are evident. Am J Hum Genet 60: 21-26.
2409A. Wieser R, Fritz B, Ullmann R, Muller I, Galhuber M, Storlazzi CT, Ramaswamy A, Christiansen H, Shimizu N, Rehder H (2005). Novel rearrangement of chromosome band 22q11.2 causing 22q11 microdeletion syndrome-like phenotype and rhabdoid tumor of the kidney. Hum Mutat 26:78-83.
2410. Wiestler OD, von Siebenthal K, Schmitt HP, Feiden W, Kleihues P (1989). Distribution and immunoreactivity of cerebral micro-hamartomas in bilateral acoustic neurofibromatosis (neurofibromatosis 2). Acta Neuropathol 79: 137-143.
2411. Wikstrand CJ, Reist CJ, Archer GE, Zalutsky MR, Bigner DD (1998). The class III variant of the epidermal growth factor receptor (EGFRvIII): characterization and utilization as an immunotherapeutic target. J Neurovirol 4: 148-158.
2412. Willis B, Ablin A, Weinberg V, Zoger S, Wara WM, Matthay KK (1996). Disease course and late sequelae of Langerhans' cell histiocytosis: 25- year experience at the University of California, San Francisco. J Clin Oncol 14: 2073-2082.
2413. Willis J, Smith C, Ironside JW, Erridge S, Whittle IR, Everington D (2005). The accuracy of meningioma grading: a 10-year retrospective audit. Neuropathol Appl Neurobiol 31: 141-149.
2414. Willman CL, Busque L, Griffith BB, Favara BE, McClain KL, Duncan MH, Gilliland DG (1994). Langerhans'-cell histiocytosis (histiocytosis X)—a clonal proliferative disease. N Engl J Med 331: 154-160.
2415. Wilson C, Bonnet C, Guy C, Idziaszczyk S, Colley J, Humphreys V, Maynard J, Sampson JR, Cheadle JP (2006). Tsc1 Haploinsufficiency without Mammalian Target of Rapamycin Activation Is Sufficient for Renal Cyst Formation in Tsc1+/- Mice. Cancer Res 66: 7934-7938.
2416. Wilson NW, Symon L, Lantos PL (1987). Gliomatosis cerebri: report of a case presenting as a focal cerebral mass. J Neurol 234: 445-447.
2417. Wimmer K, Eckart M, Meyer-Puttlitz B, Fonatsch C, Pietsch T (2002). Mutational and expression analysis of the NF1 gene argues against a role as tumor suppressor in sporadic pilocytic astrocytomas. J Neuropathol Exp Neurol 61: 896-902.
2418. Winek RR, Scheithauer BW, Wick MR (1989). Meningioma, meningeal hemangiopericytoma (angioblastic meningioma), peripheral hemangiopericytoma, and acoustic schwannoma. A comparative immunohistochemical study. Am J Surg Pathol 13: 251-261.
2419. Winger MJ, Macdonald DR, Cairncross JG (1989). Supratentorial anaplastic gliomas in adults. The prognostic importance of extent of resection and prior low-grade glioma. J Neurosurg 71: 487-493.
2420. Wippold FJ, Smirniotopoulos JG,

Pilgram TK (1997). Lesions of the cauda equina: a clinical and pathology review from the Armed Forces Institute of Pathology. Clin Neurol Neurosurg 99: 229-234.

2421. Wizigmann V, Breier G, Risau W, Plate KH (1995). Up-regulation of vascular endothelial growth factor and its receptors in von Hippel-Lindau disease-associated and sporadic hemangioblastomas. Cancer Res 55: 1358-1364.

2422. Wizigmann V, Plate KH (1996). Pathology, genetics and cell biology of hemangioblastomas. Histol Histopathol 11: 1049-1061.

2423. Woesler B, Moskopp D, Kuchelmeister K, Schul C, Wassmann H (1998). Intradural metastasis of a spinal myxopapillary ependymoma. A case report. Neurosurg Rev 21: 62-65.

2424. Wolf HK, Buslei R, Blumcke I, Wiestler OD, Pietsch T (1997). Neural antigens in oligodendrogliomas and dysembryoplastic neuroepithelial tumors. Acta Neuropathol 94: 436-443.

2425. Wolf HK, Muller MB, Spanle M, Zentner J, Schramm J, Wiestler OD (1988). Ganglioglioma: a detailed histopathological and immunohistochemical analysis of 61 cases. Acta Neuropathol 166-173.

2426. Wolf HK, Normann S, Green AJ, von Bakel I, Blumcke I, Pietsch T, Wiestler OD, von Deimling A (1997). Tuberous sclerosis-like lesions in epileptogenic human neocortex lack allelic loss at the TSC1 and TSC2 regions. Acta Neuropathol 93: 93-96.

2427. Wolf HK, Wellmer J, Muller MB, Wiestler OD, Hufnagel A, Pietsch T (1995). Glioneuronal malformative lesions and dysembryoplastic neuroepithelial tumors in patients with chronic pharmacoresistant epilepsies. J Neuropathol Exp Neurol 54: 245-254.

2428. Wolf HK, Wiestler OD (1995). Surgical pathology of chronic epileptic seizure disorders. Brain Pathol 3: 371-380.

2429. Wolf RM, Draghi N, Liang X, Dai C, Uhrbom L, Eklof C, Westermark B, Holland EC, Resh MD (2003). p190RhoGAP can act to inhibit PDGF-induced gliomas in mice: a putative tumor suppressor encoded on human chromosome 19q13.3. Genes Dev 17: 476-487.

2430. Wolff JE, Sajedi M, Brant R, Coppes MJ, Egeler RM (2002). Choroid plexus tumours. Br J Cancer 87: 1086-1091.

2431. Wolfsberger S, Fischer I, Hoftberger R, Birner P, Slavc I, Dieckmann K, Czech T, Budka H, Hainfellner J (2004). Ki-67 immunolabeling index is an accurate predictor of outcome in patients with intracranial ependymoma. Am J Surg Pathol 28: 914-920.

2432. Wolter M, Reifenberger J, Blaschke B, Ichimura K, Schmidt EE, Collins VP, Reifenberger G (2001). Oligodendroglial tumors frequently demonstrate hypermethylation of the CDKN2A (MTS1, p16INK4a), p14ARF, and CDKN2B (MTS2, p15INK4b) tumor suppressor genes. J Neuropathol Exp Neurol 60: 1170-1180.

2433. Wolter M, Reifenberger J, Sommer C, Ruzicka T, Reifenberger G (1997). Mutations in the human homologue of the Drosophila segment polarity gene patched (PTCH) in sporadic basal cell carcinomas of the skin and primitive neuroectodermal tumors of the central nervous system. Cancer Res 57: 2581-2585.

2434. Wondrusch E, Huemer M, Budka H (1991). Production of glial fibrillary acidic protein (GFAP) by neoplastic oligodendrocytes. Gliofibrillary oligodendroglioma and transitional astrocytoma revisited. Brain Tumor Pathol 8: 11-15.

2435. Wong AJ, Bigner SH, Bigner DD, Kinzler KW, Hamilton SR, Vogelstein B (1987). Increased expression of the epidermal growth factor receptor gene in malignant gliomas is invariably associated with gene amplification.

Proc Natl Acad Sci USA 84: 6899-6903.

2436. Wong K, Gyure KA, Prayson RA, Morrison AL, Le TQ, Armstrong RC (1999). Dysembryoplastic neuroepithelial tumor: in situ hybridization of proteolipid protein (PLP) messenger ribonucleic acid (mRNA). J Neuropath Exp Neurol 58: 542-542.

2437. Wong KK, Chang YM, Tsang YT, Perlaky L, Su J, Adesina A, Armstrong DL, Bhattacharjee M, Dauser R, Blaney SM, Chintagumpala M, Lau CC (2005). Expression analysis of juvenile pilocytic astrocytomas by oligonucleotide microarray reveals two potential subgroups. Cancer Res 65: 76-84.

2438. Wong TT, Ho DM, Chang KP, Yen SH, Guo WY, Chang FC, Liang ML, Pan HC, Chung WY (2005). Primary pediatric brain tumors: statistics of Taipei VGH, Taiwan (1975-2004). Cancer 104: 2156-2167.

2439. Wong TT, Ho DM, Chang TK, Yang DD, Lee LS (1995). Familial neurofibromatosis 1 with germinoma involving the basal ganglion and thalamus. Childs Nerv Syst 11: 456-458.

2440. Woodburn RT, Azzarelli B, Montebello JF, Goss IE (2001). Intense p53 staining is a valuable prognostic indicator for poor prognosis in medulloblastoma/central nervous system primitive neuroectodermal tumors. J Neurooncol 52: 57-62.

2441. Woodruff JM (1996). Pathology of major peripheral nerve sheath tumors. In: Soft Tissue Tumors (International Academy of Pathology Monograph). Weiss SW, Brooks JSJ, eds. Williams and Wilkins: Baltimore, pp. 129-161.

2442. Woodruff JM, Chernik NL, Smith MC, Millett WB, Foote FW, Jr. (1973). Peripheral nerve tumors with rhabdomyosarcomatous differentiation (malignant "Triton" tumors). Cancer 32: 426-439.

2443. Woodruff JM, Christensen WN (1993). Glandular peripheral nerve sheath tumors. Cancer 72: 3618-3628.

2444. Woodruff JM, Godwin TA, Erlandson RA, Susin M, Martini N (1981). Cellular schwannoma: a variety of schwannoma sometimes mistaken for a malignant tumor. Am J Surg Pathol 5: 733-744.

2445. Woodruff JM, Marshall ML, Godwin TA, Funkhouser JW, Thompson NJ, Erlandson RA (1983). Plexiform (multinodular) schwannoma. A tumor simulating the plexiform neurofibroma. Am J Surg Pathol 7: 691-697.

2446. Woodruff JM, Perino G (1994). Non-germ-cell or teratomatous malignant tumors showing additional rhabdomyoblastic differentiation, with emphasis on the malignant Triton tumor. Semin Diagn Pathol 11: 69-81.

2447. Woodruff JM, Selig AM, Crowley K, Allen PW (1994). Schwannoma (neurilemoma) with malignant transformation. A rare, distinctive peripheral nerve tumor. Am J Surg Pathol 18: 882-895.

2448. Wren D, Wolswijk G, Noble M (1992). In vitro analysis of origin and maintenance of O-2A adult progenitor cells. J Cell Biol 116: 167-176.

2449. Wright RA, Hermann RC, Parisi JE (1999). Neurological manifestations of Erdheim-Chester disease. J Neurol Neurosurg Psychiatry 66: 72-75.

2450. Wu R, Zhang J, Fryns JP, Cassiman JJ, Legius E (1969). Genetic heterogeneity in neurofibromatosis type 1. FASEB Summer Research Conference On Neurofibromatosis, Snowmass, Co, USA

2451. Wyatt-Ashmead J, Kleinschmidt-DeMasters B, Mierau GW, Malkin D, Orsini E, McGavran L, Foreman NK (2001). Choroid plexus carcinomas and rhabdoid tumors: phenotypic and genotypic overlap. Pediatr Dev Pathol 4: 545-549.

2452. Xiao GH, Jin F, Yeung RS (1995). Identification of tuberous sclerosis 2 messenger RNA splice variants that are conserved and differentially expressed in rat and human tissues. Cell Growth Differ 6: 1185-1191.

2453. Xu HM, Gutmann DH (1998). Merlin differentially associates with the microtubule and actin cytoskeleton. J Neurosci Res 51: 403-415.

2454. Yamada H, Haratake J, Narasaki T, Oda T (1995). Embryonal craniopharyngioma. Case report of the morphogenesis of a craniopharyngioma. Cancer 75: 2971-2977.

2455. Yamamoto K, Yamada K, Nakahara T, Ishihara A, Takaki S, Kochi M, Ushio Y (2002). Rapid regrowth of solitary subependymal giant cell astrocytoma—case report. Neurol Med Chir (Tokyo) 42: 224-227.

2456. Yamane Y, Mena H, Nakazato Y (2002). Immunohistochemical characterization of pineal parenchymal tumors using novel monoclonal antibodies to the pineal body. Neuropathology 22: 66-76.

2457. Yamashiro S, Nagahiro S, Mimata C, Kuratsu J, Ushio Y (1994). Malignant trigeminal schwannoma associated with xeroderma pigmentosum—case report. Neurol Med Chir Tokyo 34: 817-820.

2458. Yamashita Y, Handa H, Toyama M (1975). Medulloblastoma in two brothers. Surg Neurol 4: 225-227.

2459. Yang HJ, Kim JE, Paek SH, Chi JG, Jung HW, Kim DG (2003). The significance of gemistocytes in astrocytoma. Acta Neurochir 145: 1097-1103.

2460. Yang P, Kollmeyer TM, Buckner K, Bamlet W, Ballman KV, Jenkins RB (2005). Polymorphisms in GLTSCR1 and ERCC2 are associated with the development of oligodendrogliomas. Cancer 103: 2363-2372.

2461. Yang SY, Jin YJ, Park SH, Jahng TA, Kim HJ, Chung CK (2005). Paragangliomas in the cauda equina region: clinicopathoradiologic findings in four cases. J Neurooncol 72: 49-55.

2462. Yasargil MG, Curcic M, Kis M, Siegenthaler G, Teddy PJ, Roth P (1990). Total removal of craniopharyngiomas. Approaches and long-term results in 144 patients. J Neurosurg 73: 3-11.

2463. Yasargil MG, von Ammon K, von Deimling A, Valavanis A, Wichmann W, Wiestler OD (1992). Central neurocytoma: histopathological variants and therapeutic approaches. J Neurosurg 76: 32-37.

2464. Yasha TC, Mohanty A, Radhesh S, Santosh V, Das S, Shankar SK (1998). Infratentorial dysembryoplastic neuroepithelial tumor (DNT) associated with Arnold-Chiari malformation. Clin Neuropathol 17: 305-310.

2465. Yassa M, Bahary JP, Bourguoin P, Belair M, Berthelet F, Bouthillier A (2005). Intraparenchymal mesenchymal chondrosarcoma of the cerebellum: case report and review of the literature. J Neurooncol 74: 329-331.

2466. Yildiz H, Hakyemez B, Koroglu M, Yesildag A, Baykal B (2006). Intracranial lipomas: importance of localization. Neuroradiology 48: 1-7.

2467. Yin XL, Hui AB, Pang JC, Poon WS, Ng HK (2002). Genome-wide survey for chromosomal imbalances in ganglioglioma using comparative genomic hybridization. Cancer Genet Cytogenet 134: 71-76.

2468. Yin XL, Pang JC, Hui AB, Ng HK (2000). Detection of chromosomal imbalances in central neurocytomas by using comparative genomic hybridization. J Neurosurg 93: 77-81.

2469. Yokoo H, Tanaka G, Isoda K, Hirato J, Nakazato Y, Fujimaki H, Watanabe K, Saito N, Sasaki T (2003). Novel crystalloid structures in suprasellar paraganglioma. Clin Neuropathol 22: 222-228.

2470. Yokota N, Aruga J, Takai S, Yamada K,

Hamazaki M, Iwase T, Sugimura H, Mikoshiba K (1996). Predominant expression of human zic in cerebellar granule cell lineage and medulloblastoma. Cancer Res 56: 377-383.

2471. Yokota N, Mainprize TG, Taylor MD, Kohata T, Loreto M, Ueda S, Dura W, Grajkowska W, Kuo JS, Rutka JT (2004). Identification of differentially expressed and developmentally regulated genes in medulloblastoma using suppression subtraction hybridization. Oncogene 23: 3444-3453.

2472. Yokota N, Nishizawa S, Ohta S, Date H, Sugimura H, Namba H, Maekawa M (2002). Role of Wnt pathway in medulloblastoma oncogenesis. Int J Cancer 101: 198-201.

2473. Yoshimoto M, de Toledo SR, da Silva NS, Bayani J, Bertozzi AP, Stavale JN, Cavalheiro S, Andrade JA, Zielenska M, Squire JA (2004). Comparative genomic hybridization analysis of pediatric adamantinomatous craniopharyngiomas and a review of the literature. J Neurosurg 101: 85-90.

2474. You H, Kim YI, Im SY, Suh-Kim H, Paek SH, Park SH, Kim DG, Jung HW (2005). Immunohistochemical study of central neurocytoma, subependymoma, and subependymal giant cell astrocytoma. J Neurooncol 74: 1-8.

2475. Young RJ, Sills AK, Brem S, Knopp EA (2005). Neuroimaging of metastatic brain disease. Neurosurgery 57: S10-S23.

2476. Yu H, Yao TL, Spooner J, Stumph JR, Hester R, Konrad PE (2006). Delayed occurrence of multiple spinal drop metastases from a posterior fossa choroid plexus papilloma. Case report. J Neurosurg Spine 4: 494-496.

2477. Zagzag D, Krishnamachary B, Yee H, Okuyama H, Chiriboga L, Ali MA, Melamed J, Semenza GL (2005). Stromal cell-derived factor-1alpha and CXCR4 expression in hemangioblastoma and clear cell-renal cell carcinoma: von Hippel-Lindau loss-of-function induces expression of a ligand and its receptor. Cancer Res 65: 6178-6188.

2478. Zajac V, Kirchhoff T, Levy ER, Horsley SW, Miller A, Steichen-Gersdorf E, Monaco AP (1997). Characterisation of X;17(q12;p13) translocation breakpoints in a female patient with hypomelanosis of Ito and choroid plexus papilloma. Eur J Hum Genet 5: 61-68.

2479. Zak IT, Altinok D, Neilsen SS, Kish KK (2006). Xanthoma disseminatum of the central nervous system and cranium. AJNR Am J Neuroradiol 27: 919-921.

2480. Zakrzewska M, Wojcik I, Zakrzewski K, Polis L, Grajkowska W, Roszkowski M, Augelli BJ, Liberski PP, Rieske P (2005). Mutational analysis of hSNF5/INI1 and TP53 genes in choroid plexus carcinomas. Cancer Genet Cytogenet 156: 179-182.

2481. Zamecnik J, Chanova M, Kodet R (2004). Expression of thyroid transcription factor 1 in primary brain tumours. J Clin Pathol 57: 1111-1113.

2482. Zamecnik M, Michal M (2001). Perineurial cell differentiation in neurofibromas. Report of eight cases including a case with composite perineurioma-neurofibroma features. Pathol Res Pract 197: 537-544.

2483. Zang KD (2001). Meningioma: a cytogenetic model of a complex benign human tumor, including data on 394 karyotyped cases. Cytogenet Cell Genet 93: 207-220.

2484. Zarate JO, Sampaolesi R (1999). Pleomorphic xanthoastrocytoma of the retina. Am J Surg Pathol 23: 79-81.

2485. Zattara-Cannoni H, Roll P, Figarella-Branger D, Lena G, Dufour H, Grisoli F, Vagner-Capodano AM (2001). Cytogenetic study of six cases of radiation-induced meningiomas. Cancer Genet Cytogenet 126: 81-84.

2486. Zauberman A, Flusberg D, Haupt Y, Barak Y, Oren M (1995). A functional p53-

responsive intronic promoter is contained within the human mdm2 gene. Nucleic Acids Res 23: 2584-2592.

2487. Zbar B, Kishida T, Chen F, Schmidt L, Maher ER, Richards FM, Crossey PA, webster AR, Affara NA, Ferguson S, Brauch H, Glavac D, Neumann HP, Tischerman S, Mulvihill JJ, Gross DJ, Suhin T, Seizinger B, Kley N, Olschwang S, Boisson C, Richard S, Lips CHM, Linehan WM, Lerman M (1996). Germline mutations in the von Hippel-Lindau disease (VHL) gene in families from North America, Europe and Japan. Hum Mutat 8: 348-357.

2488. Zec N, Cera P, Towfighi J (1991). Extramedullary hematopoiesis in cerebellar hemangioblastoma. Neurosurgery 29: 34-37.

2489. Zein G, Yu E, Tawansy K, Berta A, Foster CS (2004). Neurofibromatosis type 1 associated with central nervous system lymphoma. Ophthalmic Genet 25: 49-51.

2490. Zevallos-Giampietri EA, Yanes HH, Orrego PJ, Barrionuevo C (2004). Primary meningeal Epstein-Barr virus-related leiomyosarcoma in a man infected with human immunodeficiency virus: review of literature, emphasizing the differential diagnosis and pathogenesis. Appl Immunohistochem Mol Morphol 12: 387-391.

2491. Zhang D, Wen L, Henning TD, Feng XY, Zhang YL, Zou LG, Zhang ZG (2006). Central neurocytoma: clinical, pathological and neuroradiological findings. Clin Radiol 61: 348-357.

2492. Zhang F, Tan L, Wainwright LM, Bartolomei MS, Biegel JA (2002). No evidence for hypermethylation of the hSNF5/INI1 promoter in pediatric rhabdoid tumors. Genes Chromosomes Cancer 34: 398-405.

2493. Zhang L, Zhang J, Lambert Q, Der CJ, Del Valle L, Miklossy J, Khalili K, Zhou V, Pagano JS (2004). Interferon regulatory factor 7 is associated with Epstein-Barr virus-transformed central nervous system lymphoma and has oncogenic properties. J Virol 78: 12987-12995.

2494. Zhang SJ, Endo S, Ichikawa T, Washiyama K, Kumanishi T (1998). Frequent deletion and 5' CpG island methylation of the p16 gene in primary malignant lymphoma of the brain. Cancer Res 58: 1231-1237.

2495. Zhang Y, Xiong Y, Yarbrough WG (1998). ARF promotes MDM2 degradation and stabilizes p53: ARF-INK4a locus deletion impairs both the Rb and p53 tumor suppression pathways. Cell 92: 725-734.

2496. Zhang YY, Vik TA, Ryder JW, Srour EF, Jacks T, Shannon K, Clapp DW (1998). Nf1 regulates hematopoietic progenitor cell growth and ras signaling in response to multiple cytokines. J Exp Med 187: 1893-1902.

2497. Zheng PP, Pang JC, Hui AB, Ng HK (2000). Comparative genomic hybridization detects losses of chromosomes 22 and 16 as the most common recurrent genetic alterations in primary ependymomas. Cancer Genet Cytogenet 122: 18-25.

2498. Zhong H, De Marzo AM, Laughner E, Lim M, Hilton DA, Zagzag D, Buechler P, Isaacs WB, Semenza GL, Simons JW (1999). Overexpression of hypoxia-inducible factor 1alpha in common human cancers and their metastases. Cancer Res 59: 5830-5835.

2499. Zhou XP, Marsh DJ, Morrison CD, Chaudhury AR, Maxwell M, Reifenberger G, Eng C (2003). Germline inactivation of PTEN and dysregulation of the phosphoinositol-3-kinase/Akt pathway cause human Lhermitte-Duclos disease in adults. Am J Hum Genet 73: 1191-1198.

2500. Zhou XP, Waite KA, Pilarski R, Hampel H, Fernandez MJ, Bos C, Dasouki M, Feldman GL, Greenberg LA, Ivanovich J, Matloff E, Patterson A, Pierpont ME, Russo D, Nassif NT, Eng C (2003). Germline PTEN promoter muta-

tions and deletions in Cowden/Bannayan-Riley-Ruvalcaba syndrome result in aberrant PTEN protein and dysregulation of the phosphoinositol-3-kinase/Akt pathway. Am J Hum Genet 73: 404-411.

2501. Zhou XP, Woodford-Richens K, Lehtonen R, Kurose K, Aldred M, Hampel H, Launonen V, Virta S, Pilarski R, Salovaara R, Bodmer WF, Conrad BA, Dunlop M, Hodgson SV, Iwama T, Jarvinen H, Kellokumpu I, Kim JC, Leggett B, Markie D, Mecklin JP, Neale K, Phillips R, Piris J, Rozen P, Houlston RS, Aaltonen LA, Tomlinson IP, Eng C (2001). Germline mutations in BMPR1A/ALK3 cause a subset of cases of juvenile polyposis syndrome and of Cowden and Bannayan-Riley-Ruvalcaba syndromes. Am J Hum Genet 69: 704-711.

2502. Zhu J, Frosch MP, Busque L, Beggs AH, Dashner K, Gilliland DG, Black PM (1995). Analysis of meningiomas by methylation- and transcription-based clonality assays. Cancer Res 55: 3865-3872.

2503. Zhu JJ, Leon SP, Folkerth RD, Guo SZ, Wu JK, Black PM (1997). Evidence for clonal origin of neoplastic neuronal and glial cells in gangliogliomas. Am J Pathol 151: 565-571.

2504. Zhu Y, Ghosh P, Charnay P, Burns DK, Parada LF (2002). Neurofibromas in NF1: Schwann cell origin and role of tumor environment. Science 296: 920-922.

2505. Zimmerman RA, Bilaniuk LT, Pahlajani H (1978). Spectrum of medulloblastomas demonstrated by computed tomography. Radiology 126: 137-141.

2506. Zimmerman RA, Bilaniuk LT, Rebsamen S (1992). Magnetic resonance imaging of pediatric posterior fossa tumors. Pediatr Neurosurg 18: 58-64.

2507. Zlatescu MC, TehraniYazdi A, Sasaki H, Megyesi JF, Betensky RA, Louis DN, Cairncross JG (2001). Tumor location and growth pattern correlate with genetic signature in oligodendroglial neoplasms. Cancer Res 61: 6713-6715.

2508. Zoller ME, Rembeck B, Oden A, Samuelsson M, Angervall L (1997). Malignant and benign tumors in patients with neurofibromatosis type 1 in a defined Swedish population. Cancer 79: 2125-2131.

2509. Zorludemir S, Scheithauer BW, Hirose T, Van Houten C, Miller G, Meyer FB (1995). Clear cell meningioma. A clinicopathologic study of a potentially aggressive variant of meningioma. Am J Surg Pathol 19: 493-505.

2510. Zu R, Varakis JN (1979). Perinatal induction of medulloblastomas in Syrian golden hamsters by a human polyoma virus (JC). NCI Monogr 51: 205-208.

2511. Zuccaro G, Taratuto AL, Monges J (1986). Intracranial neoplasms during the first year of life. Surg Neurol 26: 29-36.

2512. Zulch KJ (1957). Brain Tumours. Their Biology and Pathology. Springer-Verlag: New York.

2513. Zulch KJ (1979). Histological typing of tumours of the central nervous system. World Health Organization: Geneva.

2514. Zulch KJ (1986). Brain Tumors. Their biology and pathology. Springer Verlag: Berlin Heidelberg.

2515. Zuppan CW, Mierau GW, Weeks DA (1994). Ependymoma with signet-ring cells. Ultrastruct Pathol 18: 43-46.

2516. Zurawel RH, Allen C, Chiappa S, Cato W, Biegel J, Cogen P, de Sauvage F, Raffel C (2000). Analysis of PTCH/SMO/SHH pathway genes in medulloblastoma. Genes Chromosomes Cancer 27: 44-51.

2517. Zurawel RH, Chiappa SA, Allen C, Raffel C (1998). Sporadic medulloblastomas contain oncogenic beta-catenin mutations. Cancer Res 58: 896-899.

Subject index

C

Extraventricular neurocytoma, 95, 106, *109*

Ezrin, 105, 185, 212

F

Facial angiofibroma, 219, 220

Factor VIII, 176, 186, 195, 215

Factor VIII-related antigen, 48, 176

FAK, 42

Familial (bilateral) retinoblastoma, 127

Familial adenomatous polyposis (FAP), 127, 138, 229-231

Familial posterior fossa brain tumour syndrome of infancy, 234

Fas (CD95), 40

FasL (CD95L), 40

Fast myosin, 134

Fibrillary astrocytoma, 17, 25, 27, 29, 63, 104

Fibrohistiocytic tumour, 175

Fibrolipomatous hamartoma, 174

Fibroma, 49, 174, 205, 220, 232

Fibromatosis, 173, 174

Fibromodulin, 19

Fibromuscular dysplasia, 207

Fibronectin, 19, 217

Fibrosarcoma, 48, 160, 162, 173, 175

Fibrous meningioma, 166, 169

Fibrous xanthoma, 175

Fibroxanthoma, 175, 193

Fifth phacomatosis, 232

Flexner-Wintersteiner rosettes, 126

Flk-1, 216, 217

Fluorescence *in situ* hybridization (FISH), 28, 85, 112, 114, 136, 137, 177, 192, 208

Focal adhesion kinase (FAK), 42

Follicular lymphoma, 191

Forehead plaque, 219, 220

FSH (follicle-stimulating hormone), 238

G

G22P1, 77

Gagel's granuloma, 193

Galactolipids like galactocerebroside, 57

Galectin-3, 19, 246

GalNAcT, 45

Gangliocytic paragangliomas, 118

Gangliocytoma, 95, *103-105*, 226, 227

Ganglioglioma, 16, 23, 76, 95, 96, 102, *103-105*, 113, 149

Ganglioglioma with a tanycytic glial component, 76

Ganglioid cells, 107, 109, 113

Gangliomatosis of the cerebellum, 226

Ganglioneuroblastoma, 131, 141, 142, 160

Ganglioneuroma, 160

Gangliosides, 57

GAPD, 192

Gardner syndrome, 229

Gastrointestinal stromal tumour, 207

Gata-1, 216, 217

GD3 synthase, 45

Gefitinib, 45

Gemistocytes, 26-29, 38, 39, 55, 67, 219

Gemistocytic astrocytoma, 25, 27, 38, 88

Geographic necrosis, 79, 148, 168

Germ cell tumours, 28, 147, 175, 176, *197-204*

Germinoma, 28, *197-204*

GH (growth hormone), 238

Giant cell ependymoma, 76

Giant cell glioblastoma, 38, *46-47*, 173

Gingival fibroma, 219, 220

Glandular MPNST, 161

Gli, 137, 233

Glial hamartia, 205, 211, 212

Glioblastoma, 13, 15, 18, 19, 23, 25, 28-31, *33-49*, 58, 61, 64, 67, 76, 133, 177, 205-207, 223, 227, 229-231

Glioblastoma with oligodendroglioma component, 37

Gliofibrillary oligodendrocytes, 56, 57, 59, 61, 63

Gliofibroma, 49

Gliomatosis cerebri, 13, 37, *50-52*, 54

Gliomatosis peritonei, 51

Glioneuronal tumour with neuropil-like islands, 31

Gliosarcoma, 37, 39, 47, *48-49*, 174-176

Glomeruloid neovascularization, 133

Glomeruloid tufts, 21, 39

Glomus jugulare tumour, 117

GLTSCR1, 58

Glycerol-3-phosphate dehydrogenase 57

Gorlin syndrome, 136, 169, 205, 232

Gorlin-Goltz syndrome, 232

Granular bodies, 15, 23

Granular cell myoblastoma, 241

Granular cell neuroma, 241

Granular cell tumour, 38, 244

Granular cell tumour of the neurohypophysis, 237, *241-242*

Granular cells, 38, 159

GSK-3ß, 138

GSTP1, 192

GSTT1, 58

GTBP, 230

H

Haemangioblastoma, 75, 163, 166, *184-186*, 205, 215-217

Haemangioendothelioma, 176

Haemangioma, 173, 174, 176

Haemangiopericytoma, 161, 163, 167, 173, 176, 177, *178-180*

Haemophagocytic lymphohistiocytosis, 193, 195, 196

Hamartin, 220, 221

Hamartoma, 105, 206, 207, 210, 212, 218-221, 226, 227

Hamartomatous polyps of the colon, 205

Hamartomatous rectal polyps, 219

Hand-Schüller-Christian disease, 193

Hashimoto-Pritzker disease, 193

HCG (human chorionic gonadotropin), 199, 202

Hedgehog pathway, 137, 138

Hepatocyte growth factor, 209, 217

Hereditary non-polyposis colorectal carcinoma (HNPCC), 229-231

Herpesvirus 6 (HHV-6), 188

Herpesvirus 8 (HHV-8), 177, 188

Herring bodies, 243

Hibernoma, 173, 174

HIC-1, 77, 137

HIF-1α, *see* Hypoxia-inducible factor-1α

High-grade astrocytoma, 30, 44

High-grade glioma, 43, 44, 61, 105, 133

HIOMT, 123

Hist1H3D, 127

Low-grade diffuse astrocytoma, 25, 26, 31, 64

Low-grade intracranial lymphoma, 190

LPP, 192

Lumbosacral lipoma (leptomyelolipomas), 174

Lung cancer, 232, 248

Luse body (stromal long-spacing collagen), 155

Lymphangioleiomyomatosis, 205, 220

Lymphangiomatosis, 219

Lymphoma, 136, 177, 188-192, 230, 248

Lymphomatoid granulomatosis, 191

Lymphomatosis cerebri, 190

Lymphoplasmacyte-rich meningioma, 167

Lymphoplasmacytic lymphoma, 190

Lysosome, 118, 123, 127, 169, 237, 241

M

MAC387, 194

Macrocephaly, 14, 206, 207, 226, 232

Maffucci syndrome, 177

Malignant astrocytoma, 13, 30, 33, 230

Malignant ectomesenchymoma, 175

Malignant fibrous histiocytoma (MFH), 48, 173, 175, 177

Malignant glioma, 37, 41, 66, 147, 189

Malignant leptomeningeal melanoma, 183

Malignant lymphoma, *188-192*

Malignant melanoma, 181, 183, 187, 188, 248

Malignant meningioma, 173

Malignant peripheral nerve sheath tumour (MPNST), 151, 152, 154, 157, *160-162*, 205, 207, 208

Malignant pineocytoma, 124

Malignant rhabdoid tumour, 147, 234

Malignant schwannoma, 160

Malignant soft tissue perineurioma, 158

MALT1, 192

MAP-2, *see* Microtubule-associated protein 2

MAPK12, 77

Marginal zone B-cell lymphoma, 190

MART-1, 183

Matrilin-2, 19

Matrix metalloproteinase-9 (MMP-9), 45

Mature teratoma, 197, 201

MCM5, 77

MDM2, 24, 42, 44, 48, 49, 62, 77, 91, 225

MDM4, 62

Medullary thyroid carcinoma, 207

Medulloblastoma, 28, 110-112, 131, *132-140*, 142, 143, 145, 147, 148, 177, 183, 205, 222, 223, 229-234

Medulloblastoma with extensive nodularity, 132, 134

Medullocytoma, 110

Medulloepithelioma, 141, *143-146*

Medullomyoblastoma, 134, 175

Megalencephaly, 205, 227

Melanin, 70, 118, 123, 134, 144, 181-183, 249, 250

Melanocytic lesions, 163, *181-183*

Melanocytic medulloblastoma, 134

Melanocytoma, 163, 181-183

Melanocytosis, 181

Melanoma, 37, 154, 163, 168, 169, 181-183, 222, 232, 234, 248, 249

Melanomatosis, 163, 181-183

Melanotic ependymoma, 76

Melanotic meningioma, 183

Melanotic neuroectodermal tumour of infancy (retinal anlage tumour), 183

Melanotic paraganglioma, 118

Melatonin, 123

Meningeal haemangiopericytoma, 178-180

Meningeal lymphoma, 190

Meningeal sarcoma, 173

Meningeal sarcomatosis, 177

Meningioangiomatosis, 205, 210-212

Meningioma, 28, 34, 48, 58, 90, 91, 104, 133, 163, *164-172*, 175, 177-180, 182, 183, 190, 191, 194, 195, 205, 210-214, 222, 227, 230, 232, 234, 242, 248

Meningocerebral astrocytoma, 96

Meningothelial meningioma, 166

Merlin (schwannomin), 91, 155, 170, 212

Mesenchymal chondrosarcoma, 173, 176

Mesenchymal tumour, 97, 163, *173-177*, 178, 193

Mesenchymal, non-meningothelial tumours, *173-177*

Mesothelioma, 73

Metaplasia, 39, 111, 240

Metaplastic meningioma, 167

Metastatic tumours, *247-251*

Metenkephalin, 118

Methionine aminopeptidase-2, 19

MFH, *see* Malignant fibrous histiocytoma

MGMT, *see* O^6-Methylguanine-DNA methyltransferase

MHC class II antigen, 39

Microarray analysis, 123, 127, 192

Microcalcification, 63, 122, 126

Microcystic adenoma of the pancreas, 215, 216

Microcystic meningioma, 165, 167, 170

Microcysts, 13-15, 29, 73, 167

Microglioma, 188

Microhamartoma, 211

Microhamartomatous rectal polyp, 220

Microphthalmia transcription factor, 183

Microsatellite instability, 44, 171

Microtubule-associated protein 2 (MAP2), 23, 56, 97, 104, 111, 116, 128, 135, 220

Minichromosome maintainance 2 (MCM2), 57

Minigemistocytes, 27, 55-57, 59, 61, 63, 67, 113, 114

Mismatch repair genes, 229, 230

Mitochondria, 97, 108, 114, 116, 118, 123, 127, 159, 245

Mixed glioma, 49, 63

Mixed glioneuronal tumour, 115

Mixed oligoastrocytoma, 63

Mixed pineocytoma, 124

MLH1, 192, 205, 229-231

MMAC1, *see* PTEN

MMP-9, 45

MMP-12, 77

MN1, 170

Moesin, 212

Monoclonal origin, 48, 49, 52, 105

Monocytic leukaemia, 193

Monomorphous angiocentric glioma, 92

Mononeuropathies, 212

Monstrocellular sarcoma, 46, 173

Subcortical glioneuronal hamartomas, 218

Subependymal astrocytoma, 70

Subependymal giant cell astrocytoma (SEGA), 13, 104, 205, *218-221*

Subependymal glial nodule, 218

Subependymal glomerate astrocytoma, 70

Subependymal hamartomatous nodule, 220

Subependymal nodule, 219, 220

Subependymoma, 69, *70-71*

Subungual fibroma, 218

SUFU, 136, 138

Supratentorial PNET, 131, 139, *141*, 143, 230

Sustentacular cells, 95, 117-119

SV40, 54, 74, 82, 132, 188

Syringomyelia, 119, 183

T

Talin, 212

Tanycytes, 76, 89, 91, 93

Tanycytic ependymoma, 74, 76

Tau protein, 92, 122

T-cell lymphoma, 191

T-cell rich B-cell lymphoma, 191

TCF, 138

TCP1, 77

Tensin, 41, 42, 226, 228

Tentorium cerebelli, 232

TEP1, 228

Teratoma, 51, 174, 175, 177, *197-202*, 204

TERT (telomerase reverse transcriptase), 127, 137, 145

TGF-α, 41, 59

TGF-ß, 34, 46, 59

THBS (thrombospondin 1), 59

Thyroid neoplasms, 205

Tie-1, 179, 185

Tie-2, 216, 217

Tissue inhibitor of metalloproteinase 2 (TIMP-2), 192, 217

Tissue inhibitor of metalloproteinases-3 (TIMP-3), 43, 44, 59, 192

Topoisomerase II, 57, 209, 219

Touton giant cells, 194, 195

Toxoplasmosis, 189, 190

TP53, 18, 20, 22, 24, 27, 28, 29, 31, 32, 41-49, 52, 57, 58, 64, 65, 67, 77, 80, 82, 84, 85, 91, 93, 98, 105, 108, 112, 127, 136, 137, 140, 149, 154, 159, 162, 171, 180, 192, 196, 203, 205, 208, 209, *222-225*, 230, 231, 242

TP73, 58

TPH1, 123

TRAIL (TNF-related apoptosis-inducing ligand), 40

Transitional meningioma, 166, 170

Translocation, 58, 84, 85, 191, 192, 231, 233

Translocation between chromosomes 1 and 19, 58

Transthyretin, 83-85, 128

Trichilemmoma, 205

Trichoepithelioma, 233

Trilateral retinoblastoma syndrome, 127

Trisomy 3, 190

Trisomy 7, 136

Triton tumour, 161, 162, 206, 207

TrkC, 140

TSC, *see* Tuberous sclerosis complex

TSC1, 105, 205, 218, 220, 221

TSC2, 105, 205, 218, 220, 221

TSH (thyroid-stimulating hormone), 238

TSLC-1, 171

TSP1, 192

TTF-1 (thyroid transcription factor 1), 76

TTR, 129

TUBA2, 77

Tuberin, 220, 221

Tuberous sclerosis, 13, 205, 218

Tuberous sclerosis complex (TSC), *218-221*

Tumour necrosis factor (TNF), 40

Turcot syndrome, 44, 58, 77, 136, 138, 205, *229-231*

TXN, 77

Type 2 astrocytes, 59

U

Ulex europaeus I agglutinin (UEA-I), 49

V

Vascular endothelial growth factor (VEGF), 40, 46, 59, 179, 185, 216

Vascular thrombosis, 13, 33

VEGFR-1, 179, 185

VEGFR-2, 179, 185

v-erbB, 41

Verocay bodies, 153

Vestibular nerve schwannoma, 133

Vestibular schwannoma, 205, 210, 213

VHL, 119, 163, 184-186, 205, *215-217*

Vincristine, 62

Visceral cysts, 205, 218

von Hippel-Lindau (VHL) disease, 108, 119, 163, 184, 205, *215-217*

von Recklinghausen disease, 206

von Recklinghausen neurofibromatosis, 206, 210

W

Waf1/p21, 127

Weber-Christian panniculitis, 193

Weibel-Palade bodies, 176, 185, 215

Well-differentiated astrocytoma, 25

White matter heterotopias, 219, 220

WHO grading, *10*, 28, 54

Wilms' tumour, 136

Wishart type, 213

Wiskott-Aldrich syndrome, 188

Wnt pathway, 136, 138-140

X

Xanthogranuloma, 193, 195, 239, 240

Xanthoma, 22, 193, 195, 240

X-chromosome inactivation, 171, 195

XYY syndrome, 102

Y

YKL-40 (chitinase-3-like-1), 19, 45

Yolk sac tumour, 197, 198, *201*

Z

Zellballen, 95, 117, 118

ZFH4, 129

ZIC, 138

ZNF342, 58